Robert A. Knuppel, M.D., M.P.H.

Professor, OB/GYN and Public Health
Director, Maternal-Fetal Medicine
University of South Florida
College of Medicine
Tampa, Florida

Joan E. Drukker, R.N.C., M.S.N.

Perinatal Consultant
Tampa, Florida
Major, U.S. Army Reserve Nurse Corps
Formerly, Perinatal Outreach Coordinator
Tampa General Hospital
University of South Florida
Tampa, Florida

HIGH-RISK PREGNANCY

A TEAM APPROACH

1986

W. B. Saunders Company

Philadelphia / London / Toronto / Mexico City / Rio de Janeiro / Sydney / Tokyo / Hong Kong

W. B. Saunders Company: West Washington Square
Philadelphia, PA 19105

#125833010

64532

R G
5 7 1
H 45
1 9 8 6

Library of Congress Cataloging-in-Publication Data

Main entry under title:

High-risk pregnancy.

1. Pregnancy, Complications of.   2. Labor, Complicated.
I. Knuppel, Robert A.   II. Drukker, Joan E. [DNLM: 1.
Labor Complications. 2. Pregnancy Complications. WQ 240
H6375]

RG571.H45 1986   618.3   85–22181

ISBN 0–7216–5503–3

Disclaimer:

The opinions or assertions contained herein are the private views of
the authors and are not to be construed as official or as reflecting the
views of the Department of the Army or the Department of Defense.

Editor: Ilze Rader
Developmental Editor: Alan Sorkowitz
Designer: Karen O'Keefe
Production Manager: Bob Butler
Manuscript Editor: Erika Shapiro
Illustrators: Karen McGarry and Philip Ashley
Indexer: Ellen Murray

High-Risk Pregnancy: A Team Approach   ISBN 0–7216–5503–3

Last digit is the print number: 9   8   7   6   5   4   3   2   1

TO

Catherine V. O'Shaughnessey Stearns, the oldest of
thirteen and the greatest grandmother in the world.

—R.A.K.

David Heilig, D.O., who encouraged me to undertake
a career in nursing, and who allowed me to give
him my first injection.

—J.E.D.

CONTRIBUTORS

CYDNEY I. AFRIAT, B.S.N., C.N.M., M.S.N.
Assistant Clinical Professor, School of Midwifery, University of Southern California, Los Angeles, CA; Private Practice, Monterey, CA.

GRETCHEN M.-E. AUMANN, B.S.N., R.N.
Perinatal Clinical Specialist, Institute for the Medical Humanities, University of Texas Medical Branch, Galveston, TX.

MARGARET M. BAIRD, R.N., M.N.
Major, Army Nurse Corps; Head Nurse, Postpartum; Tripler Army Medical Center, Honolulu, HI.

JANE L. BERRY, R.N.C., M.S.N.
Acting Clinical Director, Department of Obstetrics and Neonatal Nursing, University of Pennsylvania, Hospital of the University of Pennsylvania, Woman's Hospital Division, Philadelphia, PA.

FRANK H. BOEHM, M.D.
Professor and Director, Maternal-Fetal Division, Department of Obstetrics and Gynecology, Vanderbilt School of Medicine, Nashville, TN.

REBECCA L. BROWN, R.N.
Charter Lakeside Hospital, Memphis, TN.

WINSTON A. CAMPBELL, M.D.
Division of Maternal-Fetal Medicine, Department of Obstetrics and Gynecology, University of Connecticut Health Center, Farmington, CT.

MARIA S. CASTILLO, R.N., B.S.N.
Department of Obstetrics and Gynecology, University of Texas, Health Science Center, San Antonio, TX.

ROBERT C. CEFALO, M.D., Ph.D.
Professor of Obstetrics and Gynecology; Director, Division of Maternal-Fetal Medicine; Assistant Dean, Head of Office of Graduate Medical Education; School of Medicine, University of North Carolina at Chapel Hill, Chapel Hill, NC.

VICKI COLBURN, R.N., B.S.N., M.Ed.
Clinical Education, Labor and Delivery, Coordinator of Perinatal Bereavement Team, University of Miami, Jackson Memorial Hospital; Private Practice, Nurse/Consultant; Miami, FL.

M. DOUGLAS CUNNINGHAM, M.D.
Professor of Pediatrics; Chief, Division of Neonatology; Director, Neonatal Intensive Care; University of Kentucky, Lexington, KY.

JOAN E. DRUKKER, R.N.C., M.S.N.
Perinatal Consultant, Tampa, FL; Major, U.S. Army Reserve Nurse Corps; formerly Perinatal Outreach Coordinator, Tampa General Hospital, University of South Florida; Tampa, FL.

SEBASTIAN FARO, M.D., Ph.D.
Associate Professor; Director, Section of Infectious Diseases; Department of Obstetrics and Gynecology, Baylor College of Medicine, Texas Medical Center, Houston, TX.

STEVEN G. GABBE, M.D.
Professor of Obstetrics and Gynecology, Pediatrics, School of Medicine; Director of Jerrold R. Golding Division of Fetal Medicine; University of Pennsylvania, Hospital of the University of Pennsylvania, Woman's Hospital Division, Philadelphia, PA.

CHARLES P. GIBBS, M.D.
Assistant Dean for Curriculum, Department of Anesthesiology, College of Medicine, University of Florida, J. Hillis Miller Health Center, Gainesville, FL.

STUART Z. GROSSMAN, J.D.
Attorney, Spence, Payne, Masington, Grossman & Needle, P.A., Miami, FL.

MARY F. HAIRE, R.N., M.S.N.
Associate in Obstetrics and Administrative Coordinator, Maternal-Fetal Division, Department of Obstetrics and Gynecology, Vanderbilt School of Medicine, Nashville, TN.

ROBERT H. HAYASHI, M.D.
Professor; Director of Maternal-Fetal Medicine; Department of Obstetrics and Gynecology, University of Michigan, Ann Arbor, MI.

WILLIAM N. P. HERBERT, M.D.
Associate Professor, Division of Maternal-Fetal Medicine, Department of Obstetrics and Gynecology, School of Medicine, University of North Carolina at Chapel Hill, Chapel Hill, NC.

CHARLES W. HOHLER, M.D., F.A.C.O.G.
Director of Perinatal Ultrasound, Co-Director of Prenatal Diagnostic Center, St. Joseph's Hospital and Medical Center; Board-Certified OB/GYN and Maternal-Fetal Medicine, Private Practice; Phoenix, AZ.

JOHN F. HUDDLESTON, M.D.
Professor and Director, Division of Maternal-Fetal Medicine, Department of Obstetrics and Gynecology, University of Alabama at Birmingham, Birmingham, AL.

CHARLES J. INGARDIA, M.D.
Director of Maternal-Fetal Medicine and Obstetrics, Hartford Hospital, Hartford, CT.

THOMAS M. JOHNSON, Ph.D
Department of Anthropology, Southern Methodist University; Adjunct Clinical Assistant Professor, Psychiatry Health Science, University of Texas at Dallas; Dallas, TX.

KENNETH A. KAPPY, M.D.
Division of Maternal-Fetal Medicine, Department of Obstetrics and Gynecology, Newark Beth Israel Medical Center, Newark, NJ.

MILDRED KAUFMAN, R.D., M.S.
Associate Professor, Department of Nutrition, School of Public Health, University of North Carolina at Chapel Hill, Chapel Hill, NC.

KENNETH R. KELLNER, M.D., Ph.D.
Associate Professor, Division of Maternal-Fetal Medicine, University of Florida, College of Medicine, Gainesville, FL.

JOHN H. KENNELL, M.D.
Professor of Pediatrics, Case Western Reserve University, School of Medicine, Rainbow Babies and Children's Hospital, Cleveland, OH.

MARSHALL H. KLAUS, M.D.
Professor and Chairman, Department of Pediatrics and Human Development, Michigan State University, East Lansing, MI.

ROBERT A. KNUPPEL, M.D., M.P.H.
Professor, OB/GYN and Public Health; Director, Maternal-Fetal Medicine; University of South Florida, College of Medicine, Tampa, FL.

MARIAN LAKE, R.N.C., M.P.H.
Division of Maternal-Fetal Medicine, Department of Obstetrics and Gynecology, University of South Florida, Tampa, FL.

JEFFREY LIPSHITZ, M.B., Ch.B., M.R.C.O.G., F.A.C.O.G.
Professor and Chief of Obstetrics, The University of Calgary, Calgary, Alberta, Canada.

ABBE LOVEMAN, R.N., M.B.A.
Assistant Director of Nursing, Women's Hospital Center, University of Miami, Jackson Memorial Hospital, Miami, FL.

DONALD E. MARSDEN, B.Med.Sc., M.B., B.S., M.R.C.O.G., F.R.A.C.O.G.
Consultant Gynaecologist, Royal Hobart Hospital, Hobart, Tasmania, Australia.

JAMES N. MARTIN, Jr., M.D.
Associate Professor, Department of Obstetrics and Gynecology, Division of Maternal-Fetal Medicine, University of Mississippi Medical Center, Jackson, MS.

ANNE L. MATTHEWS, R.N., M.S., Ph.D.
University of Colorado Health Sciences Center, School of Nursing, Denver, CO.

MARCELLA L. McKAY, R.N., M.S.N., M.Ed.
Executive Director, Mississippi Board of Nursing, Jackson, MS.

FRANK C. MILLER, M.D.
Chairman, Department of Obstetrics and Gynecology, University of Arkansas Medical Sciences, Little Rock, AR.

JOHN C. MORRISON, M.D.
Professor and Director, Department of Obstetrics and Gynecology, Division of Maternal-Fetal Medicine, University of Mississippi Medical Center, Jackson, MS.

JANE M. MURPHY, M.P.A., A.C.C.E.
Women's Hospital, Tampa, FL.

DAVID J. NOCHIMSON, M.D.
Director, Division of Maternal-Fetal Medicine, Department of Obstetrics and Gynecology, University of Connecticut Health Center, Farmington, CT.

HOWARD J. OSOFSKY, M.D., Ph.D.
Psychiatry Discipline Chief, Menninger Foundation, Topeka, KS.

MARY JO O'SULLIVAN, M.D.
Professor, Department of Obstetrics and Gynecology, University of Miami, Jackson Memorial Hospital, Miami, FL.

JOSEPH G. PASTOREK, II, M.D.
Assistant Professor, Section of Infectious Diseases, Department of Obstetrics and Gynecology, Louisiana State University School of Medicine, New Orleans, LA.

ROY H. PETRIE, M.D., Sc.D.
Professor of Obstetrics and Gynecology; Director, Division of Maternal-Fetal Medicine; Washington University School of Medicine, St. Louis, MO.

PAWAN RATTAN, M.D.
Assistant Professor, Department of Ob-Gyn, Division of Maternal-Fetal Medicine, Jefferson Medical College of Thomas Jefferson University, Philadelphia, PA.

JOSE C. SCERBO, M.D.
Private Practice; formerly Assistant Professor, Ob/Gyn, Division of Maternal-Fetal Medicine, University of South Florida, College of Medicine; Tampa, FL.

ANN C. M. SMITH, M.A.
Instructor, Department of Pediatrics, University of Colorado Health Sciences Center; Clinical Director, Genetic Services, The Children's Hospital; Denver, CO.

J. B. SPENCE, J.D.
Senior Partner, Spence, Payne, Masington, Grossman & Needle, P.A., Miami, FL.

JANIS GAIL SUTLIFF, B.S.N.
Director, Antepartum Testing Facility, Division of Maternal-Fetal Medicine, Department of Obstetrics and Gynecology, University of Alabama at Birmingham, Birmingham, AL.

KATHRYN E. TePAS, M.S.N., N.N.P.
Assistant Director of Nursing, Maternal Child Health, Charleston Area Medical Center, Charleston, WV.

FRED UELAND
Research Assistant, Department of Obstetrics and Gynecology, Stanford University School of Medicine, Stanford, CA.

KENT UELAND, M.D.
Professor and Chairman, Department of Obstetrics and Gynecology, Stanford University School of Medicine, Stanford, CA.

ANTHONY M. VINTZILEOS, M.D.
Division of Maternal-Fetal Medicine, Department of Obstetrics and Gynecology, University of Connecticut Health Center, Farmington, CT.

ATHANASIA M. WILLIAMS, R.N., B.S.N.
Columbia Presbyterian Medical Center, Department of Obstetrics and Gynecology, New York, NY.

FOREWORD

Today, in this age of high technology covering all aspects of the perinatal period, the health care professional, whether physician or nurse, cannot stand alone and adequately and comfortably provide health care services for the high-risk pregnant population. This book, *High-Risk Pregnancy: A Team Approach* is innovative in that the management of the pregnant woman, fetus, and newborn is considered from a collegial viewpoint.

Nurses and physicians formerly practiced their professions in adversarial roles; that is to say, the "physician-handmaiden" philosophy prevailed. However, today the socialization process has moved us to the team approach in providing perinatal services.

The richness of this book is that nurses who read it will not only have a solid scientific base for the nursing management of the patient but will also be able to understand the rationale for physician management, enabling them to collaborate fully on patient care and management.

Likewise, physicians who read this timely book will not only advance their knowledge of the practice of obstetrics but will also gain a fuller understanding and appreciation of the role and function of the nurse as a collaborator in patient care.

Every important aspect of high-risk pregnancy management is well developed and presented by the nurse-physician teams in this innovative book. The reader is fortunate to have such topics presented as Psychological Implications in High-Risk Pregnancy, Sexual Intimacy in Pregnancy, DIC, ITP, and Hemoglobinopathies, as so often these topics are not presented from the standpoint of a team approach.

As the horizons of perinatal care are continuing to expand, such important chapters as Genetic Counseling, Parent Counseling, Grief Counseling and Legal Implications as they relate to high-risk pregnancy are a powerful armamentarium to the physician-nurse team in high-risk obstetrics.

The time is now for such a comprehensive book as *High-Risk Pregnancy: A Team Approach*. John Donne stated "No man is an island." Certainly no physician or nurse can practice alone, but rather together as a team, working, studying, and practicing. Only then will the outcome of our collaborative practice improve.

SISTER JEANNE MEURER, C.N.M., M.S.
Assistant Professor
College of Public Health
University of South Florida
Tampa, Florida

PREFACE

High-Risk Pregnancy: A Team Approach is a new publication spanning the controversial and expanding areas of our specialty. This text emanated from a combination of courses that were begun more than six years ago at the University of South Florida. During those six years it became obvious to us that a true team approach to high-risk perinatal care was essential. Our assumption was that it was critically important that nurses and physicians who worked in the same practice settings have the same knowledge base in perinatal practice. Critiques of the courses demonstrated the ease with which identical didactic information could be presented and comprehended by both physicians and nurses. Consequently, we felt compelled to develop a text to support this collegial approach to learning and practice.

This text, prepared by a group of nationally respected perinatal team specialists, addresses the current status of many controversial areas in high-risk obstetrics. During the preparation of this publication we have been heartened by the willingness of all contributors to take part in this new venture, which addressed the "team approach" to perinatal care.

Robert Knuppel would like to take this opportunity to thank Nancy Barnett for her secretarial support; perinatal associate Marian Lake for her professional assistance; Evelyn Knuppel for her editorial assistance; and Denis Cavanagh, M.D., for his constant flagellation. Joan Drukker wishes to thank Margaret and Raymond Drukker for their support and encouragement. Both of us thank, most of all, the nurses and physicians who have enabled us to improve our teaching capabilities by taking time to fill out their critiques during the courses we have offered.

ROBERT A. KNUPPEL
JOAN E. DRUKKER

CONTENTS

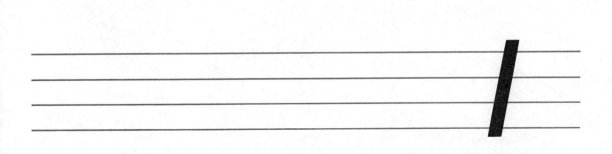

GENERAL
CONSIDERATIONS AND
ASSESSMENT

1

SCREENING FOR THE HIGH-RISK PREGNANCY

GRETCHEN M.-E. AUMANN*
MARGARET M. BAIRD*

Fifty years ago it was not uncommon to know or at least to know of someone who died in childbirth. At that time every young woman about to become a mother was realistically concerned about her safety. A healthy baby was considered an extra dividend. From the obstetric viewpoint, maternal survival was of primary importance and in some instances even living fetuses were sacrificed for the mother's safety (Burchell and Gunn, 1980).

The focus of obstetric care has changed during the past years. There has been a significant reduction in maternal mortality and morbidity as a result of advances in the management of disorders that have an adverse effect on the pregnant woman. However, there has been a less significant reduction in perinatal mortality and morbidity. In many ways, morbidity exerts a more profound economic effect than mortality (Wallace, 1971).

"The perinatal death rate is . . . like an iceberg, for we see only a portion of ill results, the deaths. But we must not forget the submerged and large fraction, the near deaths and the harm which they may cause. The correlation is suggestive because some causes of death—premature delivery, asphyxia during labor, rhesus incompatability—are known to be associated with the occurrence of mental or physical defects in some of the survivors. With a reduction in perinatal mortality there will also follow pari passu a diminution in perinatal morbidity" (Mixon, 1952).

Childbirth itself is described as part of the continuum of human development, affected by physical, biologic, psychologic, and social factors (Chez et al., 1979). The ideal time for assessment of this event is well before the antenatal period, since the majority of factors affecting perinatal outcome are present prior to conception (Hobel, 1976). However, most pregnant patients have already passed the period of fetal development most greatly affected by adverse factors by the time they first seek prenatal care. Consequently, to promote perinatal safety, it is necessary to identify those who are at risk and then to provide the specific care required to prevent death or damage.

Since the fetus in any given pregnancy is now at greater risk than the mother, the concept of "at risk" is applied to both maternal and fetal outcome. A "high-risk" pregnancy is defined as one in which the mother or the fetus has a significantly increased chance of death or disability, when compared with a "low-risk" pregnancy in which an optimal outcome is expected for both (Chez et al., 1979). The perinatal period, as a stage on the continuum, is unique in that outcome is reliant upon the early recognition and management of problems. Assessment of the existence of risks, together with appropriate and timely intervention, can help prevent disabling conditions both during the neonatal period and in future stages along this linear continuum.

The aim of obstetric care is to concentrate resources on improving perinatal outcome.

---

*The views of the authors do not purport to reflect the positions of the Department of the Army or the Department of Defense.

A multidisciplinary approach—an expensive form of health care requiring highly skilled manpower, equipment, and specialized facilities—is necessary to achieve this aim. The concept of regionalization of perinatal care implies the concentration of personnel and equipment in designated medical centers, where care is provided for all high-risk pregnancies in a defined geographic area. This approach to care of the obstetric patient is cost-effective and makes better use of highly skilled personnel, contributing to improved perinatal outcome.

This chapter will discuss the philosophy and history of screening for the high-risk pregnancy. Standards of normal prenatal care will be presented. Definitions and classifications of high risk pregnancy will be discussed, including socioeconomic, demographic, maternal medical, and fetal factors contributing toward increased risk in pregnancy. Recommendations for prevention of perinatal morbidity will be presented, along with a summary of goals for improvement in outcome.

History And Philosophy Of Risk Assessment In Obstetric Care

The idea that certain events that occur during the antenatal and intrapartum periods can have an adverse effect on the infant in later life is not a new one. As early as 1862, the association between abnormal labor and premature birth, and the child's subsequent mental and physical status was noted by London physician W. J. Little. It was not until the 1950s, nearly 100 years later, that significant work was done on even one specific abnormal neonatal outcome, that of cerebral palsy. In 1951, a retrospective study by Lilienfeld and Pasamanick showed that five factors—prematurity, multiple birth, previous stillbirths, toxemia, and placental abnormalities—were associated with later development of cerebral palsy in the infant (Hobel, 1976).

These investigators also found that prematurity or other neonatal conditions alone were associated with an increased incidence of epilepsy. They noted that the combination of a neonatal condition with maternal complications was associated with a twofold increase in the incidence of epilepsy. By 1955 it was clear that the five factors were related to perinatal morbidity and mortality.

In 1957 and 1958, Donnelly et al. and Wells et al., respectively, identified socioeconomic status, maternal age, and birth interval to be significant factors in perinatal mortality, particularly in conjunction with the previously identified factors. These studies served to validate a later study by Prechtl (1967), whose data suggested that nonoptimal conditions occur in association with each other (Hobel, 1976).

Two major prospective studies published in the 1960s and 1970s furthered progress in identification of risk factors. These were the British Perinatal Mortality Survey (Butler and Bonham, 1963), which reviewed all births in Great Britain during a short period, and the Collaborative Perinatal Study, *The Women and Their Pregnancies* (Niswander and Gordon, 1972), which examined a small population for several years. These studies clearly implicated the interrelationship between perinatal factors, and made an early attempt to identify factors responsible for later morbidity in children up to age 7 years. They also identified 13 additional factors adversely affecting perinatal outcome, including lack of prenatal care, length of labor, and smoking (Table 1–1).

Table 1–1. Literature Survey of Determinants of Perinatal Morbidity and Mortality

Investigators	Factors
Lilienfeld and Parkhurst (1951) and Lilienfeld and Passamanick (1955)	1. Prematurity 2. Multiple birth 3. Previous stillbirth or infant death 4. Toxemia 5. Placental abnormalities
Donnelly et al. (1957) and Wells et al. (1958)	6. Socioeconomic status 7. Maternal age 8. Birth interval
Butler and Bonham (1963) and Butler and Alberman (1969)	9. Parity 10. No prenatal care 11. Prolonged labor 12. Short labor 13. Breech 14. Smoking
Niswander and Gordon (1972)	15. History of infertility 16. Organic heart disease 17. Diabetes 18. Urinary tract infection 19. History of vaginal bleeding 20. Incompetent cervix 21. Hydramnios

Data from Hobel, C. J., *In* Spellacy, W. (ed.): Management of the High Risk Pregnancy. Baltimore, University Park Press, 1976.

Table 1–2. Summary of Risk Assessment Systems

Author(s)	System	Year[a]	Population Studied	Type of Study[b]	Purpose	Period Assessed[c]			When Used	High-Risk	Pregnancy at Risk[f] (%)
						Pre-natal	Intra-partum	Neonatal/Infancy			
Rogers	Risk register	1959 1964	13,020	R	Detect handicapped children	↓	22	↑	Birth to 1 month	One or more factors	26
Prechtl	Obstetrical score	1967	1378	R	Predict continuing abnormalities	↓	76	↑	Day 2 to day 14	Seven or more factors	12
Nesbitt & Aubry	Semiobjective grading system	1969	1001	R	Identify patient's poor outcome	29			Prenatally	Sum of factors (100)	29(p)
Effer	Prognostic risk score	1967 1968	211 350	P	Identify high-risk prenatal patients	↓	155	↑	Onset of labor	Sum of factors (50)	46(p) 11(p)
Goodwin	Antepartum fetal risk score	1969	936	R	Predict fetal risk	54			Onset of labor	Sum of factors (6)	10
Stembera	Identification of high-risk factors	1969 1972	3500	P	Predict high-risk neonate and infant	↓	123	→[d]	Pre-, intra-, and neonatally	Sum of factors (40)	23(p) 20(i)
Hobel	Screening to predict high-risk neonate	1969 1971	1417	P	Predict high-risk neonate	↓	126	→[e]	Pre-, intra-, and neonatally	Sum of factors (10)	32(p) 23(i)

[a]Refers to year(s) data were collected.
[b]R, retrospective; P, prospective.
[c]Numbers in column refer to number of factors used in assessment; arrows indicate risk factors in all categories; entries with no arrows indicate that only prenatal risk factors were assessed.
[d]All infants assessed during infancy.
[e]Only high-risk infants followed, with matched controls.
[f]p, prenatal patient at risk; i, intrapartum patient at risk.
From Hobel, C. J. In Spellacy, W. (ed.): Management of High Risk Pregnancy. Baltimore, University Park Press, 1976. © 1976 University Park Press, Baltimore.

In total, there are 21 factors identified in these studies as significantly contributing to increased perinatal mortality and morbidity. All of these are almost evenly divided between historical and pregnancy-related factors. These studies, therefore, provided the criteria necessary for the development of specific risk assessment techniques.

Thus, the concept of risk assessment in pregnancy grew out of the need to identify handicapped children early on in order to intervene and lessen long-term morbidity. This aim has subsequently focused prediction on a prevention of pregnancy- and birth-related morbidity and mortality of women and their infants. To this end, several studies have attempted more sophisticated prospective assessment techniques beginning as early as the prenatal period and extending throughout the continuum. A summary of these techniques can be seen in Table 1–2.

At present, no one particular assessment tool has been identified as ideal. It is generally recognized, however, that a combination of preconception, prenatal, and intrapartum factors contribute to placing the mother/infant dyad at risk. These factors and their potential for risk will be identified and discussed in light of present research.

Standards Of Prenatal Care

The prenatal period involves complex physiologic changes and emotional adjustments for the pregnant woman. These changes affect not only the woman and the fetus but also her family and the significant others in her social environment. Whatever happens to mother and fetus during the antepartum period is of critical importance to both. Adaptation is demanded of both in an ongoing sequence of events designed to prepare the fetus for life outside the uterus.

The growth of the fetus and the accompanying physical changes that occur during gestation are relatively predictable. However, the feelings and behaviors accompanying these changes may be more diverse, depending upon the unique characteristics and situation of the individual woman. Through early and continuous prenatal health care the pregnant woman and her family can be assisted in successfully adapting to these changes. Health care includes the ongoing assessment of the mother's

physical and emotional health and assessment of fetal health and development. Pregnancy provides an optimal opportunity for preventive health care, maintenance, and education. While the primary goal of antepartum care is to ensure a healthy mother and baby, a goal of equal importance is to promote an optimal physical and emotional experience for the family.

The physiologic process of pregnancy itself is normal. This process, however, imposes stresses to which both mother and fetus must adapt. Ideally, a woman will be in an optimal state of health and free from exposure to harmful substances prior to conception. As this is not always the situation, health care, if not already begun, should begin as soon as pregnancy is suspected. Prenatal care, therefore, becomes a screening process to differentiate those babies and mothers at jeopardy (high risk) from those in little danger (low risk). To be effective, such a screening system must be based on a thorough and uncompromising search for those factors that may endanger the pregnancy. Obviously, the participation of the woman in prenatal care is essential in identifying and treating problems that may threaten her or her fetus.

With the advent of regionalization, perinatal care is now, in many cases, being provided by an interdisciplinary team that includes an obstetrician, a nurse, a nurse-midwife, a nutritionist and a social worker. Each of these professionals has a distinct function and collectively can assist the patient and her family in achieving an optimal pregnancy experience. This team approach can also be more cost-effective through better utilization of health care providers.

The primary health care provider for the pregnant woman is in an ideal position to assess (1) the way in which the patient is adapting to the pregnancy, (2) the supports and resources available to her, and (3) the lifestyle and personal belief system subscribed to by the woman and her family (Becker, 1982). Early, frequent, and continuing contact with the pregnant woman provides an ideal opportunity to screen for and identify existing and potential problems that may place the woman and/or her fetus at risk.

Becker (1982) has developed a prenatal assessment guide that can assist health care providers in gathering a more comprehensive data base from which care specific to the needs of the individual patient can be

Table 1–3. Prenatal Assessment Guide*

I. Aspects of Adaptation
Age
Initial response to this pregnancy
Planned or unplanned pregnancy
Feelings about this pregnancy
Desired family size
Perception of pregnancy affecting present activities and responsibilities
Perception of parenthood affecting future activities and plans
Current developmental tasks of pregnancy: how coping with pregnancy; fantasies about pregnancy; changes in mood and effect on others
Sexual functioning during pregnancy: changes in; feelings about and/or problems with
Nature of verbal interest expressed about self and fetus
Preparation for: prenatal classes (type, when completed series?); place of delivery; care for other children in mother's absence; care for new sibling
Menstrual history: problems with; last normal menstrual period; expected date of confinement
Height and prepregnancy weight
Obstetric status: course, abdominal assessment, quickening, fetal heart sound, blood pressure, urinalysis, weight and pattern of gain, signs of any major complications of pregnancy
Medical history: illness (date)—treatment, outcome, surgery: childhood diseases; current immunization status; allergies; venereal disease; emotional problems
Family medical history: illnesses, emotional problems, genetic defects (both sides of family)
Loss of significant other in past year
Food intolerances (lactose, nausea/vomiting); food cravings; pica
Iron, vitamin, and/or mineral dietary supplements used
Elimination patterns: changes/problems with remedies used
Pattern of rest, sleep: difficulties with; remedies used

II. Aspects of Personal Belief System and Lifestyle
Date first sought prenatal care this pregnancy and in prior pregnancies
Reasons for seeking and receiving prenatal care
Beliefs about pregnancy and childbirth; cultural beliefs subscribed to with regard to childbearing (antepartum, intrapartum, postpartum)
Racial–ethnic group
Beliefs about role of father during pregnancy and labor, and role in child care
Perception of needs of fetus
Perception of needs of infant and proposed methods to meet those needs
Contraceptive history: methods used; failures and/or problems with; knowledge of alternate methods; willingness to use
Patterns of use of tobacco, alcohol, prescription and nonprescription drugs, illegal drugs; perception of effects of these substances on health of self and fetus
Patterns of nutrient intake: food dislikes; history of/method(s) of dieting
Planned method of infant feeding; why chosen
Occupation: Present, former, hours of duty per day, work requirements, hazards, amenities, plans regarding current occupation
Recreational activities: Plans to continue with; use of seat belt in car; pets in home
Community activities
Perception of health care personnel and agencies; prior experiences with
Date of last physical examination including breast exam, Pap smear, chest x-ray, and dental checkup
Breast self examination; done regularly?; if not, interested in learning about?

III. Aspects of Support
Address: How long there, housing accommodations, phone, plans to move (if so, when, where to, why?)
Level of education and future plans regarding
Religious preference; nominal or active involvement?
Marital status; how long married
Father of baby: age, occupation, educational level, racial–ethnic group, religious preference
Family composition; household members
Communication patterns with significant others
Communication patterns with health personnel
Perception of support system (mate, family, friends, community agencies): how available? how willing to use?
Perception of meaning of this pregnancy to significant others; mate's response to news of pregnancy
Type of prenatal service receiving; perception of adequacy of available transportation to receive medical care
Social service/community agencies involved with: how long? name of contact person?
Self concept and perceived ability to cope with life situations
Body image: prepregnancy; currently; response to physiologic changes of pregnancy
Mate's response to body changes in pregnancy
Feelings about parenting that woman received as a child; history of separation from mother—what age?
Prior experiences with infants; knowledge of infant care
Feelings about previous pregnancies, labor, puerperium, and mothering skills
Knowledge of reproduction, labor and delivery, and puerperium

*From Becker, C. H.: Comprehensive assessment of the healthy gravida. JOGN Nurs. 11:375, 1982.

planned and implemented. This prenatal assessment guide consists of three parts (Table 1–3). The first deals with aspects of physical and psychologic adaptation to pregnancy. The second focuses on aspects of the woman's personal belief system and lifestyle that may affect her health and the health of the fetus. The third aims to identify the support systems and resources available to the patient that may influence the course and outcome of her pregnancy.

DIAGNOSIS OF PREGNANCY

Of fundamental importance is establishment of the diagnosis of pregnancy. If this is confirmed by correlation of historical information, physical examination, and laboratory tests, the estimation of gestational age and estimated date of birth (EDB) at this early visit will minimize confusion as the pregnancy continues. Estimation of gestational age is most accurate in the early first trimester and becomes subject to increasing error as the pregnancy develops.

There are many presumptive signs of pregnancy. The most frequent is amenorrhea, which is often the first evidence to the patient of possible conception. Some patients may not be aware of pregnancy until other symptoms appear. These include nausea, vomiting, breast fullness, urinary frequency, constipation, fatigue, and enlarging abdomen.

Certain signs of pregnancy are highly suggestive of the diagnosis. These include uterine enlargement, softening of the uterine isthmus (Hegar's sign), and vaginal and cervical cyanosis (Chadwick's sign). Also, a positive laboratory test for human chorionic gonadotropin (HCG) is indicative of pregnancy (Brunel, 1980). Estimation of gestational age by uterine size is one of the most important elements of the first examination. The detection of fetal heart tones at about 10 to 12 weeks of gestation is possible with an ultrasonic Doppler, whereas the fetal heart rate cannot be heard until about 17 weeks with a DeLee stethoscope; most pregnancies will be heard by at least 19 weeks' gestation (Pritchard and MacDonald, 1980). The estimated date of birth (EDB) can be calculated by Nägele's rule: Add 7 days to the first day of the last menstrual period (LMP) and subtract 3 months. However, irregular or prolonged menstrual cycles, or a known single sexual exposure can cause variations from this calculation.

INITIAL PRENATAL CARE

Once there is a confirmed diagnosis of pregnancy, an initial visit should be scheduled as soon as it is feasible. During the initial interview with the woman, careful attention to detail is necessary. This first visit is to assess risk and establish a plan of care, and should include:

1. A careful screening history.
2. A general to specific physical examination designed to exclude risk factors.
3. Routine laboratory screening (Table 1–4).
4. Individually indicated maternal laboratory evaluation (Table 1–5).
5. Careful fetal assessment.
6. Specialized studies to ascertain fetal well-being and/or fetal maturity as individually indicated.

Patient biographic data—age, race, religion, marital status, and social and economic factors—must be carefully considered at this time. Historical data should include obstetric history (gravidity, parity, and details of previous pregnancies), menstrual history, and contraceptive history. A complete medical history must be obtained to screen for medical problems that may cause complications or be aggravated by the pregnancy. These include diabetes mellitus, hypertension, thyroid disorders, cardiac disease, and seizure disorders. The initial history must also note hospitalization, prior surgery, medications taken, allergies, smoking, alcohol, and drug usage. A conventional review of all organ systems should be done. Items of significance from the family history are multiple gestation, diabetes mellitus, bleeding disorders, and hereditary illnesses (e.g., hemophilia, Down's syndrome, and Tay-Sachs disease). During the physical exam, attention should be directed to specific organ systems as a positive history is elicited. A general examination should especially evaluate the blood pressure, weight, height, optic fundi, thyroid, lungs, heart, abdomen, and extremities.

LABORATORY DATA

Pregnancy induces dramatic changes in maternal body systems. Laboratory findings must be evaluated in terms of pregnancy

Table 1–4. General Laboratory Examinations

Tests	Initial Visit	26–30 Weeks	36 Weeks	Findings that Signal Further Assessment
Blood Tests				
1. Complete Blood Count (CBC)				
(a) Hemoglobin (Hgb)[a] or	X	X	X	Hgb <10 g/dl[d]
(b) Hematocrit (Hct)[a]				Hct 32% or less
(c) White blood cell count (WBC)	X			15,000 mm or more
(d) Differential smear (Diff)	X			Cellular abnormalities and/or decreased platelets
2. Blood Group	X			
3. Rh Factor	X			Mother: Rh-negative Mate: Rh-positive or unknown
4. Antibody Screen	X			A titer defined by the laboratory
5. Serology for Syphilis	X		Repeat[b]	Positive
6. Rubella Screen (titer)	X			A titer of 1:8 or less, or a significant rise in titer
7. Two-Hour Postprandial Blood Sugar	Obtain[c]	X	X	145 mg/dl[d] or more
Urine Tests				
1. Urine Bacteria Screen	X	X		Positive
2. Urine Glucose and Protein	AT EACH VISIT			Protein 1+ or more Glucose 1+ or more
Cervical Tests				
1. Papanicolaou smear (Pap smear)	X			Positive
2. Culture for gonorrhea	X		Repeat[b]	Positive

[a]Usually one or the other is needed, not both.
[b]Repeat test if woman is at risk for reinfection.
[c]Obtain specimen if high-risk pregnancy or if history is inadequate.
[d]Note that in current literature mg/dl may be used instead of the more traditional mg/100 ml; 1 deciliter (dl) = 100 ml. Norms may be different depending on laboratory variability.

norms rather than nonpregnancy norms. *Individual laboratories determine their own pregnancy norms, and normal values vary with the technique used.* Also, considerations such as climate and altitude may influence the norm for that population (Schneider, 1978).

Table 1–4 identifies tests for the low-risk pregnant woman. Abnormalities in these routine tests or positive findings in the history and physical examination may indicate the need for further specific tests (Table 1–5).

SUBSEQUENT PRENATAL CARE

The recommended frequency of prenatal visits is monthly, starting at the first indication of pregnancy, until 28 to 30 weeks, a visit every 2 weeks until 36 weeks, and weekly from 37 weeks until delivery. It is beneficial to see the patient weekly starting at the 18th week to gather information about fetal heart tones, uterine size, and quickening, in order to more firmly establish the correct gestational age. Once fetal heart tones are heard and quickening occurs, the patient

Table 1–5. Specific Laboratory Examinations

Tests	Initial Visit	24–28 Weeks	36 Weeks	Findings that Signal Further Assessment
Blood Tests				
Antibody screen (Rh-negative woman)	X	X	X	Significant, as defined by the local laboratory*
Sickle Cell Screen	X			Positive for trait or anemia*
Tay-Sachs Screen	X			Carrier*
Cervical Test				
Herpesvirus hominis, type 2	When physical findings indicate at any prenatal visit		X	Positive
Skin Test				
Tuberculosis	X			Positive

*Test the woman's male partner.

can again be seen monthly until 30 weeks' gestation.

SUBSEQUENT HISTORY

Information regarding changes in the woman's physical, emotional, and social status should be reviewed and noted at each visit. Problems and concerns identified previously should be followed up. Information regarding prenatal education, prenatal education classes, child care classes, Lamaze classes, and other helpful programs should be provided, along with encouragement for the woman to utilize these resources. Ongoing assessment, counseling, and education in several areas are necessary (Table 1–6).

Table 1–6. Prenatal Assessment/Teaching Guide*

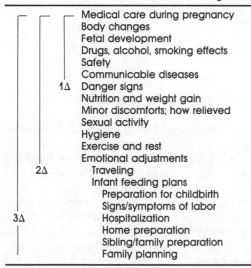

		Medical care during pregnancy
		Body changes
		Fetal development
		Drugs, alcohol, smoking effects
		Safety
		Communicable diseases
	1Δ	Danger signs
		Nutrition and weight gain
		Minor discomforts; how relieved
		Sexual activity
		Hygiene
		Exercise and rest
		Emotional adjustments
	2Δ	Traveling
		Infant feeding plans
		Preparation for childbirth
		Signs/symptoms of labor
3Δ		Hospitalization
		Home preparation
		Sibling/family preparation
		Family planning

*1Δ = 1st trimester; 2Δ = 2nd trimester; 3Δ = 3rd trimester.

SUBSEQUENT PHYSICAL ASSESSMENT

At each subsequent prenatal visit the following physical parameters should be assessed:

Maternal
1. Weight
2. Blood pressure
3. Urinalysis
4. Edema
5. Uterine growth
6. Laboratory tests as indicated (Table 1–4)

Fetal
1. Quickening and presence of daily fetal movements
2. Fetal heart tones
3. Fundal height
4. Specific assessments as indicated:
   A. Ultrasound (biophysical profile)
   B. Amniocentesis
   C. Electronic fetal heart rate (FHR); nonstress test (NST)/ contraction stress test (CST)

PARENTING ASSESSMENT

Allen and Mantz (1981) report that being "normal," that is, medically and obstetrically healthy, may carry an underestimated risk factor. Being labeled as normal may cause health care providers to overlook this group of patients, who may not be coping well with childbearing, but whose clues are often too subtle and thus overlooked until an acute emotional or social crisis occurs.

Over the course of 2 years, 180 families were studied in a project designed to provide appropriate nursing care to patients potentially at risk, although designated as normal. These criteria were as follows:

1. Significant ambivalent or negative feelings toward pregnancy after 20 weeks' gestation.

2. Insecure or negative feelings about her own mothering skills.

3. Inappropriate positive feelings about pregnancy or mothering.

4. Inadequate nuclear family support.

5. Inadequate extended support system.

6. Current or historically significant psychiatric problems (Allen and Mantz, 1981).

Therefore, in addition to the ongoing physical assessment, counseling, and education, parenting assessment must also be a continuing process. An important concern of health care providers who are committed to the promotion of healthy parenting is the prevention of child abuse and neglect. Early identification and treatment during pregnancy of those parents who are at high risk for becoming neglectful or abusive toward their children is the responsibility of all members of the health care delivery team.

Josten (1981) has devised a "prenatal assessment of parenting" guide, offering health care providers a framework for the prenatal identification of women who need assistance with their parenting skills and attitudes. On the subject of identifying parents at risk, Josten states: "It would be unethical to evaluate women prenatally on their parenting ability unless the intention was to offer them assistance. Those women identified at high risk need help so that child abuse and neglect can be prevented. I suggest using an intervention approach that focuses initially on the woman's difficulties with the developmental task of pregnancy and then the problems present in her life situation."

CONTINUING ASSESSMENT OF RISK

As pregnancy progresses, the woman should have all risk factors reassessed. At times, patients initially identified as being "low risk" develop problems later in gestation (Table 1–7). In fact, it has been suggested that the current concept and definition of the term "low risk" needs to be reexamined: As Wilson and Schifrin (1980) have noted, "In labeling a small group of patients "high risk" we may paradoxically be creating an elite class of obstetric patients destined to receive the best care the specialty has to offer. The emphasis on "high risk" may convince both physicians and lay individuals alike that a patient not considered "high risk" is "low risk." "Low risk" in turn may be interpreted to mean negligible risk—an unfortunate conclusion."

Identification Of A High-Risk Pregnancy

A high-risk pregnancy is one in which the mother or fetus has a significantly increased chance of death or disability. In order to achieve optimal perinatal outcome, all factors contributing to mortality and morbidity in a particular pregnancy must be identified and acted upon early. This section will identify and categorize high-risk pregnancy factors and outline the reasons for each factor's being so designated. The factors may be divided into the categories of socioeconomic, demographic, and medical (Table 1–8). There is considerable overlap of the various categories, and it will become apparent that the first category, socioeconomic, achieves more importance as control or improvement occurs within the purely medical category (Chez et al., 1979).

SOCIOECONOMIC FACTORS

Socioeconomic Status. The many social factors that place a fetus at greater risk are interrelated. Such conditions as overcrowding, poor standards of housing and hygiene, and poor nutrition are closely associated with high rates of infant and child morbidity and mortality. Poverty and low educational status are at the root of these problems, and in countries where social and economic improvement has occurred, there has also been a decrease in perinatal mortality (Chez et al., 1979).

Parental Occupation. Occupation of the father, as a reflection of socioeconomic status, is related to profound differences in the incidence of prematurity and infant mortal-

Table 1–7. Risk Factors in Early and Late Stages of Pregnancy

Stage	High-Risk Factors	Moderate-Risk Factors
Early Pregnancy	Failure of uterine growth or disproportionate uterine growth	Unresponsive urinary tract infection
	Exposure to teratogens (radiation, infection, chemicals)	Suspected ectopic pregnancy
	Pregnancy complicated by isoimmunization	Suspected missed abortion
	Need for antenatal genetic diagnosis	Severe hyperemesis gravidarum
	Severe anemia (9 g or less hemoglobin)	Positive VDRL test
		Positive gonorrhea screening
		Anemia not responsive to iron treatment
		Viral illness
		Vaginal bleeding
		Mild anemia (9–10.9 g hemoglobin)
Late Pregnancy	Failure of uterine growth or disproportionate uterine growth	Hypertensive states of pregnancy (mild)
	Severe anemia (less than 9 g hemoglobin)	Breech, if cesarean section is planned
	More than 42½ weeks' gestation	Uncertain presentations
	Severe preeclampsia	Need for fetal maturity studies
	Eclampsia	
	Breech, if vaginal delivery is planned	Postdate pregnancy (41–42½ weeks' gestation)
	Moderate to severe isoimmunization (necessitating intrauterine transfusion or neonatal exchange transfusion)	
	Placenta previa	
	Hydramnios or oligohydramnios	Induction of labor
	Antepartum fetal death	Suspected fetopelvic disproportion at term
	Thromboembolic disease	
	Premature labor (less than 37 weeks' gestation)	Floating presentations 2 weeks or less from the EDC
	Premature rupture of membranes (less than 38 weeks' gestation)	
	Tumor or other obstruction of birth canal	
	Abruptio placenta	
	Chronic or acute pyelonephritis	
	Multiple gestation	
	Abnormal oxytocin challenge test	
	Falling urinary estriols	
	Prolonged rupture of membranes	
	Diabetes	

Adapted from Babson, S. G., Pernoll, M. L., and Benda, G. I. (with the assistance of Simpson, K.): Diagnosis and Management of the Fetus and Neonate at Risk, 4th ed. St. Louis, C. V. Mosby, 1980.

Table 1–8. Categorization of High Risk Pregnancy Factors

Socioeconomic factors
1. Inadequate finances
2. Poor housing
3. Severe social problems
4. Unwed, especially adolescent
5. Minority status
6. Nutritional deprivation
7. Parental occupation

Demographic Factors
1. Maternal age under 16 or over 35 years
2. Overweight or underweight prior to pregnancy
3. Height less than 5 feet
4. Maternal education less than 11 years
5. Family history of severe inherited disorders

Medical Factors
A. Obstetric History
1. History of infertility
2. Previous ectopic pregnancy or spontaneous abortion
3. Grandmultiparity
4. Previous stillborn or neonatal death
5. Uterine/cervical abnormality
6. Previous multiple gestation
7. Previous premature labor/delivery
8. Previous prolonged labor
9. Previous cesarean section
10. Previous low-birth-weight infant
11. Previous macrosomic infant
12. Previous midforceps delivery
13. Previous baby with neurologic deficit, birth injury, or malformation
14. Previous hydatidiform mole or choriocarcinoma

B. Maternal Medical History/Status
1. Maternal cardiac disease
2. Maternal pulmonary disease
3. Maternal metabolic disease—particularly diabetes mellitus, thyroid disease
4. Chronic renal disease, repeated urinary tract infections, repeated bacteriuria
5. Maternal gastrointestinal disease
6. Maternal endocrine disorders (pituitary, adrenal)
7. Chronic hypertension
8. Maternal hemoglobinopathies
9. Seizure disorder
10. Venereal and other infectious diseases
11. Weight loss greater than 5 pounds
12. Malignancy
13. Surgery during pregnancy
14. Major congenital anomalies of the reproductive tract
15. Maternal mental retardation, major emotional disorders

C. Current OB Status
1. Late or no prenatal care
2. Rh sensitization
3. Fetus inappropriately large or small for gestation
4. Premature labor
5. Pregnancy-induced hypertension
6. Multiple gestation
7. Polyhydramnios
8. Premature rupture of the membranes
9. Antepartum bleeding
   a. Placenta previa
   b. Abruptio placenta
10. Abnormal presentation
11. Postmaturity
12. Abnormality in tests for fetal well-being
13. Maternal anemia

D. Habits/Habituation
1. Smoking during pregnancy
2. Regular alcohol intake
3. Drug use/abuse

ity. Kessner et al. (1973) have reported that the lowest incidence of perinatal loss occurs in cases in which the father is in a professional or managerial position, whereas the highest rates of loss are seen in situations in which the father is absent altogether. Between these two extremes, the incidence of loss gets higher as one goes down the socioeconomic spectrum, with the rate increasing through the ranks of sales/clerical workers and skilled craftsman, until it has doubled in families in which the father is in a semi-skilled or manual labor occupation.

It has further been demonstrated that a correlation exists between the occupation of the mother's father and the incidence of perinatal loss; that is, women from a higher socioeconomic background have a lower incidence of perinatal loss than those from a less affluent one (Kessner et al., 1973).

Social Environment. The effects of maternal social environment on the outcome of pregnancy are recognized to be both multiple and profound. "Social environment" itself is described as the summation of numerous factors, including the family's standards of health and hygiene, housing and financial status, emotional and social support, and so on. The effects may be direct or indirect and may be difficult to separate within the context of socioeconomic status. It is the interrelationship of these factors, rather than any single factor, that works to affect the outcome of pregnancy.

A pilot study in 1966 from a health care unit in South Philadelphia (Fed. Res. Grant IR 18-H 50 1135-01) provides some interesting observations: The majority of the families came from a deprived family background and low socioeconomic group. If the pregnant patient was married, there frequently was marital disharmony and disruption, wife and child abuse, and little help or support from relatives. The environment itself was grossly unhygienic. Recurrent infections and "poor health" were frequently noted within the family. Educational needs were, for the most part, unmet and ignored. Single-parent families were commonplace and accepted. Financial support was, at best, inadequate, with the pregnant patient frequently being the main wage earner. The adverse influences of this history of social, emotional, nutritional and financial deprivation on reproductive outcome were numerous. Reproductive histories obtained from female relatives of the pregnant patient included a high rate of reproductive loss, significant evidence of premature labor, low-birth-weight infants, and a high proportion of children with mental retardation or learning disabilities. These types of outcomes were traced through one or more generations and could be repeated in the next.

Marital Status. The frequency of cases of low-birth-weight infants and the perinatal mortality rates of infants born to unmarried mothers are double those of the children of married women. Marital status alone is not necessarily an indicator of potential risk for mother and fetus so much as it is an indicator of an unwanted/unplanned pregnancy. These pregnant women, especially if unwed or teenagers, tend to neglect antenatal care and leave advice unheeded. Statistically, pregnancy complications occur more frequently in unmarried than in married women.

Psychologic High-Risk Factors. When a woman becomes pregnant the entire family prepares for change. The support and guidance that the family receives during this preparation period will influence the family's ability to cope with the stress of this pregnancy and with its changes in family structure, as well as with other life stresses in the future. Therefore, it is important to identify psychologic maladaptation to pregnancy. Maladaptations may increase anxiety, and it has been suggested that increased anxiety can cause physical complications during pregnancy, including preterm labor (Creasy, 1981). It is also recognized that child battering, mental illness, and many psychosomatic illnesses result from unhealthy mother-infant-family relationships.

DEMOGRAPHIC FACTORS

Maternal Age. The relationship between maternal age and pregnancy outcome has long been recognized. Studies have shown that the optimal age for childbearing is between 20 and 30 years, with a steadily increasing risk of perinatal mortality when the woman is over 30 years of age. Children of mothers 19 years and younger and the firstborn of mothers 35 years of age and older are at an increased risk for prematurity and other pregnancy complications such as toxemia and congenital anomalies (Niswander and Gordon, 1972).

Maternal Education. Correlations have been indicated between the number of years of schooling completed by a pregnant woman and perinatal death rate, birth weight, and the rate of neurologic abnormalities seen in the child at 1 year of age. As the length of the mother's education increases, perinatal morbidity and mortality rates drop significantly. It is thought that this association occurs not because education in itself decreases problems in pregnancy but that length of education is a useful index of general socioeconomic status.

Maternal Height. Short stature of the mother (less than 5 ft.) has been connected with increased perinatal morbidity and mortality in several studies. The primary reason suspected for this association is that short maternal stature may be a reflection of adverse environmental conditions and poor nutrition as a child. Because stature relates to pelvic dimensions, short women have a higher incidence of operative delivery, including cesarean section because of cephalopelvic disproportion.

Maternal Weight and Weight Gain. Women who are underweight or overweight for height and age at the beginning of pregnancy are at risk for poor perinatal outcome. Both of these parameters reflect previous nutritional status of the mother. Women who are underweight and/or fail to gain the recommended 20 to 30 pounds during pregnancy are at risk for having low-birth-weight infants. Women who are overweight and/or gain more than 30 pounds during pregnancy are at risk for developing preeclampsia and having large-for-gestational-age babies. Fetuses weighing more than 4000 grams (9 pounds) are frequently associated with an increased likelihood of dystocia during labor, fetal distress, maternal and infant birth trauma, and consequently, an increased incidence of perinatal morbidity and mortality.

PREVIOUS OBSTETRIC PROBLEMS

In women who have had an obstetric complication or a perinatal loss, there is a tendency for the problem to "repeat" in a subsequent pregnancy (Shapiro et al., 1968). This is true for all of the factors listed in the high-risk pregnancy classification (Table 1–8).

History of Infertility. Conceptions following medical or surgical treatment of infertility carry a considerable high-risk factor. There is a high prevalence of spontaneous abortion, premature labor, and multiple gestation in women treated for infertility, and there is a significant increase in the perinatal mortality rate.

Previous Ectopic Pregnancy and Spontaneous Abortion. For women of any parity who have had an abortion or ectopic pregnancy, there is a significantly higher perinatal mortality rate in subsequent pregnancies. The incidence of infertility in patients who have had an ectopic pregnancy is high, as is the chance of a repeat ectopic conception. In women who have had two or more spontaneous abortions, the risk of a repeat abortion is significantly increased. However, should the pregnancy proceed beyond the second trimester, a history of previous abortion does not predispose the woman to premature labor (Cavanagh and Talisman, 1969).

Previous Stillbirth or Neonatal Death. A history of a previous perinatal death, especially if the cause is unknown, is an absolute indication of high-risk status. The perinatal mortality rate in these women is even higher than in those who have had a previous spontaneous abortion or a premature live birth (Butler and Bonham, 1963).

Uterine/Cervical Abnormality. Abnormalities of the uterus/cervix such as a bicornuate uterus, uterine septum, and incompetent cervix are frequently associated with repeated spontaneous abortions and premature labor. A large number of abnormalities of the genital tract remain undetected unless a complication of pregnancy or delivery alerts the health care provider to the need for a thorough investigation. Congenital uterine malformation should be suspected if there is a history of repeated spontaneous abortions, malpresentations, and malpositions during labor.

Previous Premature Labor/Delivery. Premature labor is one of the most challenging problems facing perinatal health care providers. Despite recent clinical advances, premature birth is still associated with up to 85 percent of nonanomalous neonatal deaths and is the cause of handicaps in at least 10 percent of the survivors (Dweck, 1977; Marriage and Davies, 1976). A woman who has had a previous premature labor and/or delivery has a significantly higher chance of delivering prematurely with a subsequent pregnancy. Depending on the etiology of the preterm birth, the history of one previous preterm birth is associated with a risk of recurrence of 25 to 50 percent, and the risk increases with each subsequent preterm birth (Creasy and Herron, 1981). There is also an increased chance that the patient will have a stillbirth or neonatal death (Cavanagh and Talisman, 1969).

The etiology of premature labor remains somewhat of a mystery, although certain risk factors have been identified (Fig. 1–1) (Creasy and Herron, 1981). Because prediction of premature labor is the first step toward prevention, several authors have attempted to develop risk assessment systems, with varying success. Most recently, a risk prediction system for preterm labor was outlined by Creasy and Herron (1981) (Table 1–9). This system reinforces the importance of both past reproductive history and current pregnancy conditions in the prediction and prevention of premature labor.

Previous Macrosomic Infant. A macrosomic infant is one who, at term, weighs more than 4000 grams or is large for his or her gestational age. A woman who has previously

had, or is suspected of carrying, a large infant is at risk for having or developing diabetes during pregnancy, with all its concomitant problems. The infants themselves are at increased risk for morbidity (including low newborn blood sugars) and mortality as a result of unstable maternal metabolic condition, placental insufficiency, and, even if the mother is not diabetic, birth trauma due to difficult delivery, shoulder dystocia, etc.

Grandmultiparity. Increasing parity increases the risk of pregnancy wastage both in terms of higher mortality rates and an increased risk of neurologic and congenital anomaly. In general, the lowest perinatal mortality rate and incidence of obstetric complication occurs in second and third pregnancies, and the highest in fifth and subsequent pregnancies. The frequency of anemia, hypertensive disease of pregnancy, antepartum hemorrhage, placenta previa, premature placental separation, and postpartum hemorrhage, as well as the number of cesarean sections, almost doubles for each of these complications in women of increasing parity (greater than para 4) compared with women of lower parity.

Maternal Medical History/Status. Certain maternal disease states diagnosed either prior to pregnancy or at the time of initial physical exam or at any time during the pregnancy may have a significant influence on the outcome of the pregnancy for both fetus and mother (see Table 1–8). These are discussed in the following paragraphs.

Maternal cardiac disease. The diagnosis of organic heart disease includes rheumatic heart disease, hypertensive heart disease, and congenital heart disease. Fetal death rates are substantially increased in women with any of these diagnoses; in fact, the stillbirth rate is doubled compared with that in women without organic heart disease. The presence of organic heart disease also significantly increases the risk of delivery of a low-birth-weight infant (less than 2500 grams).

Maternal pulmonary disease. Bronchial asthma is a rather common respiratory disease; pregnancy does not seem to have any consistent effect on it. Most women will do fairly well throughout the pregnancy. The fetuses, however, may be at increased risk

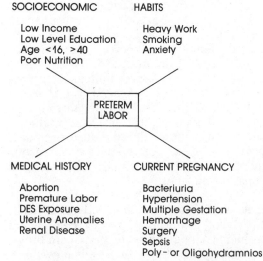

EPIDEMIOLOGY OF PRETERM LABOR

SOCIOECONOMIC

Low Income
Low Level Education
Age <16, >40
Poor Nutrition

HABITS

Heavy Work
Smoking
Anxiety

PRETERM LABOR

MEDICAL HISTORY

Abortion
Premature Labor
DES Exposure
Uterine Anomalies
Renal Disease

CURRENT PREGNANCY

Bacteriuria
Hypertension
Multiple Gestation
Hemorrhage
Surgery
Sepsis
Poly- or Oligohydramnios

Figure 1–1. Summary of risk factors for premature labor. (From Creasy, R. K., and Herron, M. A.: Prevention of premature birth. Semin. Perinatol. 5:297, 1981.)

Table 1–9. Risk of Preterm Delivery

Score	Socioeconomic Status	Past History	Daily Habits	Current Pregnancy
1	2 children at home Low socioeconomic status	1 abortion <1 yr since last birth	Work outside home	Unusual fatigue
2	<20 yr >40 yr Single parent	2 abortions	More than 10 cigarettes per day	Weight gain of 12 lb by 32 wk Albuminuria Hypertension Bacteriuria
3	Very low socioeconomic status <5 ft <100 lb	3 abortions	Heavy work Long tiring trip	Breech at 32 wk Weight loss of 5 lb Head engaged Febrile illness
4	<18 yr	Pyelonephritis		Metrorrhagia after 12 wk Effacement Dilatation Uterine irritability
5		Uterine anomaly Second trimester abortion DES exposure		Placenta previa Hydramnios Uterine myoma
10		Premature delivery Repeated second trimester abortion		Twins Abdominal surgery

EDB (estimated date of birth): _____

HIGH-RISK: Yes   No

From Creasy, R. K., and Herron, M. A.: Prevention of preterm birth. Semin. Perinatol. 5:299, 1981.

for intrauterine growth retardation, still-birth, or neonatal death.

Diabetes mellitus. Diabetes is deleterious to pregnancy in a number of ways. The adverse maternal effects that are likely to be encountered are as follows:

1. The likelihood of preeclampsia/eclampsia is increased fourfold.

2. Infection occurs more often and is likely to be more severe.

3. The fetus frequently is macrosomic, and its size may lead to difficult delivery with injury to the infant and the birth canal.

4. The tendency for fetal condition to substantially deteriorate prior to the onset of labor, as well as the possibility of dystocia, increases the frequency of cesarean section with its incumbent maternal risks.

5. Postpartum hemorrhage is more common.

6. Polyhydramnios is common.
Maternal diabetes also affects the fetus/neonate in a variety of ways:

1. Perinatal death rate is considerably higher.

2. Morbidity as a result of birth trauma or respiratory distress syndrome is common.

3. Congenital anomalies, particularly cardiac anomalies, are more frequent.

4. The infant is more likely to inherit diabetes.

5. Maternal diabetes may lead to neurologic and psychologic deficits in the child, possibly as a result of ketosis during pregnancy.

Maternal thyroid dysfunction. Thyroid disease appears to have an adverse effect on pregnancy outcome. Hypothyroidism results primarily in an increase in the stillbirth rate. Hyperthyroidism shows a slight association with increased neonatal mortality rate, a significant increase in the frequency of delivery of low-birth-weight infants, and an overall drop in the mean birth weight. Once the diagnosis of thyroid disease is made in pregnancy, therapy may be complicated by the presence of the fetus. Drugs that may be beneficial to the mother can be harmful to the fetus, and this must be taken into account when a therapeutic decision is made (Burrow and Ferris, 1982).

Gastrointestinal/hepatic system diseases. With the exception of hepatitis and appendicitis, maternal GI disease does not generally cause any increased risk in pregnancy. Hepatitis appears to be associated with an increase in low-birth-weight infants and an increased incidence of infection of the infant. Appendicitis appears to increase the rate of premature labor, fetal death and low-birth-weight infants, most probably as a result of infection, regardless of whether surgery is performed.

Chronic hypertension. In most cases of chronic hypertension, high blood pressure is the only demonstrable finding. A few patients, however, show secondary alterations that are often grave, not only in relation to pregnancy but also with regard to maternal life expectancy. These include hypertensive cardiac disease, arteriosclerotic renal disease, and retinal hemorrhages and exudate. Frequently the babies of mothers with chronic hypertension show evidence of intrauterine growth retardation. The incidence of abruptio placentae and pregnancy-induced hypertension (PIH) has been noted to be increased also.

Renal disease/UTI. Renal diseases such as glomerulonephritis, nephrotic syndrome, polycystic disease of the kidney, and previous nephrectomy/renal transplant vary in their effect on pregnancy outcome, depending on the severity of the disease. Most commonly they are associated with increased risk for premature labor, intrauterine growth retardation, and placental insufficiency leading to antepartum fetal distress.

Acute urinary tract infection (UTI), if undiagnosed or untreated, may lead to premature labor (Pritchard et al., 1985).

Current OB Status. Ideally, if a woman participates in prenatal care, identification and treatment of problems that may threaten her or her fetus will be accomplished. Prenatal care, therefore, is a screening process that incorporates the historical and social factors mentioned previously with constant surveillance of the mother and fetus as the pregnancy continues. Some of the factors contributing to poor perinatal outcome in relation to the current pregnancy are discussed below (see also Table 1–8).

Late or no prenatal care. In two groups of women matched for age, parity, and risk assessment, studies at the University of Tennessee (Ryan et al., 1980) demonstrated that perinatal outcome was substantially altered by amount of prenatal care. Analysis of outcomes revealed marked differences in pregnancy outcome between the group of women who had less than four prenatal visits and those who had four or more visits. Women with late or no prenatal care had a significantly higher rate of premature labor, premature delivery, low-birth-weight infants, and stillborns.

Antepartum bleeding. Antepartum bleeding is defined as bleeding from the vagina after the 28th week of gestation and prior to the onset of labor. The etiology includes (1) placenta previa, (2) abruptio placentae, (3) local causes such as cervical polyps or erosions, and (4) unknown etiology in which a specific cause cannot be found.

Placenta previa, and consequent bleeding from a placenta partly or wholly attached to the lower uterine segment, is a complication frequently associated with multiparity and older gravidas. Women who have had a placenta previa tend to repeat this complication in subsequent pregnancies. Maternal mortality associated with placenta previa has been reduced to less than 1 percent, but maternal morbidity from this complication is still as high as 20 percent (Cavanagh et al., 1982).

Prematurity is the prevalent cause of perinatal mortality associated with placenta previa. Despite the availability of neonatal intensive care, the perinatal mortality rate remains as high as 20 percent, with intrauterine hypoxia and developmental anomalies also complicating the situation.

Abruptio placentae is described as the premature separation of a normally situated placenta from the uterine implantation site with ensuing retroplacental bleeding, which may or may not cause vaginal bleeding. Abruption of the placenta is most commonly caused by hypertension of any origin, including preeclampsia. High parity and a history of previous abruption have also been implicated. In a study by Pritchard et al. (1970), 47 percent of women with abruptions severe enough to cause fetal death were hypertensive. Women having their 7th child were 6 times more likely to have an abruption than were primiparous women. Other factors implicated as possible causes of abruption are trauma, sudden uterine decompression (particularly with polyhydramnios), short umbilical cord, and uterine leiomyomas and anomalies.

Maternal mortality in abruptio placentae ranges from 2 to 10 percent in severe cases with associated fetal death. Perinatal mortality approaches 50 percent primarily because of the acuteness of the insult.

In general, antepartum bleeding is associated with significantly increased risks for premature labor and delivery, intrauterine growth retardation, fetal and maternal anemia, and perinatal death.

Multiple gestation. Perinatal mortality in twins is 2 to 3 times higher than in single births. The predominant cause of perinatal death is prematurity. Other major complications include placenta previa, intrauterine growth retardation, twin-to-twin transfusion, prolapsed cord, premature separation of the second placenta, and malformations. Women with a multiple gestation have an increased incidence of preeclampsia, anemia, polyhydramnios, and postpartum hemorrhage.

Pregnancy-induced hypertension (PIH). Also known as preeclampsia/eclampsia or toxemia, PIH occurs usually late in pregnancy and is characterized by hypertension, edema, and proteinuria. The differentiating feature in this disease is the presence or absence of maternal convulsions: Once a seizure occurs, the patient has proceeded from preeclampsia to eclampsia.

The incidence of PIH in the United States is approximately 5 percent. PIH seems to be higher in blacks for each age and parity group, and it runs in families. The incidence is also higher in young, primiparous women and in multiparous women over 35. It is frequent in women with twins, diabetes, chronic hypertension, polyhydramnios, and hydatidiform mole. Approximately one third of women who have had PIH previously will develop it in subsequent pregnancies (Burrow and Ferris, 1982).

Maternal effects of PIH range from relatively transient to serious morbidity, such as renal damage or cerebral vascular accident, to death of the mother or fetus, or both. Fetal problems include increased incidence of intrauterine growth retardation, abruptio placentae, preterm birth, stillbirth, and mental retardation in surviving offspring.

PIH is a major cause of perinatal mortality and is the second leading cause of maternal death in the United States (Cavanagh et al., 1982).

At present, it is not possible to prevent PIH. It is possible, however, to identify patients who are especially prone to develop the disease. Conditions that predispose a woman to develop PIH include:

1. First pregnancy
2. Multiple pregnancy
3. Chronic hypertension
4. Hydatidiform mole
5. Chronic renal disease
6. Malnutrition
7. Diabetes
8. Hydrops fetalis
9. History of PIH in family or in previous pregnancy
10. Age <20 or >30
11. Patient's developing polyhydramnios

Premature rupture of the membranes. Premature rupture of the membranes (PROM), that is, rupture more than 2 hours prior to the onset of labor, is a major perinatal complication. It is associated with a high perinatal mortality rate, attributable primarily to delivery of premature, low-birth-weight infants. Depending on management, PROM can also be associated with significant perinatal morbidity, including premature delivery, maternal and/or fetal infection, and fetal respiratory distress syndrome. Other problems, such as breech presentation, prolapsed cord, transverse lie, aplastic lungs, and positional limb deformities of the fetus due to the lack of "cushioning" normally provided by amniotic fluid, have also been reported. It is felt by several authors that preexisting infection may contribute significantly to PROM.

Intrauterine growth retardation. Intrauterine growth retardation (IUGR) complicates approximately 3 to 7 percent of all pregnancies. Babies born in or below the 10th percentile of mean weight for gestation are at greater risk of antepartum death, perinatal asphyxia, neonatal morbidity, and later developmental problems. Babies with IUGR have a perinatal mortality rate that is 8 times that of normal infants (Butler and Alberman, 1969).

Two types of fetal growth retardation—asymmetric and symmetric—have been described. In asymmetric IUGR, there is increasing disproportion in head-to-body ratios. This type of IUGR is the more common and is known as "brain sparing," because the last organ to be deprived of essential nutrients is the brain. Asymmetric IUGR is most commonly caused by placental insufficiency resulting from such conditions as PIH, chronic hypertension, multiple gestation, chronic abruption, smoking, and alcoholism. Symmetric IUGR is non–brain sparing, occurs less commonly, and can be the result of an acute maternal infection, chromosomal abnormalities in the fetus, maternal drug addiction, or maternal malnutrition.

Whatever the cause and type of IUGR, affected babies are at increased risk for death or damage during both the antepartum and intrapartum periods. Prompt identification and continued follow-up of the fetuses during pregnancy can mean the difference between life and death for these babies, as well as affecting the quality of life in those that survive.

At present, diagnostic accuracy of IUGR is only about 50 percent; that is, half of the babies identified as having IUGR will actually be above the 10th percentile of mean weight for gestational age; and half of all IUGR babies will remain undiagnosed until birth. Diagnostic screening for IUGR infants includes meticulous use of McDonald measurements between 20 and 34 weeks, accurate assessment of gestational age, and serial ultrasonography as appropriate, along with a review of the patient's history to look for factors predisposing her baby to IUGR.

Rh isoimmunization. In the early 1960s, Rh hemolytic disease of the newborn was responsible for 5000 to 6000 perinatal deaths annually. Medical science, in the space of one generation, has elucidated the pathogenesis of the disease, outlined a plan for prenatal diagnosis and intrauterine and neonatal treatment, and developed a method for prevention of the disease that has resulted in total prevention of the severe form now being within reach. With optimal management at a tertiary level perinatal center, perinatal mortality from Rh erythroblastosis

has been reduced from 14.3 to 1.5 percent (Bowman, 1978).

The simple step of determining a woman's Rh status should be done at the initial exam for all pregnant women. Every Rh-negative woman carrying a child fathered by an Rh-positive man should be tested for antibodies in every pregnancy, starting with the first prenatal visit. Past history should be elicited from the woman and should include the following:

1. History of transfusion of incompatible blood
2. Outcome of previous pregnancies
   a. Rh factors of infants
   b. Severity of hemolytic disease
   c. Gestational age at intrauterine death, if any
   d. Questionable autopsy confirmation of erythroblastosis
3. Existing conditions implicated in predisposition to Rh isoimmunization
   a. PIH
   b. External version
   c. Abruptio placentae

Once this information is obtained, appropriate measures—including amniocentesis, intrauterine fetal transfusion, and planning for possible early delivery—can be instituted.

Prevention is the key to eradicating this disease. With assiduous attention to detail in caring for all Rh-negative women (regardless of outcome of pregnancy) and appropriate use of Rh immunoglobulin, this goal may be possible.

Prolonged pregnancy. Prolonged pregnancy is a common obstetric problem with potentially profound consequences. Three definitions are important at the outset:

1. *Postdatism*—the pregnancy has gone beyond the expected date of birth.
2. *Prolonged pregnancy*—the length of gestation has exceeded 42 weeks.
3. *Postmaturity*—a pediatric diagnosis based on neonatal examination.

The incidence of prolonged pregnancy ranges from 7 to 12 percent, with an average of approximately 10 percent. The diagnosis of prolonged pregnancy starts at the first prenatal visit with an accurate and meticulous estimation of gestational age, taking into account the last menstrual period, last normal period, dates of negative and positive pregnancy tests, history of oral contraceptive use, history of menstrual irregularity, and pelvic exams. Later important determinations are based on hearing fetal heart tones with a fetoscope at 20 weeks, fundal height measurements, and ultrasonography when appropriate. All of these are necessary in order to "date" the pregnancy and to later differentiate between postdatism and prolonged pregnancy should the need arise.

The perinatal impact of prolonged pregnancy may be severe: Perinatal mortality for these infants is increased 2 to 3 times and, in small-for-gestational-age infants, 7 times. Morbidity includes birth trauma, meconium aspiration, and hypoglycemia. Developmental defects in surviving infants have been identified.

The vast majority of prolonged pregnancies are idiopathic; however, anencephaly, trisomy 18, and placental sulfatase deficiency have all been implicated in the etiology of this syndrome.

Habits/Habituation

Smoking during pregnancy. Cigarette smoking during pregnancy has been demonstrated to be detrimental to the fetus. The mechanism of the effect of smoking on the outcome of pregnancy is still obscure, but it is felt to be related to decreased placental perfusion of the smoker. Studies have shown that among pregnant women who smoke, particularly those who smoke more than 20 cigarettes per day, the incidence of premature labor and delivery is significantly increased. There is also a strong correlation between smoking and low birth weight, premature infants, and stillbirths. Evidence has also been presented that smoking during pregnancy increases the incidence of bleeding, abruptio placentae, placenta previa, and premature and prolonged rupture of the membranes. In addition, infants of smoking mothers tend to continue to be smaller at 1 year of age when compared with offspring of nonsmoking mothers. Women who cannot stop smoking should be urged to at least reduce the number of cigarettes smoked to 10 or fewer per day (Smith, 1979).

Alcohol. Infants born to mothers who drink alcohol on a regular basis are at risk for fetal alcohol syndrome (FAS), a combination of FAS facies, mental retardation, intrauterine growth retardation, and developmental failure. The actual amount of alcohol ingested that will cause the syndrome is unclear in light of present studies.

Drugs (see also Chapter 6). Although some animal studies have implied teratogenic effects from certain drugs, these studies cannot always be applied to humans, and some drugs have not been tested at all. The best recommendation is that no medication be taken during pregnancy unless absolutely necessary (Drukker, 1983). See Chapter 6 for a more detailed discussion.

Conclusion

"If we are interested in quality then let us know what can assure it; likewise let us understand those events which are responsible for developmental delay" (Hobel, 1977).

At conception, every fetus receives his or her own genetic potential through his or her parents. This genetic potential for intelligence, development, and quality of life is subjected to numerous environmental, physical, social, and psychologic obstacles along the continuum of pregnancy. How or if the fetus survives depends a great deal on the health care provided the mother.

To be born too soon, too small, unwanted, or uncared for has dire consequences for the child not only in terms of physical problems but also in terms of mental and emotional development. Problems during pregnancy, labor, and delivery have too often affected the fetus in ways that may make the achievement of his or her genetic potential impossible.

We therefore see two major goals. The first is to ensure accessibility to the appropriate health care system for all women, preferably through the extension of a regionalized system of maternal-child care. With this approach, neonatal mortality in participating states has been reduced to 10/1000 deliveries (Eisner, 1978).

Our second goal is to reduce the number of low-birth-weight infants born. Although this group represents only 1 percent of all liveborn infants, it contributes to over half the neonatal mortality in parts of the United States.

"Low-risk" pregnancy is a diagnosis made only in retrospect. Continuous and thorough assessment of and intervention for mother and fetus prenatally, during the intrapartum period, and neonatally is a means of contributing toward the quality of life for them as individuals and for all of us.

REFERENCES

Allen E., and Mantz, M. L.: Are normal patients at risk during pregnancy? JOGN Nurs. 10:348, 1981.

Arsenault, P. S.: Maternal and antenatal factors in the risk of sudden infant death syndrome. Am. J. Epidemiol. 111:279, 1981.

Babson, C., and Benson, R.: Management of the High Risk Pregnancy and Intensive Care of the Neonate. St. Louis, C. V. Mosby Co. 1975, pp. 1–21, 276–281.

Becker, C. H.: Comprehensive assessment of the healthy gravida. JOGN Nurs. 11:375, 1982.

Bowman, J. M.: The management of Rh-isoimmunization. Obstet. Gynecol. 52:1, 1978.

Brewer, D.W., and Aubry, R.H.: Physiology of pregnancy, clinical pathologic correlations. Postgrad. Med. 52:110, 1972.

Brewer, D. W., and Aubry R. H.: Physiology of pregnancy, clinical pathologic correlations. Postgrad. Med. 53:221, 1973.

Brunel, L. E.: Prenatal care. In Niswander, K. R. (ed.): Manual of Obstetrics: Diagnosis and Management. Boston, Little, Brown & Co. 1979, pp. 27–35.

Burrow, G. N., and Ferris, T. F.: Medical Complications During Pregnancy, 2nd ed. Philadelphia, W. B. Saunders Co., 1982.

Burchell, R. C., and Gunn, J.: The new birth experience. JOGN Nurs. 9:250, 1980.

Butler, N. R., and Bonham, D. G.: Perinatal Mortality: The First Report of the 1958 British Perinatal Survey. Edinburgh and London, E. & S. Livingstone, Ltd., 1969.

Butler, N. R., and Alberman, E. D.: Perinatal Problems: The Second Report of the 1958 British Perinatal Mortality Survey. Edinburgh and London, E. & S. Livingstone, Ltd., 1969.

Cavanagh, D., O'Connor, T. C. F., and Knuppel, R. A. K.: Obstetric Emergencies. Philadelphia, J. B. Lippincott Co., 1982, Chapters 1,2,6,9,11.

Cavanagh, D., and Talisman, F. R.: Interval between pregnancies. In Cavanagh, D. (ed.): Prematurity and the Obstetrician. New York, Appleton-Century-Crofts, 1969.

Cetrulo, C. L., and Freeman, R.: Bioelectric evaluation in intrauterine growth retardation. Clin. Obstet. Gynecol. 20:137, 1977.

Creasy, R. K., and Herron, M. A.: Prevention of preterm birth. Semin. Perinatol., 5:295, 1981.

Degeorge, F. V., Nesbitt, R. L., and Aubry, R. H.: High risk obstetrics. VI. An evaluation of the effects of intensified care on pregnancy outcome. Am. J. Obstet. Gynecol. 111:650, 1971.

Donnelly, F. J., Flowers, C. E., Creadice, R. N., et al.: Parental, fetal, and environmental factors in perinatal mortality. Am. J. Obstet. Gynecol. 74:1245, 1957.

Douglas, C. P.: Prenatal risks: an obstetrician's point of view. In Aladjem, S. (ed.): Risks in the Practice of Modern Obstetrics, 2nd ed. St. Louis, C. V. Mosby Co., 1975.

Drukker, J.: Antenatal Assessment. Part I. Maternal profile. NAACOG Update Series, Continuing Professional Education Center, Inc., Princeton, NJ, 1983.

Dweck, H. S.: The tiny baby: past, present, and future. Clin. Perinatol. 4:425, 1977.

Eisner, V., Pratt, M. W., Hexter, A., et al.: Improvement in infant and perinatal mortality in the United States, 1965–1973. I. Priorities for intervention. Am. J. Public Health 68:359, 1978.

Goodwin, J. W., Dunne, J. T., and Thomas, B. W.: Antepartum identification of the fetus at risk. Can. Med. Assoc. J. 101:458, 1969.

Halliday, H. L., Jones, P. K., Jones, S. L., et al.: Method of screening obstetrics patients to prevent reproductive wastage. Obstet. Gynecol. 55:656, 1980.

Hobel, C. J.: Recognition of the high risk pregnant woman. In Spellacy, W. (ed.): Management of the High Risk Pregnancy. Baltimore, University Park Press, 1976, pp. 1–28.

Hobel, C. J.: Identification of the patient at risk. In Bolognese, R. J. (ed.): Perinatal Medicine: Clinical Management of the High Risk Fetus and Neonate. Baltimore, Williams & Wilkins, 1977, pp. 1–25.

Hobel, C. J., Hyvarinen, M. A., Okada, D. M., et al.: Prenatal and intrapartum high-risk screening. 1. Prediction of the high-risk neonate. Am. J. Obstet. Gynecol. 117:1, 1973.

Josten, L.: Prenatal assessment guide for illuminating possible problems with parenting. MCN 6:113, 1981.

Kappy, K. A., Cetrulo, C. L., Knuppel, R. A., et al.: Premature rupture of the membranes: a conservative approach. Am. J. Obstet. Gynecol. 134:655, 1979.

Kessner, D. M., Singer, J., Kalk, C. E., et al.: A selected review of the epidemiology of infant mortality. In Contrasts on Health Status, Vol. 1: Infant Death: An Analysis by Maternal Risk and Health Care. Washington, D.C., Institute of Medicine, National Academy of Sciences, 1973, pp. 110–113.

Lilienfeld, A. M., and Parkhurst, E.: A study of the association of factors of pregnancy and parturition with the development of cerebral palsy. A preliminary report. Am. J. Hyg. 53:262, 1951.

Lilienfeld, A. M., and Pasamanick, B.: The association of maternal and fetal factors with the development of cerebral palsy and epilepsy. Am. J. Obstet. Gynecol. 70:93, 1955.

Little, W. J.: On the influence of abnormal parturition, difficult labours, premature birth and asphyxia neonatorum, on the mental and physical condition of the child, especially in relation to deformities. Trans. Obstet. Soc. London 3:293, 1862.

Marriage, K. J., and Davies, P. A.: Neurological sequelae in children surviving mechanical ventilation in the neonatal period. Arch. Dis. Child. 52:176, 1977.

Mixon, W. C. W., and Hickson, E. B.: A Guide to Obstetrics in General Practice. Staples Press, London, 1952.

Naeye, R. L., and Blank, W. A.: Influences of pregnancy risk factors on fetal and newborn disorders. Clin. Perinatol. 1:187, 1974.

Niswander, K. R., and Gordon, M.: The Women and Their Pregnancies. Philadelphia, W. B. Saunders Co., 1972.

Paul, R. H., and Hon, E. H.: Clinical fetal monitoring. V. Effect on perinatal outcome. Am. J. Obstet. Gynecol. 114:529, 1974.

Peabody, F. W.: The care of the patient. J. Am. Med. Assoc. 88:877, 1927.

Prechtl, H. F. R.: Neurological sequelae of prenatal and perinatal complications. Br. Med. J. 34:763, 1967.

Pritchard, J. A., and MacDonald, P. C.: Hypertensive disorders in pregnancy. In Williams Obstetrics, 15th ed. New York, Appleton-Century-Crofts, 1978, p. 552.

Pritchard, J. A., MacDonald, P. C., and Gant, W. F.: Preterm and postterm pregnancy and fetal growth retardation. In Williams Obstetrics, 17th ed. Norwalk, CT, Appleton-Century-Crofts, 1985.

Ryan, G. M., Sweeney, P., and Solola, A.: Prenatal care and pregnancy outcome. Am. J. Obstet. Gynecol. 129:876, 1980.

Scott, D. E., and Pritchard, J. A.: Anemia in pregnancy. *In* Milunsky, A. (ed.): Clinics in Perinatology. Philadelphia, W. B. Saunders Co., 1974.

Schneider, K. D.: Primary care of the pregnant woman: laboratory tests. A Staff Development Program in Perinatal Nursing Care. White Plains, NY, National Foundation–March of Dimes, 1978.

Shapiro, S., Schlesinger, E. R., and Nesbitt, R. E. L.: Infant, Perinatal, Maternal, and Childhood Mortality in the United States. Cambridge, MA, Harvard University Press, 1968.

Smith, D.: Mothering Your Unborn Baby. Philadelphia, W. B. Saunders Co., 1979.

Trotter, C. W., Chang, P.-N., Thompson, T., et al.: Perinatal factors and the developmental outcome of preterm infants. JOGN Nurs., 11:83, 1982.

Wallace, H. M.: Factors associated with perinatal mortality and morbidity. Clin. Obstet. Gynecol. 13:38, 1971.

Wells, H. B., Greenberg, B. G., and Donnelly, J. F.: North Carolina fetal and neonatal death study. I. Study design and some preliminary results. Am. J. Publ. Health 48:1583, 1958.

Wilson, R. W., and Schifrin, B. S.: Is any pregnancy low risk? Obstet. Gynecol. 55:653, 1980.

2

REGIONALIZATION AND THE TEAM CONCEPT OF HIGH-RISK OBSTETRICS

FRANK H. BOEHM
MARY F. HAIRE

Background Events

In 1976 the National Foundation–March of Dimes published a document entitled *Toward Improving the Outcome of Pregnancy: Recommendations for the Regional Development of Maternal and Perinatal Health Services* (Committee on Perinatal Health, 1976). This very important publication was prepared jointly by the American College of Obstetricians and Gynecologists, The American Medical Association, The American Association of Family Practitioners, and The American Academy of Pediatrics, and helped lead the way to regionalization of perinatal health care in this country.

Regionalization of perinatal health care can be described as *the organization of a region in which there are defined levels of perinatal care consisting of at least one tertiary care hospital whose primary concerns are education, consultation, and transportation.* Since publication of the work by the National Foundation, numerous states have developed regionalization plans to aid in the refinement of perinatal health care so as to reduce morbidity and mortality and also to reduce the costs of perinatal health care in a region. In August of 1976, Berger et al. reported that 28 states had regionalization programs in operation, with 15 of these being on a state-wide basis. Sixteen other states indicated plans to implement a program within the next few years, and only four states reported no plan for regionalization of perinatal health care by 1976.

In 1980, the Wisconsin Association for Perinatal Care contacted the directors of maternal-child health in each of the 50 states and asked them to respond to the following questions: (1) Does your state have a set of perinatal guidelines? (2) What process does your state use to designate hospitals? (3) Has your state designed a regionalization system to deliver perinatal care services? (Organization of Perinatal Services throughout the United States, 1980). Of the 50 states, 37 responded. Twenty-seven reported having perinatal care regions; 23 had perinatal guidelines; 7 had designated hospitals by level of care; and 20 had state perinatal advisory committees to assist in coordinating and developing activities at the state level.

In most states today, whether programs are well organized or not, regionalization has become a modality for perinatal health care. Most states have followed the three-tiered model recommended by the Committee on Perinatal Health (see References), which classifies hospitals as *Level I*—care solely for normal obstetric patients or normal newborns; *Level II*—care for more complicated pregnancies and neonatal illnesses, with referral of newborns to other hospitals if they require mechanical ventilation, surgery, or other complex procedures; or *Level III*—care at a regional center accepting referrals and providing the entire spectrum of medical and surgical services for pregnant women and newborns.

In 1974 the Tennessee State Legislature passed a bill designed to help develop a plan to implement a program for the diagnosis and treatment of certain life-threatening conditions present in the newborn, and to establish a Newborn Advisory Committee. In 1977, through further legislation, this committee was expanded to encompass obstetric concerns and is now known as the Perinatal Advisory Committee. This committee has been extremely active and has adopted guidelines, distributed grants throughout the state, and been an integral part of the process of reducing perinatal mortality in Tennessee. Perinatal mortality in Tennessee, which was 31.2 per 1000 in 1970, steadily declined to 15.8 per 1000 in 1983. Maternal deaths have also been noted to decline, with a maternal death rate of 2.9/10,000 live births reported during the years 1970 and 1975, and 1.3/10,000 during the years 1979 through 1983.

Other states have also shown a decreased neonatal mortality with regionalization, as evidenced by the statistics shown at the bottom of this page.

Arizona (Harris, 1980) and Ohio (Cordero, 1982) have also noted decreases in perinatal mortality with regionalization.

Many states have also described a decrease in neonatal mortality with maternal in utero transports over neonatal transports. (Cho et al., 1982; Harris et al., 1978; Harris, 1980; Modanlou, 1980; Knuppel et al., 1979; Levy et al., 1981; Sachs et al., 1983; Souma, 1979). A report from Nova Scotia indicates that a regionalized care system could result in perinatal mortality rates in small hospitals that approach the low mortality rates of non-referral patients in sophisticated Level II units (Peddle et al., 1983). Regional care systems, through periodic reviews, may identify potentially preventable deaths in small hospitals in which normally low neonatal death rates may mask previously unconsidered problems (Hein et al., 1981).

These dramatic reductions in perinatal mortality have come about in part because of the regionalization of perinatal health care, as well as improvements in neonatal and obstetric medicine. By the process of making medical advances in perinatal medicine readily available to individuals in areas where such care did not previously exist, the benefits of superior health care have become more widespread, and regionalization certainly deserves a major part of the credit.

Economic Considerations

One of the more important aspects of the regionalization of perinatal health care is its prevention of duplication of services. Because personnel and equipment in perinatal health care are becoming extremely expensive, it seems obvious that hospitals providing community-type care for normal obstetric and newborn patients cannot be staffed and equipped to handle all of the more complicated and expensive procedures. Therefore, the centralization of personnel and equipment can result in a reduction in perinatal health care dollars in the local communities. Furthermore, by establishing educational services as a responsibility of the tertiary center, a reduction in duplication of these services can and does result.

The ability to provide early intervention in a high-risk pregnancy may substantially reduce or minimize the potential complications in the mother, fetus, or newborn infant. It also follows that the provision of improved perinatal health care to mothers and babies can significantly reduce morbidity (Johnson, 1982).

It has been estimated in Tennessee to cost an average of $5500 to identify and manage a high-risk pregnancy. At Vanderbilt University Hospital the average cost in 1980 for a surviving infant weighing less than 1000 grams at birth during the initial admission to the neonatal intensive care unit was

State	Before Regionalization	After Regionalization	Source of Data
Kansas	1974 12.0/1000	1979 7.7/1000	Cho et al., 1982
Minnesota	1978 9/1000	1980 5.5/1000	Hoekstra et al., 1981
Mississippi	1965 41.5/1000	1977 18.3/1000	Morrison and Rhodes, 1980
Colorado	1971 13.4/1000	1978 6.9/1000	Bowes, 1981

$33,019.00 (Killam et al., 1981), while Pomerance and coworkers (1978) estimated a total cost of $88,000.00. Obviously, the number of complications and length of stay will determine costs for most patients. These estimated costs should be balanced by the knowledge that a damaged infant requiring life-long institutional care will cost society approximately one million dollars over the course of an average 45-year life expectancy. Clearly, it makes both fiscal and humanitarian sense to try to prevent damage to newborn infants.

Statistics compiled for the state of Illinois by Anderson (1981) showed that the mean cost of survivors was $6473 for those babies transported in utero and $12,208 for those transported after delivery (p = <0.05). The mean length of stay for these infants was 19 days for in-utero transports and 27 days for neonatal transports (p = <0.05). Obviously this mean-stay difference contributed to the cost difference. Levy et al. (1981) in Louisiana and Harris (1980) in Arizona also found a lower mean length of stay in those babies transported in utero. Jung and Bose (1983) found that using the Level I and II hospitals for back transports also decreased the cost of care.

Prevention of perinatal health care problems will result in improved outcomes. By administering early prenatal and competent intrapartum care, morbidity and mortality can be reduced. With regionalized systems in which early detection of complications is the rule, and with outpatient management of many of these complications, care providers and receivers will notice a reduction in health care dollars.

Third-party response over the past 10 years to regionalization of perinatal health care has generally been good. While slow at the outset, third-party payment has been improved in newborn care by legislation as well as in obstetric care by choice.

Data are available, however, that suggest that perinatal health care is a low priority in our society for investment of resources (Harris, 1980). Maternal and child health care is grossly underfinanced when one considers total health care expenditures. Whereas general health care expenditures have continued to increase in this country, the proportion reserved for maternal and child health care seems to have further declined in terms of real dollars. Because of a concentration of high-risk pregnancies and

newborns in the lower socioeconomic groups, it has also been noted that tertiary centers offering care to these patients are accepting an ever-increasing deficit spending, thereby assuming some of the greatest financial burdens for health care in this country.

Unfortunately, studies of cost-benefit ratios are, for the most part, short-term outcome measures rather than long-term morbidity evaluations (Anderson et al., 1981). The effectiveness of perinatal health care is further in question, owing to lack of randomized control studies, leading to a significant bias in reporting, and reliance on faith rather than science. The closest the medical community has come to cost-benefit analyses are descriptive reports rather than comparative studies. According to Johnson (1982), the complexities of looking at costs—including direct and indirect; immediate and long-term—may preclude clear-cut means of proving cost-effectiveness of regionalized care systems in dollar figures. The greatest benefit of such systems may well be in providing means of improving standards of care and in assuring access to complex care for all mothers and babies who may require it.

Regionalization programs must assume the burden of proving effectiveness, both financially and medically, if costs are to be justified and eventually contained (Boyle et al., 1983; Donabedian, 1984). For this reason, many state systems are attempting to develop standardized data bases and follow-up programs.

In developing both maternal and neonatal regional transport systems, preplanning to provide for additional nursing and other personnel at the tertiary care centers is essential. Since these systems will increase the number of patients as well as the complexity of care at Level II centers, the impact on the nursery personnel should also be taken into account (Kanto et al., 1982, 1983).

Maternal-Fetal Transport

One of the outgrowths of regionalized systems of perinatal care has been the development of maternal-fetal transport systems. Newborn transport had been developed earlier by neonatologists to provide rapid access to intensive care for high-risk infants born in community hospitals. Over the years, however, it was shown in numerous studies that maternal transport not only was more practical but perhaps more beneficial (Harris et al., 1978; Harris et al., 1981; Merenstein et al., 1977; Modanlou et al., 1979 and 1980).

One example was the Vanderbilt Hospital's experience following development of a maternal transport system. A reduction in neonatal mortality rates when babies were delivered in the tertiary center rather than in the community hospital was observed (Table 2–1). As can be seen in Table 2–1, the percentage of inborns admitted to the neonatal intensive care unit increased from 1975 through 1981, with a decrease observed in the outborn admissions, reflecting an increased number of maternal transports to Level III institutions. Interestingly, mortality rates of inborn admissions to the intensive care unit decreased over the years from 16.5 to 4 percent, although outborn mortality did not reveal these dramatic declines. In addition, the mean birth weights of inborns in 1980 and 1981 were significantly lower than the mean weights of those in the outborn group, further emphasizing the dramatic reduction in infant mortality rates for high-risk babies born at the tertiary center.

Further evidence that neonatal mortality rates can be reduced by having the mother deliver at a Level III hospital was noted by Paneth et al. (1982), who examined neonatal mortality rates of low-birth-weight infants (501 to 2250 grams) born between 1976 and 1978 at three levels of hospitals in New York City. Among 13,560 singleton, low-birth-weight infants the adjusted neonatal mortality rate for Level III hospitals was 128.5 per 1000 live births, significantly lower ($p<0.0001$) than the rates for both Level II (168.1) and Level I units (163.0).

Based on these data and others (Cordero, 1982; Elliott et al., 1982; Giles et al., 1977;

Kanto et al., 1982) it is generally believed that the ideal situation is to transport pregnant women to a tertiary center for complicated deliveries, especially in cases in which a preterm baby is expected. When maternal transport is not possible, immediately available transport by a neonatal team to the tertiary center should be arranged, either in standard emergency vehicles or in neonatal intensive care vans, which are available in a number of regions.

This neonatal team should include at least two experienced personnel, one being a physician or physician extender (neonatal nurse clinician or specialist, or neonatal transport nurse) and one a nurse experienced in managing sick neonates (Cook and Kattwinkel, 1983; Johnson, D. E., 1982; Johnson and Boros, 1979; Johnson et al., 1974; Meyer, 1974; Ostrea, 1975; Pettet et al., 1975; Slovis and Comerci, 1974). Nurse participation in the transport team can improve response time to transport requests, improve consistency of care provided to the newborns during transport, maximize utilization of skilled perinatal health care professionals, and enhance perinatal educational opportunities for physicians and nurses (Thompson, 1980).

If a high-risk baby is expected but there is no time for maternal transport, the neonatal team can be present for the delivery or shortly after the birth. However, if the distressed infant was not expected, a delay of several hours may occur before transport can occur. During this time it is important to stabilize the infant. If the referring hospital has had very little experience with high-risk infants, frequent communication with an intensive care unit will be necessary. One region even used two-way television to increase this communication (Jones et al., 1980).

Once the neonatal team arrives, continued stabilization is necessary. Many authors, including the American Academy of Pediatrics, think that stabilization before transport, while awaiting the team, produces better results (Chance et al., 1978; Cunningham and Smith, 1973; Fanaroff and Klaus, 1973; Feldman and Sauve, 1976; Pettet et al., 1974; Storrs and Taylor, 1970).

Maintenance of the transport equipment and vans is very important. Equipment failure can be disastrous en route. Many transport teams carry extra batteries and other equipment in case of failures.

Table 2–1. Vanderbilt University Hospital Neonatal Intensive Care Unit Admissions

Year	Inborn (%)	Mortality (%)	Outborn (%)	Mortality (%)
1975	20.9	16.5	78.8	15.4
1976	32.9	10.8	67.1	15.2
1077	36.3	8.8	63.7	15.3
1978	37.2	8.9	62.8	12.0
1979	45.8	8.3	53.7	11.2
1980	52.0	5.0	48.0	7.0
1981	51.0	4.0	49.0	7.0

In larger regions, fixed-wing and helicopter service is also available for transport (Elliott et al., 1982). These aircraft are equipped much like the vans. For high-altitude flying, special transport incubators are needed to protect the neonate from hypothermia and pressure changes (Parsons and Bobechko, 1982). Sudden decompression during air transport can decrease oxygen supply to the fetus or neonate, and so must be avoided (Parer, 1982). However, the rapid transportation that is afforded by air certainly is advantageous.

Development of a maternal-transport system is not as simple as it may sound, because of the reluctance of numerous physicians to refer patients to a specific tertiary center. Ryan and coworkers (1982) surveyed five regionalized systems across the nation and found that initial fears that regionalization would result in closure of large numbers of hospitals, with subsequent loss of patients to other areas, were generally unfounded. The fault of many regionalization programs seems to be poor communication among the institutions involved. An initial visit from the health care team to each hospital offering obstetric care, for the purpose of identifying specific needs and problems in the area and to open lines of communication, can significantly reduce the threatening aspects of regionalized programs (Wirth, 1980). Getting the health care team out of the tertiary center setting to visit each of the hospitals in a region, and to meet with the various people involved in perinatal health care within the hospitals, results in better assessments being made of the needs and concerns of these institutions (Boehm and Haire, 1979; Boehm et al., 1979). This individualized approach contributed to the development of a working system in middle Tennessee, as can be seen by the increasing number of maternal transports to Vanderbilt University Hospital carried out over the years (Table 2–2).

Care for the high-risk mother and neonate, particularly that type of care requiring use of complex technology, should be available to every patient within a regional system but need not be available within each hospital. Levels of care deliverable by individual hospitals are determined by the availability of technology and skilled personnel, both medical and nursing. *Quality* of care is not the issue, since quality should be consistent throughout the region regardless of designated level of technology.

A formalized referral system that takes advantage of existing referral patterns, regional resources, and geographic proximity ensures that each patient has access to the level of care required (Boehm and Haire, 1979; Bowes, 1981; Giles, 1977; Mayer, 1983). Names of specialists at the tertiary center and 24-hour telephone access for consultation should be available to each physician and hospital within a region. If the regional system is set up to include functioning Level II units, appropriate referrals to these units should be clearly designated, based on the expertise available in individual hospitals. Harvey and Bowes (1981) looked at their experiences in Colorado and found that of all *appropriately* referred maternal transport patients, 36 percent delivered infants who did not require Level III neonatal care, and 44 percent of the mothers did not require Level III perinatal care. Therefore, the development of Level II centers should reduce the burden on Level III units.

Maternal-fetal transport refers to the movement of patients from one institution to another prior to delivery in order to take advantage of higher levels of technology and advanced training of personnel. Patients may be referred for treatment of real or potential complications of either the mother or the fetus. Depending on the facilities available, the distance and terrain to be covered, and the resources and philosophies of the region involved, such transport may be either one-way or two-way.

One-way transport originates at the referring hospital and usually involves local emergency transport vehicles and staff; occasionally, private automobiles are used, but only in carefully selected instances. The responsibility for safety during transport rests with the referring hospital and physician until the patient arrives at the regional center.

Table 2–2. Number of Maternal Referrals by Year to Vanderbilt University Hospital

	Inpatient	Outpatient
1976 (6 months)	77	—
1977	246	140
1978	301	193
1979	397	239
1980	431	280
1981	443	369
1982	495	381

Two-way transport refers to the use of a designated team and vehicle from the receiving hospital traveling to the referring hospital for stabilization and transport of the mother or the neonate, or both. Responsibility for safety during transport is generally considered to rest with the transport team from the moment their care begins, whether this is in the referring hospital or in the transport vehicle.

Neonatal transport refers to the movement of babies after delivery to specialized units, in order to take advantage of the higher level of technology and advanced training of personnel. *Maternal transport* encompasses not only movement of patients to be directly admitted to an intensive care facility *within* the region but also referrals *into* the regionalized system for outpatient care or evaluation. Some of these patients may be delivered in the tertiary setting if they remain at risk. However, some of these women may be referred back to their referring hospitals if their condition is stable or resolved, as in premature labor once fetal maturity is identified.

To use the regionalization system to its optimum, transport should also be available to bring babies who are at lower risk back to the referring (i.e., Level I or II) hospital. Protocols unique to each regionalized system should be developed to identify which babies should be back transported. Moving these lower-risk babies back to the Level I or II hospital has several advantages. It has a positive effect on the personnel at the Level I and II hospitals by increasing their management skills, showing trust in their competency, and giving the primary physician at the Level I and II nursery a chance to become familiar with the infant before hospital discharge (Jung and Bose, 1983). From an economic standpoint, it frees beds for sicker neonates at the Level III center, decreases the cost of care, and increases the efficiency of the transport service, personnel, and equipment. Another advantage of back transport is that it allows the baby to be in a hospital setting closer to the parents, so that the parents can perform caretaking tasks for their infant and thus promote attachment.

Potential disadvantages of this system of back transport are lack of appropriate care in the Level I and II hospitals or need for readmission to the Level III nursery. (Although information on this is limited, gen-erally speaking, readmission has not been much of a problem with hospitals that have established appropriate protocols [Jung and Bose, 1983]). Another potential problem is that of the parents' acceptance of a new care provider. Joint decision-making regarding the choice of physician and hospital by the parents and Level III center can be helpful in this regard. Introduction of the concept of back transport to the parents early in the care of their infants may also facilitate acceptance.

INDICATIONS FOR MATERNAL/FETAL TRANSPORT

Decisions concerning transport are best made in consultation with a specialist at the receiving hospital. In cases in which referral is made for outpatient testing or counseling, careful scheduling is required to decrease the amount of time the patient and her family must spend at the regional center. Specialized testing for the purpose of evaluating fetal well-being accounts for most of the outpatient referrals (Table 2–3). In the majority of outpatient referrals, once testing is completed, the patient is referred back to her clinic or private physician for further management. A small number of patients will require joint management with regional center personnel, and an even smaller number will be transferred to the care of the specialist at the regional center for management throughout the remainder of the pregnancy.

Referred outpatients may arrive by private automobile, public transportation, or clinic vans, so instructions to the patient should include directions to the hospital clinic/office, and instructions for parking while there. If overnight accommodations are required, suggestions based on distance of the hotel or motel from the regional center and

Table 2–3. Outpatient Referrals

Reason for Referral	Percentage
Genetic counseling	56%
Infertility history	5%
Diabetes	3%
Antepartum testing	3%
Hypertension	3%
Postdates	2%
Other	28%
TOTAL	100%

room costs should also be available. Some patients come a long distance on public transportation. Every effort should be made to see these patients promptly and to carry out all examinations and testing as efficiently as possible, so that the patient can meet her transportation schedules and be seen in one day. If the patient cannot afford to stay overnight, arrangements should be made ahead of time with local family members. If this is not possible, a social worker should be assigned to find accomodations for these patients.

Prompt follow-up to the referring physician and/or clinic may be by phone call, a letter, or both. Follow-up includes descriptions of test results, physical findings, recommendations for further management, and any other information that was shared with the patient. Every effort should be made by regional center personnel to maintain positive relationships with referring physicians and to encourage the patient's trust in her physician's management. Whether the mother is referred as an outpatient or is transported as an inpatient, periodic phone calls or letters will aid in communication and help keep the referring physician and clinic informed of the patient's progress. This information is especially vital if the patient is under the care of the Level III hospital for a long time. It is also helpful to notify the nursing staff from the referring hospital about the transport. They are interested in their patient's well-being and calling to notify them can also serve as an opportunity to give suggestions for improving outcome and to offer praise for a job well done.

Inpatient referrals should begin with a phone call from the referring physician to confirm bed space for both mother and neonate, and to alert receiving hospital personnel about potential problems that may require immediate action on arrival. Preterm labor, or the possible necessity for preterm delivery in medically complicated pregnancies, accounts for the majority of inpatient referrals (Table 2–4). The nursery census must be considered when maternal transports are accepted. However, as the time of delivery may not occur until a few days to a week after admission, the identification of those mothers who are expected to deliver immediately versus those for whom the likelihood of imminent delivery is remote can be helpful for nursery assessment, and may

Table 2–4. Inpatient Referrals

Reason for Referral	Percentage
Premature labor	53%
Hypertension	15%
Bleeding	7%
Rh disease	3%
Diabetes	2%
Other	20%
TOTAL	100%

allow for some maternal transports even when there is a full nursery census.

Evaluation and stabilization of the patient prior to transport are vital to reducing the likelihood of emergencies developing en route. Laboring patients (including those on tocolytic drugs) or very ill mothers (e.g., preeclamptic patients requiring $MgSO_4$) or infants should be accompanied by a team of specialists. Since in many instances ambulance regulations prohibit family members from accompanying the patient, a familiar face from the referring hospital can be of tremendous support to the woman during this trying experience.

Since even in the best of circumstances emergencies may arise that require treatment during transport, equipment and drugs carried in the ambulance should allow for appropriate treatment of these conditions (Subcommittee on Perinatal Transportation of the Perinatal Advisory Committee, 1979). Procedures requiring a high degree of dexterity may necessitate stopping the vehicle (or landing an air vehicle) for safety. Alternative hospitals along the route should be identified for those situations that may require emergency measures.

PREPARATION FOR TRANSPORT

Patient preparation prior to referral should include, in addition to medical stabilization for physical safety, emotional preparation of the patient and her family. Fear of the unknown medical situation, coupled with the feeling that events have moved completely out of their control, adds to the feelings of unreality and helplessness experienced by parents at this time. The excitement of impending birth or recent delivery is overshadowed by the knowledge that something has gone wrong. Feelings of guilt concerning the possible cause of the complication are common and require considerable understanding and patience on the part of health care personnel.

Patient education prior to transport should also provide specific information on the reasons for transport, including an accurate discussion of both the risks and the benefits to the mother and her baby. Since many patients have known of friends who were referred to a medical center for any number of reasons, and who may have died or had their babies die while there, the association, frequently on a subconscious level, is that people are referred to these centers when death is imminent. Explanations regarding the benefits derived from advanced technologic expertise and handling by specialized personnel, including information on survival statistics for the regional center, can significantly reduce parents' anxiety regarding the need for transport of the mother or infant.

Most patients find it helpful to know in advance the nature of the tests or procedures that might be ordered at the regional center. Receiving this information from their own health care professionals not only helps to reduce anxiety but also reaffirms the patient's sense of faith in the health care workers' judgment and knowledge. When the baby is transported it is important for the patients to know what to expect upon arrival at the intensive care unit. This preparation should be done before transport, but can be done before the patients first visit the unit.

Although at many regional centers a number of resident physicians will be involved with patient care, most patients prefer identifying with one physician. Knowing that an attending physician supervises their care, and wherever possible, knowing his or her name in advance, is reassuring. It is highly recommended that maternal transport patients be admitted to the private service of the attending physician on call at the regional center; this will ensure that the advantages gained by delivering at a regional center are not lost through the mistakes of inexperienced personnel providing unsupervised care (Donabedian et al., 1984).

In addition, designating specific members of the nursing staff at the regional center to serve as advocates for transport patients promotes a sense of continuity of care (Boehm and Haire, 1979). These nurses see the patient on a daily basis to answer questions concerning treatment, outcomes, and long-term consequences; to provide support for the family; and to maintain contact with the referring physician and hospital staff.

One advantage of a well-designed regional referral system is that regional center personnel become particularly attuned to the emotional needs of high-risk patients, and to problems encountered when these patients are separated from their usual support systems and care providers. If patients are from a low-income family, this separation may be compounded by the inability of family and friends to visit or even call the regional center at frequent intervals. This is true for the antepartum mother as well as the neonate. Sometimes, because of the distance involved, it is difficult for the parents to visit their child, which adds more stress to the situation. Therefore, referral back to a Level I or II hospital closer to the family, when feasible, is very important. Consequently, regional center personnel should be prepared to serve as "family surrogates" for transport patients and their spouses. Primary nursing of the neonate is important not only to support the parents but also to parent the newborn. If the baby dies or is transported, these primary nurses and other staff often experience great separation anxiety and grief for their loss.

Intraregional Communication

Communication between referring and receiving physicians and between referring and receiving hospitals should follow a systematic approach, designed both to provide information about the current patient and to serve as a source of education regarding future patient complications. Immediate follow-up by phone provides the referring physician/clinic with up-to-date information about the woman's and/or the infant's status, information that is helpful to the physician (or clinic staff) in dealing with questions from family members who remain in the community.

A follow-up letter outlining the care given, the outcome, and instructions given to the patient on discharge, as well as a copy of the hospital discharge summary, provides further continuity for the patient and her care giver. Except in rare instances, patients should be referred back to their own physician/clinic following discharge from the regional center (Boehm and Haire, 1979).

VANDERBILT REGIONAL REFERRAL CENTER MATERNAL TRANSPORT FORM

Please complete this form and send with patient, along with copies of pertinent clinical records (prenatal records when available, hospital record, laboratory data, etc.)

Patient's Name_____ Age_____ G____ P____ AB_____

LMP_____ EDC_____ Blood Type & Rh_____ Allergies_____

Date_____ Referring Hospital_____

Hospital's Address_____

M.D. & Address_____

MATERNAL COMPLICATIONS
____ Premature Labor   ____ Post Term Pregnancy
____ Premature Rupture of Membranes   ____ Diabetes
____ Hypertension   ____ Intrauterine Fetal Demise
____ Bleeding   ____ IUGR
____ Other_____

_____

Medication 24 Hours Prior to Transport (drug, dosage, time, etc.)_____

_____

TRANSPORT INFORMATION	TREATMENT & OUTCOME (completed by the OB Regionalization Coordinator)
____ Ambulance ____ Private Auto ____ Air Transport ____ Other	Hospital_____ Attending M.D._____ Treatment_____
Time of Referring Call_____ Departure Time_____ Arrival Time_____	Delivery Information: Date_____
Accompanied by_____	Time_____ Sex_____ Weight_____
Problems in Route_____	C/S_____ Vaginal___ Breech_____
_____	Apgar_____ 1 Min.____ 5 Min._____
	Admitted to ___ NICU _____ NNB
QUESTIONS OR COMMENTS CONCERNING THE TRANSPORT:	COMMENTS:

ATTENTION REGIONAL REFERRAL CENTER PERSONNEL: THIS FORM IS NOT PART OF THE VANDERBILT HOSPITAL MEDICAL RECORD. PLEASE HOLD FOR THE OBSTETRIC REGIONALIZATION COORDINATOR.

Figure 2–1. Maternal transport form. (Courtesy of Mary F. Haire, Nashville, TN.)

Nursing follow-up can be provided by using a two-page carbon referral form as shown in Figure 2–1. The first page is maintained at the regional center as part of transport system statistics. The second page is returned to the referring hospital to provide an outcome record for the hospital. Other forms have been described for transport (Bowen, 1980; Reedy et al., 1984).

In many communities, the relationship between patients and their care providers is longstanding and includes other family members as well. This is not only true of private physicians and their staff but is often the case in the clinic system as well. Frequently, less mobile low-income patients have greater difficulty with referrals, as they may never have traveled outside their community before. Not only is it difficult for the patient to trust her care to strangers, it is difficult for the local-community physicians and nurses to relinquish care of their patients to providers they may not know. A well-defined two-way system of communication, based on recognition of these relationships, benefits all concerned.

Legal Implications

In most states, legal responsibility during one-way transport rests with the referring hospital until the patient arrives at the receiving hospital. Careful evaluation of the patient's status to determine the safety of transport, and to designate appropriate personnel to accompany the patient, require on-site information that is best provided by those care givers who have the most knowledge of the patient and her condition.

In two-way transports, responsibility for patient safety rests with the transport team from the time they assume care of the patient. If further stabilization is required by the transport team before the patient is moved from the original hospital, the recommended procedure is to involve the patient's own physician and team in the process as much as possible, both for educational purposes and for patient reassurance.

Regardless of whether the system is one-way or two-way, record-keeping should continue during the trip. Progress notes should indicate the reason for referral, the type of vehicle (ambulance, private automobile, aircraft), the time of departure from the referring hospital and arrival at the regional center, who accompanied the patient, and any pertinent events that occurred during transport. Ideally, these forms should include a carbon copy, to provide both institutions with a record of the transport.

Regionalization and Education

As can be seen in an overall schematic of a regionalized system (Fig. 2–2), education is the most important aspect of a tertiary care center's responsibility (Boehm et al., 1978). Tennessee has developed state-wide perinatal educational guidelines for nurses, physicians, social workers, and paramedics to promote consistency of information. These guidelines are used by outreach education personnel to design education programs based on the level of care expected of individual hospitals and personnel (Level I, II, or III). Other states, including South Carolina, Illinois, Missouri, Iowa, Virginia, and Georgia, have developed similar programs (Ellenberger et al., 1979; Hein and Brown, 1981; Kanto et al., 1979; Nowacek et al., 1983; Winegar et al., 1983).

Regionalization offers significant educational advantages to the professional staff at a tertiary center. While the process of regionalization was and is primarily intended

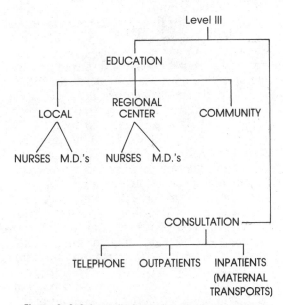

Figure 2–2. Schematic for regionalization of perinatal health care. (From Boehm, F. H., Haire, M. F., Davidson, K., et al.: Maternal-fetal transport: inpatient and outpatient care. J. Tenn. Med. Assoc. 72:829, November 1979.)

to improve perinatal health care, regionalization does provide for a concentration of high-risk patients needing care at a tertiary center. Professional staff at these centers, including attending and resident physicians, nursing staff, social workers, and nutritionists, are exposed daily to extremely high-risk perinatal patients who require a considerable amount of understanding and care. Personnel at the center are made aware of the total spectrum of perinatal complications inasmuch as they are at the receiving end of an entire region of patients.

A concentration of such patients also allows for improved research in the field of perinatal health care. As an example, prior to development of the maternal transport system at Vanderbilt University Hospital, only a few patients were sent to Vanderbilt for the care of preterm labor. In 1982, over half of those transported (some 250 patients) had as their reason for transport some aspect of preterm labor or delivery. It is no wonder that members of the professional staff at Level III centers develop expertise in handling these problems (because of high volume and exposure) and also are able to study the outcome of various protocols for care.

Many regional centers hire nurse educators whose specific role is to coordinate the outreach educational programs (Haire et al., 1981). Obstetric and neonatal educators should work closely together to provide a truly perinatal approach. Frequent evaluations of the effectiveness of such programs not only provide information needed for changes in approach but also allow recipients of these programs to offer input into the content offered (Ellenberger et al., 1979; Hanau-Walsh, 1982; Haire et al., 1981; Kanto et al., 1979). Programs presented at the outlying hospitals can be tailored to what the hospital needs. The Level III hospital can also establish programs to provide additional information, expose the participants to outside speakers, and allow the staff of these hospitals to share their knowledge and experiences. In Florida, the "Florida Regional Perinatal Nurses Association" was founded in 1980 to bring together all the Level III hospitals in the state to share information on regionalization. Once this group became functional, the Level I and II hospitals were invited to join to give input to this organization. In 1984 they presented their first annual 2-day educational meeting, which was developed to meet the needs identified by this group. In 1985 this group

was absorbed into the Florida Perinatal Association.

Physician education is coordinated by a member of the regional center faculty and may also include outreach and regional programs. Another common approach is to develop either "mini-residencies" of several weeks' duration, or to provide frequent 1-day workshops to cover a variety of health care topics.

Intensive consumer education is also important to the regionalization system. Through mass media using advocacy groups, as well as health educators in public health settings, physician's offices, and hospital settings, consumer education can take place. This education may include information on nutrition, medical risks, contraception, smoking, drinking and drugs, general preventive health care, and regionalization. This instruction should not just be available for the indigent patient. Because of complacency and decreased knowledge about availability of proper health care, private patients often receive less than adequate health care (Morrison and Rhodes, 1980).

Summary

With education of nurses, physicians, and other team members, in settings that include the outlying community hospitals, tertiary centers, and the community at large, comes improved patient care and, as a spin-off, an increased number of consultations, either by telephone or by outpatient or inpatient visits. After a number of years of regionalizing perinatal health care in this country, we have witnessed a reduction in mortality rates and an increased number of state-based perinatal guidelines being put into effect. We have seen an increase in the number of maternal transports and an overall change in attitude toward the high-risk obstetric patient as well as the preterm infant. Physicians are now more accepting of the regionalization concept. This change in attitude is reflected in a recent survey on regional planning sent to members of the American College of Obstetrics and Gynecology in Massachusetts. As can be seen in Table 2–5, most responses were favorable concerning the outcome of regionalization of perinatal health care (Harris et al., 1978).

Much of the success of these programs is due to the development of a team concept of health care. In each region this perinatal

Table 2–5. Effects of Regional Planning on Your Hospital

	Yes	No
Better coordination with other facilities in the region	146 (62%)	46 (20%)
Better fetal monitoring	133 (57%)	60 (20%)
Improved facilities or equipment	128 (54%)	67 (29%)
Better OB nursing personnel	120 (51%)	75 (32%)
Better OB anesthesia	86 (37%)	105 (45%)

Do you believe regional planning is an effective way to approach problems of:	Yes	No
Perinatal mortality	182 (91%)	18 (9%)
Accessability of care	155 (72%)	60 (28%)
High cost	91 (46%)	107 (54%)

From Ryan G. M., and Fielden J. G.: Obstetrics and Gynecology 53:187, 1979. *Reprinted* with permission from the American College of Obstetricians and Gynecologists.

team is made up of physicians, nurses, hospital administrators, patients and their families, and, wherever possible, social workers, dieticians, and supporting staff. No one specialty should attempt to function without involving others in the care required. Future health care planning must be designed to meet long-range community needs and must continue to involve all health-related agencies. Review systems must be established for frequent evaluations of the systems for cost-effectiveness, efficiency of health delivery, and outcome statistics (Bowes, 1981; Thompson, 1982; Winegar, 1983).

Such a team concept is also necessary at the organizational and coordinating levels of a regional network. Most networks function best with medical directors and nurse coordinators of both newborn and obstetric teams. It is the responsibility of these two teams to maintain the communication and transport systems, to serve as troubleshooters for problems within the system, and to serve as resource personnel for the professionals within the region.

REFERENCES

American Academy of Pediatrics: Committee on Fetus and Newborn Standards and Recommendations for Hospital Care of Newborn Infants, 6th ed. Evanston, IL, American Academy of Pediatrics, 1977.

Anderson, C. L., Aladjem, S., Ayuste, O., et al.: An analysis of maternal transport within a suburban metropolitan region. Am. J. Obstet. Gynecol. 140:499, 1981.

Barr, P. A., Suthers, J. A., and Leslie, G. I.: Newborn transport in metropolitan Sydney: experience with a newborn intensive care unit based regional transport service. Aust. Paediatr. J. 17:95, 1981.

Berger, G. S., Gillings, D. B., and Siegel, E.: The evaluation of regionalized perinatal health care programs. Am. J. Obstet. Gynecol. 125:924, 1976.

Boehm, F. H., and Haire, M. F.: One-way transport: an evolving concept. Am. J. Obstet. Gynecol. 134:484, 1979.

Boehm, F. H., Haire, M. F., Davidson, K., et al.: Maternal-fetal transport: inpatient and outpatient care. J. Tenn. Med. Assoc. 72:829, November 1979.

Bowen, P. A.: Regional centers. Part II. The newborn transport system. Health Care of Women, 2:5, 1980.

Bowes, W. A., Jr.: A review of perinatal mortality in Colorado, 1971 to 1978, and its relationship to the regionalization of perinatal services. Am. J. Obstet. Gynecol. 141:1045, 1981.

Boyle, M. H., Torrance, G. W., Sinclair, J. C., et al.: Economic evaluation of neonatal care of very-low-birth-weight infants. N. Engl. J. Med. 308:1330, 1983.

Chance, G. W., Matthew, J. D., Gash, J., et al.: Neonatal transport. A controlled study of skilled assistance. J. Pediatr. 93:662, 1978.

Cho, S., Christman, C. M., Floyd, P. S., et al.: Outcome of 201 maternal transports compared with newborn transports and infants born at the tertiary perinatal center. Birth Defects: Original Article Series, Vol. 18, Number 3A, pp. 199–201, 1982.

Committee on Perinatal Health: Toward Improving the Outcome of Pregnancy: Recommendations for the Regional Development of Maternal and Perinatal Health Services. White Plains, NY, The National Foundation–March of Dimes, 1976.

Cook, L. J., and Kattwinkel, J.: A prospective study of nurse-supervised versus physician-supervised neonatal transports. JOGN Nurs. 12:371, 1983.

Cordero, L., Backes, C. R., Zuspan, F. P.: Very low–birth weight infant: influence of place of birth on survival. Am. J. Obstet. Gynecol., 143:533, 1982.

Crenshaw, C., Jr., Payne, P., Blackmon, L., et al.: Prematurity and the Obstetrician. Am. J. Obstet. Gynecol. 147:125, 1983.

Cunningham, M., and Smith, F. R.: Stabilization and transport of severely ill infants. Pediatr. Clin. North Am. 20:359, 1973.

Donabedian, A.: Volume, quality, and the regionalization of health care services. Med. Care 22:95, 1984.

Ellenberger, D., Kennedy, A. H., and Chase, C.: An education program for nurses from referring hospitals in a perinatal regionalization system. JOGN Nurs. 8:158, 1979.

Elliott, J. P., O'Keefe, D. F., and Freeman, R. K.: Helicopter transportation of patients with obstetric emergencies in an urban area. Am. J. Obstet. Gynecol. 143:157, 1982.

Fanaroff, A., and Klaus, M.: Transportation of the high-risk infant. In Klaus, M. H., and Fanaroff, A.: Care of the High-Risk Neonate. Philadelphia, W. B. Saunders Co., 1973, p. 90.

Feldman, B. H., and Sauve, R. S.: The infant transport service. Clin. Perinatol., 3:469, 1976.

Giles, H. R., Isaman, J., Moore, N. J., et al.: The Arizona high-risk maternal transport system: an initial view. Am. J. Obstet. Gynecol. 28:400, 1977.

Haire, M. F., Davidson, K., and Boehm, F. H.: Perinatal nursing education in Tennessee: a regional approach. JOGN Nurs. 10:451, 1981.

Hanau-Walsh, J.: Evaluating the effectiveness of a perinatal outreach education program. JOGN Nurs. 11:226, 1982.

Harris, B. A., Jr., Wirtschafter, D. D., Huddleston, J. F., et al.: In utero versus neonatal transportation of high-risk perinates: a comparison. Obstet. Gynecol. 57:496, 1981.

Harris, T. R., Isaman, J., and Giles, H. R.: Improved neonatal survival through maternal transport. Obstet. Gynecol. 52:294, 1978.

Harris, T. R., Isaman, J., and Giles, H. R.: Improved survival in very low birth weight premature and postmature neonates through maternal transport (Abstract). Clin. Res. 26:180A, 1978.

Harris, T. R.: Influence of newborn and maternal transport programs of neonatal mortality in the state of Arizona. In Sell, E. J. (ed.): Follow-up of the High Risk Newborn: A Practical Approach. Springfield, IL, Charles C Thomas, 1980, p. 14.

Harvey, K., and Bowes, W. A., Jr.: Maternal-fetal transport. Perinatol. Neonatol. 5:53, 1981.

Hawkins, M. M.: Nursing and regionalization of perinatal services. JOGN Nurs. 9:215, 1980.

Hein, H. A., and Brown, C. J.: Neonatal mortality review: a basis for improving care. Pediatrics 68:504, 1981.

Hoekstra, R., Fangman, J., Perkett, E., et al.: Regionalization of perinatal care. Perinatal Care, October 1981.

Johnson, D. E., and Thompson, T. R.: Resuscitation, stabilization and transport of the ill newborn infant. II. Stabilization and transport. Pediatrics, April 1982.

Johnson, K. G.: The promise of regional perinatal care as a national strategy for improved maternal and infant care. Publ. Health Rep. 97:134, 1982.

Johnson, P. J., and Boros, S. J.: Implementation of a new expanded nursing role. II. Perinatol. Neonatol. 3:25, 1979.

Johnson, P. J., Jung, A. C., and Boros, S. J.: Neonatal nurse practitioners. I. A new expanded nursing role. Perinatol. Neonatol. 3:34, 1979.

Jones, P. K., Jones, S. L., and Halliday, H. L.: Evaluation of television consultations between a large neonatal care hospital and a community hospital. Medical Care 18:110, 1980.

Jung, A. L., and Bose, C. L.: Back transport of neonates: improved efficiency of tertiary nursery bed utilization. Pediatrics 71:918, 1983.

Kanto, W. P., Jr., Bryant, J., Thigpen, J., et al.: Impact of a maternal transport program on a newborn service. South. Med. J. 76:834, 1983.

Kanto, W. P., Jr., Johnson, G., Sturgill, C., et al.: Performance of a level II nursery in a neonatal regional program. Part I. Patient population and role of the general pediatrician. Part II. Analysis of transferred patients and criteria for maternal transport. South. Med. J. 75:1043, 1982.

Kanto, W. P., Maples, J. C., Goldberg, G. H., et al.: Evaluation and need of education programs for community hospital nurses providing neonatal care. JOGN Nurs. 8:98, 1979.

Killam, A. P., Barrett, J. M., and Cotton, R. B.: The impact of a tertiary perinatal center on survival of the very low birth weight infant. J. Tenn. Med. Assoc. 74:870, 1981.

Knox, G. E., Schnitker, K. A.: In-utero transport. Clin. Obstet. Gynecol. 27:11, 1984.

Knox, G. E., and Hoekstra, R.: Regionalization pact increases revenue. Hospitals, 57:38, 1983.

Knuppel, R. A., Cetrulo, C. L., Ingardia, C. J., et al.: Experience of a Massachusetts Perinatal Center. N. Engl. J. Med. 300:560, 1979.

Lane, J. C., and Jarosch, G.: Mercy flights. Med. J. Aust. 2:311, 1983.

Levy, D. L., Noelke, K., and Goldsmith, J. P.: Maternal and infant transport program in Louisiana. Obstet. Gynecol. 37:300, 1981.

Mayer, J. D.: The distance behavior of hospital patients: a disaggregated analysis. Soc. Sci. Med. 17:819, 1983.

Merenstein, G. B., Pettett, G., Woodall, J., et al.: An analysis of air transport results in the sick newborn. II. Antenatal and neonatal referrals. Am. J. Obstet. Gynecol. 128:520, 1977.

Meyer, H. P. B.: Transport of high-risk infants in Arizona. In Sunshine, P. (ed.): Report of the 66th Ross Conference on Pediatric Research. Columbus, OH, Ross Laboratories, 1974, p. 65.

Minckley, B. B.: Nursing Research and Regionalization in the Midwest. Rep. Reg. Res. Develop. 29:193, 1980.

Modanlou, H. D., Dorchester, W. L., Freeman, R. K., et al.: Perinatal transport to a regional perinatal center in a metropolitan area: maternal versus neonatal transport. Am. J. Obstet. Gynecol. 138:1157, 1980.

Modanlou, H. D., Dorchester, W. L., Thorosian, A., et al.: Antenatal versus neonatal transport to a regional perinatal center: a comparison between matched pairs. Obstet. Gynecol. 53:725, 1979.

Morrison, J. C., and Rhodes, P. G.: Perinatal regionalization: it works for all of us. J. Miss. State Med. Assoc. 21:137, 1980.

Nowacek, G. A., Cook, L. J., and Kattwinkel, J.: Assessment of transportability of a perinatal education system. South. Med. J. 76:1490, 1983.

Organization of Perinatal Services throughout the United States. Unpublished document compiled by the Wisconsin Association for Perinatal Care, 1980.

Ostrea, E. M., and Schuman, H.: The role of the pediatric nurse practitioner in a neonatal unit. J. Pediatr. 86:628, 1975.

Paneth, N., Kiely, J. L., Phil, M., et al.: Newborn intensive care and neonatal mortality in low-birth-weight infants. N. Engl. J. Med. 307:149, 1982.

Parer, J. T.: Effects of hypoxia on the mother and fetus with emphasis on maternal air transport. Am. J. Obstet. Gynecol. 142:967, 1982.

Parsons, C. J., and Bobechko, W. P.: Aeromedical transport: its hidden problems. Can. Med. Assoc. J. 126:237, 1982.

Peddle, L. J., Brown, H., Buckley, J., et al.: Voluntary regionalization and associated trends in perinatal care: the Nova Scotia reproductive care program. Am. J. Obstet. Gynecol. 145:170, 1983.

Pettet, G., Merenstein, G. B., Baltaglia, F. C., et al.: An analysis of air transport results in the sick newborn infant. 1. The transport team. Pediatrics 55:774, 1975.

Pomerance, J. J., Ukrainski, C. T., Ukra, T., et al.: Cost of living for infants weighing 1000 grams or less at birth. Pediatrics 61:908, 1978.

Reedy, N. J., Alonso, B. K., Bozzelli, J. E., et al.: Maternal-fetal transport: a nurse team (forms). JOGN Nurs. 13:91, 1984.

Ryan, G. M., Jr., and Fielden, J. A.: The impact of regionalization programs on patterns of perinatal care. Obstet. Gynecol. 53:187, 1979.

Ryan, G. M., Jr., Fielden, J. G., and Pearse, W. H.: Regional planning—effects on the obstetrician-gynecologist. Obstet. Gynecol. 59:202, 1982.

Sachs, B. P., Marks, J. S., McCarthy, B. J., et al.: Neonatal transport in Georgia: implications for maternal transport in high-risk pregnancies. South. Med. J. 76:1397, 1983.

Slovis, T. L., and Comerci, G. D.: The neonatal nurse practitioner. Am. J. Dis. Child. 128:310, 1974.

Souma, J. L.: Maternal transport: behind the drama. Obstet. Gynecol. 134:904, 1979.

Storrs, C. N., and Taylor, M. R. H.: Transport of sick newborn babies. Br. Med. J. 3:328, 1970.

Subcommittee on Perinatal Transportation of the Perinatal Advisory Committee: Tennessee Perinatal Care System Guidelines for Transportation. Nashville, Tennessee Department of Health and Environment, September 1979.

Thompson, J. D.: One application of the DRG planning model. Top. Health Care Finan. 8:51, Summer, 1982.

Thompson, T. R.: Neonatal transport nurses: an analysis of their role in the transport of newborn infants. Pediatrics 65:887, 1980.

Winegar, A., Spellacy, W. N., Vidyasagar, D., et al.: A system to monitor patient care in a perinatal region. Am. J. Obstet. Gynecol. 145:39, 1983.

Wirth, F. H.: A community-directed perinatal regional system. Perinatol. Neonatol. 4:13, 1980.

3

ANTEPARTUM BIOELECTRIC AND BIOCHEMICAL FETAL EVALUATION

JANIS GAIL SUTLIFF
JOHN F. HUDDLESTON

Although there has been steady and respectable improvement in perinatal outcome during recent years, a small percentage of pregnancies continue to terminate in either fetal mortality or serious morbidity. Although not all potentially disastrous outcomes can be predicted, a majority of pregnancies with such potential can be identified through screening methods (such as the history, the physical examination, and laboratory tests) and thus be labeled as "high-risk" (Aubry and Pennington, 1973; Goodwin et al., 1969; Hoebel et al., 1973). Over the last two decades, several surveillance methods have been developed and utilized in managing these high-risk pregnancies—pregnancies that because of factors justifying the high-risk label would be expected, without effective surveillance methods and selective intervention, to produce the majority of cases of perinatal morbidity and mortality.

Pregnancies can be designated as high-risk for any of several undesirable outcomes. For instance, the woman who has lost several babies because of recurrent preterm labor in the midtrimester presents a management problem different from the woman with longstanding diabetes mellitus who has had several stillbirths near term. Another pregnancy in the diabetic woman would be at risk for the inadequate provision of nutrients and of oxygen—that is, uteroplacental insufficiency.

Pregnancies considered to be at risk for uteroplacental insufficiency carry a serious threat for fetal growth retardation, intrauterine fetal demise, intrapartum fetal distress, and various types of neonatal morbidity. Factors such as insulin-requiring diabetes and hypertensive disorders can interfere with uterine blood flow, intervillous-space perfusion, and placental exchange, thereby possibly interfering with fetal nutrition and oxygenation (Parer, 1976). The potential for perinatal morbidity or mortality is thereby increased. Of the general types of surveillance methods that have been developed, those using electronic monitoring of the fetal heart rate have become the most widely used and accepted for fetal assessment in the management of those pregnancies at risk for uteroplacental insufficiency (Resnik et al., 1982). Through assessment of the at-risk fetus with antepartum heart-rate (and at times biochemical and sonographic) monitoring, those pregnancies with normal uteroplacental exchange, as evidenced by repetitively normal tests, can confidently be managed with a "hands-off" policy. Of this large majority with normal tests, most can be carefully followed to term and can undergo spontaneous labor and delivery. For those few babies whose tests are abnormal—and thus suggest decreased uteroplacental function—corrective efforts can be effected either to improve uterine blood flow or to remove the fetus from its unfavorable environment.

Indications for Testing
(Table 3–1)

Maternal factors that place a pregnancy at risk for uteroplacental insufficiency include chronic and pregnancy-induced hypertension, chronic renal disease, insulin-requiring diabetes mellitus, cyanotic congenital heart

38

Table 3–1. Suggested indications for Antepartum Fetal Assessment

Chronic hypertension/pregnancy-induced
  hypertension
Chronic renal disease
Diabetes mellitus (insulin-requiring)
Cyanotic congenital heart disease
Rhesus (or other) isoimmunization
Homozygous hemoglobinopathies
Maternal abuse of cigarettes/alcohol/drugs
Previous unexplained stillbirth
Fetal growth retardation
Postdatism
Hydramnios/oligohydramnios
Decreased fetal movement
Multiple gestation
Premature rupture of membranes (PROM)
Third trimester bleeding
Arrhythmias
Sickle cell anemia
Maternal collagen vascular disease

disease, isoimmunization, sickle-cell diseases, maternal cigarette abuse, and history of a previous pregnancy that terminated with an unexplained stillbirth. Other obstetric problems that also place a pregnancy at such risk include fetal growth retardation, postdatism (42 or more gestational weeks), hydramnios, and oligohydramnios. Testing should also be considered when there are maternal sensations of decreased fetal movement and in cases of multiple gestation near term.

Primary emphasis in this chapter will be given to bioelectric testing, as it is used more extensively. For the sake of completeness, biochemical testing methods will be outlined.

Bioelectrical Testing Methods

Any fetus at risk for uteroplacental insufficiency is a candidate, as early as the 26th to 28th gestational week, for bioelectric fetal evaluation. The time chosen to begin testing will depend upon the circumstances surrounding the individual pregnancy and the neonatal survival data for tiny babies at a particular hospital or referral center. Generally, for at-risk pregnancies that are progressing well by clinical criteria, testing is started at about 32 to 34 weeks of gestation. The lower gestational-age limit to begin testing is defined as that at which, after consultation with the patient and her husband, one would do a cesarean operation for fetal indications.

In tertiary referral centers, this lower limit currently is about 26 weeks.

Two types of bioelectric fetal evaluation have achieved widespread acceptance for antepartum surveillance. The first described was the contraction stress test (CST), which relies for its interpretation on the fetal-heart-rate response to uterine contractions (Pose et al., 1969; Ray et al., 1972). Since even normal uterine contractions will exert some hypoxic stresses to the fetus through impairment of uterine blood flow (Poseiro et al., 1969), uteroplacental function can be assessed through performance of the CST. If function (and thus fetal oxygenation) has been normal, these temporary interruptions of uterine blood flow will not disturb fetal oxygenation sufficiently to affect the heart rate (Parer, 1976). However, contractions may cause repetitive late decelerations if fetal basal oxygenation is low, a finding that implies impairment in uteroplacental exchange (Martin, 1978; Myers et al., 1973; Pose et al., 1969). A finding of a negative CST (no late decelerations with a contraction frequency of 3 in 10 minutes) has been found highly predictive of intrauterine survival for 7 subsequent days (Freeman et al., 1982; Huddleston and Freeman, 1982). Gabbe et al. (1978) have found CST results to be reliable even early in the third trimester.

The second of these bioelectric tests is the nonstress test (NST), which relies for its interpretation on fetal-heart-rate reactivity: accelerations of the heart rate found in response to fetal movements (Evertson et al., 1979; Rochard et al., 1976). As with the negative CST, a reactive NST is also highly predictive of intrauterine survival for 7 subsequent days (Freeman et al., 1982; Martin and Schifrin, 1977). However, a finding of a nonreactive pattern may imply that the fetus is acidotic, as a result of prolonged suboptimal oxygenation. In the evolution of fetal deterioration due to hypoxia, we consider that the appearance of late decelerations in response to contractions (positive CST) will precede loss of heart-rate reactivity (nonreactive NST) (Huddleston and Freeman, 1982; Huddleston et al., 1984) (see Fig. 3–1). On the other hand, since a nonreactive pattern frequently exists for other reasons, a follow-up CST is generally performed to explain a nonreactive pattern. A positive CST suggests that this pattern is due to protracted fetal hypoxia; a negative CST suggests that the nonreactivity exists because of

	Metabolically Normal Fetus ⇌	Critical Hypoxia During Contractions ⇢	Fetus With Asphyxia
Basal Oxygenation	Normal	Subnormal	Subnormal
Contraction Stress Test	Negative	Positive	Positive
Acid-Base Status	Normal	Normal	Acidotic
Nonstress Test	Reactive	Reactive	Nonreactive

Figure 3–1. Evolution of fetal deterioration due to hypoxia. Loss of reactivity, when due to hypoxia, is usually preceded by late decelerations, if the uterus is contracting. If this is the correct sequence of events, then the CST is a better indicator of fetal reserve, whereas the NST defines better acute fetal condition.

some other factor, such as fetal sleep or maternal ingestion of narcotic or sedative drugs (Martin and Schifrin, 1977).

Of these two bioelectric tests used for fetal surveillance, the NST has become the primary test in many institutions, because it is simpler, requires less time, and is less costly than the CST (Resnik et al., 1982). In the authors' opinion, there do remain, however, definite indications for the CST. Not only is it used to define fetal status when a nonreactive NST is found, but some institutions rely on the CST for primary testing of their pregnancies at highest risk. (At our institution, four conditions qualify: severe chronic hypertension, insulin-requiring diabetes, fetal growth retardation substantiated by ultrasound, and oligohydramnios) (Huddleston and Freeman, 1982). Moreover, data now available from the CST/NST Collaborative Study suggest that the CST may be a better predictor of fetal reserve, as its use for primary fetal surveillance seems to be associated with fewer stillbirths when compared with primary use of the NST (Freeman et al., 1982). Moreover, recent methods employing maternal nipple stimulation to produce uterine contractions may encourage more widespread use of the CST, as this test now compares favorably with the NST with regard to simplicity and, therefore, cost (Freeman, 1982; Huddleston et al., 1984).

THE CONTRACTION STRESS TEST

CST Methodology

The gravida is placed in the left-lateral position, in an attempt to prevent aortic vena caval compression (Scott and Kerr, 1963) (such compression can reduce uterine blood flow and result in temporary fetal hypoxia and an abnormal test, independent of the reason for which the pregnancy is being tested). External fetal monitoring equipment is then applied. Blood pressure is measured initially and at 10- to 15-minute intervals throughout testing. Any hypotension is noted and corrected by maternal positional change. Baseline fetal heart rate and spontaneous uterine contractions are assessed for 15 to 20 minutes after application of the external fetal heart rate transducer (ultrasonic Doppler, phonotransducer, or abdominal ECG) and the tocotransducer. Care must be taken in positioning and tightly securing the tocotransducer to ensure that uterine activity (and fetal movements) will be recorded on the monitor strip. After the baseline recording has been obtained, uterine activity is assessed as to adequacy and, if spontaneous activity is inadequate (arbitrarily defined as less than three palpable 40- to 60-second contractions in a 10-minute period), either oxytocin delivery is begun with an intravenous infusion pump, or contractions are initiated by intermittent nipple stimulation.

Some relative contraindications should be considered when administering the CST. These include placenta previa, previous uterine rupture, previous vertical cesarean section, premature labor, incompetent cervix, and premature rupture of the membranes.

Oxytocin Release via Intravenous Infusion Pump. If spontaneous uterine activity is deemed inadequate following the 15- to 20-minute baseline period, a small, slow intravenous infusion is begun (generally with either normal saline or Ringer's lactate solution). A controlled-rate infusion pump is used to regulate the infusion, which is administered in a "piggy-backed" fashion into the intravenous line for oxytocin delivery. Oxytocin, diluted in normal saline, is begun initially at a rate of 0.5 to 1.0 milliunits/minute and then increased (per protocol described in the oxytocin product literature) approximately every 15 to 30 minutes until an adequate contraction frequency is achieved. The typical rate of oxytocin delivery required to elicit adequate uterine activity is 4 to 5 milliunits/minute; rarely will a gravida require more than 8 milliunits/minute to achieve this activity (Huddleston et al., 1979; Huddleston and Freeman, 1982). The average duration of a CST employing this method of oxytocin delivery is reported to be 80 to 90 minutes (Schifrin, 1977).

Oxytocin Release via Intermittent Nipple Stimulation. As a result of impulses transmitted via thoracic sensory nerve roots, breast stimulation in the lactating woman causes the posterior pituitary to release oxytocin (Cobo, 1974). It has been suggested that nipple stimulation in the gravida is an alternative for achieving uterine contractions for CSTs, in lieu of intravenous oxytocin delivery (Freeman, 1982; Huddleston et al., 1984). However, the mechanism by which nipple stimulation causes contractions is not clear. Women wearing light clothing are instructed to rub one nipple, through their clothes and with the palmar surfaces of their fingertips, for 2 minutes, and then to stop nipple stimulation for 5 minutes. If a woman has several layers of clothing on, she is instructed to stimulate one nipple through the brassiere. Stimulation is stopped immediately if a contraction commences during the 2 minutes of stimulation, as we found uterine hyperstimulation occasionally to occur with prolonged stimulation (Huddleston et al., 1984). A gravida may alternate nipples during stimulation, in order to decrease the chances of producing nipple tenderness. A 7-minute cycle is composed of the 2 minutes of stimulation plus the 5 minutes of rest. On average, 2 or 3 nipple-stimulation cycles are required to elicit adequate uterine activity, with the average length of a CST using intermittent nipple stimulation being 40 to 45 minutes (including the 15 to 20-minute observation period (Huddleston et al., 1984).

CST Interpretations

Negative. CST results are interpreted in the classic manner (Freeman, 1975). The CST is defined as negative when there are no late decelerations present on the tracing and uterine contractions have been adequate to sufficiently stress the fetus (three 40- to 60-second palpable contractions in a 10-minute period or a tetanic contraction lasting ≥90 seconds). Usually, but not always, fetal heart-rate reactivity is seen (Figs. 3–2 and 3–3). The negative CST is repeated every 7 days until delivery, unless severe clinical decompensation occurs (e.g., diabetic ketoacidosis or exacerbation of hypertensive disease). However, some researchers are advocating testing patients with insulin-requir-

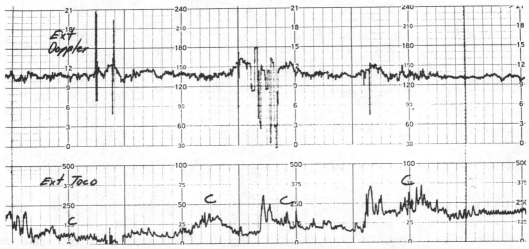

Figure 3–2. Negative CST. No late decelerations with a contraction frequency of at least 3/10 min.

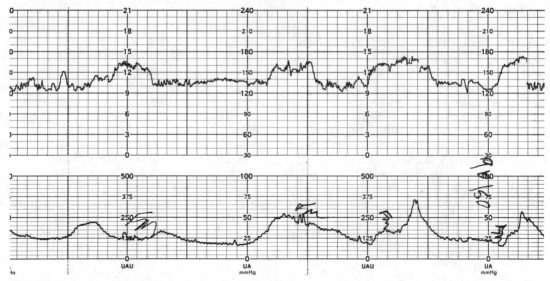

Figure 3–3. Negative CST. Reactivity associated with fetal movements (FM) is so pronounced as to perhaps cause confusion in interpretation. However, the baseline heart rate is 130 to 140 beats/min, and the return of the heart rate to baseline following the accelerations does not represent late deceleration.

ing diabetes, gestational diabetes with a previous stillborn, postdate pregnancy, or intrauterine fetal growth retardation (IUGR) twice a week. With this strict, classic interpretation for the negative test, we and others have found a false-negative CST (fetal death occurring with 7 days of a negative test) rate of only 1 to 2 per 1000 cases (Freeman et al., 1982; Huddleston and Freeman, 1982). Thus, we have not seen reason to shorten the time interval between tests. About 80 to 85 percent of tests will be negative.

Positive. In the absence of uterine hy-

perstimulation or supine hypotension, the presence of late decelerations with 50 percent or more of the contractions during a period of adequate uterine activity constitutes a positive CST (Huddleston and Freeman, 1982). However, it is unnecessary and actually undesirable to continue efforts to achieve three contractions in a 10-minute period if recurrent late decelerations are evident with contractions occurring less frequently. Reactivity may or may not be present (Figs. 3–4 and 3–5).

From 3 to 5 percent of CSTs will be classified as positive. The fetus with a positive

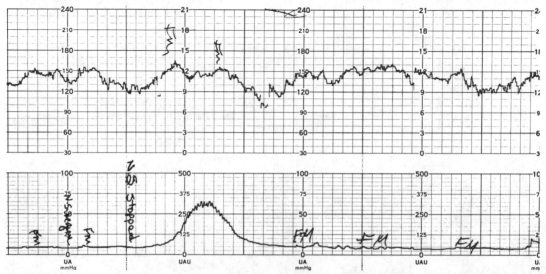

Figure 3–4. Positive, reactive CST. Only one contraction, with one late deceleration is seen in this particular frame, which was chosen to display the obvious reactivity in response to fetal movements (FM).

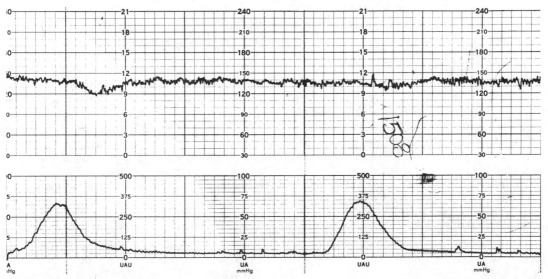

Figure 3–5. Positive, nonreactive CST. Recurrent late decelerations with no reactivity. This fetus stands a high likelihood of intrapartum distress and neonatal morbidity.

CST is probably suboptimally oxygenated, at least at the time of testing (Freeman et al., 1976). Therefore, management of the positive-CST fetus generally will include prompt intervention. The fetus at term or postterm most frequently is delivered. The route of delivery is predicated on the presence of concurrent heart-rate reactivity and on obstetric factors, such as cervical "ripeness" (assessed by the Bishop score [Bishop, 1964]) and fetal lie. It has been found that, if such conditions are favorable and the fetus is treated prophylactically for fetal distress (i.e., mother placed in the left-lateral position, hydrated intravenously, and given oxygen by mask), about half of these fetuses can safely endure the induction of labor with oxytocin (Braly and Freeman, 1977; Huddleston et al., 1979). However, if the positive CST is also nonreactive, the fetal condition is generally such that labor cannot be tolerated; cesarean delivery is generally employed in a preemptive manner for these patients. However, some institutions do give these patients a trial of labor. If fetal maturity is in doubt *and* if heart-rate reactivity* is present on the positive CST tracing, an amniocentesis typically is done for studies of pulmonary maturity. If such studies suggest that the fetus is quite immature *and* if the frequently assessed heart-rate reactivity remains reassuring, such a patient temporarily

*Heart-rate reactivity being defined as 2 accelerations in a 20-minute period increasing 15 beats above the baseline and lasting 15 seconds (reactive NST).

may be managed by having the gravida remain at bedrest in the left-lateral position (Huddleston and Freeman, 1982). Some physicians consider in these patients the use of glucocorticoids, in an attempt to hasten fetal pulmonary maturity (Liggins and Howie, 1972). The management of such an immature fetus includes *daily* assessments for reactivity (NST) and/or daily estriol determinations. (A discussion of these tests appears later in this chapter.) However, if the NST is nonreactive and/or the estriol determinations are low, the fetus generally is transferred from its hostile intrauterine environment to a neonatal intensive care unit.

Equivocal. About 15 to 20 percent of CSTs will not be interpretable as either negative or positive. These tests are designated as equivocal and impart little useful information concerning fetal well-being. They should be repeated within 24 hours, in an attempt to achieve a definitive result concerning fetal well-being. Equivocal tests may be further categorized as suspicious, hyperstimulation, and unsatisfactory (Huddleston and Freeman, 1982).

A CST is considered suspicious when late decelerations only intermittently are present with an adequate (but not excessive) contraction frequency (e.g., present with fewer than half of contractions) Usually, but not always, heart-rate reactivity is present. As only about one-fifth of these suspicious tests will become positive on repeat testing, and since a delay of 24 hours to repeat a suspicious test has not resulted in fetal loss at this institution, such repeat testing is almost always employed (Bruce et al., 1978; Huddleston et al., 1979).

In the presence of excessive uterine activity (contractions occurring more often than every 2 minutes and/or lasting more than 90 seconds) with associated late deceleration(s), a CST is labeled hyperstimulation. As uterine sensitivity to oxytocin varies with each gravida, extreme care must be taken when introducing intravenous oxytocin, or when beginning the intermittent nipple stimulation. Excessive uterine activity may even occur in the gravida who is contracting spontaneously.

Occasionally, the quality of a tracing will be such that an interpretation of the CST cannot be made confidently; such tests are termed unsatisfactory. Factors that may increase the chances for an unsatisfactory CST include extreme obesity, hydramnios, and a very active fetus. The effect of these factors can be reduced if the tester remains with the patient and monitors the tracing. Uncommonly, an adequate contraction frequency may not be obtainable, and such a CST is also classified as unsatisfactory. This latter type of unsatisfactory result seems limited to those tests stimulated by exogenous oxytocin; our experience to date with the CST by intermittent nipple stimulation is that adequate uterine activity can be achieved in all cases (Huddleston et al., 1984). Most of these gravidas on follow-up testing within 24 hours will readily achieve an adequate frequency of contractions.

THE NONSTRESS TEST

NST Methodology

The NST is conducted much the same as the CST, except that there is no need for a means to elicit uterine contractions. The gravida is placed in the left-lateral or semi-Fowler's position, and the external fetal monitoring equipment is applied. Blood pressure is measured initially and at 10- to 15-minute intervals during testing, and any maternal hypotension is noted and corrected with maternal positional change. Observation is made of the baseline fetal heart rate, of any spontaneous contractions occurring, and of any decelerations (most commonly of the variable type) evident on the monitor strip. Not infrequently, the gravida undergoing an NST will be spontaneously contracting at a frequency sufficient to give a "bonus": the added reassurance of a negative CST. Fetal movements are annotated on the monitor strip, either through a marker pressed by the patient or by writing "FM" on the strip. Fetal movements usually are manifested as a spike on the tocotransducer tracing and are generally audible over the monitor's speaker. Since some gravidas in late pregnancy are unaware of any but the strongest fetal movements, it is important that both patient and nurse seek to determine fetal activity.

As it is considered that sleep/rest cycles occur at 20-minute intervals (Evertson et al., 1979), the sleeping fetus may be encountered during an NST. Usually, gentle manipulation of the fetus by the mother or the nurse or an external stimulus such as loud noise (Read and Miller, 1977) will awaken the healthy but sleeping fetus and elicit fetal movements with reactivity. Such fetal stimulation will generally serve to differentiate between a sleeping fetus and a fetus that is hypoactive because of reduced uteroplacental exchange.

NST Interpretations

Disturbances of autonomic influences on the fetal heart rate—and thus fetal metabolic health—can be evaluated through heart-rate patterns of beat-to-beat variability and accelerations associated with fetal movements. With chronic suboptimal oxygenation, both a reduction of heart-rate reactivity and a flattening of normal beat-to-beat variability will be exhibited. The latter assessment is generally valid only during the intrapartum period, when the fetal heart rate is derived from a scalp electrode. Evaluation of apparent beat-to-beat variability is many times misleading with external Doppler transducers. Therefore, interpretation of the antepartum NST is based upon the grosser changes of heart-rate reactivity, which are of sufficient magnitude and duration so as not to be confused with the smaller heart-rate changes (beat-to-beat variability), which may be spurious. This reactivity implies that, at the time of testing, the fetus (from an acid-base perspective) is metabolically normal (Parer, 1976; Resnik et al., 1982).

Reactive. The NST is defined as reactive when there are accelerations of the fetal

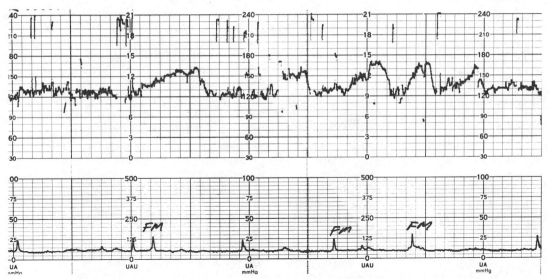

Figure 3–6. Reactive NST. Impressive accelerations of the fetal heart rate, occurring in response to fetal movements (FM).

heart rate, in response to fetal movements, of at least 15 beats/minute and lasting at least 15 seconds (Fig. 3–6). Much has been published concerning the number of heart-rate accelerations within a certain time frame required to justify a designation of reactive (Evertson et al., 1979; Mendenhall et al., 1980; Resnik et al., 1982). We have considered that two accelerations meeting the above criteria within a 20-minute period suffice as a reactive test (Resnik et al., 1982). Fetal movements may occur (a) spontaneously, (b) following abdominal palpation,

(c) in response to spontaneous contractions, or (d) as a result of sonic stimulation (Read and Miller, 1977) or ingestion of fruit juice. A reactive NST, without variable decelerations, using whatever criteria one elects for the required number of accelerations, is a good predictor of fetal well-being for 1 week (unless severe clinical decompensation occurs) (Resnik et al., 1982). Some researchers are advocating testing twice a week for insulin-dependent diabetics, gestational diabetics with a previous stillborn, cases of postdatism, or IUGR. However, if variable

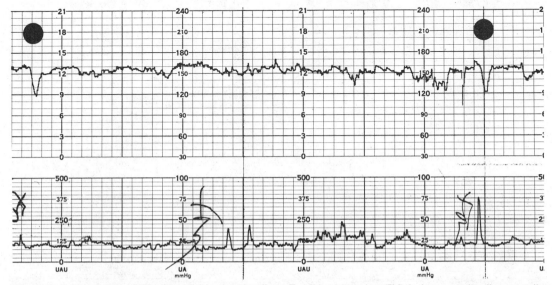

Figure 3–7. Nonreactive NST with variable decelerations. The fetus is moving (FM), but no accelerations meeting the criterion of 15 beats/min for 15 sec are seen. Several variable decelerations (dots) suggest vulnerability of the umbilical cord, most commonly due to oligohydramnios.

decelerations are present (Fig. 3–7), one should suspect oligohydramnios, and further evaluation (generally ultrasound and a CST) should be pursued (Freeman et al., 1983).

Nonreactive. If the criteria for reactivity are not met, the NST is termed nonreactive. It must be ascertained, however, whether fetal sleep or a sedative drug (including ones that may have been obtained illicitly) may have been responsible for the nonreactivity. In such cases, prolonging the NST for an additional 20 minutes may provide a reactive test (Evertson et al., 1979; Resnik et al., 1982). As a nonreactive NST in and of itself provides little or no useful information as to fetal well-being, a CST should then be performed to provide a definitive answer. At the time of the CST, produced either by intravenous oxytocin or through intermittent nipple stimulation, the fetus may begin to stir and the tracing may become reactive. In these cases, it is not necessary to continue with oxytocin delivery or nipple stimulation, unless there is some other clinical indication for the CST besides the transiently nonreactive NST.

Keegan and coworkers (1980) found that if the nonreactive NST was repeated later in the day, 98 percent of those tests became reactive. Therefore, some hospitals are now repeating the NST the same day before proceeding to the CST.

Sinusoidal. Sinusoidal patterns (Fig. 3–8) are seen as baseline oscillations at a frequency of 2 to 5 per minute, varying from 5 to 15 beats per minute, with an absence of heart-rate reactivity (Rochard et al., 1976). Thus, the sinusoidal pattern is a variant of the nonreactive test, and the presence of good reactivity on any adjacent part of the tracing should preclude serious consideration of its being truly sinusoidal. These patterns are found usually in Rhesus-sensitized fetuses or in fetuses with severe fetomaternal bleeding; they are rare and are an ominous sign (Modanlou et al., 1977; Rochard et al., 1976).

PATIENT EDUCATION AND CONSIDERATIONS FOR THE NST/CST

Prior to initiating NST/CST testing, the procedure is fully explained to the patient by a member of the high-risk team. In some hospitals a consent form, which will cover a single test or the series of tests, is obtained before testing (Table 3–2). A thorough explanation of the reasons for and methods of testing is essential and will help prevent most anxieties otherwise common in these patients. Testing on a weekly basis (or more often if required) will be necessary for most women until delivery. These rare exceptions (for which testing is not repeated) include gravidas whose complaint is decreased fetal movement and whose initial test is normal (as long as fetal movements continue), and those few patients who no longer have an

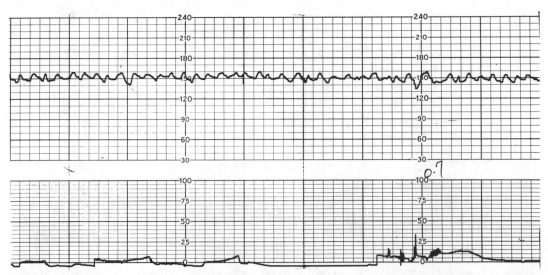

Figure 3–8. Sinusoidal pattern. Narrow, sine-wave–like undulations with no heart rate reactivity. An ominous tracing, most likely indicative of severe fetal anemia.

Table 3–2 Informed Consent for NST and CST

Because my pregnancy is complicated, it has been recommended that I have periodic evaluations of my baby's heartbeat (NST and/or CST) during the rest of my pregnancy. I understand that this will be done by placing small, painless, and (as far as is known) harmless devices on my abdomen to pick up the heartbeat and any of my baby's body movements (NST), as well as to pick up any contractions. I also understand that, because of my particular complication or because the NST may not be able to give a definite answer, I may be asked to rub one of my nipples, which will cause me to have a few contractions (CST). This has not been found to cause premature labor. I further understand that the response of the heartbeat, either to the baby's movements or to contractions, will determine whether the test is normal or not: (1) if normal (which most are), this is reassuring, but the test must be repeated every 7 days; (2) if slightly abnormal, the test will have to be repeated in a day or so; (3) if quite abnormal (which very few tests are), this will indicate that my baby may be in serious trouble and that I may need to be hospitalized for further tests or delivery.

It has been explained to me that these procedures have been performed thousands of times, both here and at other hospitals, and no ill effects on the baby have been related to the procedures.

I understand the above statements; I have been given the opportunity to ask questions, and the answers to my questions (if any) have been satisfactory. By signing this permit, I hereby agree to have these tests (NST and/or CST) performed for the remainder of my pregnancy.

Witness_____

Date_____

Signature_____

Date_____

indication for testing. The majority of these are patients who on initial testing were considered to have exhibited signs of fetal growth retardation but for whom subsequent careful ultrasonic assessment has shown no evidence of this problem. Patients are encouraged to eat prior to testing, as this promotes greater activity by the fetus (Miller et al., 1978). The anticipated time requirement for testing should be explained and, when feasible, testing should be scheduled on the same day as the patient's medical appointment. This coordination helps alleviate problems such as transportation and is especially appreciated by those women who might be working or who have small children at home. Some fetuses seem to be active at particular times of the day. If the mother notes that the fetus is active in the morning, it would be best to schedule her appointment for that time, in order to facilitate testing. Decreasing maternal anxiety by em-

phasizing that testing is not painful and that very few tests are abnormal is extremely important and will also help alleviate the problem of "no shows" or cancellations. A well-informed patient will be a more cooperative and willing patient for testing. It is also possible that allaying fears might even reduce chances for a positive test result. Patients should be encouraged to participate in the testing by pushing the button to mark fetal movement, or verbally indicating when fetal movement has occurred. Since all of these mothers have been labeled "high-risk," most are relieved when the test indicates fetal well-being. Involving the mother in the testing also helps to decrease the number of "no shows" and cancellations. Patients may resume their previous level of activity immediately following testing.

Testing of multiple gestations can be accomplished by doing separate testing on each fetus, making certain that different heart-rate baselines are distinguishable. With some multiple gestations, two recordings can be detected at the same time, which can shorten the duration of the test. This is usually done with ultrasound and a phonotransducer. Two ultrasound signals may interfere with each other, making the test difficult.

Since antepartum fetal heart rate testing usually takes a minimum of 10 to 15 minutes and may take an hour or so, it is an excellent time to educate the patient about what to expect during the prenatal period, labor and delivery, and the postpartum period. Not only is education easily accomplished during the testing period but the rapport it develops offers an excellent opportunity for counseling. Therefore, the nurses doing the NST/CST testing are an integral part of the team, because they can provide much education, patient information, and counseling.

Inpatient testing is performed in the same manner as outpatient testing. However, although the NST has been performed in the office setting, most CST tests have been performed in the hospital setting or in offices adjacent to the hospital due to the administration of intravenous oxytocin.

The cost of NST/CST testing will probably vary from facility to facility, with an average NST cost range of $35 to $50, and an average CST range of $50 to $100. Factors included in figuring cost are the expenses of intravenous supplies (this is not needed for the NST and is the reason for its lower cost), the time required for testing, and the time of a nurse specialist and his or her medical backup. In addition, equivocal tests will need to be repeated until a definitive test result can be obtained. Consideration should be given to charging less for CSTs by nipple stimulation, as intravenous infusion equipment is not necessary and length of testing is shorter. Most insurance carriers will defray at least part of the expense involved in NSTs/CSTs.

Biophysical Profile*

The biophysical profile was developed by Drs. Manning and Platt to help discriminate between fetuses that are well and those that are in distress (Manning et al., 1980).

The biophysical profile is based on five observations. The first assessment is the NST; the other four, which are diagnosed by ultrasound, are (1) the presence of fetal body movements (3 movements in 10 minutes); (2) the presence of fetal chest wall movements, i.e., fetal breathing (30 seconds of continual breathing in 30 minutes); (3) the observation of good fetal tone (one extension/flexion cycle of a fetal limb with rapid return to the flexed posture in 30 minutes); and (4) the presence of a normal amount of amniotic fluid (the presence of a "pocket" of fluid that is greater than 1 cm).

Each parameter receives 2 points if present and 0 points if absent (or nonreactive); the maximum best score is 10, and the worst score is 0. Scores of 8 to 10 are considered reassuring, and testing can be repeated in a week unless fetal or maternal circumstances change. A score of 4 to 6 is considered equivocal and requires that testing be repeated within 24 hours. Scores of 0 to 2 are abnormal and worrisome and indicate immediate evaluation for delivery.

A theoretical concern with the biophysical profile is that it measures only steady-state conditions and therefore might not be as predictive of uteroplacental reserve as a test requiring a fetal stress, such as the CST. A study comparing the relative efficacies of the biophysical profile and the CST has not been reported.

---

*See also Chapter 4.

PATIENT EDUCATION AND CONSIDERATIONS

Most of the ultrasound component of the biophysical profile can be completed within 30 minutes. It is important to make the mother comfortable during that part of the examination. Education of the mother and her support person regarding the test is very important. Educational materials should be presented to the couple prior to the test to prepare them for it. Photographs of other ultrasonic scans may help with the explanation. An explanation that the procedure is not painful is also helpful.

Biochemical Fetal Evaluation

Biochemical assays of estriol and human placental lactogen (HPL) are still used by some obstetricians in assessing fetal well-being and placental function. The most common situation for current use of these tests is when the fetal-monitoring test results are nonreassuring and the pregnancy is preterm. Even for those physicians regularly ordering estriol or HPL assays, fetal monitoring tests are generally performed concurrently. The serum or plasma concentrations of both hormones increase as pregnancy progresses, and sharp or progressive decreases in concentration may indicate fetal jeopardy. Serial sampling, therefore, is essential for determining sequential changes and assessing fetal well-being. Estriol values correlate with fetal weight in the third trimester, and increasing HPL values parallel increasing placental mass.

MATERNAL ESTRIOL MEASUREMENT

Production of the steroid hormone estriol by the placenta is dependent on proper functioning of the fetal adrenal gland and liver, and the amount produced is influenced by several factors. Length of gestation, multiple gestation, fetal and placental size, certain drugs (particularly glucocorticoids), maternal activity, maternal renal function, and glycosuria may affect either urinary or serum estriol levels and must be considered when interpreting values. In addition, maternal disease may affect test results. Low values from assays in a diabetic gravida are generally more ominous than low values in a hypertensive patient. A single assay is essentially worthless in terms of assuring fetal condition, unless the value is so low as to suspect that fetal demise is imminent. Either urinary or plasma radioimmunoassays should be done 2 to 3 times weekly, so that any impending fetal disaster may be determined and delivery affected if indicated. Any sharp (50 to 60 percent less than preceding value) or progressive decrease in serial values is suggestive of fetal jeopardy. The normal range of daily estriol excretion at term is from 10 to 30 mg, and the range for plasma estriol is 9 to 22 mcg/dl. Results of 24-hour urinary estriol excretion are generally available in about 12 hours, and measurement of blood estriol levels may be returned within approximately 1 hour (Green and Touchstone, 1963; Kochenour, 1982).

HUMAN PLACENTAL LACTOGEN LEVELS

Human placental lactogen (HPL) is a single-chain protein hormone released by the cytotrophoblast into the maternal circulation, where it can be detected as early as 20 to 40 days after implantation. Production slowly increases until 37 weeks' gestation, after which it remains the same or decreases slightly. By 42 weeks' gestation, an impressive decrease is seen (Zlatnik et al., 1979). As a result of associated increases in placental volume, higher HPL values are seen in multiple gestation, erythroblastosis, and poorly controlled diabetes. With these conditions, prediction of fetal well-being by HPL seems to be particularly inaccurate (Varner and Hauser, 1982). Conversely, lower values have been reported by some in pregnancies complicated both by fetal growth retardation and maternal hypertension. Radioimmunoassays for HPL generally are performed weekly, and the range for normal maternal-serum values near term is 5.4 to 7.0 mcg per ml. Values lower than 4 mcg per ml may represent fetal compromise after 30 weeks' gestation, and consistently low values may be as ominous as decreasing values (Spellacy, 1973). It has been suggested that HPL radioimmunoassays be done serially on specific high-risk pregnancies as an adjunct to other fetal surveillance methods.

INDICATIONS FOR ESTRIOL AND HPL RADIOIMMUNOASSAYS

Some fetuses at risk for uteroplacental insufficiency may be candidates for estriol and/or HPL radioimmunoassays. Both estriol and HPL assays have been claimed to be helpful in identifying possible postmaturity in postdate pregnancies if values are low, and both may be of some benefit in the management of hypertensive disorders of pregnancy. However, doubt has been cast over the value of HPL in predicting postmaturity (Berkowitz and Hobbins, 1977). Estriol assays may be beneficial for fetal surveillance when maternal diabetes is present; HPL assays, however, have been reported to be of limited value in the management of this disorder (Spellacy, 1973). The diagnosis of fetal growth retardation may be suspected from HPL determinations, but probably not as readily from serum assays for estriol. Moreover, neither assay has been shown to be of great benefit in the management of Rh isoimmunization. *Although these fetal surveillance methods are still practiced in some obstetric centers, there has been a progressive decrease in their clinical use over the last several years.*

PATIENT EDUCATION AND CONSIDERATIONS

As serial estriol assays must be performed 2 to 3 times weekly for reasonable surveillance of fetal well-being, a patient must be sufficiently motivated and concerned with her pregnancy to undertake the 24-hour urine collections and/or blood samplings that are required several times weekly (Kochenour, 1982). Patients who have transportation problems, who are working, or who do not have the money to cover the cost of serial assays will probably be unwilling or find it impossible to comply with this testing. Furthermore, outpatient management might be difficult for even the most compliant patient. Other factors that might affect the accuracy of results are the collection of an accurate 24-hour urine specimen, variations in fluid intake, the amount of bedrest, concurrent drug administration, and renal function. While serial plasma assays would certainly be less time consuming for the gravida, blood sampling must still be done 2 to 3 times weekly (daily for diabetics) (Goebelsmann et al., 1973) for any impending disastrous changes to be appreciated and intervention effected. However, HPL measurements may require only weekly blood sampling, but may not be as helpful.

Inpatient management results in more accurate results for the 24-hour urine collections for estriol excretion assays, as well as providing more control over factors such as fluid intake and bedrest. Transportation to and from the clinic or office, working schedules, and problems with small children at home are all eliminated when the gravida is treated as an inpatient. Cost, however, is increased and, unless a patient's insurance coverage is excellent, could prove a financial burden for the patient and her family. Also, child care expenses and loss of wages if the mother works would further increase the burden. Therefore, management should be accomplished in the outpatient setting if at all possible. Motivation and reliability of the patient can effect accurate and therefore beneficial test results. Also, thorough patient education on collection of a 24-hour urine sample is essential. If, however, adequate teaching fails, or if the patient is unreliable or noncompliant, another means for assessing fetal well-being should be considered, rather than resorting to hospitalization. Even noncompliant and unreliable patients might be most willing to have weekly NSTs or CSTs for fetal surveillance, especially if these tests are performed on the same day as their medical appointment.

Summary

Approximately 15 percent of pregnancies in a referral center will have indications that place them at risk for uteroplacental insufficiency, and antepartum fetal surveillance methods play an important role in the obstetric management of these women. Although bioelectric fetal evaluations are the more commonly used, some clinicians do rely on estriol and/or HPL radioimmunoassays in managing these pregnancies, and the use of the biophysical profile is gaining acceptance. Biochemical fetal evaluations, when performed serially, may be of benefit in differentiating between the well fetus and the fetus tolerating its environment poorly. Any sharp or progressive decrease in values

is suggestive of fetal jeopardy, and intervention (or further evaluation) should be considered; normal values justify a policy of nonintervention. However, estriol assays must be performed at least 2 to 3 times weekly to be of any benefit, results are not immediately available to the clinician, and even the most compliant patients might have difficulty managing 2 to 3 visits weekly to the physician or laboratory. Moreover, neither estrogen nor HPL assays are satisfactory for the surveillance of every high-risk pregnancy.

Bioelectric fetal evaluations have achieved the most widespread acceptance for antepartum fetal surveillance. These tests of the fetal heart rate can identify accurately, within these high-risk pregnancies, those fetuses (with negative CSTs and/or reactive NSTs) tolerating their intrauterine environments acceptably, and these normal tests usually need be repeated only weekly. These reassuring tests are of great comfort to both the patient and the clinician, and test results are available immediately. Those few fetuses whose test result is abnormal and who are in possible jeopardy can be identified immediately, and corrective measures can be undertaken. Moreover, a policy of nonintervention can be followed in approximately 95 percent of these high-risk pregnancies undergoing fetal-heart-rate testing, as only a small percentage (those with positive CSTs) will be at serious risk for impending disaster (Huddleston and Freeman, 1982).

REFERENCES

Aubry, R. A., and Pennington, J. C.: Identification and evaluation of high-risk pregnancy: the perinatal concept. Clin. Obstet. Gynecol. 16:3, 1973.

Berkowitz, R. L., and Hobbins, J. C.: A reevaluation of the value of hCS determination in the management of prolonged pregnancy. Obstet. Gynecol. 49:156, 1977.

Bishop, E. H.: Pelvic scoring for elective induction. Obstet. Gynecol. 24:266, 1964.

Braly, P., and Freeman, R. K.: The significance of fetal heart rate reactivity with a positive oxytocin challenge test. Obstet. Gynecol. 50:689, 1977.

Braly, P. S., Freeman, R. K., Garite, T. J., et al.: Incidence of premature delivery following the oxytocin challenge test. Am. J. Obstet. Gynecol. 141:5, 1981.

Bruce, S. L., Petrie, R. H., and Yeh, S. Y.: The suspicious contraction stress test. Obstet. Gynecol. 51:415, 1978.

Cobo, E.: Neuroendocrine control of milk injection in women. In Josimovich, J. F., Reynolds, M., and Cobo, E. (eds.): Lactogenic Hormones, Fetal Nutrition, and Lactation. New York, John Wiley & Sons, 1974, p. 433.

Evertson, L. R., Gauthier, R. J., Schifrin, B. S., et al.: Antepartum fetal heart rate testing. I. Evolution of the nonstress test. Am. J. Obstet. Gynecol. 133:29, 1979.

Freeman, R. K.: The use of the oxytocin challenge test for antepartum clinical evaluation of uteroplacental respiratory function. Am. J. Obstet. Gynecol. 121:481, 1975.

Freeman, R. K.: Contraction stress testing for primary fetal surveillance in patients at high risk for uteroplacental insufficiency. Clin. Perinatol. 9:265, 1982.

Freeman, R. K., Anderson, G., and Dorchester, W.: A prospective multi-institutional study of antepartum fetal heart rate monitoring. I. Risk of perinatal mortality and morbidity according to antepartum fetal heart rate test results. Am. J. Obstet. Gynecol. 143:771, 1982.

Freeman, R. K., Anderson, G., and Dorchester, W.: A prospective multi-institutional study of antepartum fetal heart rate monitoring. II. Contraction stress test versus nonstress test for primary surveillance. Am. J. Obstet. Gynecol. 143:778, 1982.

Freeman, R. K., Goebelsmann, U., Nochimson, D., et al.: An evaluation of the significance of a positive oxytocin challenge test. Obstet. Gynecol. 47:8, 1976.

Freeman, R. K., Huddleston, J. F., Petrie, R. H., et al.: Ensuring optimum outcome for postdate pregnancy. Contemp. Ob/Gyn 22(6):187, 1983.

Gabbe, S. G., Freeman, R. K., and Goebelsmann, U.: Evaluation of the contraction stress test before 33 weeks' gestation. Obstet. Gynecol. 52:649, 1978.

Goebelsmann, U., Freeman, R. K., Mestman, J. H., et al.: Estriol in pregnancy. II. Daily urinary estriol assays in the management of the pregnant diabetic woman. Am J. Obstet. Gynecol. 115:795, 1973.

Goodwin, J. W., Dunne, J. T., and Thomas, B. W.: Antepartum identification of the fetus at risk. Can. Med. Assoc. J. 101:458, 1969.

Green, J. W., Jr., and Touchstone, J. C.: Urinary estriol as an index of placental function. Am. J. Obstet. Gynecol. 85:1, 1963.

Hoebel, C. H., Hyvarinen, M. A., Okada, D. M., et al.: Prenatal and intrapartum high-risk screening. I. Prediction of the high-risk neonate. Am. J. Obstet. Gynecol. 117:1, 1973.

Huddleston, J. F., Sutliff, G., Carney, F. E., Jr., et al.: Oxytocin challenge test for antepartum fetal assessment: report of a clinical experience. Am. J. Obstet. Gynecol. 135:609, 1979.

Huddleston, J. F., and Freeman, R. K.: Assessment of fetal well-being by antepartum fetal heart rate testing. In Bolognese, R. J., Schwarz, R. H., Schneider, J. (eds.): Perinatal Medicine: Management of the High Risk Fetus and Neonate, 2nd ed. Baltimore, Williams and Wilkins, 1982, p. 129.

Huddleston, J. F., Sutliff, G., and Robinson, D.: Contraction stress test by intermittent nipple stimulation. Obstet. Gynecol. 63:669, 1984.

Keegan, K. A., Paul, R. H., Broussard, P. M., et al.: Antepartum fetal heart rate testing. V. The nonstress test—An outpatient approach. Am. J. Obstet. Gynecol. 136:81, 1980.

Kochenour, N. K.: Estrogen assay during pregnancy. Clin. Obstet. Gynecol. 25:659, 1982.

Liggins, G. C., and Howie, R. N.: A controlled trial of antepartum glucocorticoid treatment for prevention of the respiratory distress syndrome in premature infants. Pediatrics 50:515, 1972.

Manning, F. A., Platt, L. D., and Sipos, L.: Antepartum fetal evaluation: development of a fetal biophysical profile. Am. J. Obstet. Gynecol. 136:787, 1980.

Martin, C. B., Jr.: Regulation of the fetal heart rate and genesis of FHR patterns. Semin. Perinatol. 2:131, 1978.

Martin, C. B., Jr., Schifrin, B. S.: Prenatal monitoring. In Aladjem, S., and Brown, A. K. (ed.): Perinatal Intensive Care. St. Louis, C. V. Mosby Co., 1977, p. 155.

Mendenhall, H. W., O'Leary, J. A., and Phillips, K. O.: The nonstress test: the value of a single acceleration in evaluating the fetus at risk. Am. J. Obstet. Gynecol. 136:87, 1980.

Miller, F. C., Skiba, H., and Klapholz H: The effect of maternal blood sugar levels on fetal activity. Obstet. Gynecol. 52:662, 1978.

Modanlou, H. D., Freeman, R. K., Ortiz, O., et al.: Sinusoidal FHR pattern and severe anemia. Obstet. Gynecol. 49:537, 1977.

Myers, R. E., Mueller-Heubach, E., and Adamsons, K.: Predictability of the state of fetal oxygenation from the quantitative analysis of the components of late deceleration. Am. J. Obstet. Gynecol. 115:1083, 1973.

Parer, J. T.: Normal and impaired placental exchange. Contemp. Ob/Gyn 7(2):117, 1976.

Platt, L. D., Eglinton, G. S., Sipos, L., et al.: Further experience with the fetal biophysical profile. Obstet. Gynecol. 61:480, 1983.

Pose, S. V., Castillo, J. B., Nora-Rojas, E. O., et al.: Test of fetal tolerance to induced uterine contractions for the diagnosis of chronic distress. In Perinatal Factors Affecting Human Development. Washington, D. C., Pan American Health Organization, 1969, p. 96.

Poseiro, J. J., Mendez-Bauer, C., Pose, S. V., et al.: Effect of uterine contractions on maternal blood flow through the placenta. In Perinatal Factors Affecting Human Development. Washington, D. C., Pan American Health Organization, 1969, p. 161.

Ray, M., Freeman, R. K., Pine, S., et al.: Clinical experience with the oxytocin challenge test. Am. J. Obstet. Gynecol. 114:1, 1972.

Read, J. A., and Miller, F. C.: Fetal heart rate acceleration in response to acoustic stimulation as a measure of fetal well-being. Am. J. Obstet. Gynecol. 129:512, 1977.

Resnik, R., Huddleston, J. F., Freeman, R. K., et al.: NST or CST? What's best for spotting the high-risk fetus? Contemp. Ob/Gyn 19(4):92, 1982.

Rochard, F., Schifrin, B. S., Goupil, F., et al.: Nonstressed fetal heart rate monitoring in the antepartum period. Am. J. Obstet. Gynecol. 126:699, 1976.

Schifrin, B. S.: Antepartum fetal heart rate monitoring. In Gluck, L. (ed.): Intrauterine Asphyxia and the Developing Fetal Brain. Chicago, Yearbook, 1977, p. 205.

Scott, D. B., and Kerr, M. G.: Inferior vena caval pressure in late pregnancy. J. Obstet. Gynaecol. Br. Commonw. 70:1044, 1963.

Spellacy, W. N.: Human placental lactogen in high-risk pregnancy. Clin. Obstet. Gynecol. 16:298, 1973.

Varner, M. W., and Hauser, K. S.: Human placental lactogen and other placental hormones as indicators of fetal well-being. Clin. Obstet. Gynecol. 25:673, 1982.

Zlatnik, F. J., Varner, M. W., and Hauser, K. S.: HPL: physiologic and pathophysiologic observations. Obstet. Gynecol. 54:314, 1979.

4

ULTRASOUND AND HIGH-RISK OBSTETRICS

CHARLES W. HOHLER

The Role of Obstetric Ultrasound Today

Diagnostic ultrasound is now a fundamental tool used in high-risk obstetric practice. Over the past decade, it has developed from a research center tool into a common presence in virtually all hospitals with over 100 beds and in approximately one third of all private obstetric offices in the United States (Fig. 4–1) (Hohler, 1980).

Static B-scan imaging instruments, mainly used in hospital-based radiology laboratories, have given way to the rapid deployment of dynamic imaging or "real-time" B-scan (RTBS) imaging instruments, either of linear array or sector design (Fig. 4–2) in obstetricians' offices. Such RTBS instruments, because of their relatively low cost, ease of operation, and high resolution and reliability, have become an important part of the diagnostic capabilities of modern obstetrics (Hohler, 1981). But this is a rapidly developing, rapidly changing technology that places clinicians and their assistants alike at the leading edge of both medical understanding of the pathophysiology of pregnancy complications and electronic and ultrasound technologic capability. With increasing reliance upon diagnostic ultrasound for basic information about fetal status, new indications for its use are arising, while older obstetric "rituals" and dictums are being modified or replaced in light of new knowledge.

In short, diagnostic ultrasound has provided those interested in perinatal care the ability to approach the developing fetus as a separate patient with an identifiable set of reflexes, activity patterns, and reactions to outside stimuli.

Who Should Be Scanned?

In the 1980s we face the exciting possibility of intrauterine surgery on the fetus to correct or at least ameliorate the effects of many types of congenital anomalies of the central nervous system and genitourinary and gastrointestinal tracts (Table 4–1). At the same time, detection capacities are being refined for many other types of congenital anomalies such as those that affect the car-

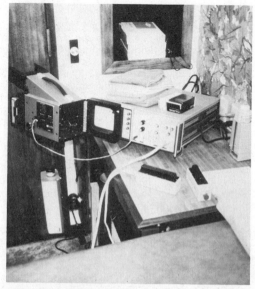

Figure 4–1. Diagnostic ultrasound equipment is now a common tool in obstetric practice.

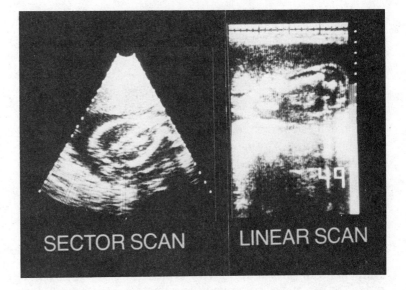

SECTOR SCAN   LINEAR SCAN

Figure 4–2. Measurement of a fetal femur by both sector and linear array ultrasound equipment.

diovascular system (Clewell et al., 1982; Kirkinen et al., 1982; Kleinman et al., 1980).

Since many such lesions can and should be treated immediately upon birth in order to minimize residual motor, mental, or developmental damage to the fetus, diagnostic ultrasound is beginning to play a vital role in the regionalization of perinatal care (Sabbagha et al., 1982). The ability that ultrasound affords to detect the type and etiology of many potentially correctable fetal congenital anomalies early in pregnancy can allow planning time and organization of the requisite team so that each child can be born at the right place, at the right time, and with the right support equipment and personnel available to maximize the chances for intact survival of high quality in as many cases as possible.

Thus, the regionalization of perinatal care, care that is both expensive and labor intensive, can make ultrasound available to those who need it the most. For this reason, among others, I am in favor of a single ultrasound examination of every fetus at 16 to 20 weeks of gestation. Ultrasound screening can offer the following benefits:

1. Increased early detection of twins
2. Increased detection of growth retardation
3. Better early detection of congenital anomalies
4. Improved accuracy of pregnancy dating
5. Decreased patient anxiety
6. Decreased total cost of perinatal care

Unless an anomaly is detected during pregnancy, it cannot be treated until discovery at birth—which in many cases is too late to effect any treatment (Hohler, 1982c).

Not only can many fetal structural anomalies now be detected but also functional disturbances of fetal heart rate and rhythm, respiration, and growth can all be observed. The standard obstetric ultrasound examination provides, at a minimum, the following information:

1. Fetal number
2. Fetal cardiac activity
3. Fetal lie
4. Placental location
5. Amount of amniotic fluid

Table 4–1. Common Representative Anomalies Detectable with Diagnostic Ultrasound

CNS and Skull	Spine
Hydrocephaly	Meningomyelocele
Anencephaly	Spina bifida
Holoprosencephaly	
Microcephaly	**Abdomen**
Encephalocele	Omphalocele
Arachnoid cysts	Gastroschisis
Vein of Galen	Atresias of bowel
aneurysm	Renal agenesis
Cystic hygroma	(unilateral or bilateral)
Craniosynostosis	Ascites
	Bladder outlet obstruction
Thorax	Ovarian cysts
Diaphragmatic hernia	Hydronephrosis
Pleural effusions	Hydroureter
Pericardial effusions	Persistent cloaca
Hypoplastic heart	
Arrhythmias	**Limbs**
Teratomas	Short-limbed dwarfism
Esophageal atresia	Osteogenesis imperfecta
Ventricular septal	(I–IV)
defects	Phocomelia
Valvular atresias	Thanatophoric dysplasia
	Achondroplasia

6. Estimated gestational age (by multiple parameters)

7. Major fetal anatomical landmarks

8. Description of uterus and adnexae

So many uses have been found for ultrasound, especially for dynamic-imaging B-scan ultrasound, that it is probably only a matter of time before all of the roughly 3½ million babies born in the United States each year will receive at least one diagnostic ultrasound examination.

The consensus Development Committee on Diagnostic Imaging in Pregnancy established by the National Institutes of Health (NIH) reviewed the literature and had discussions with the nation's leading experts on ultrasound at a conference held February 6–8, 1984. In their review they did not recommend routine scanning. *However,* they did draw up a list of reasons to consider ultrasound screening:

- Estimation of gestational age for patients with uncertain clinical dates, or verification of dates for patients who are to undergo scheduled elective repeat cesarean delivery, indicated induction of labor, or other elective termination of pregnancy
- Evaluation of fetal growth
- Vaginal bleeding of undetermined etiology in pregnancy
- Determination of fetal presentation
- Suspected multiple gestation
- Adjunct to amniocentesis
- Significant uterine size/clinical dates discrepancy
- Pelvic mass
- Suspected hydatidform mole
- Adjunct to cervical cerclage placement
- Suspected ectopic pregnancy
- Adjunct to special procedures
- Suspected fetal death
- Suspected uterine abnormality
- Intrauterine contraceptive device localization
- Ovarian follicle development surveillance
- Biophysical evaluation for fetal well-being after 28 weeks of gestation
- Observation of intrapartum events
- Suspected polyhydramnios or oliogohydramnios
- Suspected abruptio placentae
- Adjunct to external version from breech to vertex presentation
- Estimation of fetal weight and/or presentation in premature rupture of membranes and/or premature labor
- Abnormal serum α-fetoprotein value
- Follow-up observation of identified fetal anomaly
- Follow-up evaluation of placenta location for identified placenta previa
- History of previous congenital anomaly

- Serial evaluation of fetal growth in multiple gestation
- Evaluation of fetal condition in late registrants for prenatal care (Eastman, 1984)

The NIH stressed the importance of proper training and suggests "minimum training requirements and uniform credentialing for all physicians and sonographers performing ultrasound examinations" (Eastman, 1984). The American College of Obstetricians and Gynecologists (ACOG) supported this need for training in ACOG Technical Bulletin No. 63, which stated, "the use of this technique (ultrasound) without proper training could result in false diagnosis and reduce cost-effectiveness." Many postgraduate courses are now available at medical centers to make the education more readily available.

The NIH recommended that pregnant women *not* be scanned merely for fetal sex determination or for pictures for their baby books.

The Nursing Responsibility*

It is apparent that nurses are increasingly being called upon to understand at least the rudiments of diagnostic ultrasound theory and use, to answer patient questions about examination technique and safety, and, most important, to help patients understand the limitation of the technique so that unrealistic patient expectations do not develop. It is axiomatic with diagnostic ultrasound that the experience and skill of the ultrasonologist determine to a major degree the value of the examination. Reliance on obstetric ultrasound "data" should never be total and must always be tempered with this realization. Ultrasound data must always be integrated with clinical observations to reach accurate conclusions about fetal status.

Patient education is very important to the ultrasonic procedure. Many members of the high-risk team should be involved in this teaching. Preparation for the procedure can provide realistic expectations for the patient and can reduce patient anxiety. This information can include an explanation of the safety of the procedure, what can be seen, how it is done, and that it is not painful.

---

*As nurses increase their responsibilities, they should be aware of the legal implications of taking on advanced skills. If nurses participate in the additional skill of reading ultrasound scans, they should be educated through advanced courses.

Often handouts or photographs can be very helpful for this teaching.

Observing the fetus in utero can foster prenatal bonding for the mother and her family. If possible, the partner should be allowed to accompany the woman during her ultrasound. In some circumstances siblings may also be invited to see the scan. As the ultrasound is performed, the patient and her family can watch the screen and can be educated as to the location of fetal parts, the placenta, the cord, and so on. If anomalies are present, the scan can be very helpful in increasing the patient's understanding of the anomaly and its consequences. However, it must be mentioned that with this increased prenatal bonding resulting from the visualization of the fetus, patients can be expected to grieve more if the baby is stillborn.

The nurse should accompany the physician when the ultrasound report is given to the patient. This enables the nurse to answer questions and provide further explanation of the results consistently at a later time if necessary.

The patient should be made comfortable during the procedure, as it may take up to 30 minutes to be completed. A pillow under the patient's knees may make her more comfortable, and a firm pillow beneath her buttocks may help to elevate the presenting part. Loose-fitting clothing is advised for reasons of comfort; slacks and a top will make the mother's abdomen more accessible and may be a more modest outfit for the procedure.

A full bladder aids in increasing ultrasonic resolution, elevating the presenting head for biparietal diameter measurements; a full bladder also serves as a landmark for the scan. (Variations in the requirement for a full bladder are discussed on p. 59, under Patient Preparation.) The patient should be encouraged not to void for 3 hours before the ultrasonic examination. It has been suggested that fluids be encouraged starting about 1½ hours before the procedure. The mother should be forewarned that her full bladder will probably be uncomfortable, but that it is important. Explaining the rationale may help her comply. Instillation of solutions into the bladder by a catheter is discouraged, as this predisposes to bladder infections. The patient is provided an opportunity to void as soon as the procedure is completed.

Theory and Principles of Diagnostic Ultrasound

PHYSICAL PRINCIPLES IN BRIEF

Ultrasound is sound energy above the frequency range of human hearing (i.e., greater than 20,000 hertz or cycles per second). For obstetric diagnosis, the most commonly used frequencies are between 3 and 7.5 megahertz (i.e., 3 to 7.5 million cycles per second). At these very high frequencies, the sound energy becomes very directional. An ultrasound beam can be pictured, then, as being similar to a flashlight beam being directed into the pregnant uterus (Fig. 4–3).

Ultrasound energy directed into the pregnant uterus is of extremely low intensity (on the order of 10 milliwatts per square centimeter spatial peak, temporal average intensity, or less), well below any recognized intensity level associated with tissue damage or destruction. For imaging, such energy is introduced into the tissues in short bursts, or pulses, approximately 1000 times per second, with each pulse lasting on the order of one millionth of a second. Thus, over 99 percent of the time, the ultrasound transducer is turned "off" and is available to

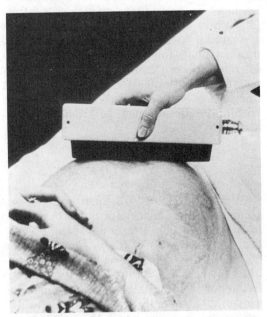

Figure 4–3. The ultrasound transducer produces a beam of sound energy that is directed into the pregnant uterus.

detect returning echoes from energy reflected from structures within the tissues.

A *transducer* is used to produce the ultrasound energy. This is a dipolar crystal that either (a) expands when an electric current is passed through it, thus producing mechanical ultrasound longitudinal pressure waves, or (b) produces an electric current when mechanically compressed by ultrasound waves returning from the tissues. This capacity to transduce electrical into mechanical energy, and vice versa, is known as the *piezoelectric effect*. Reflected energy returning to the transducer is electronically collected, amplified, and then displayed on a television screen as a two-dimensional, cross-sectional image.

In order for pulsed ultrasound to be useful for producing diagnostic images, the sound waves sent out from the transducer must be reflected from either stationary or moving boundaries, called *interfaces*, between tissues of different acoustic impedence. *Acoustic impedance* is a property of tissues that depends on their density and the velocity of sound in each. In general, the greater the differences between the acoustic impedences of tissues, the greater the amount of ultrasound energy that will be reflected at such a boundary or interface. A computer, built into the ultrasound instrument, keeps track of the time between electrical stimulation of the transducer crystal to the time ultrasound echoes return to the transducer crystal (the "time of flight" of an ultrasound pulse). Since *the speed of ultrasound is assumed to be a constant 1540 meters per second in soft tissues*, the distance to a given interface or between successive interfaces within the tissues can be calculated and 'displayed.

TERMINOLOGY AND WHAT IT MEANS

Ultrasound waves are longitudinal pressure waves that move molecules to and fro in the axis of the ultrasound beam. Resolution along the axis of (i.e., in the direction of) the ultrasound beam is called *axial resolution* and is dependent primarily upon the frequency of the ultrasound transducer employed (Fig. 4–4). In general, the higher the frequency used, the better the axial resolution of the ultrasound image. Resolution across the beam is called *lateral resolution* and is dependent primarily upon transducer

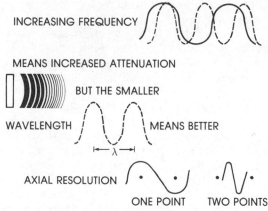

Figure 4–4. Relationship between frequency and axial resolution.

size, effective aperture, and various electronic and mechanical focusing techniques used to reduce the cross-sectional size of the beam at various distances away from the transducer (Fig. 4–5).

The higher the frequency of a sound beam, the more quickly the energy within the beam becomes dissipated as a result of tissue absorption and reflection away from the beam axis. This property is called *attenuation* (Fig. 4–6). Attenuation is approximately one db/mHz/cm in human tissues. A decrease of three db in ultrasound intensity is equivalent to approximately a 50 percent decrease in ultrasound intensity as compared with the amount of energy that left the transducer crystal. Attenuation of ultrasound energy is felt to be an important factor in the safety of fetal ultrasound exposure, since the fetus, lying 10 to 12 cm from the transducer, is thus being exposed to perhaps as little as one one-hundredth of the amount of energy leaving the transducer face.

Returning amplified ultrasound signals are displayed using an image processing technique called "gray scaling." The amplitude (strength) of each returning echo is examined and displayed as one of several shades of gray on a TV screen, depending on the

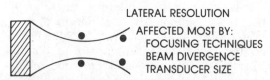

Figure 4–5. Lateral resolution is affected most by focusing techniques, beam divergence, and transducer size.

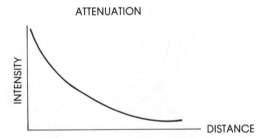

Figure 4–6. Attenuation is a reduction in the beam's intensity, as a function of distance, as the sound travels through a medium. It is caused by reflection, scattering, beam divergence, and absorption.

range of intensity into which each echo falls. Usually, between 10 and 256 gray levels are employed to produce obstetric diagnostic ultrasound images.

The "raw" signals returning to the transducer can be processed as A-scan, B-scan, or M-mode displays. *A-scan* is a display of the amplitude of returning echos along a time baseline. *B-scan* display requires that A-scan information be ordered to a two-dimensional array and stored in digital format for display in a matrix, usually 256 by 512 pixels in size. Echo amplitude information is retained by gray scaling in this fashion while position data on a time line is also maintained. More detailed information about ultrasound physics and instrumentation can be obtained from any one of several excellent sources in the ultrasound literature (Bushong, 1981; Kremkau, 1980; McDicken, 1981).

M-mode is the display of A-mode output onto a strip-chart recorder. This allows plotting of the movement of an interface, such as a fetal cardiac valve, over time. In this way, much important diagnostic information can be gained about normal physiologic functioning.

In order to form an ultrasound image, several types of instruments can be employed: (1) static B-scanners, which "paint" a static image on a TV screen as a single transducer is moved over the maternal abdomen; (2) dynamic-imaging scanners, which form "real-time" B-scan images by grouping ultrasound transducer crystals into linear rays, or which form images by moving a single transducer very rapidly within a housing so that 20 to 60 pictures per second are displayed so rapidly that movement appears simultaneous with its actual occurrence.

Various instruments have advantages and disadvantages for specific obstetric indications and gestational ages. In general, most obstetric scanning, up until the 12th week of gestation, is done with sector scanners; after the 12th week, a linear array is employed. Static B-scanning is used when a large field of view is desired and is usually done by radiologists, whereas obstetricians rely primarily on dynamic imaging when doing ultrasound examinations during labor and delivery, or in the office or an outpatient setting. In the future, however, it is anticipated that more radiologists will begin to do real-time B-scanning in addition to static B-scanning for complete fetal evaluation.

Biologic Effects

In over 25 years of use worldwide, no harmful effects have been reported from the use of pulsed echo or continuous wave (Doppler) ultrasound on the human body at intensities used in present-day diagnostic ultrasound instruments. However, use of any energy form must produce some effects when applied, even if only transient and subtle (Hohler, 1982b).

To the practicing clinician, the possible existence of any short- or long-term multigenerational biologic effects of a deleterious sort that would necessitate limitations of ultrasound exposure at any gestational age and, hence, even contraindications to its use, are of concern. As of this writing, no such limitations or contraindications to the use of either diagnostic B-scan pulsed ultrasound or Doppler ultrasound exist. This is reflected in the American Institute of Ultrasound in Medicine (AIUM) Safety Statement (Table 4–2).

The ultimate, complete safety of ultrasound use in pregnancy has not been, and may never be, established. This incomplete understanding of ultrasound–tissue interactions should inject a degree of caution into its clinical use, but not nihilism. Much is already known, and vigilance and research are keen in this important field. In any case, biologic effects should never be, a priori, equated with biologic hazards until proved.

Any biologic effect that might occur through the clinical use of diagnostic ultrasound could be beneficial, harmful, or neutral; transient or permanent; biologically significant or insignificant; immediate or delayed. This could alter physical structure

Table 4–2. American Institute of Ultrasound in Medicine Safety Statement*

Diagnostic ultrasound has been in use for over 25 years. Given its known benefits and recognized efficacy for medical diagnosis, including use during human pregnancy, the American Institute of Ultrasound in Medicine herein addresses the clinical safety of such use: No confirmed biological effects on patients or instrument operators caused by exposures at intensities typical of present diagnostic instruments have ever been reported. Although the possibility exists that such biological effects may be identified in the future, current data indicate that the benefits to patients of the prudent use of diagnostic ultrasound outweigh the risks, if any, that may be present.

October, 1983

*Adopted by the Board of Governors of the American Institute of Ultrasound in Medicine, October, 1983.

and change physiologic function or later behavior of an entire organism or of its cells, tissues, or organ systems. Current measurement techniques may permit only partial identification of the presence of biologic changes produced by ultrasound, or there may be nothing else to find. The effects we do know about, however, have been and are being carefully assessed. It must be anticipated that new biologic effects will be identified in the future. The National Science Foundation Survey 18 in 1973 did not find any biologic hazard in animals or plants with use of continuous-wave (Doppler) ultrasound at levels below 100 mW/cm average intensity at frequencies between 0.5 and 10 mHz (National Science Foundation Survey Team, 1973). Most Doppler fetal heart monitors use a frequency of about 2.5 mHz.

For pulse systems, during as much as 99 percent of the examination time, the transducer is "off" or passively "listening" for returning echos from the tissues sent out by the transducer. The author has calculated that with one popular linear ray (ADR Model 2130AA)*, for every half hour of examination time, the fetus is exposed to approximately one second of ultrasound. This pulsed energy emission pattern makes dosimetry analysis very complex. Comparison with data derived from continuous-wave experiments is, therefore, not direct.

Two broad categories of ultrasound interactions with tissues have been defined: (1) cavitational and other effects and (2) thermal changes dependent on sound energy absorp-

*ADR Corporation, Tempe, Arizona

tion and the properties of the ultrasound field.

Cavitation is a phenomenon in which bubbles form during the rarefaction phase of an ultrasound wave. During the succeeding compression phase, these bubbles can collapse, with the subsequent release of larger amounts of energy into the cytoplasm. This produces a violent disturbance inside the cell. In liquids, in the 1- to 4-mHz range, stable cavitation has been observed only under experimental conditions at intensities above 200 mW/cm². The intensity levels required for the production of cavitation in organized tissues are much larger, on the order of 2000–5000 W/cm². These intensity levels are not possible with currently manufactured diagnostic equipment and are some 10,000 times greater than the intensity levels used for clinical examinations. Furthermore, cavitation may be a phenomenon seen only with continuous-wave ultrasound, not with pulsed ultrasound.

In the future, some other observed effects may actually prove to be cavitational or heating phenomena. Reports about such effects have raised some concerns, especially in the press, but have not as yet been independently confirmed. Some controversy even exists about the relevance of these other, so-called "direct" biologic, effects to the clinical application of ultrasound to the pregnant woman. Some of these postulated direct effects are changes in the speed of chemical reactions, activation or deactivation of enzymes, particle agglomeration, changes in cell surface and surface charges, changes in membrane permeability, and increase in the incidence of sister chromatid exchange, which has been seen in vitro. For many of these effects a clear-cut dose-response relationship has yet to be demonstrated.

Among the properties of the target tissues with regard to ultrasound exposure that are important and relevant for evaluation of tissue effects are ultrasound exposure, time, heat dissipation capacity, vascularization, gas content, density, proportion of extracellular fluid to cell mass, and cell cohesiveness.

Of all of the above considerations, the heat dissipation capability of the human gravid uterus is one of the most important factors to understand. The effects caused by elevation of tissue temperature are predictable. They are a function of the ultrasound intensity, frequency, and exposure time, as well as of the absorption coefficient of the tissue being insonated. The temperature threshold for tissue damage by heat is time dependent. Such destruction thresholds seem to be independent of the source or type of energy used to create the temperature rise. A laser, a blow torch, or high-intensity ultrasound exposure can lead to a common "endpoint" of thermal denaturation. The cytotoxic threshold of many different types of somatic cells to thermal injury are known.

It has been estimated by Lele (1979) that continuous-wave ultrasound exposure at intensity levels of 1.5 W/cm² at 2.5 mHz for about 5 minutes is necessary to raise the tissue temperature to 44°C. He further estimates that such exposure levels would have to be maintained for at least 15 minutes for permanent damage to occur. While still not accepted by all investigators, the conclusion is emerging that no significant biologic effects of ultrasound exposure occur in organized mammalian tissues without concomitant elevation of temperature. It is assumed that temperature elevations of less than 1°C (i.e., the approximate normal diurnal variation) are of no consequence. Furthermore, pulsed ultrasound at intensities as high as 250 W/cm² have demonstrated no significant thermal effects.

WHAT TO TELL PATIENTS

The current understanding of ultrasound interactions and dosimetry is only partial and tentative. The relevance of data obtained on different species and other classes of organisms is not always immediately apparent. Prudence dictates caution in the face of the unknown or at least the obscure. This message must be communicated to the patients in a way that does not provoke anxiety or lead to refusal to accept ultrasound examination when it will be beneficial for obstetric management, because as far as is now known, any risk that may exist must be infinitesimally minute and beyond our current ability to discern. Diagnostic ultrasound has an unparalleled safety record. Nothing currently known about ultrasound–tissue interactions at the intensities being used clinically threatens this status. However, since no drug is completely safe under all circumstances of use, vigilance in this field is widespread and ongoing. It is a consensus now

Table 4–3. Indications for Obstetric Ultrasound Examinations

1. Estimation of gestational age (by multiple parameters)
2. Evaluation of fetal growth (for growth retardation or macrosomia)
3. Placental localization when vaginal bleeding occurs
4. Determination of fetal lie
5. Fetal number confirmation
6. Adjunct to *all* amniocenteses
7. Uterus size/clinical dates discrepancy
8. Estimation of fetal size in breech presentation
9. Suspected congenital anomaly
10. Pelvic masses
11. Suspected hydatidiform mole
12. Adjunct to cervical cerclage
13. Suspected ectopic/abdominal pregnancy
14. Adjunct to special procedures such as fetoscopy and intrauterine transfusion
15. Fetal demise
16. Uterine pathology (e.g., leiomyoma or bicornuate uterus)
17. Postpartum evaluation of uterus and adnexae
18. Intrauterine contraceptive device localization
19. Ovarian follicle development surveillance
20. Evaluation of postdate pregnancy
21. Fetal activity studies to assess fetal well-being
22. Monitoring intrapartum labor/delivery events (e.g., version/extraction of second twin)
23. Evaluation of amount of amniotic fluid (when oligohydramnios or polyhydramnios suspected)

that ultrasound is safe enough to use in any pregnant woman at any gestational age as often as the clinical indications (Table 4–3) are present, without need for informed consent, since this would imply much more hazard than is felt to be potentially present.

Patient Preparation

All patients who are to undergo an ultrasound examination should have a full urinary bladder if they have been pregnant for 20 weeks or less. After 20 weeks, in most cases, the requirement of a full urinary bladder is not necessary for technical completion of the examination and just causes much unnecessary patient discomfort.

There are several exceptions to the above rule. One would be the patient who is being examined for placenta previa after 20 weeks of gestation. In these patients, both pre- and postvoid views in the longitudinal and transverse planes are needed to completely and satisfactorily determine the location of the placental margin with reference to the internal cervical os. It should be noted in this regard, however, that overfilling of the urinary bladder can sometimes compress and elongate the cervix so that the apparent position of the internal cervical os under these abnormal circumstances may bear no relation to the actual situation. It is to avoid this problem that the postvoiding scans are done. They are most important to avoid misdiagnosis, which, in many cases, may lead to the patient's being hospitalized, or even to delivery of an immature fetus, with an attendant unfortunate outcome.

A second exception is the patient about to undergo a genetic amniocentesis between 16 and 18 weeks of gestation. In fact, for these patients it is a good idea to have the bladder empty, to avoid the possibility of an inadvertent tap of the bladder rather than the amniotic sac, especially by an inexperienced physician. In this regard, the fluid removed at the time of amniocentesis can always be checked for the presence of glucose and protein. The presence of both of these substances in the amniotic fluid will distinguish it from maternal urine whenever there is a question as to where the needle tip ended up. Real-time B-scan (RTBS) guidance of the needle into the amniotic fluid can also help to avoid this mistake.

Likewise, at the time of amniocentesis later in pregnancy, to check for the severity of suspected Rh sensitization or to document fetal lung maturity, a full bladder is neither necessary nor a good idea, especially if the superpubic approach is to be used to obtain the amniotic fluid, because the maternal urinary bladder may be inadvertently sampled.

Other than the provision of a full urinary bladder for routine diagnostic ultrasound examinations prior to 20 weeks, no other patient preparations are necessary. The patient may eat or drink as much and as often as she would like.

The patient should be instructed to expect that she will be asked to lie on an examining table or cot and expose her abdomen (Fig. 4–7). Therefore, it is advisable for her to wear slacks and a loose fitting top, as in most laboratories it is not the routine for the patient to have to undress completely for obstetric ultrasound examinations. A water-soluble gel will be spread over her abdomen to ensure proper contact of the ultrasound transducer or transducer array to the abdomen. Mineral oil may be used for this function as well, but gel is preferable, since mineral oil stains the patient's and the technologist's clothes. It also does not possess the ultrasound transmission qualities of the water-soluble gels. Mineral oil is cheap, but it transmits approximately only 25 percent of the ultrasound energy emitted by the transducer or transducer array, whereas the gels transmit virtually 100 percent of emitted energy. Theoretically, then, images should be somewhat better if a gel is used, undiluted, rather than the more messy mineral oil (Reid, 1977). RTBS diagnostic ultrasound examinations usually take a shorter amount

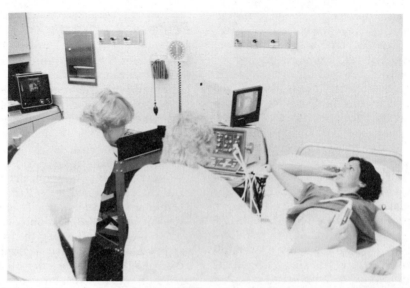

Figure 4–7. For an ultrasound examination the patient is asked to lie on an examining table or cot and to expose her abdomen. For this reason, she should be advised to wear slacks and a loose-fitting top.

of time than static B-scan ultrasound examinations. They average about 15 minutes and are completely painless. Patient scheduling at 30-minute intervals is usually sufficient in a busy ultrasound department for proper assessment and performance of obstetric ultrasound examinations.

Representative pictures of portions of the ultrasound examinations are taken using either videotape, Polaroid film, or x-ray multiformat film, which is somewhat less expensive. In some cases, the patient will be given a picture of the baby, but this is not done in all locations. My feeling, however, is that this picture can be important psychologically to the mother and father of the baby, and therefore a picture is always provided in our laboratory. The patient should understand that the rest of the pictures are an important part of the permanent record of the ultrasound examination. Relevant measurements (Table 4–4) are documented in these pictures, as well as pertinent views of important placental and fetal anatomic landmarks, such as the kidneys, stomach, and bladder, to name but a few such structures. In some cases, the examination may be stored on videotape for later analysis by other physicians or for instructional purposes.

Once the pictures and measurements have been taken, the patient is usually asked to remain while the results are analyzed. This usually takes only a few minutes and can avoid the need for a "recall" examination should the responsible physician deem the examination technically deficient and ask for more views to be taken.

The patient should be told that the technologist will usually not be in a position to discuss the results of the examination, since it places the technologist in a difficult position to be asked by the patient to do so. Once the complete analysis of an ultrasound examination has been carried out by the physician responsible for overseeing ultrasound examinations in that facility, the patient's physician will be notified of the results or the responsible physician will discuss the findings with the patient if that is the wish of the patient's doctor.

It is part of the nurse's role to reassure the patient that such procedures are for the patient's own protection from information that might be erroneously supplied by a technologist who may have the best of intentions but who has inadequate knowledge of the patient's complete medical and obstetric history. Lawsuits have resulted when information provided in such a fashion proved to be incorrect after complete analysis of the ultrasound findings. Therefore, caution is advised in this regard.

In many offices and laboratories, husbands and significant other individuals are allowed in the examination room to view the obstetric ultrasound examination. This should be encouraged provided that the physical plant of the hospital or physician's office allows for complete privacy for all patients; in no case should any patient's privacy be violated by the presence of another patient's family members.

Complications From Obstetric Ultrasound

Some women cannot tolerate lying in the supine position for the length of time necessary to complete an ultrasound examination. This situation does not occur just at term but at any gestational age. However, women in advanced stages of pregnancy and those carrying twins are most likely to experience difficulty with the supine position for examination.

When a woman lies supine, flat in bed, the uterus presses upon the inferior vena cava and the aorta, restricting blood flow to and from the lower extremities and the uterus, which can lead to a drastic reduction in cardiac output and a decrease in blood flow. The resultant hypotension can be severe enough to cause several serious complications. Supine hypotension can lead to

Table 4–4. Fetal Ultrasound Measurements

A. *Crown-Rump Length* (CRL)
B. *Head*
  - Biparietal diameter (BPD)
  - Occipitofrontal diameter (OFD)
  - Lateral ventricle/hemisphere ratio (LVR)
  - Head circumference (HC)
C. *Abdomen*
  - AP abdominal diameter (APAD)
  - Transverse abdominal diameter (TAD)
  - Abdominal circumference (AC)
  - Kidney circumference (KC)
D. *Limbs*
  - Femur length (FL)
  - Thigh diameters (TDs)
  - Thigh circumference (TC)

abruption of the placenta from the uterine wall through change in the blood-flow characteristics in the placental bed attendant to rapid fluctuation in the intravascular mean arterial pressure. This, in turn, can lead to fetal demise. Another complication, which is more common, is syncope in the mother from the hypotension and resultant acute decrease in cerebral blood flow during the time of reduced blood flow from the extremities. Both of these problems can usually be avoided by early recognition of the presence of the problem, and by proper patient positioning.

When a patient becomes hypotensive from the pressure of the pregnant uterus on the aorta and/or inferior vena cava, she usually experiences some "nervousness" or restlessness in the first moment of the hypotensive episode. If the patient is turned on to her left side at this point, the supine hypotensive episode can usually be aborted. Rarely, oxygen may be necessary to assist with proper fetal oxygenation, but usually positioning is all that is required.

If the patient complains of restlessness, anxiety, shortness of breath, or states that she feels "lightheaded" (and especially if the patient becomes diaphoretic or feels like she may faint), she is probably suffering from supine hypotension. The patient should be positioned on her left side, and her blood pressure should be taken. Should syncope occur, the patient is positioned on her left side, "smelling salts" can be used to arouse her, and help should be summoned to assist with proper airway maintenance and cardiovascular support as necessary. It is important to remember that although supine hypotension is the most likely problem being addressed, other causes for the patient's distress should be investigated if repositioning and routine supportive measures do not bring about an immediate positive response, including improvement in the blood pressure, decrease in the pulse rate back to normal rates, and improvement in the patient's subjective feelings of well-being.

It is important to remember that a patient may be examined with RTBS linear arrays or sector scanners quite adequately when she is in the left lateral recumbent position. Obese women, those carrying multiple gestations, those with polyhydramnios, and many women in late pregnancy are most at risk for the supine hypotension syndrome. Fast action by the attendant in recognizing

the early warning signs for this condition may help prevent major problems.

At present, there are *no contraindications* to the performance of a Doppler or diagnostic B-scan ultrasound examination on any pregnant woman at any gestational age. There are no medical complications of pregnancy that preclude the use of diagnostic ultrasound at any gestational age.

Psychologic Issues Related to Use of Ultrasound

Diagnostic ultrasound is a great anxiety reliever in pregnancy. It is apparent that women are reassured by seeing movement of their babies at even the earliest stages of pregnancy.

In the first trimester of pregnancy, bleeding from the vagina occurs in 10 to 15 percent of women. Such bleeding is an indication for diagnostic ultrasound examination. Since the presence of fetal heart and body motion is of great prognostic significance (Heitz et al., 1980), ultrasound evidence of such motion can do much to relieve the anxiety of the patient. If such cardiac motion is not present after 7 weeks from the last menstrual period (LMF) (Table 4–5), a definitive diagnosis of missed abortion–blighted ovum can often be established immediately so that, in many cases, a treatment plan can be initiated without delay, thus avoiding several days or weeks of bleeding, cramping, and worry. In experienced hands, the diagnosis of missed abortion, blighted ovum, and definite fetal demise will allow a suction curettage that can be accomplished the same day as the diagnosis is made. This, in turn,

Table 4–5. Real-Time Milestones in the First Trimester

Age (from LMP)	Milestone
6 weeks	Gestational sac appears in the uterus
7 weeks	Fetal heart motion can first be detected
8 weeks	Spontaneous fetal body movements begin
9 weeks	Definite fetal heart and body movements present
12 weeks	Biparietal diameter can be measured

can reduce maternal morbidity. It is important to recognize, however, that this diagnosis is not always easy, and repeat examination, within a few days, to verify the findings of the initial scan is usually advantageous (Fig. 4–8).

For women over the age of 35 years who are about to undergo genetic amniocentesis, there is good evidence that an ultrasound examination done just prior to the amniocentesis not only makes the entire procedure safer but also allays maternal anxiety about the well-being of the fetus. Such an ultrasound examination is also important in mothers who are having a second-opinion consultation ultrasound examination when the maternal serum alpha-fetoprotein is elevated beyond 2.5 standard deviations above the mean on two separate specimens between 16 and 20 weeks' gestation. If a congenital anomaly is found, it is now becoming possible not only to assess the extent of the defect but also to discover the specific etiology of such defects. Termination of pregnancy has been, until now, the only alternative to carrying the anomalous fetus. In the 1980s, however, fetal surgery can provide a chance for repair of certain defects. For example, bladder outlet obstruction or hydrocephalus can be treated by the placement of shunts that drain the urine or the excessive spinal fluid from these defects into the amniotic fluid, thus preventing further tissue damage (Golbus et al., 1982; Birnholtz

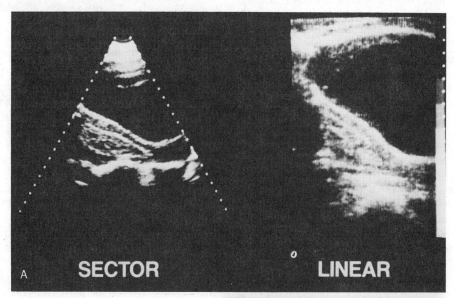

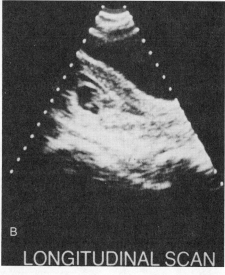

Figure 4–8. *A,* A missed abortion of 4 months' duration is shown on both a sector and a linear scan. *B,* A longitudinal scan shows early implantation in the posterior wall of the endometrium.

and Frigoletto, 1981). Certain potentially salvageable anomalies can thus lead to planning as to the proper location, timing, and route of delivery in order to minimize fetal risk of permanent or lethal deformity. Such planning must of necessity include the parents and other appropriate maternal and fetal advocates.

Maternal-infant attachment is a complex interaction between parent and child that begins to take place long before birth. Each day in a pregnancy leads to new sensations of fetal life for the pregnant woman. Diagnostic ultrasound viewing of fetal motions can in many cases actually lead to maternal recognition of certain specific fetal behaviors such as hiccoughing, fetal·chest wall movements (i.e., "breathing"), and limb motions. This maternal learning process is an important and positive factor in the bonding of mother and child. Personality traits begin to be attributed to the child as a separate, complete, and sensate human being. For both the mother and the father, this can be a source of great personal joy and satisfaction. Such an opportunity to view a future child can be an important part of parenting and sharing of responsibility between the parents and even siblings.

Once the baby has been seen with real-time B-scan ultrasound, the common question comes up, "Is it a boy or a girl?" No comprehensive research has been carried out to find out whether such knowledge acquired before birth is a positive or negative factor in parent-child bonding. Historical data from other countries indicate that female children are aborted much more readily than are male children. Parents with two children of the same sex are much more likely to have a third child than are parents who have two children of the opposite sex. What would happen in the United States if it were possible to accurately predict fetal sex at 16 to 20 weeks with diagnostic ultrasound alone is purely conjectural.

It has been my personal experience that there are some parents who wish to know the fetal sex, some who definitely do not, and some who do not particularly care whether they know or not. It is important to point out that ultrasound diagnosis of fetal sex is not always accurate before the 24th week of gestation (Scholly et al., 1980), especially in the diagnosis of a female fetus. The male has clearly visible external genitalia (Fig. 4–9). While the fetal female peri-

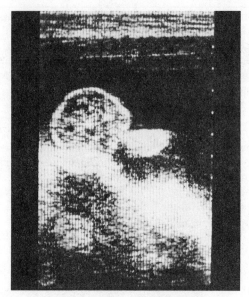

Figure 4–9. Fetal male genitalia.

neum can sometimes be easily seen (Fig. 4–10), at other times it is impossible to view. In some cases, the male genitalia cannot be seen either. Such "shy" male fetuses can cause errors in a very important diagnosis. To avoid this problem, one should avoid getting into the situation of having to state what the fetal sex is in an unequivocal fashion. Instead it is probably better to speak in terms of probabilities and always leave clear room for doubt and "hope" in the parents' minds.

From unpublished research studies carried out at the University of Rochester in New York by this author and others in the mid 1970s, it is apparent that the opportunity to see the fetus with diagnostic ultrasound is a positive factor for *paternal* bonding to the infant. Such fathers definitely show greater attention to the actual developmental stages of the fetus and seem much more inclined to attribute personality traits to the fetus than do fathers who have not had the opportunity to view the developing fetus on ultrasound.

In late pregnancy, diagnostic ultrasound and, in particular, real-time B-scan ultrasound, can allow the patient and the physician, together with the husband, to "see" many situations that may require hospitalization, cesarean section, prolonged bedrest, or other therapies (Wetrich, 1982). Patient compliance with such management regimens, family understanding of the pregnant woman's plight, and lessened chances for

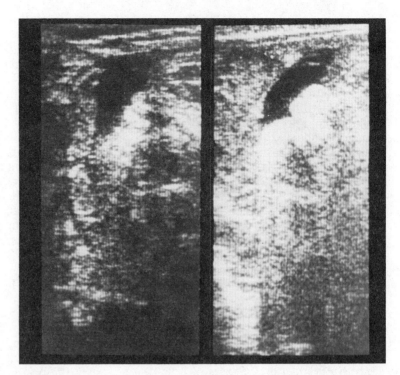

Figure 4–10. Fetal female perineum.

patient-physician misunderstandings are all very much promoted by the availability of the ultrasound to help as a "visual aid" in the physician's explanation of specific medical and obstetric complications that call for the pregnancy to be considered at "high risk" for fetal jeopardy from whatever cause. The measurements from ultrasound examinations, together with all other pertinent observations taken in such a procedure, can also help to allay physician concern when clinical factors are discrepant. For all of these reasons, this technology tends to draw the parents closer to their child, the physician closer to the patient and her family, and physicians closer to each other in providing optimal regionalized perinatal care.

Types of Specialized Obstetric Ultrasound Examinations

BIOPHYSICAL PROFILE

This type of examination is done to document the well-being of the fetus. It was developed by Drs. Manning and Platt to assist perinatologists in discriminating between fetuses that are well adapted to their intrauterine environment and those in danger of intrauterine fetal demise, which might fare better by being delivered (Manning et al., 1980).

The biophysical profile (BPP) consists of a set of five observations (Table 4–6). It is based on the interpretation of a fetal heart rate monitor tracing of the resting fetus (i.e., the nonstress test or NST) and four observations of diagnostic ultrasound findings: the presence of fetal body movement (3 movements in 30 minutes), the presence of fetal chest wall movements (30 seconds of continuous breathing in 30 minutes), the observation of good fetal tone (1 extension per flexion cycle of a fetal limb, with rapid return to the flexed posture in 30 minutes), and the presence of a normal amount of amniotic fluid (a greater-than-1-cm "pocket" of fluid).

Each observed parameter receives a "planning score" of 2 or 0 depending on whether

Table 4–6. Biophysical Profile

Parameter	Score
Nonstress test (NST)	0–2
Fetal body movement	0–2
Fetal breathing	0–2
Fetal tone	0–2
Amniotic fluid volume	0–2
TOTAL	0–10

or not it meets the criteria outlined above. A "perfect" score would thus be 10, and the worst score would be 0. It has been found that such 30-minute observations are useful in the estimation of fetal well-being and in the reduction of perinatal mortality attributable to stillbirth in a high-risk obstetric population. Furthermore, in some circumstances, such a test can be used to identify "false-positive" results from the nonstress test and/or contraction stress test, thus avoiding needless intervention for a fetus in good condition. While further research is needed to identify which of the above observations most strongly correlate with the fetal condition, this use of diagnostic ultrasound to assess fetal well-being is a promising approach to reducing the stillbirth rate that for the past 20 years has been decreasing only very grudgingly.

Some research has already been done to show that of all of the observations contained in the BPP, amniotic fluid amount and fetal tone may be the most important (Schifrin et al., 1981). Scores of 8 to 10 are interpreted as "reassuring" and normal. Such tests can then be repeated in 1 week, unless maternal circumstances change; then, the BPP should immediately be repeated. Scores of 4 to 6 are interpreted as "equivocal," and the test should be repeated in 24 hours. Scores of 0 to 2 are "abnormal and worrisome" and indicate the need for very careful fetal evaluation for delivery in an expeditious fashion, even by cesarean section in some cases.

Manning has shown that such babies rarely, if ever, revert to higher planning scores, so that if stillbirth is to be prevented, immediate delivery or maternal treatment of underlying pathologic conditions affecting the fetus should be addressed without delay (Manning et al., 1981).

AMNIOCENTESIS

Ultrasound guidance of amniocentesis is considered mandatory. Amniocentesis without ultrasound examination immediately prior to the tap, in the same examining room, could be construed as malpractice. In Europe, guidance of the needle into the amniotic sac is done almost routinely under direct vision, as the procedure is in progress. In the United States, it is more customary to find an accessible "pocket" of amniotic fluid

away from the cord insertion sight in the placenta and also away from any vital fetal organs, measure its depth, and determine the proper angle of needle entry to reach the middle of that pocket of fluid. The procedure is then done "blind" immediately thereafter, unless signs of a major shift of fetal position or presentation are noted. This approach has worked quite satisfactorily to reduce the incidence of bloody amniotic fluid specimens, the number of "dry" tap failures, and the number of fetal and maternal injuries that can result from amniocentesis at term (Galle and Meis, 1982; Hohler et al., 1978; Mennuti et al., 1980; Porreco et al., 1982; Antenatal Diagnosis, 1979).

INTRAUTERINE TRANSFUSION

Intrauterine transfusion of blood into the fetal peritoneal cavity to ameliorate the effects of severe anemia due to Rh sensitization is not a new procedure, but it is only over the past 5 years that the procedure has been transformed from one done entirely under x-ray guidance to one done entirely under ultrasound guidance from start to finish (Larkin et al., 1981). This is a great advance both in simplifying the procedure technically and in increasing fetal safety by the avoidance of x-ray exposure (Fig. 4–11). In conjunction with fetoscopy, such transfusions are even being modified so that actual exchange transfusions are being done much earlier in pregnancy than had been possible before. Such exchange transfusions are done by removal of fetal blood and exchange with O-negative blood through a fetoscopically guided needle that is introduced into one of the umbilical vessels (MacKenzie et al., 1982).

When blood is placed in the fetal abdomen, the amount that can be tolerated by the fetus can be determined by ultrasound visualization, so that babies do not die of overdistention of the abdomen or compression of the heart to such a degree that stroke volume is impeded to the danger point.

Catheter placement in the fetal abdomen can be checked and verified by the injection into the catheter of a small amount of saline or air, which will show up on ultrasound as a jet of echogenic "bubbles" in the case of saline or as an "air artifact" in the case of the air injection (which usually works the best). Since no x-ray guidance is needed, the

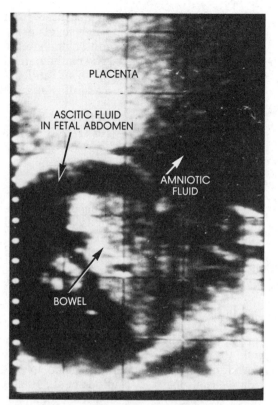

Figure 4–11. Cross-section of fetal abdomen. The use of ultrasound guidance has simplified intrauterine blood transfusion and increased its safety by eliminating the need for x-ray guidance.

intrauterine transfusion can be done in a fetal intensive care area on the labor/delivery floor or some comparable location. Thus, patient transport is minimized. In short, use of ultrasound has made the technique of intrauterine transfusion safer, more convenient, and more precise.

FETOSCOPY

This technique, devised in the mid 1970s, has been of great benefit for the identification of babies at risk for congenital anomalies, for sampling of fetal blood and skin for rapid tissue culture, for examination of chromosomes, and for new forms of intrauterine diagnosis such as fetal liver biopsy and intrauterine exchange transfusion (Rodeck, 1980). The fetoscope is a fiberoptic telescope about the diameter of a 16-gauge needle, the tip of which is placed into the amniotic sac transabdominally, under local anesthesia, using diagnostic ultrasound dynamic imaging guidance. Blood can be sampled from

the umbilical cord or vessels coursing along the fetal surface of the placenta. In some cases, fetal skin biopsies can be taken for tissue culture.

The indications for fetoscopy are changing as genetic and tissue culture methods and amniotic fluid sampling methods change. In the future, however, it seems inevitable that the fetoscope and its guiding ultrasound-imaging will play an invaluable role in the development of intrauterine fetal therapeutic regimens.

Ultrasound Measurements
(Table 4–7)

PRIOR TO 12 WEEKS' GESTATION

Pregnancy location, fetal number, gestational sac number, presence of fetal heart and/or body motion, and crown/rump length measurement of the fetus should all be carried out. Any observations of associated uterine wall pathology or pelvic masses, as well as a technical assessment of the overall quality of the ultrasound examination, should be noted.

AFTER 12 WEEKS' GESTATION

Fetal number, presentation, notation of fetal heart, body, and breathing activity, placental localization, and observation of specific fetal anatomic landmarks should be routinely carried out. The amount of amniotic fluid should be estimated, the presence of any uterine or pelvic pathology

Table 4–7. Routine Stage I Ultrasound: Appropriate Measurements at Various Gestational Ages

Age	Measurement
<12 weeks	Crown-rump length (CRL)
	Gestational sac mean diameter (GSMD)
12–24 weeks	Biparietal diameter (BPD)
	Femur length (FL)
≥24 weeks	Biparietal diameter (BPD)
	Occipitofrontal diameter (OFD)
	Anteroposterior abdominal diameter (APAD)
	Transverse abdominal diameter (TAD)
	Femur length (FL)

should be noted, and a technical quality assessment of each examination should be given.

From five major fetal measurements, namely, the biparietal diameter (BPD), the occipitofrontal diameter (OFD), the antero-posterior abdominal diameter (APAD), the transverse abdominal diameter (TAD), and the femoral length (FL), several important calculations can be carried out. Menstrual age can be calculated to within plus or minus 2 weeks of the actual gestational age in about 90 percent of cases. Estimation of fetal weight to within plus or minus 10 percent of the actual weight can be performed in approximately 60 percent of cases. In addition, the estimation of fetal head shape and the relationship between the symmetry and proportionate growth of the fetal brain, liver, and body length can be expressed as ratios that are in some cases independent of gestational age.

Biparietal diameter (BPD) is used to calculate the fetal gestational age (Sabbagha and Hughey, 1978) and to estimate the fetal weight. It is also used to calculate the cephalic index and the femoral length/BPD ratio.

The occipitofrontal diameter (OFD) is used to calculate head circumference and the cephalic index (see below). The antero-posterior diameter of the fetal abdomen (APAD) is measured at the level of the umbilical vein as it goes into the substance of the liver at the level of the ductus venosus (Fig. 4–12). Together with the transverse abdominal diameter (TAD) measured from the same picture and the same level in the abdomen, the APAD is used to calculate the abdominal circumference. The mathematical formulas for calculating the head and abdominal circumference are as follows:

HC (in cm) = 1.57 × (BPD + OFD)
AC (in cm) = 1.57 × (APAD + TAD)

General Formula

$$C = \frac{\pi}{2}(D_1 + D_2)$$

The femoral length (FL) is used to estimate the gestational age of the fetus (Hohler and Quetel, 1982) and to calculate the femoral length/biparietal diameter ratio (Hohler and Quetel, 1981).

Head circumference is used to calculate menstrual age (Hadlock et al., 1982b) and, together with the abdominal circumference, is used to calculate the head circumference/abdominal circumference ratio (Campbell, 1977).

Abdominal circumference is used to calculate gestational age (Hadlock et al., 1982a) and, together with the biparietal diameter, is also used to estimate fetal weight (Shepard et al., 1982). Abdominal circumference is also used in the calculation of the head circumference/abdominal circumference ratio. The cephalic index (CI) is the ratio of (BPD/OFD) × 100 (Hadlock et al., 1981). This ratio allows quantitation of fetal head shape as a means of verifying ultrasound dating (Fig. 4-13). The normal range for this

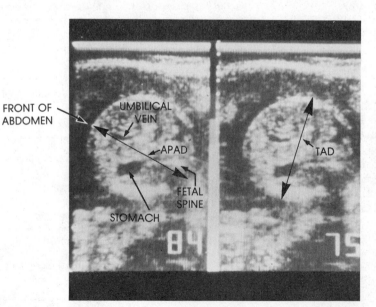

FRONT OF ABDOMEN
UMBILICAL VEIN
APAD
FETAL SPINE
STOMACH
TAD

Figure 4–12. Reference level cross-section of the fetal abdomen at the level of the umbilical vein. The circumference of the fetal trunk is calculated from the anterior-posterior abdominal diameter (APAD) and the transverse abdominal diameter (TAD), which are shown in this view. (See text for equation and details.)

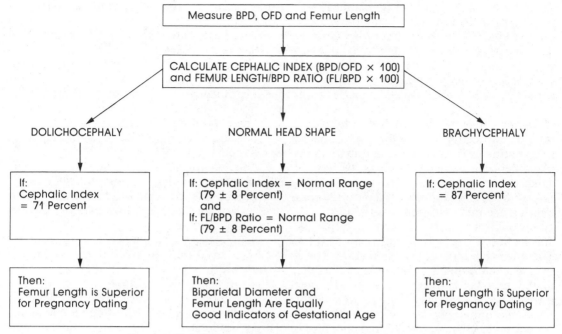

Figure 4–13. Reliability verification of ultrasound dating methods.

head shape index is 79 percent plus or minus 8 percent (plus or minus two standard deviations), from 14 weeks of gestation. CIs of less than 71 percent indicate the presence of a dolichocephalic in which the BPD is flattened in relation to the normal head shape. In such cases the BPD would underestimate rather than properly reflect menstrual age. On the other hand, a CI of over 87 percent indicates the presence of a brachycephalic head shape in which the BPD is elongated in relation to the normal head shape. In such cases the BPD would overestimate rather than properly reflect gestational age.

In cases in which the CI is out of the normal range, the BPD should not be used for gestational age at all (Law and MacRae, 1982). In addition, weight estimates, which require knowledge of an accurate BPD from a head of normal shape, will be erroneous when such BPDs are used. Caution in weight interpretation must therefore be exercised when such unusual head shapes are found. Age estimates based on head and abdomen circumferences, together with femoral length, then allow estimation of weight by substitution of the "mean BPD" for the given estimated gestational age into the formulas for weight based on knowledge of the BPD and the abdominal circumference. Such estimates, however, are likely to prove less

accurate than estimates based on accurate BPD information.

The femoral length/BPD ratio, after 22 weeks of gestation, has a normal value of 79 percent plus or minus 8 percent. Use of this ratio will allow some quality control in the consistency between measurements of the BPD and femoral length. When pictures are taken that afford technically good measurements of the femur and BPD, but the femur length/BPD ratio is too low, it is possible that hydrocephaly or a position-related brachycephaly exists, or that short-limbed dwarfism is present. However, in the vast majority of cases, when the femoral length/BPD ratio is abnormal, the reason is poor technical quality of ultrasound measurements of the femur and/or the head.

When the femur length/BPD ratio is too high, it is possible that microcephaly (i.e., a head circumference more than three standard deviations below the mean for the gestational age of the fetus) or craniosynostosis (i.e., premature closure of one or more sutures between the bones of the fetal skull) is present.

The head circumference/abdomen circumference measurement is an indirect comparison between brain size and liver size. Before 36 to 37 weeks of gestation, this ratio is almost invariably greater than 1.00. However, at about 36 to 37 weeks of gestation, this ratio becomes 1.00 and thereafter is less than 1.00 in a normally developing fetus. Low head circumference/abdominal circumference ratios are associated with technically poor measurements of the fetal abdomen and with macrosomia, as in, for example, the babies of class A and class B diabetic mothers.

On the other hand, a high or plateauing ratio is indicative of possible asymmetric intrauterine growth retardation due to uteroplacental insufficiency from a variety of causes.

The head circumference/abdominal circumference ratio cannot be used to estimate gestational age. It is, instead, a ratio that speaks to the issue of intrauterine nutrition. The adequacy of liver glycogen stores is the primary determinant of liver size and, thus, of abdominal circumference. Although some ultrasound centers have begun to use the head circumference/abdominal circumference ratio to estimate gestational age, this is not a correct utilization of this ratio. Head circumference alone, abdominal circumference alone or femur length alone in nondiabetic cases can be used effectively to estimate gestational age.

The head circumference/abdominal circumference ratio can be calculated directly without prior calculation of the separate circumferences by using the following formula:

$$HC/AC = (BPD + OFD)/(APAD + TAD)$$

The estimation of gestational age and weight from the five major measurements of every fetus after 12 weeks' gestation (outlined above) will allow thorough evaluation of any fetus in a very rapid, quite accurate, and precise manner.

A sample computer printout report form used at our hospital is shown in Fig. 4–14. All of the pertinent observations, measurements, and calculations for the complete performance of a standard obstetric ultrasound examination are shown.

Professional Organizations

There are several organizations that are involved in the development of diagnostic ultrasound for use in obstetrics and gynecology:
- The American Institute of Ultrasound in Medicine (AIUM)
- The American Registry of Diagnostic Medical Sonographers (ARDMS)
- The Society of Diagnostic Medical Sonographers (SDMS)
- The Section of OB/GYN of AIUM.
- The American College of Obstetricians and Gynecologists (ACOG)
- The American College of Radiology (ACR)

Each of these organizations is composed of professionals dedicated to the advancement of ultrasound imaging for obstetric and gynecologic patients.

The issues that relate to the use of diagnostic ultrasound in obstetrics are complex and multidisciplinary, and they encompass the full spectrum of problems from medical to economic to ethical. Such organizations have made major contributions to better patient understanding of ultrasound technology, have increased political support for the use of imaging by a variety of professionals in several traditional specialty areas of medicine, and have helped to establish guidelines for the safe implementation of ultrasound in obstetrics. Physicians, technologists, and nurses performing or interested in the performance of diagnostic ultrasound examinations in the obstetric patient are urged to join the AIUM or the SDMS, especially since these are multispecialty, "umbrella" organizations formed solely to promote cooperation and education across traditional specialty lines. The address and telephone numbers of the AIUM and the Society of Diagnostic Medical Sonographers (SDMS) are listed below:

American Institute of Ultrasound in Medicine
4405 E.-W. Highway, Suite 504
Bethesda, MD 20814 (301) 656-6117

Society of Diagnostic Medical Sonographers
P. O. Box 35008
Dallas, TX 75235
(214) 369-4332

These organizations can provide the interested reader with more information about specific subjects relevant to obstetric ultrasound. Resource personnel within the organizations have expert knowledge of all facets of diagnostic ultrasound and are available for consultation should the need arise.

ST. JOSEPH'S

ROOM NO.

Hospital and Medical Center
350 WEST THOMAS ROAD • PHOENIX

PT. ID NO.: 52232358
PT. NAME   DIXON,PATRICIA
HOSP. NO.
DATE   1/24/85
DOCTOR   C.HOHLER

STANDARD EXAM

PT. BIRTHDATE: 3/31/53   AGE @ VISIT: 31
GRAVIDITY: 1   RACE: C
MATERNAL HEIGHT: 5 FT, 4 IN   MATERNAL WEIGHT: 154 LBS
NON-SMOKER   FETAL NUMBER: 1
INDICATION FOR SCAN: ESTIMATION OF GESTATIONAL AGE FOR REPEAT
    C-SECTION OR INDUCTION OF LABOR
MEDICAL COMPLICATION(S): NONE KNOWN

FETAL DESCRIPTION   FETAL MOVEMENTS
================   ================
ANATOMY SURVEY: NORMAL
PRESENTATION: VERTEX   HEART: YES
GENDER: MALE   BODY/LIMBS: YES
EST. WEIGHT: 3172 GRAMS   BREATHING: YES

              FETAL AGE AND SIZE ESTIMATE
              ===========================
LMP: 5/15/84 36   WEEKS
PHYSICIAN'S ESTIMATE: 36   WEEKS
BEST ESTIMATE FROM PRIOR U/S (9/4/84)... 36 WEEKS
ULTRASOUND BPD SIZE: .... 37.0 WEEKS
ULTRASOUND FEMUR SIZE: .... 36.7 WEEKS
ULTRASOUND HEAD CIRCUMFERENCE SIZE: ... 35.7 WEEKS
ULTRASOUND ABDOMEN CIRCUMFERENCE SIZE: . 37.9 WEEKS

FETAL SIZE AVERAGE FOR: .... 36.8 (+/-2) WEEKS

           PLACENTA AND AMNIOTIC FLUID DESCRIPTION
           =======================================

PLACENTA LOCATION: POSTERIOR   PLACENTA HEIGHT: HIGH
PLACENTA GRADE: 2   AMNIOTIC FLUID AMOUNT: NORMAL
UTERINE ABNORMALITY: NO   AMNIOCENTESIS PERFORMED: NO
EXAM QUALITY: GOOD   ADNEXAL MASS: NO

==
 BPD   OFD   APAD   TAD   FL   TD-1   TD-2
 9.1   11.3   11.0   10.5   7.2   4.3   3.5
==
HC/AC   FL/BPD   FL/AC   FL/HC   CI   HC   AC   TC

 95%   79%   21%   22%   80%   32.0   33.8   12.2

REMARKS:

EXAM PERFORMED BY: REVIEWED BY:
CC
DD
DT 1/24/85   ┌───┐
BY   │ TITLE OF REPORT OBSTETRIC ULTRASOUND REPORT │
MR-522-0   └───┘
                          CHART

Figure 4–14. Sample obstetric ultrasound report. (Courtesy of the Prenatal Diagnostic Center at St. Joseph's Hospital and Medical Center, 350 West Thomas Road, Phoenix, Arizona.)

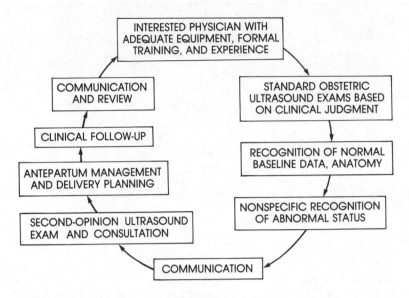

Figure 4–15. Diagram showing the ideal functioning of regionalized ultrasound consultation.

Future Trends in Obstetric Ultrasound

The 1980s are seeing many advances in obstetric ultrasound imaging. The equivalent of an ultrasound "CAT" scanner will probably become available in the next few years. In addition, magnetic resonance imaging will allow study of both the structure and function of the fetoplacental unit simultaneously. This will give us a 3-D capability for fetal evaluation that will open up vast new areas for research into the world of the developing fetus. Color image-processing will, in some limited situations, replace gray scaling and make imaging interpretation easier and less subtle. Increasing reliance upon computers—not only for image enhancement and processing but also for data acquisition, calculation, and comparison—will take much of the computational "drudgery" out of ultrasound examinations (Hohler, 1982a). Indirect information about the functional maturity of various fetal organs will probably become possible through the analysis of signal processing from tissue characterization work now being done. In some cases, direct operator interaction with the display screen by use of a light pen or digitizer marker "mouse" will make transcription of data unnecessary. Computer "networking" for the purpose of data collection, storage, retrieval, and regional consultations will become commonplace. Perinatal regionalization of standard obstetric ultrasound examinations in obstetricians' offices, together with second-opinion consultation ultrasound examinations over the telephone, will allow instant image transfer anywhere in the world. How such regionalized ultrasound consultation ideally should work is shown in Figure 4–15.

In short, the electronic wonders that confront us daily in our offices and homes will continue to influence the development of diagnostic ultrasound image construction, transmission, interpretation, and storage. Thus the "art" of ultrasound diagnosis will continue to become more objective and accurate, which will, in turn, protect the patient from inadvertent error in measurement. In the last analysis, however, it will remain essential that the clinician use diagnostic ultrasound as a confirmatory tool that provides information to be integrated into *all* of the clinical information about the patient in any given case. All of those using diagnostic ultrasound information would do well to heed the oath of all physicians to "first, do no harm" and to interpret ultrasound information with caution, seek adequate training, and seek the advice of consultants whenever uncertainty about ultrasound findings exists.

REFERENCES

Antenatal Diagnosis. NIH Publication No. 79-1973. II. Predictors of Fetal Maturation, Appendix, II–61, April 1979.

Birnholz, J. C., and Frigoletto, F. D.: Antenatal treatment of hydrocephalus. N. Engl. J. Med. 304:1021, 1981.

Bundy, A., and James, A. E.: How wrongful death actions may arise. Contemp. Ob/Gyn 23:209, May 1984.

Bushong, S. C.: The physics and biology of diagnostic ultrasound. *In* Athey, P. A., and Hadlock, F. P. (eds.): Ultrasound in Obstetrics and Gynecology. St. Louis, C. V. Mosby Co., 1981, p. 247.

Campbell, S.: Ultrasound measurement of the fetal head to abdomen circumference ratio in assessment of growth retardation. Br. J. Obstet. Gynecol. 84:165, 1977.

Clewell, W. H., Johnson, M. L., Meier, P. R., et al.: A surgical approach to the treatment of fetal hydrocephalus. N. Engl. J. Med. 306:1320, 1982.

Eastman, P.: The NIH Consensus Report: a closer look. Contemp. Ob/Gyn 23:164, May 1984.

Galle, P. C., and Meis, P. J.: Complications of amniocentesis: a review. J. Reprod. Med. 27:149, 1982.

Golbus, M. S., Harrison, M. R., Filly, R. A., et al.: In utero treatment of urinary tract obstruction. Am. J. Obstet. Gynecol. 142:383, 1982.

Hadlock, F. P., Deter, R. L., Carpenter, R. J., et al.: Estimating fetal age: effect of head shape on BPD. Am. J. Roentgenol. 137:83, 1981.

Hadlock, F. P., Deter, R. L., Harriet, R. B., et al.: Fetal abdominal circumference as a predictor of menstrual age. Am. J. Roentgenol. 139:367, 1982a.

Hadlock, F. P., Deter, R. L., Harriet, R. B., et al.: Fetal head circumference: relation to menstrual age. Am. J. Roentgenol. 138:649, 1982b.

Heitz, J. B., Mantoni, M., and Svenstrup, B.: Threatened abortion studied by estradiol-17 in serum and ultrasound. Obstet. Gynecol. 55:324, 1980.

Hohler, C. W.: How microcomputers will improve your OB ultrasound exams. Contemp. Ob/Gyn 20(special issue):98, 1982a.

Hohler, C. W.: Ultrasound bioeffects for the perinatologist. *In* Sciaira, J. (ed.): Gynecology and Obstetrics, Vol IV. Philadelphia, Harper and Row, 1982b, Chapter 71.

Hohler, C. W.: Use of ultrasound. *In* Ingram, J. M. (ed.): The Collected Letters of the International Correspondence Society of Obstetricians and Gynecologists, 23:26, 1982c.

Hohler, C. W.: Update on real-time ultrasound equipment for the OB-GYN office. Contemp. Ob/Gyn 18:13, 1981.

Hohler, C. W.: Real-time ultrasound moves into the OB office. Contemp. Ob/Gyn 16:75, 1980.

Hohler, C. W., Doherty, R. A., Lea, J., et al.: Ultrasound placental site in relation to bloody taps in midtrimester amniocentesis. Obstet. Gynecol. 52:555, 1978.

Hohler, C. W., and Quetel, T. A.: Fetal femur length: equations for computer calculation of gestational age from ultrasound measurements. Am. J. Obstet. Gynecol. 143:479, 1982.

Hohler, C. W., and Quetel, T. A.: Comparison of ultrasound femur length and biparietal diameter in late pregnancy. Am. J. Obstet. Gynecol. 141:759, 1981.

Kirkinen, P., Jouppila, P., Tuononen, S., et al.: Repeated transabdominal renocenteses in a case of fetal hydronephrotic kidney. Am. J. Obstet. Gynecol. 142:1049, 1982.

Kleinman, C. S., Hobbins, J. C., Jaffe, C. C., et al.: Echocardiographic studies of the human fetus: prenatal diagnosis of congenital heart disease and cardiac arrhythmias. Pediatrics 65:1059, 1980.

Kremkau, F. W.: Diagnostic Ultrasound: Physical Principles and Exercises. New York, Grune & Stratton, 1980.

Larkin, R. M., Knochel, J. Q., Kochenour, N. K., et al.: Ultrasound air contrast transfusion technique: an aid to managing the Rh-affected fetus with ascites. Obstet. Gynecol. 57:225, 1981.

Law, R. G., and MacRae, K. D.: Head circumference as an index of fetal age. J. Ultrasound Med. 1:281, 1982.

Lele, P. P.: Safety and potential hazards in the current applications of ultrasound in obstetrics and gynecology. Ultrasound Med. Biol. 5:307, 1979.

McDicken, W. N.: Diagnostic Ultrasonics: Principles and Use of Instruments, 2nd ed., New York, John Wiley & Sons, 1981.

MacKenzie, I. Z., MacLean, D. A., Fry, A., et al.: Midtrimester intrauterine exchange transfusion of the fetus. Am. J. Obstet. Gynecol. 143:555, 1982.

Manning, F. A., Baskett, T. F., Morrison, I., et al.: Fetal biophysical profile scoring: a prospective study in 1,184 high-risk patients. Am. J. Obstet. Gynecol. 140:289, 1981.

Manning, F. A., Platt, L. D., and Sipes, L.: Antepartum fetal evaluation: development of a fetal biophysical profile. Am. J. Obstet. Gynecol. 136:787, 1980.

Mennuti, M. T., Brummond, W., Cromblaholme, W. R., et al.: Fetal-maternal bleeding associated with genetic amniocentesis. Obstet. Gynecol. 55:48, 1980.

Moore, M. L.: Realities in Childbearing, 2nd ed. Philadelphia, W. B. Saunders Co., 1983.

National Science Foundation Survey Team on Ultrasonic Imaging: Prospectives for Ultrasonic Imaging in Medical Diagnosis. Washington, D. C., National Science Foundation, 1973.

Perez, R. H.: Protocols for Perinatal Nursing Practice. St. Louis, C. V. Mosby Co., 1981.

Porreco, R. P., Young, P. E., Resnick, R., et al.: Reproductive outcome following amniocentesis for genetic indications. Am. J. Obstet. Gynecol. 143:653, 1982.

Reid, D. C.: Efficiency of ultrasound coupling agents. Physiotherapy 63:255, 1977.

Rodeck, C. H.: Fetoscopy guided by real-time ultrasound for pure fetal blood samples, fetal skin samples, and examination of the fetus *in utero*. Br. J. Obstet. Gynaecol. 87:449, 1980.

Sabbagha, R. E., and Hughey, M.: Standardization of sonar cephalometry and gestational age. Obstet. Gynecol. 52:402, 1978.

Sabbagha, R. E., Tamura, R. K., Dal Campo, S.: Obstetric ultrasonography in perspective. Perinatol. Neonatol. 6:53, 1982.

Schifrin, B. S., Guntes, V., Gergely, R. C., et al.: The role of real-time scanning in antenatal fetal surveillance. Am. J. Obstet. Gynecol. 140:525, 1981.

Scholly, T. A., Sutphen, J. H., Hitchcock, D. A., et al.: Sonographic determination of fetal gender. Am. J. Roentgenol. 135:1161, 1980.

Shepard, M. J., Richards, V. A., Berkowitz, R. L., et al.: An evaluation of two equations for predicting fetal weight by ultrasound. Am. J. Obstet. Gynecol. 142:47, 1982.

Tucker, S. M., and Bryant, S.: Fetal Monitoring and Fetal Assessment in High Risk Pregnancy. St. Louis, C. V. Mosby Co., 1978.

Wetrich, D. A.: Routine ultrasound in midpregnancy. Obstet. Gynecol. 60:309, 1982.

PERINATAL INFECTIONS

SEBASTIAN FARO
JOSEPH G. PASTOREK II

Infection continues to be a major problem for the high-risk team, even though a plethora of antimicrobial agents are available. The practitioner must be familiar with those potential pathogenic microorganisms that exist in the environment, as well as with the patient's endogenous microflora. There must also be a basic understanding of both the mechanisms of action and the strengths and weaknesses of individual classes of antibiotics. All antibiotics, especially the newer broad-spectrum antibiotics, can exert selective pressure on microorganisms, thereby selecting out resistant strains. The obstetrician is further challenged because it is often difficult to make a diagnosis of an acute infection, since some infections may be chronic or asymptomatic. The pregnant female poses a special problem in that the presence of the fetus often prohibits the use of many antimicrobial agents.

Viral Infections

AIDS

For the most recent information available, see "Update on AIDS," p. 111.

HERPES

Epidemiology

Genital herpes has become one of the most common sexually transmitted diseases, ranking in prevalence with gonorrhea and syphilis. The Centers for Disease Control (CDC) estimates that there are approximately 300,000 new cases of genital herpes per year, occurring more frequently in the 15- to 24-year-old age group. Data collected from venereal disease clinics show that the ratio of gonorrhea to herpes is 10:1. However, data obtained from the UCLA Student Health Clinic indicated that genital herpes is more prevalent than gonorrhea, with a ratio of 1:10 (gonorrhea/herpes). These two sources of information imply that herpes may be more common among the middle and upper socioeconomic classes.

Microbiology

Genital herpes is caused by either herpesvirus serotype I or serotype II (HSV-I or HSV-II). HSV-I and HSV-II both contain a central core of DNA that is surrounded by an icosahedral protein capsid. The protein capsid is enveloped by an impermeable membrane made up of lipids, polyamines, and glycoproteins. The two serotypes can be distinguished by serologic, biologic, and biochemical analysis.

These viruses are unique in that they have evolved to develop a complex relationship with their adult hosts. Humans are the only known natural host, and the virus can cause an active infection, a latent infection, or cell transformation.

Infection

Genital herpes occurs either as a primary infection or as recurrent disease. Primary genital infection may be asymptomatic, mild, or severe. Inoculation of the host by the virus occurs by contact with infectious material, usually via sexual intercourse or orogenital sex. Vesicles appear at the site of inoculation (e.g., the vulva, vagina, or cervix) 2 to 10 days after inoculation. An individual with a primary infection may experience a prodrome of general malaise that precedes the development of genital lesions. Before the formation of vesicles, the area may become edematous, erythematous, and painful. Bilateral inguinal lymphadenopathy is common in those individuals who develop numerous lesions. The vesicles may be grouped close together and may coalesce to form large bullous lesions. The vesicles contain clear serum and tend to disrupt spontaneously, forming shallow ulcers with clean margins and red bases. If the vulva is not kept clean, the lesions easily become secondarily infected. The lesions persist for 7 to 21 days and resolve spontaneously. Viral shedding continues until the lesions become reepithelialized. The patient with herpetic cervicitis and no other lesions will not experience pain; she may be totally asymptomatic or have a watery discharge.

During the symptomatic phase, the virus invades the epithelial cells, replicates, and ultimately destroys the host cell. Upon entering the host cell, viral DNA is exposed and host DNA-dependent RNA polymerase transcribes viral DNA, thereby coding for viral proteins and viral DNA, resulting in the synthesis of new herpesviruses. It is estimated that well over 100,000 copies of viral DNA are made per host cell, with approximately 20,000 being encapsulated, resulting in intact virus.

Resolution of the lesion is associated with the latent stage of the virus. Latency is thought to be accomplished by viral migration along sensory nerves, with ultimate residence in the sensory ganglion.

Diagnosis

Approximately half the infants exposed to herpes during vaginal delivery will become infected. Approximately half of these infected infants will die, and half of the survivors will have severe sequelae.

Primary infection occurs in those individuals who have not been exposed to HSV-I or HSV-II. An individual can be primarily infected with HSV-I and HSV-II simultaneously. Clinical symptoms and signs of infection usually appear within 3 to 7 days after exposure; however, the incubation period may be 20 days. Lesions are usually multiple and are generally preceded by a prodromal phase characterized by headache, generalized aching, malaise, low-grade fever, paresthesia, and burning in the area where the vesicles are destined to appear. The patient may develop inguinal and pelvic lymphadenopathy, giving rise to pelvic and inguinal pain. Micturition may be accompanied by severe pain, resulting in urinary retention. Lesions may develop on the labia majora and minora, the perianal region, and the vaginal and ectocervical epithelium. The lesions appear as small vesicles, often in clusters, on an erythematous base. In moist areas such as the labial folds and introitus, the vesicles become unroofed within 48 hours and easily become secondarily infected (Fig. 5–1). Lesions on the drier areas of the vulva tend to remain vesicular for longer periods. The entire vulva may become edematous and erythematous.

If the cervix is involved there may be a profuse watery discharge. The lesions may be few in number, usually appearing as small erythematous shallow ulcers. Occasionally, the cervix may be covered by a large fungating, necrotic mass that may be mistaken for a malignancy. The lesions may last from 2 to 6 weeks. When healing has occurred there is usually no residual scarring.

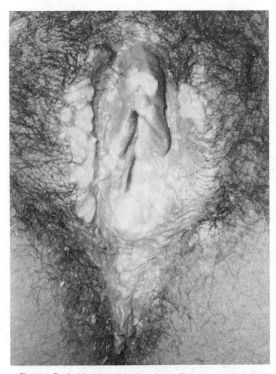

Figure 5–1. Herpes simplex type II. Large ulcerated lesions that have a thick purulent exudate. Lesions have become secondarily infected. Note white discharge exiting from introitus (patient also had *T. vaginalis* vaginitis).

Recurrent episodes of genital herpes occur in approximately 66 percent of the patients during the first 12 months following the primary episode. Recurrent lesions are usually fewer in number, less severe, and restricted to small areas, and usually develop near the site of the primary lesions. Patients experiencing recurrent herpes may note a prodromal period beginning 24 hours before the appearance of lesions. The prodromal symptoms may consist of localized itching, burning, or hypersensitivity of the skin, as well as neuralgia and severe pruritus. Recurrent lesions may be minute and inconspicuous and, therefore, difficult to identify. The vesicles may become pustular and develop a crust. Reepithelization occurs in a few days to 3 weeks. Recurrences are less likely with HSV-I than with HSV-II. The frequency of recurrence tends to decrease with the passage of time.

The presumptive diagnosis of herpes can be established by Papanicolaou smear, serology, or direct fluorescent antibody staining technique. A definitive diagnosis can be established only by isolation of the virus from a lesion. Fluid can be aspirated from a vesicle, or the base of an unroofed vesicle can be touched with a sterile swab and the specimen placed in transport medium. The specimen should be taken to the laboratory immediately or temporarily kept at 4°C. If it is to be stored for a prolonged period, it should be kept at −70°C. Rabbit kidney cells or similar tissue can be inoculated to determine if herpes virus is present.

If the capability to culture HSV-I or HSV-II does not exist, then the Pap smear, fluorescent antibody studies, or antibody titer determination can be done. The Pap smear or Giemsa stain can be used to detect the presence of multinucleated giant cells or intranuclear inclusions in host cells. These tests will detect from 60 to 80 percent of genital infections. Serum antibody test can be performed to determine if an acute infection has occurred; however, there is cross-reactivity between HSV-I and HSV-II. Antibody to HSV-I is usually acquired in childhood, and approximately 60 percent of pregnant women will have antibody to HSV-II; therefore, it is often difficult to establish the existence of an acute infection. Acute and convalescent sera should be obtained for determination of the presence of herpes antibody using paired sera. Herpes-specific IgM will remain elevated for several months.

The presence of type-specific antibody does not offer the patient protection against recurrent infection. Serum antibody determinations are of no value in the face of recurrent infection, since there will be no elevation during the convalescent period.

Treatment

The patient must be reassured that even though she has contracted a herpetic infection, she is not a social outcast; she can have a normal sex life and bear children, barring any infertility problem. The disease is manageable, and new agents are available that are promising.

The patient and her husband (or sex partner) must be educated about herpes. They should be taught to recognize prodromal symptoms and signs of recurrent lesions. The male partner must also be made aware of how to examine himself. Patients should not engage in sexual activity if genital or oral lesions (Fig. 5–2) are present. Intercourse should be avoided for 10 to 14 days after the lesions subside.

When lesions are present, it is important that the vulva be kept clean and dry. If a vaginal discharge is present, this should be examined microscopically. Endocervical and urethral specimens should be obtained for the possible isolation of *Neisseria gonorrhoeae*, since sexually transmitted dis-

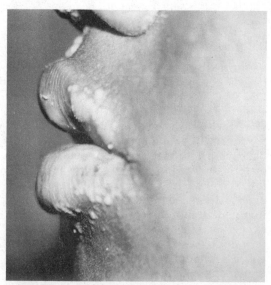

Figure 5–2. Herpes simplex. Note multiple vesicles on the lips; lesions are individual, and on upper lip have coalesced.

eases tend to occur in conjunction. A serum VDRL test should also be obtained. If the lesion is solitary, or if there are only two to three lesions and they are not really painful, then a dark-field microscopic examination and Gram stain should be performed.

If the patient is having difficulty voiding, she should be advised to take sitz baths and void in the water. This will dramatically reduce the discomfort. If there is severe edema and urinary retention, a Foley catheter should be inserted. The vulva can be washed with povidone-iodine solution, which may also be used to douche, provided the patient is not pregnant. Such treatment will not facilitate resolution of the viral infection, but it will help reduce the possibility of secondary infection.

A number of treatment modalities have been tried, such as iodine, idoxuridine, neutral red dye and light, lysine, zinc, and 2-doxy-D-glucose; however, all have been shown to be worthless. Acycloguanosine (acyclovir [Zovirax]) and vidarabine are two newer agents that appear to be very promising. Acyclovir inhibits virus-specific thymidine kinase, blocking DNA synthesis. The drug has been shown to reduce the durations of lesions and viral shedding during acute primary infection. Acyclovir does not eliminate latent infection, but it can reduce the intensity of recurrent attacks.

Pregnant women with a history of herpes antedating the pregnancy, or who have their initial infection during the pregnancy, should be examined every 2 weeks during the last 2 months for the presence of active infection. It is best to obtain specimens for culture; if this not possible, Pap smears or fluorescent antibody studies can be done. If there is clinical or laboratory evidence of herpes within the last 2 weeks of pregnancy, the infant should be delivered by cesarean section. If the patient's amniotic membranes have been ruptured for up to 12 hours, cesarean section should still be considered. If the membranes have been ruptured for more than 12 hours, however, the patient should be allowed to deliver vaginally, if possible. The infant may then be treated with acyclovir.

If the patient has lesions on the abdomen, thigh, or buttock at the time she goes into labor, cervical and vulval specimens can be obtained for fluorescent antibody test. If the cervix and vulva are found to be free of virus, vaginal delivery should be attempted.

Postpartum management should be directed at preventing infection of the infant, as well as all individuals coming in contact with the mother. The mother should be isolated until her lesions begin to heal. Premature and newborn infants are at risk for developing serious infection. If a patient understands the risks and wishes to handle her infant, she should cover all lesions, wash her hands and put on a surgical gown and gloves. The infant should then remain with the mother and not be taken back to the nursery. All personnel should practice good aseptic technique while tending to patients with active herpes lesions. All bandages, dressings, perineal pads, etc., should be double-bagged and disposed of properly.

RUBELLA

Epidemiology

Rubella virus has no known animal vector. Transmission is from human to human, usually via the respiratory route. However, rubella is not as highly contagious as varicella or the rhinoviruses; therefore, a sizable population of susceptible individuals exists among unvaccinated women of childbearing age. This is perhaps the major reason for the high incidence of congenital rubella infection in an unvaccinated population.

Microbiology

Rubella is a member of the family Togaviridae. It is an RNA virus with a characteristic protein capsid and lipoprotein envelope. Immunologically, rubella possesses a complement-fixing antigen and two precipitins. Of paramount medical importance is the hemagglutinating antigen on the viral envelope, which is the basis for laboratory antibody testing.

Infection

Postnatal rubella infection is usually a benign disease. The hallmark of acute infection is the characteristic nonconfluent maculopapular rash that starts on the face and migrates caudally, lasting roughly 3 to 5 days. Desquamation may occur. In 30 percent of infections, however, the rash may be absent or clinically inapparent.

Concomitant findings include fever, malaise, posterior auricular and occipital adenopathy, and anorexia; arthritis/arthralgia also may develop, especially in adults. Viral shedding may occur up to 10 days before onset of the rash and for up to 15 days after its onset. The fact that the rash does not correspond with the peak viremia indicates that a possible immunologic mechanism is involved.

Maternal rubella infection in the absence of maternal immunity may be transmitted transplacentally with devastating results to the fetus, depending upon gestational age at the time of infection.

It is estimated that 50 to 90 percent of fetuses are affected by rubella if exposure occurs during the 1st trimester. Approximately one third of these cases will result in spontaneous abortions, while the surviving affected fetuses may be severely compromised. Abnormalities such as deafness, psychomotor retardation, and microcephaly have been reported in offspring of mothers infected up to 21 weeks' gestation. A fetus exposed to rubella in the 2nd or 3rd trimester appears relatively safe. However, those exposed in the 2nd or 3rd trimester may develop subtle abnormalities that may be manifested later in life in a child who seemed normal at birth, such as childhood diabetes, thyroid disorders, precocious puberty, progressive panencephalitis, and "soft" neurologic defects.

Diagnosis

Postnatal rubella infection is such a mild disease that clinical diagnosis is difficult. Many other viruses may cause similar signs and symptoms. The virus may be isolated from respiratory secretions or from the pharynx. Seroconversion, however, is the chief diagnostic modality. Hemagglutination inhibition (HI) is an easy-to-perform and sensitive method, commonly used in most laboratories. HI antibody is long-lasting and is therefore a useful indication of previous infection and immunity. It is first necessary to document acute infection conversion from negative to positive HI serology. If the initial (acute) sample is drawn too late, i.e., after HI antibodies have had time to develop, rubella-specific IgM may be measured, or complement-fixing (CF) antibodies may be utilized, since they arise later in the infection (4 to 8 weeks) than do HI antibodies.

The clinical manifestations of congenital (intrauterine) rubella infection (Table 5–1) are not unique to this virus. Therefore, doc-

Table 5–1. Clinical Manifestations of Congenital Rubella Infection

Intrauterine growth retardation	Seizures
Failure to thrive	Radiolucent long bone lesions
Cataracts	Bulging fontanelles
Glaucoma	CSF pleocytosis
Patent ductus	Deafness
Valvular lesions	Vestibular dysfunction
Septal defects	Mental retardation
Thrombocytopenic purpura	Microphthalmia
Hepatosplenomegaly	Chorioretinitis
Hepatitis	Iridocyclitis
Motor delay	Chronic meningitis

umentation of intrauterine fetal infection is derived from detection of rubella-specific IgM or viral isolation from the infant.

Treatment

Prenatal rubella is treated symptomatically. Immune serum globulin (ISG) may attenuate maternal symptoms but will not alter fetal infection. ISG may be administered as a desperation measure (in the hope that it might alter fetal infection) should a woman decide against abortion after documented rubella infection early in gestation.

Immunization is the cornerstone of therapy. Vaccination is recommended at age 15 months for all children. Any nonimmune woman of childbearing age should be immunized if not pregnant, or vaccinated after delivery if susceptibility is discovered during pregnancy. It is recommended that a woman not become pregnant for 3 months following vaccination, since there is a theoretical risk to the fetus from the live-virus vaccine. In practice, however, no congenital rubella abnormalities have been documented in children exposed to vaccine in utero, although vaccine virus has been recovered from the conceptus in cases in which the mother opted for abortion.

Vaccination has reduced the incidence of congenital rubella syndrome in the United States. In 1982 the CDC reported 2325 cases of rubella in the United States, including 9 cases of congenital rubella.

CYTOMEGALOVIRUS

Epidemiology

Cytomegalovirus (CMV) can be isolated from many body fluids, including blood, saliva, semen, breast milk, endocervical mucus, urine, and feces. In the United States, 0.5 to 2.5 percent of newborns may be infected at birth. In the neonatal period, 2 to 5 percent of infants are colonized with CMV by handling, breastfeeding, and other means of contact. By age 10 years, 10 to 30 percent of children show evidence of exposure to CMV. This figure rises to 20 to 50 percent for women during the childbearing years and 60 to 90 percent for individuals over 60 years of age.

Microbiology

Cytomegalovirus is a member of the herpesvirus group, which includes herpes simplex virus types I and II, Epstein-Barr virus, and varicella-zoster virus, as well as numerous animal herpesviruses. CMV is a DNA virus that may invade the host's cells and insert its DNA into the host's nucleus, remaining latent only to be reactivated under the influence of, as yet, poorly understood stimuli.

Human CMV exists as many different serotypes, some quite antigenically diverse. Antigenic cross-reactivity usually exists between strains. Occasionally a strain will be unique enough to confound routine serologic tests. Additionally, a person may be primarily infected with one strain of CMV only to contract a separate strain of virus against which he or she has little or no protective antibody from the first infection. It is important to note that a woman may have more than one affected infant owing to infection by antigenetically different strains during different pregnancies.

Infection

Primary CMV infection in adults is usually asymptomatic and clinically inapparent. Symptomatic primary infection in adults may take the form of a heterophil-negative mononucleosis syndrome, resembling Epstein-Barr virus infectious mononucleosis. There is usually less adenopathy and pharyngitis with CMV disease than with the latter infection; however, the epidemiology of the two syndromes is similar, with each being spread as a "kissing disease" among a fairly young population.

CMV infection may occur after blood transfusion. Seven per cent of CMV seronegative individuals will become seropositive following transfusion, resulting in a syndrome of fever, splenomegaly, and atypical lymphocytosis. Immunocompromised individuals, including transplant recipients, are at risk for a fulminating systemic form of the disease that may include chorioretinitis, encephalitis, and pneumonitis. A fatality rate of 80 percent or more is not uncommon. The source of the virus may be latent disease in the patient, transmission in the transplanted organ (especially with kidney transplants), or infection via blood transfusion.

Congenital CMV infection is a significant neonatal problem. Ninety-five percent of infants infected in utero are asymptomatic at birth. However, 5 to 10 percent of these infants go on to develop significant neurologic difficulties, such as hearing deficit, lower IQs, and chronic CMV shedding (usually up to 2 years, although cases of shedding for as long as 8 years have been reported).

In the minority of infants symptomatic from CMV infection at birth, the outlook is grave. There may be intrauterine growth retardation (IUGR), jaundice, hepatosplenomegaly, microcephaly with severe mental retardation, chorioretinitis, and optic atrophy, intracranial calcification, seizures, and numerous other disorders. If the infant acquires CMV after birth, however, there is little ill effect other than occasional mild liver dysfunction, pneumonitis, and/or skin lesions.

Diagnosis

Viral culture is the best method of viral isolation and identification. Nearly any body fluid may be cultured, and specimens may successfully be stored and transferred at 4°C (refrigerator temperature) for a week. Results must be interpreted cautiously, however. The virus isolated may be merely an agent of colonization, and not the organism responsible for the particular illness.

Serology for CMV is difficult to interpret. Although seroconversion in the face of characteristic clinical illness may make a good case for primary infection, there may be a significant number of false-positives and false-negatives, especially when different techniques are used. Other herpesviruses may cross-react with CMV. Also, if the infecting strain is antigenically distinct from the testing strains, there may appear to be no seropositivity. Additionally, viral shedding may wax and wane (as in pregnancy) with no change in antibody titer.

Treatment

Treatment for CMV is still essentially in the research stage. Chemotherapy with nucleic acid analogs has been shown to decrease viral shedding, but not the clinical course, in infected infants. Interferon has been shown to have little clinical benefit.

Active immunization with live attenuated strains (AD-169, Towne strain) has been shown to induce both humoral and cell-mediated immunity in volunteers. The risks of such vaccination (and colonization with live vaccine DNA virus) are as yet unknown. The subjects did not excrete virus, however. Passive immunization with large doses of human immune globulin has been anecdotally reported to help immunosuppressed patients with severe systemic disease. No extensive studies have conclusively documented consistent efficacy.

The mainstay of therapy is thus avoidance. Isolation of pregnant women from known CMV excretors seems to be indicated. However, the effect on the whole picture is probably minimal, since the virus seems to be a remarkably successful parasite living in a large reservoir of usually asymptomatic hosts, with no known animal vector to be controlled and no way to break the chain of transmission.

VARICELLA-ZOSTER

Epidemiology

Varicella (chickenpox) is a highly contagious disease, frequently occurring in children. Humans are the only natural host, and transmission is via droplets or direct contact. Zoster infections (shingles) may occur at any age but are more frequent in the older population. Upon reactivation of the varicella-zoster virus, migration occurs along a nerve, vesicles are produced along a well-demarcated dermatome, and the virus does not cross the midline.

Pregnant women who contract varicella infection during the first trimester have a 2 percent risk of having a child with congenital defects. However, data collected by the Collaborative Perinatal Research Study revealed a prevalence rate of only 1 in 7500 pregnancies. A total of 8 cases were found in 60,000 pregnancies, and none of these infants had evidence of congenital disease.

Sequelae from congenital infection include scarring from skin lesions, hypotrophy of limbs, atrophy of digits, psychomotor and growth retardation, and cortical atrophy. Maternal infection appearing in the last 4 days of gestation, including 48 hours postpartum, can result in severe, often fatal infection of the newborn.

Microbiology

Chickenpox and herpes zoster are caused by the varicella-zoster virus, which is a member of the herpesvirus group. The varicella-zoster has a central core of DNA surrounded by a protein capsid that in turn is covered by a lipid-protein envelope. Unlike herpes simplex, there is only one serotype of the varicella-zoster virus.

Infection

The incubation period following exposure to the varicella virus is from 12 to 18 days. A prodrome occurs in which the patient develops fever (from 38.3 to 39.4°C), myalgia, and malaise. Following the prodromal phase, a rash develops on the skin and mucous membranes that becomes vesicular. These vesicles appear in clusters and are pruritic. The exanthem is asynchronous in that all stages can be found—unlike variola, in which the lesions are synchronous.

The lesions seen in varicella and herpes zoster are indistinguishable; morphologically they are identical to the lesions seen in herpes simplex infection. The vesicles of varicella and herpes zoster are surrounded by an intense erythema of inflammation (Fig. 5–3) and contain straw-colored fluid. The vesicles of varicella appear in successive crops, first on the trunk; followed by the neck, face, and finally the extremities (Fig. 5–4). Vesicles appearing on the skin are usually painless, whereas those occurring on the tympanum, cornea, or mucous membranes are often painful. The rash may be mild or severe, as determined by the number of lesions.

The illness may be limited to several vesicles appearing in a simple crop, or the individual may experience recurring crops of lesions. Serious systemic disease may occur in the form of pneumonia, encephalitis, Reye's syndrome, glomerulonephritis, myocarditis, or thrombocytopenia.

Varicella pneumonia is an uncommon occurrence in children but occurs in up to 35

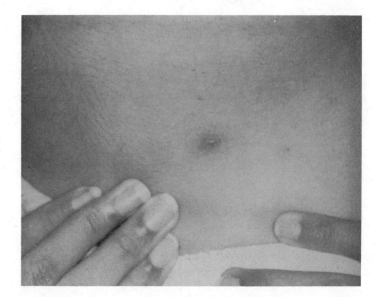

Figure 5–3. Varicella lesion. Note erythematous margin surrounding a pustule.

percent of adults who are infected with the varicella virus. Pulmonary symptoms begin with the onset of the exanthem. These may consist of nothing more than a mild, nonproductive cough that resolves spontaneously; in more severe cases, a high fever, chills, chest pain, nonproductive cough, hemoptysis, dyspnea, and cyanosis may develop. Approximately 10 percent of the patients who develop varicella pneumonia will have pleural effusions. Severely ill patients may also develop pulmonary edema, subcutaneous emphysema, secondary bacterial infection, and abscesses. Varicella pneumonia may result in pulmonary fibrosis and diffusion defects. The patient may develop

calcific nodules that resemble healed tuberculosis lesions.

Varicella may involve the central nervous system, producing encephalitis, transverse myelitis, neuritis, and aseptic meningitis. Encephalitis is the most common neurologic complication, occurring more frequently in males than in females. Reye's syndrome (acute encephalopathy and visceral fatty degeneration) primarily occurs in children. The syndrome develops following many viral infections and may occur in up to 10 percent of the cases of varicella.

Congenital varicella is rare, and antepartum maternal infection has not been associated with an increase in fetal mortality or

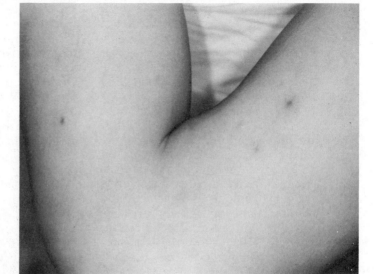

Figure 5–4. Varicella lesions that have formed a scab. Note also older healed lesions.

prematurity. Neonatal varicella occurring within the first 28 days of life is seen in 25 percent of neonates whose mothers acquire varicella 1 to 16 days before delivery. Approximately 20 percent of neonates who develop a rash 5 to 10 days after birth will die; however, no deaths have been reported among those infants who develop a rash within the first 4 days of life.

Diagnosis

The diagnosis is usually made by the clinical presentation, especially if there has been exposure within the previous 3 weeks. Giemsa- or Wright-stained preparations from the base of a fresh vesicle will often reveal the presence of multinucleated giant cells characteristic of herpes and varicella-zoster infection. Direct fluorescent antibody staining of cellular material from a new vesicle is useful. Measurement of serum antibody, demonstrating a fourfold increase in varicella-zoster antibody titer is useful, especially in mild or atypical cases. Complement-fixing antibodies appear within 4 days after the onset of the exanthem, and it is within this time period that acute-phase serum should be obtained; convalescent serum should be obtained 2 to 6 weeks later.

Treatment

There is no specific therapy for varicella, and treatment is directed to alleviating the symptoms. Measures should be taken to prevent bacterial infection of the skin lesions; this can be achieved by having the patient bathe daily in warm water with an antibacterial detergent. Mild sedation and relief from pruritus can be accomplished by administering histamines.

There is no varicella-zoster vaccine available. Human immune serum globulin (HISG) can be administered within 3 days of exposure. HISG will not prevent manifestation of the disease, but it may reduce the severity. Zoster immune globulin (ZIG) administered within 3 days of exposure prevents varicella in normal children and attenuates the disease in compromised individuals. However, ZIG has been shown to be of no value in the treatment of pregnant women with varicella-zoster infection to prevent fetal infection, congenital defects, or abortion. ZIG is prepared from sera obtained from individuals 2 to 28 days after the onset of the zoster rash.

HEPATITIS

There are three distinct viruses responsible for acute viral hepatitis: hepatitis A, also known as infectious hepatitis; hepatitis B, which is referred to as serum hepatitis; and non-A, non-B hepatitis, which is commonly referred to as posttransfusion hepatitis and also is designated hepatitis C. Hepatitis B is of major concern in pregnancy because of the possibility of genital infection and the risk of maternal chronic hepatitis.

Epidemiology

It is estimated that the hepatitis A virus has an attack rate of approximately 80 cases per 100,000 population, with the highest frequency seen in individuals less than 20 years old. The hepatitis A antibody is present in approximately 24 to 64 percent of the adult population. The virus is transmitted by serum and feces, with the fecal-oral route being the most common.

Hepatitis B has been estimated to affect more than 300,000 individuals annually. The peak incidence occurs in the 15- to 24-year age group. The hepatitis B virus is prevalent among percutaneous drug users, individuals receiving blood transfusion, those requiring hemodialysis, and individuals who handle human blood, serum, and blood products. The virus can gain entrance to the body through any open skin or mucous membrane, or it may be transmitted via oral ingestion of infected material. The virus is rather hardy and may be transmitted on toothbrushes, baby bottles, toys, razors, eating utensils, or respirators and other equipment.

Non-A, non-B hepatitis has been observed more frequently over the last 10 years. The incidence of non-A, non-B hepatitis is higher when blood is obtained from paid donors. However, it has been found that not all cases of non-A, non-B hepatitis are related to blood transfusions, but a route of transmission remains unknown.

Microbiology

The hepatitis A virus is an RNA virus measuring 28 nm in diameter and is similar to the picornaviruses; the genome is a single strand of RNA enveloped by three polypeptides.

The hepatitis B virus is quite different

from the hepatitis A virus. It is a DNA virus which measures 42 nm in diameter. The hepatitis B virus is antigenically complex. There are three main antigens, the surface antigen, HB_sAg; the core antigen, HB_cAg; and the "e" antigen, HB_eAg. The surface antigen (HB_sAg) is complex and consists of eight subtypes that are clinically important. The core antigen (HB_cAg) is associated with the Dane particle, which consists of the surface antigen, a lipid-containing outer envelope, and an internal nucleocapsid. The HB_eAg is distinct from HB_sAg and HB_cAg, and is present only in HB_sAg-positive sera.

The non-A, non-B hepatitis virion has not yet been isolated, although preliminary data suggest that a specific virus is responsible for non-A, non-B hepatitis. Controversy exists as to whether or not more than one etiologic agent is responsible for non-A, non-B hepatitis.

Infection

The incubation period for hepatitis A virus (HAV) is between 14 and 49 days, with a mean of 28 days. Infection with HAV results in lasting immunity against reinfection with HAV but offers no protection against hepatitis B or non-A, non-B hepatitis infection. The likelihood of percutaneous transmission of HAV occurring is low and is due to the relatively short incubation period and short duration of viremia. Approximately 2 to 3 weeks after infection, hepatitis A antigen (HAA_g) particles can be detected in feces. The titer of HAA particles peaks coincidently with the elevation of SGOT, and HAA_g excretion becomes negative at about the time SGOT concentration peaks. Antibody to HAA_g (anti-HAA_g) begins at approximately 5 weeks following infection and peaks at 8 weeks post infection. Anti-HA can be detected in the serum for many years following infection.

Hepatitis B infection may follow one of three courses: self-limited infection with transient serum surface antigenemia; self-limited infection without surface antigenemia; and persistent infection with chronic HB_sAg carriage. Hepatitis B has an incubation period of 28 to 196 days. Individuals who develop a self-limited HB_sAg-positive infection usually have antigen detectable 42 to 84 days after infection. The HB_sAg titer peaks at about 56 days after infection and begins to decline with the onset of clinical

symptoms. Core antibody (anti-HB_c) becomes detectable with onset of clinical illness, and as the anti-HB_c titer rises, the HB_sAg titer falls. Anti-HB_s becomes detectable approximately 2 to 3 weeks after HB_sAg disappears. However, the anti-HB_c rises and reaches its peak at this time and remains elevated for many years. Approximately 11 weeks following infection, HB_eAg appears and the serum remains positive until the clinical illness resolves. Anti-HB_e appears shortly after anti-HB_s appears. Individuals with self-limited disease without surface antigenemia can manifest serum antibody (anti-HB_s) 24 to 84 days after exposure to HBV. The anti-HB_s titer rises rapidly and may be detected for several years. Coincident with the rise in anti-HB_s, the serum becomes positive for anti-HB_c. Individuals who remain HB_sAg-positive for 20 weeks or longer are likely to develop persistent hepatitis and remain HG_sAg-positive indefinitely. Anti-HB_c is present in all patients with persistent infection, and HB_eAg is present in up to 50 per cent of these individuals.

In non-A, non-B hepatitis the time between transfusion and abnormal liver function is about 8 weeks. The infection does not result in manifestation of detectable antibodies.

Diagnosis

Clinically it is not possible to distinguish between the various causes of viral hepatitis, although there may be subtle differences. Initially the patient experiences fever, malaise, headache, anorexia, nausea, and vomiting. Patients who smoke usually develop an aversion to tobacco. The patient may develop hepatosplenomegaly, which is followed by scleral icterus, generalized jaundice, and pruritus, as well as cervical lymphadenopathy.

Prior to the onset of symptoms, the serum glutamic-pyruvic and serum glutamic-oxaloacetic transaminases become elevated, with the SGPT reaching greater than 1000 units/ml. The SGOT usually rises first and precedes the onset of jaundice by approximately 5 days, peaking prior to the onset of jaundice. The total serum bilirubin rarely exceeds 10 mg/100 ml and gradually falls over a 2- to 4-week period. The hematocrit and hemoglobin are usually not significantly affected. There may be a mild lymphocytosis. Urobilinogen and bilirubin are found in the urine.

The diagnosis of the specific viral hepatitis is established by the presence or absence of specific antigens and/or antibodies, in conjunction with the clinical and laboratory findings. The diagnosis of hepatitis A may be established on finding hepatitis A antigen (HAA$_g$) in the stool. However, a more common method is to demonstrate in serum the presence of antibody to hepatitis A antigen (anti-HAA$_g$) during the acute phase of the disease. The presence of anti-HAA$_g$ in the absence of jaundice excludes HAV as the cause of illness. Serum should be obtained also during the convalescent phase and titers determined in conjunction with the initial specimen. A fourfold or greater rise in titer is indicative of active disease.

The diagnosis of hepatitis B can be established by serologic determination of HB$_s$Ag, anti-HB$_s$, and anti-HB$_c$. Serum that is positive for HB$_s$Ag is indicative of active infection except in cases of conversion following blood transfusion. Serum that is positive for HB$_s$Ag and negative for anti-HB$_c$ in conjunction with the absence of HB$_s$Ag indicates past infection and immunity to HBV. Individuals who are seropositive for HB$_e$Ag are considered to be more likely to transmit infection.

Individuals who have HB$_s$Ag-positive sera for greater than 20 weeks are at risk to develop persistent hepatitis. Chronic persistent hepatitis is usually asymptomatic. The SGOT and SGPT may be either persistently or intermittently elevated, and usually there is no jaundice. These patients have persistent mild hepatosplenomegaly and usually show no progression of their disease. However, patients with persistent hepatitis associated with chronic or episodic jaundice have chronic active hepatitis. These individuals have a guarded prognosis in that they may develop cirrhosis with hepatic failure and succumb to the disease.

Non-A, non-B hepatitis does not produce a detectable antigen or antibody in the patient's serum. The diagnosis is usually based on clinical findings, as well as the elevation of SGOT and SGPT and the absence of antibodies or antigens to HAV or HBV.

Treatment

There is no specific therapy for acute viral hepatitis in either the nonpregnant or the pregnant patient. However, the liver of a pregnant patient in her 2nd or 3rd trimester is thought to be more susceptible to noxious liver stimuli. Therefore, if a pregnant patient is found to have a rising SGOT and SGPT, it is recommended that she be hospitalized with restricted activity until her liver functions begin to return to normal. Isolation procedures should be followed to prevent transmission of the virus.

Immune globulin, immune serum globulin (ISG) for hepatitis A exposure, and hepatitis B immune serum globulin (HBIG) should be administered shortly after exposure. Early administration of ISG or HBIG is capable of modifying or arresting the infection. HBIG should be given when direct exposure to HBV occurs via a needle stick or broken skin contact with blood, following sexual intercourse, or by exchange of saliva through kissing. The dosage of ISG is 0.02 ml/kg of body weight, with a repeat dose in 28 days. Prior to administering HBIG, blood studies should be obtained for measurement of SGOT and SGPT and presence of HB$_s$Ag and anti-HB$_s$. If the individual is negative for HB$_s$Ag and anti-HB$_s$, then HBIG should be administered. Sera should be obtained at 2 and 6 months after exposure for testing of SGOT, SGPT, HB$_s$Ag, and anti-HB$_s$. Individuals who were initially positive for HB$_s$Ag and anti-HB$_s$ do not need HBIG.

Pregnant patients with antigenemia, i.e., those who are positive for HB$_s$Ag and HB$_e$Ag, have a greater than 50 percent chance of infecting their offspring. Infants born to these women should receive HBIG. Mothers positive for HB$_s$Ag and anti-HB$_e$ have a 10 percent chance of infecting their infants; however, their infants should also receive HBIG. HB$_s$Ag-positive mothers should be advised not to breastfeed their infants. These women should be instructed in handwashing and other precautionary techniques to be used when coming in contact with their infants. There is no need to separate the infant and the mother; however, the infant should not be placed in the nursery with the other infants.

MUMPS (PAROTITIS)

Epidemiology

Man is the only known natural host of mumps virus. The virus is spread via respiratory droplets, direct contact, or fomites. The peak contagious period is just prior to or during the initial attack of parotitis.

Ninety percent of mumps cases occur in individuals less than 14 years of age, although infants less than 12 months old are usually protected by transplacentally acquired immunity. Women of childbearing age are unlikely to be susceptible, and the problem of prenatal exposure to mumps virus is not very common.

Microbiology

Mumps is caused by a member of the paramyxovirus family, which includes the paramyxoviruses (mumps, parainfluenza, and Newcastle disease virus), the morbilliviruses (measles), and the pneumoviruses (respiratory syncytial virus). The virus consists of a nucleocapsid made up of a single strand of RNA surrounded by protein units that have RNA-polymerase activity. The nucleocapsid is surrounded by a complex envelope of glycoprotein, lipid, and nonglycosylated protein structures exhibiting various characteristic viral antigens.

Infection

A nonspecific prodrome of fever, headache, malaise, and anorexia heralds the onset of clinical mumps after an incubation period of 2 to 4 weeks (usually 16 to 18 days). Parotid tenderness follows within a day or two. Over the next 2 or 3 days, the parotid glands enlarge rapidly, causing severe pain, with an accompanying fever as high as 40°C. Thereafter, signs and symptoms rapidly resolve over the next week or so.

Parotitis occurs in 60 to 70 percent of persons with mumps. Other salivary glands are affected perhaps 10 percent of the time. In addition, epididymo-orchitis may occur in up to 25 percent of postpubertal males and oophoritis in 5 percent of postpubertal females. The next most common manifestation of mumps is central nervous system infection. Approximately half of patients exhibit CSF pleocytosis, while up to 10 percent have actual aseptic meningitis. Rarely encephalitis occurs.

Mumps infection during pregnancy has been a mildly controversial topic. Most reports of congenital malformations are anecdotal and not supported by findings of large cohort studies, which demonstrate a slight increase in fetal deaths associated with first-trimester maternal infection. Fetuses infected in the first trimester who do not abort are usually of low birth weight.

There is a suggestion that intrauterine mumps infection may be associated with endocardial fibroelastosis (EFE) in the neonate. A high incidence of positive mumps skin test has been demonstrated in children with EFE. This is supported to some extent by chick embryo studies. However, since EFE and intrauterine mumps infection are both uncommon entities, the association is still very tenuous.

Diagnosis

Mumps is commonly diagnosed by clinical examination. This is especially easy in cases of appropriate prodrome followed by obvious parotitis in a person with a history of exposure. If a case is atypical, or if extraparotid infection occurs that may be due to other viruses, virus may be isolated from saliva, urine, or CSF (if indicated) during the period from several days before until 4 to 5 days after the onset of clinical illness.

Serologic mumps testing demonstrates a fourfold rise in antibody titer, measured by hemagglutination inhibition (HI), complement fixation, or neutralization tests. The HI test has a high rate of cross-reactivity with parainfluenza viral infections, and hence must be used cautiously.

Treatment

Therapy of mumps infection is purely supportive. There have been reports that injection of mumps immunoglobulin may reduce the incidence of orchitis in men. The patient should, of course, be isolated from susceptible individuals to prevent spread of the disease.

The cornerstone of mumps therapy is active immunization with live attenuated mumps virus vaccine. This is usually given to infants at age 15 months, in combination with measles and rubella vaccine. A single inoculation produces an antibody response in 95 percent of subjects. The vaccine should not be administered to pregnant patients, since it is a live virus.

CONDYLOMA ACUMINATUM

Epidemiology

Warts in humans present either as condyloma acuminatum, verruca vulgaris, verruca plana, or verruca plantaris. The verruca varieties usually occur on the skin, whereas the condylomas tend to occur on mucous membranes. Although these lesions are seen world-wide and know no age, sex, or racial barriers, the obstetrician-gynecologist is the physician who usually treats patients with condyloma acuminatum. The specific concerns are the presence, number, and distribution of genital lesions, infection of the newborn, treatment of the pregnant patient, and possible long-term maternal sequelae.

Microorganism

The human papillomavirus (HPV) belongs to the group papovaviridae, which causes condyloma acuminatum. The HPV is a small icosahedral DNA virus. The virus gains entrance to the host cell and enters the nucleus, gaining control of nucleic acid and protein synthesis. HPV can produce latent, chronic, and proliferative infection.

Infection

Condyloma acuminatum is transmitted via direct contact, but fomites can also serve as a source of infection. However, the most common route of transmission is sexual in-tercourse. The incubation period is thought to be from 2 to 6 months.

The lesions begin as small verrucous or pyriform growths on the labia, fourchette, urethral meatus, vagina, cervix, perineum, or anus. The lesions may appear as flat or endophytic growths, with the verrucose form being the most easily recognized. Spread of the disease is accomplished by the formation of small seedling-like growths adjacent to the initial lesions. These verrucose-like growths enlarge, proliferate, and may coalesce to form large lesions that may replace the labia (Fig. 5–5). Proliferation is often associated with concomitant vaginitis, poor personal hygiene, use of oral contraceptives, pregnancy, and altered cell-mediated immunity. Condylomatous lesions occur more frequently in moist areas and thus have a predilection for mucosa or mucosa-like surfaces; they are rarely seen on the normally drier dermal areas.

Two problems have been raised in conjunction with condyloma acuminatum: the development of malignant change and the formation of laryngeal papillomatosis. Once the virus infects the cell, the host cell undergoes marked alterations, including alterations of the nucleus. An association has been

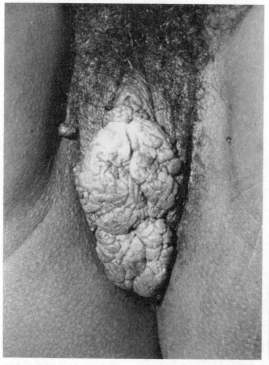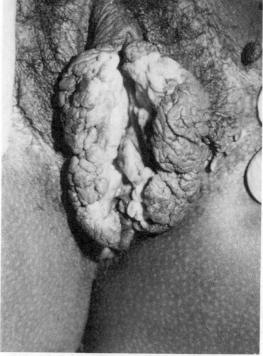

Figure 5–5. Condyloma acuminatum lesions have replaced the labia. This patient was delivered by cesarean section.

made between the occurrence of vulvar carcinoma and condyloma acuminatum, but although vulvar carcinoma has been reported in some individuals with condyloma acuminatum, this association has not been substantiated by epidemiologic data. The second problem that has surfaced is the development of laryngeal papillomatosis in offspring born to mothers with genital condyloma acuminatum at the time of delivery.

Diagnosis

The greatest difficulty in making a diagnosis of condyloma acuminatum is realizing that not all lesions are exophytic, pyriform, or soft. The lesion may be flat or endophytic, and therefore may go unrecognized by the naked eye. The exophytic lesions are usually white, whereas the flat and endophytic lesions may not appear different from the surrounding tissue on gross examination.

The presence of condyloma acuminatum in the female should alert the physician to have her male partner examined. However, if the male patient is sent to a urologist who has no real interest in sexually transmitted diseases, he will conduct a gross examination that will more than likely be unrewarding. The male penis must be examined colposcopically, since the lesions are usually minute and are on the penile shaft. It should be remembered that if the female develops condyloma acuminatum, the virus must have been transmitted to her, and the most likely route is via sexual intercourse.

If the lesion becomes indurated or ulcerated or does not respond to treatment, a biopsy is warranted. If the lesions are flat, sessile, red or white, and generally do not resemble condylomata acuminata, a biopsy is indicated. It is important that the abnormal-appearing areas be biopsied before any treatment is begun, because agents such as podophyllin will cause atypical changes.

Treatment

The pregnant patient with condyloma acuminatum poses several interesting challenges for the obstetrician. What modality should be used for treatment? Should the patient with genital condyloma acuminatum in labor be delivered by cesarean section?

The initial procedure in the treatment of the patient with condyloma acuminatum is the taking of a detailed sexual history. It is important to determine whether the patient practices oral-genital sex or anal intercourse, since the virus attacks any mucosal epithelium. If extragenital sites are involved but remain undetected, they will serve as foci for viral shedding.

If the pregnant patient has lesions on the cervix or vagina, they should *not* be treated with podophyllin. It should first be determined whether or not the lesions are secondarily infected. If they are, antibiotics should be employed. A culture should be obtained and Gram-stained; commonly S. *aureus*, S. *epidermidis*, or perhaps a gram-negative bacterium will be involved. An initial choice would be a first-generation cephalosporin. If there are a few small isolated lesions on the vulva, then podophyllin can be used. It should be noted that the chemical composition of podophyllin preparations varies from one batch to another. The half-life of podophyllin is from 1 to 4.5 hours. The toxic effects range from local irritation to acute systemic toxicity. The patient may experience dizziness, general weakness, emesis, diarrhea, hypotension, bradycardia, stupor, depressed respirations, progressive peripheral neuropathy, and depression of the bone marrow. Small lesions on the vulva, vagina, and cervix may be treated with either bichloroacetic or trichloroacetic acid. The lesions in the pregnant patient are more vascular than in the nonpregnant patient, so if topical therapy is used, bleeding may occur. Small lesions on the vulva may be treated with electrocoagulation.

Patients who are pregnant tend to develop large cauliflower-like lesions that sometimes fill the vagina or replace the labia. In such cases, it is best to allow the patient to reach term and deliver by cesarean section. Following the termination of the pregnancy, the lesions will become reduced in size over a short period of time and can be managed more easily.

Bacterial Infections

SYPHILIS

Epidemiology

Syphilis, caused by *Treponema pallidum*, continues to be a major sexually transmitted disease. The infection is transmitted by direct contact with an infected lesion, by accidental inoculation, or by blood transfusion from a syphilitic donor. Congenital syphilis occurs when there is maternal bacteremia and *T. pallidum* crosses the placenta and infects the fetus.

Syphilis is most prevalent among those in the reproductive age group. The Centers for Disease Control estimates that there are probably more than 400,000 cases of untreated syphilis and only about 80,000 reported cases yearly.

Microbiology

Treponema pallidum is a spiral bacterium that is 0.25 μm in diameter and up to 15 μm long. The bacterium moves by an undulating motion as well as by a corkscrew-like rotation about its long axis. Identification of the bacterium is accomplished by dark-field microscopy of a serum sample obtained from a chancre, which enables the examiner to note the organism's morphology as well as its characteristic motion.

T. pallidum was once considered an anaerobic bacterium but is now known to utilize oxygen for growth and reproduction. The spirochetes require moisture and tissue for survival. The treponemes are destroyed by drying, water, heat, and disinfectants.

Infection

T. pallidum gains entrance to the body through minute abrasions or by penetration of intact mucous membranes. Once the treponemes have entered the body, they enter the lymphatic and vascular systems. The incubation period from infection to development of the chancre is approximately 10 to 90 days and is dependent upon the number of organisms present. An ulcerative lesion forms at the point of contact—usually the genital organs—but it may occur at other sites, such as the lips, oral mucosa, fingers, or anus.

Diagnosis

The diagnosis of syphilis can be difficult at times. Syphilis has been referred to as the "great mimic." There are three stages of syphilis—primary, secondary, and tertiary—which are related to the time of onset of the infection.

Primary syphilis is characterized by the appearance of a nontender, indurated, clean ulcer known as a chancre (Fig. 5–6). The

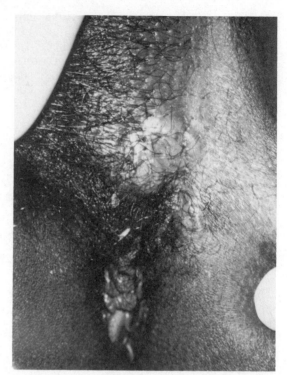

Figure 5–6. Primary chancre of syphilis. Note that ulcers appear clean with erythematous base.

ulcer contains numerous spirochetes and, therefore, is highly infectious. Primary syphilis is best diagnosed by the identification of spirochetes in serum obtained by scraping the surface of an ulcer, which is examined by dark-field microscopy. In the female patient, the primary chancre may go unnoticed because it is painless and may form between labial folds or on the cervix. Therefore a careful examination of the vulva, vagina, and cervix must be performed on all patients.

Secondary syphilis occurs after the spirochetes invade the tissues of the host—usually 8 to 10 weeks after the appearance of the primary chancre, which generally disappears before the onset of secondary syphilis. The disease may affect every organ of the body, but the diagnosis is usually made on the basis of skin lesions. The cutaneous lesions may be quite varied, manifesting as macular, papular, papulosquamous, pustular, follicular, or nodular lesions (Fig. 5–7). It is because of this great variety of presentations that syphilis is referred to as the "great mimic." The lesions often appear on the trunk and extremities as well as on the palms and soles (Fig. 5–8).

The patient may develop alopecia, which occurs in a random fashion, leaving patches

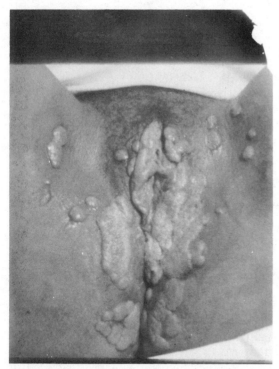

Figure 5–7. Secondary syphilis: anogenital condylomata lata.

of hair. The alopecia is temporary and resolves whether treatment is begun or not. In addition, the patient may develop symptoms of systemic illness. She may present with malaise, anorexia, headache, sore throat, arthralgia, and low-grade fever. She may also develop lymphodenopathy with large non-tender, discrete lymph nodes.

Latent syphilis is categorized as either *early* latent syphilis, referring to disease of less than 4 years, or *late* latent syphilis, denoting disease of more than 4 years. Early latent syphilis is associated with relapses of mucocutaneous lesions if the patient is not treated and is infectious. Latent syphilis is present when the patient has serologic evidence of disease but has no clinical signs or symptoms of syphilis. She may or may not have a history of primary or secondary syphilis, and the cerebrospinal fluid may be normal. The diagnosis is established by obtaining positive results with the reagin serum test when repeated several times, together with a positive fluorescent treponemal antibody-absorption test. Diseases known to produce false-positive reagin tests, such as infectious mononucleosis, hepatitis, leprosy, systemic lupus erythematous, rheumatoid arthritis, and sarcoidosis, should be ruled out. Late latent syphilis may be transmitted to a fetus in utero or to transfusion recipients.

Tertiary syphilis is a noninfectious destructive stage of the disease, manifested by gummatous (late benign) syphilis, cardiovascular syphilis, and neurosyphilis. The difficulty with this stage of the disease is that it can be present even though the serologic tests for syphilis are nonreactive. Gummatous syphilis is characterized by lesions that appear mainly on the skin but which may also develop in bone, liver, and the cardiovascular and central nervous systems. The cutaneous gummas appear as superficial nodules or punched-out ulcers. This stage of the disease appears in untreated individuals from 1 to 10 years after the initial lesions.

Cardiovascular syphilis occurs 10 or more years after the initial infection. The primary lesion is aortitis. The elastic tissue of the aorta is destroyed and replaced by fibrous tissue. The ascending and transverse segments of the aorta are primarily affected.

Neurosyphilis occurs within 5 to 35 years after the initial infection in untreated individuals. Early central nervous system involvement is usually asymptomatic. Because nontreponemal tests are nonreactive in one

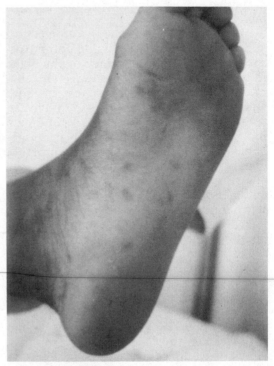

Figure 5–8. Rash of secondary syphilis: papular rash on sole of foot.

third of patients with neurosyphilis, a specific treponemal test should be done in patients suspected of having neurosyphilis. In asymptomatic neurosyphilis the cerebrospinal fluid is abnormal (i.e., >5 mononuclear cells/mm^3), total protein is >40 mg/100 ml, and there is a reactive (positive) VDRL.

Neurosyphilis may present as a meningovascular and parenchymatous syphilis. Meningovascular syphilis includes meningitis and central nervous system involvement resulting from cerebrovascular occlusion, infarction, and encephalomalacia. Parenchymatous syphilis includes syphilitic pareses and tabes dorsalis.

Pregnant women who contract syphilis may transmit the disease to their fetus at any time during the pregnancy. If the pregnant patient is untreated, approximately 25 percent of the fetuses will die in utero, 30 percent will die shortly after birth, and 40 percent of the survivors will develop late syphilis. The clinical manifestations of congenital syphilis can be divided into early disease (occurring before age 2) and late congenital syphilis (occurring after age 2). The earlier the onset of signs and symptoms, the poorer the prognosis. Active disease at birth is associated with a higher neonatal death rate.

Serologic diagnosis of syphilis can be established by reactive reagin or treponemal tests. The reagin tests are nontreponemal and are based on a modification of the Wasserman cardiolipin test; they include the following: Venereal Disease Research Laboratory (VDRL), rapid plasma reagin (RPR), automated reagin (ART), and unheated serum reagin (USR). The VDRL and RPR are the two most widely diagnostic nontreponemal tests employed in the United States. The treponemal tests use *T. pallidum* as the antigen and detect specific antitreponemal antibodies; these tests are performed for verification procedures. The standard test used today is the fluorescent treponemal antibody–absorption (FTA-ABS) test.

The nontreponemal reagin tests are the most commonly used diagnostic tests. The VDRL becomes positive 1 to 3 weeks after the appearance of the primary chancre. The titer rises rapidly and reaches a peak dilution of 1:256. The titer then falls as the patient enters the latent stage of syphilis. After 10 to 20 years the VDRL begins to plateau and may remain at a dilution of 1:4 to 1:8. However, some individuals may develop nonreactive sera even in the absence of treatment. The FTA-ABS becomes especially important in those individuals who are suspected of having syphilis but in whom the VDRL is nonreactive.

Treatment

Penicillin remains the treatment of choice for syphilis. Primary, secondary, and early latent syphilis can be treated with benzathine penicillin G, 2.4 million units given intramuscularly, or with aqueous procaine penicillin G, 4.8 million units, given as 600,000 units by intramuscular injection daily for 8 days. Patients who are allergic to penicillin can be treated with erythromycin, 500 mg orally 4 times daily for 15 days.

Late syphilis is best treated with benzathine penicillin G, 7.2 million units given in doses of 2.4 million units intramuscularly weekly for 3 weeks, or aqueous procaine penicillin G, 600,000 units intramuscularly daily for 15 days. Pregnant patients who are allergic to penicillin may be treated with erythromycin, 500 mg orally 4 times a day for 30 days.

Penicillin is highly effective in the treatment of syphilis; however, treatment failures do occur, and posttreatment follow-up is extremely important. Posttreatment follow-up is more important when an antibiotic other than penicillin is used. Individuals treated for primary and secondary syphilis should be monitored with quantitative VDRL measurements at 1, 3, 6, 9, and 12 months. Those patients with latent and late syphilis should be followed at 1, 3, 6, 9, 12, 18, and 24 months. Patients with primary syphilis who were adequately treated will have a negative titer within 2 years. Of those individuals with secondary syphilis, 25 per cent will remain VDRL-positive 2 years after treatment. In syphilis of less than 2 years' duration, the VDRL titer will decrease or stabilize at a low titer. Individuals with syphilis of more than 2 years' duration who are successfully treated will be seropositive and have a reactive VDRL.

TUBERCULOSIS

Epidemiology

Tuberculosis results from infection by *Mycobacterium tuberculosis*. Transmission is by aerosolized droplets of liquid containing the bacteria, which are inhaled by a noninfected individual and taken into the lung. The bacteria become lodged in the alveoli, where they implant and cause infection.

Most individuals who contract tuberculosis are asymptomatic. Infected individuals are frequently detected by exhibiting a hypersensitivity reaction when subjected to intradermal injection of mycobacterial protein. In adults, the disease usually remains asymptomatic after the initial infection, and it is only years later that clinical signs and symptoms of infection occur.

Microbiology

Mycobacterium tuberculosis is an obligate aerobic, nonmotile, nonencapsulated, acid-fast bacillus. The bacteria do not readily take up stains and require heat to take up basic fuchsin dye. Once the bacteria are stained, they resist decolorization by alcoholic solution of mineral acids. The bacteria are slow-growing, requiring up to 24 hours to replicate. They are also resistant to desiccation and produce no endotoxin.

Infection

Tuberculosis is primarily an infection of the pulmonary system. Infection of the female genital tract usually results from hematogenous dissemination from the pulmonary tract. However, if the gastrointestinal tract is the portal of entry, dissemination follows involvement of the lymphatics in the area of the cecum and terminal ileum. The fallopian tubes are the primary site of infection, which usually results in sterility. Approximately 2 to 5 percent of all cases of infertility are due to genital tuberculosis.

The pregnant patient with tuberculosis will most likely be asymptomatic. A noninfected pregnant or nonpregnant patient, who subsequently becomes infected, inhales droplets containing *M. tuberculosis*, which then become lodged on the surface of alveoli and are phagocytized by macrophages. It is within the macrophages that the bacteria multiply. Once the inflammatory response has begun, bacteria outside the macrophages also begin to reproduce and migrate into the pulmonary bloodstream, through which they are disseminated and may lodge anywhere in the body. Progression of the disease is noted by the development of tubercles and caseation necrosis.

Symptomatic patients may present with malaise, fatigue, loss of appetite, weight loss, and temperatures of 103° to 104°F (39.4° to 40°C). An increase in body temperature occurs in late afternoon and evening and is accompanied by night sweats. Patients in the initial stages of disease usually have no cough and produce little sputum. When the disease has progressed to the cavitary stage, the patient has a chronic cough and produces a mucopurulent sputum containing streaks of blood.

Congenital infection is rare but may occur following maternal bacillemia. Fetal infection follows thrombin formation in the intervillous spaces, which stimulates an inflammatory response in the adjacent placental tissue. Infection of placental tissue leads to fetal infection. The primary focus of infection in the congenitally infected fetus is the liver or regional lymph nodes.

Diagnosis

The diagnosis of *M. tuberculosis* infection is established by isolating and identifying the bacteria. A tentative diagnosis can be established if typical acid-fast bacilli are found in smears of sputum. Infection may go unnoticed, since the primary infection is normally asymptomatic. The tuberculin skin test can be used as a screening procedure. A positive skin test indicates a history of tuberculosis and not necessarily active disease. The purified protein derivative skin test (PPD intradermal skin test, also known as the Mantoux test) is administered by injecting 0.1 ml in the dermis of a patient. A positive tuberculin reaction is characterized by an area of erythema and induration more than 10 mm in diameter forming within 48 hours. Patients with a positive PPD should have a chest roentgenogram if they are known converters, or if the time of conversion is unknown and if the history or physical examination suggests disease.

Treatment

Treatment of tuberculosis is based on the administration of one or more antibicrobial agents to prevent the growth of resistant organisms, and the therapy must be continued for a prolonged period of time. Chemotherapy for established or suspected active tuberculosis in the pregnant woman is similar to that in the nonpregnant woman. Prophylactic chemotherapy should be withheld during pregnancy and administered following delivery.

The recommended therapy regimen is isoniazid (INH), 300 mg/day, plus ethambutol, 15 mg/kg/day. INH has been shown to be associated with a twofold increase in fetal malformations when administered to those with active disease. Pyridoxine should be administered concomitantly with INH to prevent fetal neurotoxicity. Ethambutol is not contraindicated during pregnancy.

LISTERIOSIS

Epidemiology

Listeriosis is caused by *Listeria monocytogenes*, which is found in soil, water, sewage, and animals—both domestic and wild, including birds, flies, ticks, and crustaceans. It is also transmitted via consumption of unpasteurized milk or contaminated meat. Approximately one third of the cases occur during pregnancy, and the disease can be transmitted transplacentally to the fetus. Infection in adults occurs most frequently in those over 40 years of age, and is associated with a mortality approaching 50 percent.

Microbiology

Listeria monocytogenes is a gram-positive non–spore-forming bacillus. The organism is microaerophilic and motile, and causes hemolysis when grown on blood agar. When gram-stained in clinical specimens, the organisms may appear coccoid and are easily mistaken for gram-positive cocci. Listeria may be mistaken for *Corynebacterium*, *Erysipelothrix*, beta-hemolytic streptococci, or enterococci.

Infection

Listeriosis is not manifested by any unique characteristics. The patient may be asymptomatic, have only genital colonization, or present with a flu-like or mononucleosis-like syndrome. Some patients present with high spiking temperatures accompanied by back and flank pain. Others initially present with diarrhea and subsequently develop bacteremia. A patient may be totally asymptomatic but present with intrauterine fetal de-

mise. If maternal infection is treated early, fetal infection may be averted.

Rupture of the amniotic membranes allows for ascending infection. Maternal fever is usually coincident with the onset of labor and the development of chorioamnionitis. In most instances, when the fetus is delivered and the uterus evacuated, the mother's clinical illness resolves. However, in some instances maternal infection may progress to meningitis. A careful history will usually reveal that the meningitis was preceded by gastrointestinal disturbance or mild respiratory infection. Following the initial symptoms, the patient develops headache, myalgia, fever, chills, nausea, vomiting, and a stiff neck.

Fetal infection usually results in intrauterine death. Liveborn infants that were infected in utero frequently die within a week or two of birth. They develop cardiovascular collapse and respiratory as well as CNS complications.

Diagnosis

Listeriosis is often not detected because of the lack of symptoms. Because *L. monocytogenes* is morphologically similar to *Corynebacterium*, cultures of the organism are frequently discarded under the assumption that they are diphtheroid contaminants. It would be beneficial to request that bacteriology laboratory personnel screen for listeria whenever culture arouses suspicion.

Gram-stained preparations that reveal small, short, gram-positive rods with rounded ends should arouse suspicion for listeria. The organism can be differentiated from other diphtheroids by its motility at 20° to 30°C. *L. monocytogenes* can be easily cultured from spinal fluid, blood, and urine.

Treatment

Listeria monocytogenes is sensitive to penicillin, ampicillin, cephalothin, erythromycin, chloramphenicol, and tetracycline. Therapy should be continued for 2 weeks. The drug of choice is ampicillin, 40 to 60 mg/kg/day intravenously every 6 hours; or penicillin 300,000 units/kg/day, intravenously every 6 hours. Erythromycin, 60 mg/kg/day intravenously every 6 hours, may be used in patients who are allergic to penicillin. Asymptomatic colonization may be treated with ampicillin, 40 to 60 mg/kg/day orally every 6 hours. The isolates should be tested for antibiotic sensitivities, and patients should be recultured after therapy is complete.

CHORIOAMNIONITIS

Epidemiology

Chorioamnionitis is an infection of the chorion, amnion, and amniotic fluid. Approximately 1 percent of all pregnant women are at risk of developing chorioamnionitis, which is a major cause of perinatal—as well as maternal—morbidity and mortality. The histologic evidence of chorioamnionitis far exceeds the incidence of clinically manifested chorioamnionitis. In most fatal cases of fetal intrauterine bacterial infection, histologic chorioamnionitis can be demonstrated. Although chorioamnionitis is usually associated with premature rupture of the amniotic membranes, infection of the amniotic membranes and amniotic fluid has been demonstrated in patients with intact membranes.

Chorioamnionitis occurs most frequently in patients who are in labor and whose membranes have ruptured. Intrauterine infection may occur following amniocentesis or intrauterine transfusion; however, infection is most commonly due to the invasion of the uterine contents by members of the endogenous microflora of the lower genital tract. Organisms introduced from the external environment, such as N. gonorrhoeae, have also been implicated in chorioamnionitis.

Microbiology

Infection is frequently caused by the bacteria that inhabit the genital tract; however, organisms such as N. gonorrhoeae, L. monocytogenes, herpes simplex virus, and cytomegalovirus have also been implicated in chorioamnionitis. Among the endogenous bacteria, E. coli, group B beta-hemolytic streptococci (GBBS), anaerobic streptococci, and Bacteroides are frequently involved in chorioamnionitis. The isolation of N. gonorrhoeae, Listeria monocytogenes, group A or B beta-hemolytic streptococci, or Staphylococcus aureus should be considered evidence of pathogenesis.

Infection

There are numerous gram-negative as well as gram-positive aerobic and anaerobic bacteria present in the lower genital tract. Many of these bacteria have the potential to be pathogenic. During pregnancy the physiologic environment of the lower genital tract is altered, owing to the hormonal changes that affect the pH, glycogen level, and other local environmental parameters, and these changes, in turn, will affect the normal bacterial flora with regard to growth and the ratio of one genus to another.

There are basically two barriers protecting the fetus against infection. The cervical mucus is a formidable barrier preventing the bacteria from advancing up the endocervical canal and thereby colonizing the amniotic membranes. The fetus and amniotic fluid are encased and protected by the amniotic membranes. Once the more pathogenic bacteria, e.g., E. coli or GBBS, advance up the endocervical canal, they may colonize the amniotic membranes and weaken them by enzymatic activity, thereby facilitating rupture or bacterial crossing of the membranes. Although the amniotic fluid contains bacterial inhibitors, the concentrations of these inhibitors in the second and early third trimesters are low, and therefore they may not effectively protect against the bacteria. In addition, the amniotic fluid contains glucose and amino acids, making it a good medium for the growth of bacteria.

Chorioamnionitis can lead to maternal or fetal infection. The fetus may become infected either by swallowing infected amniotic fluid, by inhaling the fluid, or by hematogenous spread from the placenta. If these organisms gain entrance to the lungs, the bacteria multiply in the intraalveolar spaces, and the fetus develops an intraalveolar pneumonia. If fetal infection begins with bacterial colonization of the fetal side of the placental circulation, venous vasculitis ensues and fetal septicemia may occur.

The development of chorioamnionitis with intact membranes has been reported with L. monocytogenes, GBBS, E. coli, and Streptobacillus moniliformis. In some instances, a hematogenous route is suspected, since the mother presents with a mild illness. However, in some instances the mother may be completely asymptomatic except for being in premature labor, and the site of origin of the bacteria is unknown.

Chorioamnionitis exposes both the mother and the fetus to serious infection. The fetus may develop pneumonia, sepsis, or meningitis. Women with chorioamnionitis who deliver vaginally are at relatively low risk of developing a postpartum infection, whereas those who deliver by cesarean section have a much greater risk of developing postpartum endometritis, peritonitis, septic pelvic vein thrombosis, and sepsis, and of dying.

Diagnosis

The diagnosis of chorioamnionitis may be difficult to establish, especially during the initial stages, since the clinical diagnostic criteria are vague. The risk of maternal infection increases with the amount of time that has passed since the membranes have ruptured.

Initially the patient may present in premature labor with intact membranes and no other findings. Often these individuals are at less than 34 weeks' gestation, and tocolytic agents are administered, as well as corticosteroids. It would be prudent to determine whether infection is present before embarking on such a course. Amniocentesis may be attempted in order to have the amniotic fluid Gram-stained and cultured for aerobic and anaerobic bacteria. If bacteria are seen in the Gram-stained preparation, a tentative diagnosis of chorioamnionitis can be established. Bacterial growth is accompanied by the release of pyrogens and endotoxins that will cause maternal fever and tachycardia. This will also be reflected in a rise in the fetal heart rate. Progression of the infection will be manifested by the development of uterine tenderness and a discharge that may or may not be purulent or malodorous. The presence of a foul odor is characteristic of an anaerobic infection.

Treatment

If amniotic fluid can be obtained via amniocentesis or by intrauterine aspiration, it should be cultured for aerobic and anaerobic bacteria. If fluid cannot be obtained, which is frequently the case when the membranes have ruptured, an endocervical specimen should be obtained for the culture and identification of N. gonorrhoeae, GBBS, L. monocytogenes, H. influenzae, and Chlamydia trachomatis.

Once the diagnosis is established, anti-biotic therapy should be instituted. If the patient is thought to have a mild case of chorioamnionitis, and vaginal delivery is imminent, then antibiotics may be withheld. Many patients who deliver vaginally with mild chorioamnionitis have spontaneous resolution of their infection following delivery. However, if the labor appears protracted or dysfunctional and delivery is not imminent, or if the infection has progressed to a more advanced stage, then antibiotics should be administered.

The newer broad-spectrum antibiotics, such as mezlocillin, piperacillin, ticarcillin, and cefoxitin, are effective against gram-positive and gram-negative aerobic and anaerobic bacteria. These antibiotics have an advantage in that they may be used as single agents that have less serious toxicity than do combinations of antibiotics that include the aminoglycosides. Antibiotics cross the placenta and achieve peak levels in the fetal circulation within an hour after parenteral administration to the mother. Antibiotics also enter the amniotic fluid, but at a slower rate. The concentration will often be below therapeutic levels.

One very critical aspect in the management of chorioamnionitis is delivery of the fetus, as this drains the uterus of infected material and allows for treatment of the fetus. The tendency is to want to deliver the patient immediately; however, this often means a cesarean section, which places the mother at a risk for serious postpartum infection. If the patient is in good labor and making progress and there is no evidence of fetal distress, then she should be allowed to deliver via the vaginal route, while being closely observed for the progression of infection during labor.

If the patient is not in strong active labor, or if she has a dysfunctional labor pattern or fails to make adequate progress, an attempt should be made to establish a good labor pattern. If this fails, or if there are additional obstetric indications, cesarean section should be performed. It should be pointed out that as the infection progresses and the myometrium is invaded, the muscle loses its capacity to contract effectively and a dysfunctional labor ensues. These patients are also at risk for severe postpartum uterine atony. In the postpartum period the patient may develop a serious endomyoparametritis, bacteremia, and sepsis. The patient who develops extensive infection, myometritis, and necrosis may require a cesarean hysterectomy.

GENITAL MYCOPLASMAS

Epidemiology

The actual epidemiology of the mycoplasmas is extremely difficult to delineate. It is known that these organisms inhabit the vagina and urethra and are sexually transmissible. However, carriage rates in asymptomatic women may be as high as 60 percent for *Mycoplasma hominis* and 80 percent for *Ureaplasma urealyticum*. Therefore, the exact relationship of carriage to disease, and the usual methods of spread, are nebulous.

Microbiology

The mycoplasmas and *U. urealyticum* are bacteria that lack cell walls. They divide by binary fission and constitute one of the smallest groups of cellular microorganisms; highly pleomorphic, they can pass through filters that retain bacteria and are considered to be gram-negative.

Infection

Genital mycoplasma infection during pregnancy is thought to take the form of chorioamnionitis, postabortal fever, and postpartal fever. In some studies, however, women who were thought to have mycoplasma infections recovered even without antibiotics. Mycoplasmas have also been isolated from the blood of pregnant women who were completely afebrile.

Diagnosis

Both *U. urealyticum* and *M. hominis* may be grown on appropriate artificial media. A patient presenting with dysuria and pyuria, but with negative routine bacterial cultures, is a prime suspect for *Mycoplasma, Ureaplasma,* or *Chylamydia* urethritis. In the absence of the capability to culture for these organisms, treatment may be initiated empirically.

Treatment

The mycoplasmas do not respond to the beta-lactam antibiotics, since they have no cell walls. Tetracycline and related drugs are usually effective against most clinically important species. Erythromycin is effective against *U. urealyticum*, whereas lincomycin is effective against *M. hominis*. Erythromycin is the antibiotic of choice for the pregnant patient.

CHLAMYDIA

Epidemiology

A variety of diseases have been associated with *C. trachomatis*. Besides trachoma and neonatal conjunctivitis, lymphogranuloma venereum (LGV) has long been known to be caused by certain serotypes of *C. trachomatis*. Recently a syndrome of infant pneumonitis and several forms of urogenital infection have been described.

The common thread in many forms of *C. trachomatis* infection is genital carriage and sexual transmission. Asymptomatic male and female carriers probably serve as a reservoir and pass the organism by sexual contact. Further, genital carriage by the pregnant woman at parturition serves to colonize the infant, leading to conjunctivitis. If the infant's tracheal tree is similarly colonized, pneumonitis may result.

Microorganism

C. trachomatis is a bacterium. It contains both DNA and RNA, divides by binary fission, stains gram-negative, and is susceptible to antibiotics. It is an obligate intracellular parasite that depends upon the host cell for a supply of ATP. *C. trachomatis* exists as multiple serotypes. Endemic trachoma is caused by types A, B, Ba, and C. Serotypes De, E, F, G, H, I, J, and K produce infant disease and the urogenital syndromes. LGV is produced by the somewhat different, more invasive serotypes L_1, L_2, and L_3.

Infection

Chlamydia preferentially infects columnar epithelial cells in the human, primarily because these cells have specific receptors that cause the chlamydial organism to bind to them. The human disease syndromes are, therefore, diseases of columnar epithelium.

Neonatal conjunctivitis has been associated with chlamydia, as well as with gonorrhea. The conjunctivitis usually begins within days of birth and is relatively self-limiting, unlike the progressive lesions of endemic trachoma. Colonization of the nasopharynx at birth may lead to the development of a characteristic diffuse pneumonitis in the infant that usually manifests by 4 to 6 weeks of age. In most cases the mother harbors the organism in the endocervix.

The urogenital syndromes associated with *C. trachomatis* include cervicitis, epididymitis, and urethritis. Many cases of the acute urethral syndrome in women, as well as nongonococcal urethritis, are apparently caused by chlamydia. Another important site of chlamydial disease is the columnar epithelium of the fallopian tubes. Acute salpingitis is said to be a major complication of chlamydial colonization in some parts of the world.

The pregnant uterus is at risk for chlamydial infection. Chlamydial colonization increases the risk of pelvic infection after elective abortion. Severe puerperal infection associated with *C. trachomatis* has been reported after cesarean delivery, and a syndrome of late (up to 6 weeks) postpartum endometritis after vaginal delivery has been attributed to the organism.

Maternal cervical carriage of *C. trachomatis* has been reported to be as high as 23 per cent in some groups of patients. Preliminary data suggest that pregnancies complicated by chlamydial infection may have a poor outcome (i.e., stillbirth, premature delivery, abortion) in up to 10 times the usual rate of cases.

Diagnosis

Since chlamydia are intracellular parasites, they can be propagated only in cell culture. After suitable growth and processing, the cells are stained with iodine, enhancing the visibility of the intracellular inclusion bodies, which are then easily seen under the light microscope.

Chlamydial infection may occasionally be documented by a Giemsa or Wright stain of clinical materials. Also a Pap smear may reveal characteristic inclusions in exfoliated cells. Both of these methods are fraught with error and are not standard diagnostic techniques. Infection may be assumed to have occurred if acute and convalescent paired sera show a fourfold rise in titer.

Treatment

In vitro and in vivo studies have shown that *C. trachomatis* is sensitive to tetracyclines, erythromycin, sulfonamides, and rifampin. The Centers for Disease Control recommend therapy with tetracycline, 500 mg orally 4 times per day for 7 days in cases of urogenital disease. Since tetracyclines are contraindicated during pregnancy, erythromycin may be used, 500 mg orally 4 times per day.

Chlamydial conjunctivitis may be prevented in the newborn by prophylaxis with erythromycin ointment at birth. The usual 1 per cent silver nitrate solution used for gonococcal prophylaxis is not effective. Established chlamydial conjunctivitis or infant pneumonitis must be treated with a 3-week course of systemic erythromycin, 50 mg/kg/day in 4 divided doses.

GONORRHEA

Epidemiology

Nearly 3 million cases of gonorrhea occur in the United States annually, an estimate based on the more than 1 million cases actually reported. The majority of cases of gonorrhea are contracted by sexual contact, including oral, genital, and rectal contact. Vertical transmission from mother to infant may also occur. The incidence of *N. gonorrhoeae* isolation during pregnancy varies from population to population and may range from less than 5 percent to over 15 to 20 percent.

Microbiology

N. gonorrhoeae is a gram-negative coccus that classically occurs within leukocytes and in pairs in clinical specimens. The organism is grown on Thayer-Martin medium, with chocolate agar combined with various antibiotics added to inhibit overgrowth by other, less fastidious organisms. The gonococcus may be differentiated from the other *Neisseria* species, such as *N. meningitidis*, by carbohydrate fermentation tests.

There may be some relation between auxotype, antibiotic sensitivity, and clinical virulence among gonococci. Evidence indicates that the strains that are most likely to be invasive are also more likely to show antibiotic resistance and have fewer requirements for the various amino acids in auxotyping.

Infection

N. *gonorrhoeae* infection during pregnancy usually consists of subclinical cervical colonization, because of blockage by the pregnancy of the usual route of access by the organism to the fallopian tubes. The gonococcus possesses surface receptors that allow it to attach to the surfaces of the columnar epithelium of the endocervix. The major areas of primary colonization of the body are the cervix, urethra, pharynx, rectum, and conjunctiva.

The pregnant woman with gonococcal cervical colonization is at risk for several different syndromes. Cervical inflammation and weakening of the neighboring fetal membranes may cause premature rupture of membranes and place the fetus at risk for premature delivery, or infection if delivery is delayed. During labor and delivery, chorioamnionitis and subsequent postpartum endomyoparametritis may develop, occasionally accompanied by bacteremia. In the era before antibiotics, deaths due to gonococcal sepsis, and such entities as gonococcal endocarditis, were common.

If the patient is colonized with N. *gonorrhoeae*, which remains relatively asymptomatic for a long period of time, she seems to be at risk for developing the syndrome known as disseminated gonococcal infection (DGI). Pregnant women seem to be especially at risk for DGI, possibly because they remain asymptomatically colonized; i.e., they are not likely to develop salpingitis. The main clinical presentation during pregnancy is infectional arthritis or tenosynovitis, accompanied by fever, malaise, and often a fine papular, erythematous rash, especially on the extremities. These women may be colonized by the organism on the cervix, urethra, rectum, or pharynx, or combinations thereof. However, it is difficult to isolate the gonococcus from the joint fluid or skin.

Diagnosis

Clinical materials suspected of harboring N. *gonorrhoeae* should be immediately plated on Thayer-Martin medium and placed in an environment enriched with carbon dioxide, e.g., a candle jar, as soon as possible. Prolonged exposure to air or cold temperatures will cause a decrease in yield. All clinical specimens should be Gram-stained in an attempt to demonstrate the gram-negative diplococci that characteristically occur within polymorphonuclear leukocytes. This not only gives immediate information upon which to initiate patient therapy but also serves to augment the results of formal cultures, should they fail to grow for the reasons mentioned above.

Treatment

N. *gonorrhoeae* that does not produce penicillinase is still very sensitive to penicillin. The recommended therapy for uncomplicated urethritis or cervicitis is aqueous procaine penicillin, 4.8 million units intramuscularly in 2 divided doses, accompanied by probenecid, 1.0 g orally. Alternate therapy is ampicillin, 3.5 g orally at one sitting, or amoxicillin, 3.0 g orally; both of these agents are given with probenecid. The patient who is allergic to penicillin is usually treated with tetracycline or doxycycline; however, both of these are contraindicated during pregnancy. The penicillin-allergic pregnant woman with uncomplicated colonization should receive spectinomycin, 2.0 g intramuscularly.

Penicillinase-producing gonococci may be treated with spectinomycin, 2.0 g intramuscularly, as well as with either cefoxitin, 2.0 g intramuscularly, or cefotaxime, 1.0 g intramuscularly, each in combination with 1.0 g of oral probenecid. These regimens are often ineffective against pharyngeal colonization, however. Pharyngeal infection with penicillinase-producing strains may be treated with 9 tablets of trimethoprim-sulfamethoxazole (80 mg/400 mg), although it should be noted that trimethoprim has not been approved for use in pregnancy.

Pregnant patients with DGI must be hospitalized for initial therapy. Several treatment regimens may be used; aqueous crystalline penicillin, 10 million units intravenously per day until improvement, followed by amoxicillin or ampicillin, 500 mg orally 4 times a day for at least a week of total antibiotic therapy; or erythromycin, 500 mg orally 4 times daily for 7 days (for penicillin-allergic patients).

Neonatal ophthalmic prophylaxis may be

accomplished with ocular deposition of 1 percent silver nitrate drops, tetracycline ointment, or erythromycin ointment. Systemic infection or actual conjunctivitis, however, should be treated with aqueous crystalline penicillin in appropriate newborn dosages, or cefotaxime if the organism is known or thought to be penicillinase-producing.

POSTPARTUM ENDOMETRITIS

Epidemiology

The vast majority of cases of postpartum endometritis occur following operative delivery, usually cesarean section. While in most populations the endometritis rate following vaginal delivery is less than 5 percent, postcesarean endometritis rates may be as high as 60 to 80 percent in selected populations of patients.

Risk factors for postpartum endometritis include both endogenous factors such as low socioeconomic status, anemia, and undernutrition (the "poor protoplasm" factors) and exogenous factors (usually associated with cesarean delivery) such as the use of general anesthesia and indwelling catheters. The risk factors for endometritis are listed in Table 5–2.

Microbiology

Multiple bacteria are usually isolated from the uterine cavity of women with postpartum endometritis. Even when care is taken to prevent cervical and vaginal contamination, specimens will usually contain three or more types of general bacteria. Both aerobes and anaerobes are isolated. Thirty per cent of cases will have only aerobic and

Table 5–2. Endometritis Risk Factors

Operative delivery
General anesthesia
Rupture of membranes (≥6 hours pre-op)
Multiple cervical exams
Prolonged labor
Indwelling catheter
Low socioeconomic status
Anemia
Poor nutrition
Cervicitis
Urinary tract infection
Amnionitis
Colonization (e.g., Group B beta-hemolytic streptococcus [GBBS])

Table 5–3. Bacteriology of Endometritis

Aerobes	Anaerobes
Escherichia coli	Peptostreptococcus spp.
Proteus mirabilis	
Streptococcus agalactae	Peptococcus spp.
Streptococcus faecalis	Bacteroides bivius
Neisseria gonorrhoeae	Bacteroides disiens
Klebsiella spp.	Bacteroides melaninogenicus
Citrobacter spp.	Bacteroides fragilis group
	Fusobacterium

30 percent only anaerobic species isolated. The remaining patients will have a mixed aerobic/anaerobic flora. The most frequently isolated bacteria are listed in Table 5–3.

Infection

Bacterial colonization of the endometrial cavity following delivery is unavoidable. However, the magnitude of colonization—i.e., the numbers of organisms present—is related to the length of labor and the amount of time elapsed between rupture of the membranes and the time of delivery; another factor is the degree of manipulation involved in delivery (e.g., use of forceps, manual removal of placenta). In addition, impairment or destruction of natural defenses, such as by immunocompromise due to poor nutrition or by breech of tissue barriers due to cesarean section, aids in the establishment of infection rather than mere surface colonization.

Bacteria are likely to colonize and infect areas of the uterus that have been denuded or damaged, notably the placental attachment site and any cervical or lower segment lacerations and abrasions. Cesarean delivery introduces additional variables: the uterine incision, a foreign body (i.e., the suture material), tissue strangulation, and relative hypoxia.

If the development of endometritis is followed by extension of infection into myometrial tissues through lymphatics and large venous channels, endomyometritis is produced. Bacteria can further disseminate, via the same pathways, into the broad ligaments, paracervical tissues, and adnexae, resulting in endomyoparametritis. At any point in this progression, but depending in large part on host factors and the virulence of the bacteria, microorganisms may gain entry into the bloodstream (bacteremia).

If untreated or improperly treated, postpartum infection, especially endomyoparametritis, may progress to diffuse pelvic cellulitis, pelvic peritonitis, pelvic abscess, and on to disseminated intraabdominal infection. In any stage of the disease after cesarean delivery, wound infection is not uncommon, in part because many of the risks and predisposing factors are the same for the two entities.

Diagnosis

Postpartum endometritis is not difficult to diagnose. Common initial findings include elevated temperature, mild to moderate tachycardia, and uterine tenderness. If pelvic peritonitis is present, lower abdominal rebound tenderness will be evident.

The initial examination is extremely important in the evaluation of a patient with fever during the puerperium. A general physical examination should be performed, with emphasis on the lungs (to rule out pneumonia, especially after general anesthesia) and the cardiovascular system (tachycardia, bounding pulse, weak pulse, elevated or decreased blood pressure). The general abdominal examination should be directed at the presence of rebound and direct tenderness, the size and firmness of the uterine fundus, and the status of the abdominal incision, if present. Specific attention should be directed to any incision that is overtly bloody or leaking any fluid (serum, pus), indurated, erythematous, or unusually tender. Needle aspiration of the wound may be attempted in an effort to locate a seroma, hematoma, or abscess in a suspicious wound.

Cultures should be obtained from the endometrium (with as little cervicovaginal contamination as possible), venous blood, catheterized urine specimen, wound exudate or discharge if present, and sputum if indicated. All specimens should be processed aerobically and anaerobically. It is important to remember that *Neisseria gonorrhoeae* is a common puerperal pathogen in certain patient populations. In such persons, it is a good idea to plate all genital specimens on Thayer-Martin medium as well as on the routine media.

Treatment

Postpartal endometritis is usually due to infection by the aerobic and anaerobic flora of the lower genital tract; therefore, antibiotic therapy should be directed against these bacteria. In the patient with moderate to severe infection, initial therapy with a broad-spectrum agent that has a reasonable anaerobic spectrum and also activity against the Enterobacteriaceae is recommended. Suitable antimicrobial agents are the second-generation cephalosporins such as cefoxitin; third-generation cephalosporins such as moxalactam, cefotaxime, and cefoperazone; and the expanded-spectrum penicillins, such as ticarcillin, mezlocillin, and piperacillin. In the case of a patient who is seriously allergic to penicillin, a combination regimen employing either clindamycin or metronidazole, plus an aminoglycoside, may be substituted. These combinations tend to be more difficult to use, since serum levels of aminoglycosides should be monitored to avoid toxicity.

Initial therapy with single antibiotic agents or the combinations listed above will cure approximately 90 percent of patients with moderate to severe infection. Failures after treatment with the cephalosporin drugs or the combinations are often due to resistant strains of enterococci, requiring the addition of penicillin or ampicillin to effect cure. Failures with the expanded-spectrum penicillins are most often due to resistant gram-negative facultative organisms and respond to the addition of an aminoglycoside. Before adding any other antibiotics, however, the physician should thoroughly reexamine the patient to rule out abscess formation and document that persistent fever and other signs are truly due to continuing endometritis, rather than to such entities as drug fever or septic pelvic vein thrombophlebitis.

PNEUMONIA

Epidemiology

Pneumonia may be caused by a number of infectious organisms, including viruses and bacteria. Most of these agents produce pneumonia in a sporadic manner, and as such there are no true epidemiologic factors to discuss with respect to the organisms themselves. However, host condition is an important predisposition to the development of pneumonia.

Whether pregnant or not, certain groups of women of childbearing age are prone to develop pneumonia. Patients who are asplenic, either iatrogenically or through autosplenectomy, as with sickle cell hemoglobinopathy, have a higher incidence of pneumonia due to encapsulated bacteria, notably *Streptococcus pneumoniae.* Patients from endemic areas are more at risk to develop active *Mycobacterium tuberculosis* pulmonary infection than are members of the usual population, as evidenced by the high incidence of this disease among Southeast Asian immigrants in this country in recent years. Finally, some studies, though not all, implicate pregnancy itself as the factor increasing the rate of pneumonia, especially some of the viral pneumonias such as varicella (chickenpox) pneumonia.

Microorganism

The most common isolate in most studies is *S. pneumoniae.* Culture-negative pneumonia, i.e., presumed viral pneumonia, and pneumonia due to *Mycoplasma pneumoniae* are the other major categories. Other bacteria isolated less frequently include *Haemophilus influenzae, Staphylococcus aureus, M. tuberculosis,* and *E. coli.*

Infection

Pneumonia, whatever the cause, is a clinical syndrome commonly defined by cough, sputum production, fever, and chest roentgenogram demonstration of either lobar consolidation or patchy infiltration of the lungs. Bacterial and viral pneumonias are generally classified by organism.

Pneumonia during pregnancy used to be associated with maternal mortality rates as high as 20 or 30 percent. Advances in antibiotics and medical support technology have decreased this rate to nearly zero in recent surveys. A concomitant rise in the level of neonatal intensive care has dropped the perinatal mortality rate from over 50 percent to less than 10 percent in infants delivered during the acute phase of the disease.

Diagnosis

The woman who presents with fever, productive cough, and possibly dyspnea should be thoroughly examined. The chest should be auscultated and percussed in order to locate any areas of decreased breath sounds, rales or rhonchi, E to A changes, or percus-

sive dullness. Pleural rubs should also be sought.

The heart should be carefully auscultated for rubs, gallops, or murmurs. Bacterial endocarditis is not so rare in pregnancy that it should not be suspected, nor should congestive heart failure be overlooked. Care must be taken not to confuse the rotation of the heart and physiologic murmur due to pregnancy with pathologic changes.

The abdomen and gravid uterus should be examined in the usual manner. The physician should be alert for any signs of premature labor. Fetal tachycardia may be the result of maternal fever. However, fetal tachycardia that is inconsistent with the mother's condition may signal chorioamnionitis, either secondary to maternal bacteremia or as a primary infection. The flanks should be examined for renal tenderness, since renal colic due to calculus or infection may mimic lower lobe pneumonia.

Laboratory examination should include a complete blood count with white cell differential, urinalysis to exclude pyelonephritis or calculus, and a chemistry panel to explore the liver transaminases and rule out acute hepatitis. Serum electrolytes should be measured, as fever, coughing, and the anorexia and nausea accompanying severe infection may cause dehydration and electrolyte disturbances.

If pneumonia is suspected, the physician should not hesitate to obtain posteroanterior and lateral chest roentgenograms, with the abdomen suitably shielded. The risk of radiation to the fetus is far outweighed by the risk of complications if a case of pneumonia is overlooked during pregnancy. If the chest x-ray supports the diagnosis, efforts should be made to isolate the microorganism responsible.

A good tracheal sputum specimen should be obtained for Gram stain and culture and sensitivity testing. If the patient fails to raise sputum, or cannot give a sputum specimen correctly without too much oral contamination, a transtracheal specimen may be aspirated. In the healthy young woman, the trachea should normally be free of leukocytes and bacteria. Sputum or nasopharyngeal specimens may be cultured for viruses if viral infection is suspected and facilities are available.

Finally, blood for acute viral serology may be collected, as well as cold agglutinin titers if *M. pneumoniae* is considered.

Treatment

Therapy for pneumonia during pregnancy is based on the organism suspected. The most common pathogen, S. pneumoniae, is still sensitive to penicillin in this country, although penicillin-tolerant strains are being reported around the world. Penicillin-allergic patients may be treated with erythromycin. If an individual is particularly susceptible to pneumococcal pneumonia because of splenectomy or some immune defect, trivalent pneumococcal vaccine may be administered for future protection. The vaccine is made from polysaccharide bacterial capsule and is not dangerous to the fetus, since there is no live virus. M. pneumoniae is best treated with erythromycin, whereas viral pneumonias are treated with supportive care and vigilance against bacterial superinfection.

URINARY TRACT INFECTION

Epidemiology

Asymptomatic bacteriuria during pregnancy occurs in up to 10 percent of gravidas, depending upon the population examined. One of the more serious possible sequelae to asymptomatic bacteriuria is pyelonephritis, which develops in perhaps 40 percent of patients who have asymptomatic bacteriuria. Intermediate in degree of seriousness of urinary infection is cystitis, which is bacterial infection of the bladder wall with resultant inflammation.

Factors that predispose certain individuals to develop urinary tract infections during pregnancy are at least partially understood and include the following: a progesterone-induced decrease in ureteral motility, leading to relative ureteral distension; partial obstruction of the ureters by the enlarging uterus and the engorged pelvic vasculature; and somewhat decreased perineal hygiene. These all aid, to some extent, in the pathophysiologic course that may lead to infection.

Microorganism

The bacterial species most frequently involved in urinary tract infection are members of the family Enterobacteriaceae. Most initial and uncomplicated urinary infections are due to Escherichia coli, Proteus mirabilis, Klebsiella pneumoniae, and various species of Citrobacter and Enterobacter. Group B beta-hemolytic streptococci may also cause bacteriuria and infection in a small percentage of pregnant patients.

Patients who have been hospitalized, catheterized, or previously treated with antibiotics have a different bacterial flora. Hospital flora tend to consist of resistant gram-negative facultative organisms, including Enterobacter species, the pseudomonads (especially Pseudomonas aeruginosa), and Serratia species. The enterococci, which are notoriously resistant to cephalosporin antibiotics, are more commonly seen in patients following instrumentation of the urinary tract. It is important, therefore, for the patient's previous history to be considered as a factor in the discussion of the possible offending organisms in urinary infections.

Infection

Asymptomatic bacteriuria is, by definition, a "noninfection." The patient has no signs or symptoms of infection, other than a positive urine culture. Cystitis, on the other hand, may be an extremely symptomatic infection. Inflammation of the bladder wall and urethra causes the subjective symptoms of dysuria (pain when the bladder is full) and urinary incontinence resulting from irritability of the detrusor muscle. Occasionally there may even be flank discomfort resembling that seen with pyelonephritis. Physical examination may reveal suprapubic tenderness, especially with the bladder full. If there is significant urethral involvement, the urethral meatus may be erythematous and swollen. The urinary sediment will contain numerous polymorphonuclear leukocytes and bacteria, and occasionally blood.

The patient with pyelonephritis presents with high fever, occasionally to 104°F (40°C), tachycardia, and hypotension if significant bacteremia or bacterial toxemia has occurred. The flank on the side of the infected kidney will be extremely tender to percussion. There may be associated nausea or vomiting.

Pyelonephritis may progress rapidly to gram-negative septic shock, leading ultimately to death. The kidney may develop microabscesses that eventually coalesce, resulting in nephric and perinephric abscess. Areas in the body seeded during the bacteremia may also develop infection and abscess.

In the pregnant patient, untreated pyelonephritis often incites premature labor, as will any severe febrile illness during pregnancy. Hypotension decreases uteroplacental perfusion, leading to fetal compromise and myometrial irritability. However, even in women without overt pyelonephritis, i.e., those with asymptomatic bacteriuria or cystitis, there may be a higher rate of premature delivery and lower birth weight babies, although this is still a matter of some debate. Maternal anemia and decrease in renal function may occur with urinary infection during pregnancy, especially after pyelonephritis.

Diagnosis

The cornerstone of diagnosis of urinary tract infection is the demonstration of bacteria in the urine. A clean-catch midstream urine specimen is considered colonized if more than 100,000 colonies of bacteria are recovered per milliliter of urine. Catheterized specimens, or specimens obtained by suprapubic bladder aspiration, are considered significantly colonized if any pathogenic bacteria are grown from the specimen.

The clinical diagnosis of either asymptomatic bacteriuria, cystitis, or pyelonephritis is made on the basis of the physical findings combined with the results of urinalysis. For instance, a patient who has many white blood cells and bacteria in a catheterized urine specimen and is spiking a temperature of 103°F (39.5°C) with severe right-sided pain is diagnosed as having acute pyelonephritis. A similar urinalysis in a patient with no fever or other symptoms, except dysuria and frequency, indicates cystitis. The diagnosis of asymptomatic bacteriuria is made when the patient has no signs or symptoms but urine culture reveals the presence of significant colonies of bacteria.

Occasionally a patient with the signs and symptoms of acute pyelonephritis will be found to have no pyuria on initial urinalysis. This is not uncommon in the patient who has partial obstruction of the ureter as a result of calculus or compression by the gravid uterus. In these cases, it is helpful to position the patient with her affected side up, e.g., on her left side if she has right flank pain, and collect another urine specimen for examination after the affected ureter has been allowed free drainage for 20 to 30 minutes. This maneuver will often allow drainage of infected urine into the bladder and thus reveal the diagnosis.

Treatment

Patients with asymptomatic bacteriuria should be started on a course of at least 7 to 10 days of oral antibiotic therapy to eradicate the organism colonizing the bladder and thus prevent possible future development of cystitis and acute pyelonephritis. The choice of antibiotic may be made based upon culture results, since these are usually available at the time the diagnosis is made. Antibiotics that produce high urinary levels but which have little systemic effect, e.g., nitrofurantoin, are of use in these patients. It may be wise to save antibiotics that have greater systemic action for use in patients with pyelonephritis. After completion of the course of therapy, the urine should be recultured to document clearing of the bacteriuria.

Patients with cystitis during pregnancy should be treated with oral antibiotics for 10 to 14 days, again, to eradicate the bacteria and prevent future infection. If symptoms are severe, a bladder anesthetic, e.g., pyrimethamine, may be included for the first few days for symptomatic relief. The patient should be encouraged to increase oral fluid intake. The physician should review the results of the culture and sensitivity tests after 48 to 72 hours, in case the organism is resistant to the initial antibiotic prescribed. Antibiotics that give high urinary levels are also useful in treating cystitis during pregnancy. Posttherapy reculture of the urine is mandatory.

Acute pyelonephritis in pregnancy is a serious disease, and patients with this entity should be hospitalized. Intravenous fluids should be given to prevent dehydration and to ensure good urine output. A large-bore intravenous line guarantees quick access in case the patient becomes shocky and unstable. Blood should be obtained initially for a complete blood count and white cell differential, serum electrolyte studies, a chemistry profile, and for the isolation of bacteria. A catheterized urine specimen should be sent for urinalysis, culture, and sensitivity testing. The fetus should be monitored and any signs of premature labor noted, since chorioamnionitis often mimics pyelonephritis and vice versa. Sustained high maternal body temperature may have a deleterious effect upon the fetus; therefore, acetaminophen should be given when the maternal temperature is greater than 102.2°F (39°C).

Initial antibiotic therapy should be based upon the patient's clinical condition and the physician's experience with the antibiotic sensitivities of those organisms most often causing pyelonephritis at the particular institution. If the patient is in septic shock, antibiotics that provide coverage against urinary pathogens should be chosen. Combinations of a semisynthetic penicillin and an aminoglycoside, for example, would provide coverage against the pseudomonads, the coliforms, and the enterococcus. In fact, synergy between these combinations of drugs has been documented for many of these pathogens.

If the patient is not in clinical shock, a single agent that is known to be active against most isolates clinically encountered in the particular institution is generally adequate. The physician must be aware of the sensitivity patterns of *E. coli, P. mirabilis,* the *Klebsiella* species and the occasional streptococci encountered. In some institutions, drugs such as ampicillin may be adequate. In many institutions antibiotic pressures have caused many of the *E. coli* and other organisms to become resistant to ampicillin, as well as to ticarcillin and carbenicillin. *Klebsiella pneumoniae* is almost universally resistant to these drugs as well. In such cases, the first-generation cephalosporins, such as cephalothin, cefazolin, and cephapirin, may be successfully used to treat these infections.

After the patient has been on therapy for 48 to 72 hours, she should show signs of response, such as defervescence and decreasing pain. At this time, the urine should be sterile. Failure to respond to antibiotics may indicate a resistant organism or some urinary tract abnormality, such as total or partial obstruction of a ureter. Such patients need a more in-depth workup, which may include renal ultrasonography or one-shot intravenous pyelography. It is advisable to evaluate creatinine clearance in these patients to determine if any profound decrease in renal function has occurred.

If a patient is treated and responds appropriately to antibiotics given for acute pyelonephritis, she may be switched to oral medication after being afebrile for approximately 48 hours. Ideally, the oral medication should be of the same type as the parenteral drug. The patient should complete a 14-day course of medication, and the urine should be recultured at the conclusion of the treatment course. Any patients with persistent bacteriuria, and patients who have had several

different episodes of urinary tract infection during the pregnancy, should probably be put on suppressive therapy for the duration of the pregnancy and monitored closely.

Parasitic Diseases

TRICHOMONIASIS

Epidemiology

The incidence of infection with *T. vaginalis* in women in the United States is estimated to be 3 million per year. The disease is more common in individuals with multiple sexual partners, and the incidence in female prostitutes is over 70 percent. Therefore, the argument for sexual transmission is very strong.

Trichomoniasis may also be acquired by nonvenereal means, since the organism may live for varying amounts of time in fresh water, semen, and urine, and even on toilet tissue, toilet seats, and damp wash cloths. The rate of infection, therefore, is expectedly high in institutionalized individuals, even when there is no sexual activity.

The newborn infant may acquire trichomoniasis by birth through an infected cervix and vagina. The infection in the neonate is short-lived, however, since the organism cannot survive in the infantile, nonestrogenized vagina.

Microbiology

T. vaginalis is a motile protozoan organism that is recognized in wet preparation by its characteristic twitching, caused by the five flagella that are distributed on the surface of the organism. The animal is anaerobic and ingests bacteria and erythrocytes by phagocytosis.

Infection

Approximately 75 percent of women with *T. vaginalis* infection are symptomatic. The usual infection consists of a vaginitis/cervicitis, accompanied by a frothy, greenish discharge that may occasionally have a disagreeable odor. There may be an associated vulvitis. Dysuria and urinary frequency are not uncommon, and trichomonads may be seen in the bladder urine. Unusual features in the infection are inguinal adenopathy and lower abdominal pain resembling pelvic inflammatory disease. None of these factors are specific for trichomoniasis.

Diagnosis

Demonstration of the organism from genital secretions is the method for diagnosis of trichomoniasis. Up to 60 to 70 percent of infections may be documented by microscopic examination of vaginal secretions. There will also be many white cells and erythrocytes, depending upon the amount of inflammation present. It is important that vaginal pool fluid be used, not endocervical mucus.

Treatment

In the nonpregnant patient, metronidazole (Flagyl) is the drug of choice for trichomoniasis. Metronidazole given in a dose of 250 mg orally 3 times daily for 7 days will cure roughly 95 percent of women. Those who fail therapy should be retreated, along with their sexual partner. A regimen of 2.0 g orally at one sitting gives reasonably comparable rates of cure.

Metronidazole has been shown to be tumorigenic in laboratory animals given large doses for long periods of time. However, no adverse reports have been described in humans, other than mild nausea, bitter taste, and an Antabuse-like reaction if taken with alcohol. Still, usage in pregnancy during the first trimester is probably contraindicated. During the last two trimesters the use of metronidazole must be weighed against the risk from severe cervicitis and vaginitis. In lieu of metronidazole therapy, nonspecific local care, such as douches or suppositories, may be helpful.

TOXOPLASMOSIS

Epidemiology

Toxoplasmosis results from infection by the parasite *Toxoplasma gondii*, which is found in herbivorous, omnivorous, and carnivorous animals. The domestic cat is the only known animal known to shed oocysts. Therefore, cats serve as vectors of transmission to other animals and humans. Invertebrates that feed on feces can transport oocysts and thus serve as intermediate hosts.

The disease can also be contracted by the ingestion of raw meat or by transplacental infection.

Toxoplasmosis occurs more frequently in tropical areas. In addition to geographical location being a factor, there is also an increased incidence of seropositivity with increasing age. Approximately 20 to 25 percent of women in the reproductive age group in the United States are seropositive for *T. gondii*. The incidence of primary infection in pregnancy is estimated to range between 0.5 and 1.5 percent, with a third of these women giving birth to infected neonates.

There is an inverse relationship between the time of infection in pregnancy and the incidence of fetal infection. Pregnant women who contract *T. gondii* in their first trimester will transmit the disease to their fetuses in 15 percent of cases. If the disease is contracted in the second trimester, the incidence of fetal infection increases to 25 percent, and 60 percent of fetuses will contract the disease if the mother acquires it during the third trimester. However, the manifestations of congenital toxoplasmosis are more severe with earlier infection. Infection that occurs early in the first trimester may result in abortion, whereas infection acquired in the third trimester may be asymptomatic.

Microorganism

Toxoplasma gondii exists in three forms during its life cycle: trophozoites, tissue cysts, and oocysts. The trophozoite is the proliferative form, which invades the mammalian cells. Once within the host cells, the trophozoites multiply until the cells are disrupted, thereby liberating more trophozoites or tissue cysts.

Tissue cysts have an outer wall that protects against the host defense mechanisms. This form of the disease is the latent stage and may also serve to transmit the disease. Disruption of the cell wall results in the liberation of viable parasites that are capable of invading host epithelial cells.

Oocysts have been found only in members of the cat family. The cat ingests tissue cysts or oocysts, which enter the cat's gut; here, dissolution of the cyst wall occurs, releasing viable *T. gondii*. The parasite then invades the epithelial cells lining the intestine and begins the asexual phase of its life cycle. This is shortly followed by a sexual phase, which results in the formation of noninfectious unsporulated oocysts. These oocysts are shed in the cat's feces. Once outside the body, each oocyst undergoes sporogeny, forming two sporocysts. Each sporocyst matures, forming four sporozoites. Ingestion of the oocysts containing the sporozoites results in liberation of trophozoites, thereby completing the life cycle.

Infection

Toxoplasmosis is a unique disease in that infection by *T. gondii* is often asymptomatic, but may be fulminant. Infection acquired by the mother during pregnancy is often asymptomatic, but congenital infection can result in serious sequelae. The disease is seen in the following four forms: congenital, acquired, ocular, and in the immunocompromised patient. Infection in the adult is frequently asymptomatic, although the patient may present with lymphadenopathy, chorioretinitis, myocarditis, meningoencephalitis and/or a rash resembling the exanthem seen in typhus.

Toxoplasmosis acquired during pregnancy may range from asymptomatic to fatal acute fulminant disease. The most common manifestation during pregnancy is cervical lymphadenopathy, which may be associated with supraclavicular and inguinal lymphadenopathy. The patient may also have fever, myalgias, pharyngitis, and headache. The presentation mimics that seen in mononucleosis or cytomegalovirus infection. In addition, some individuals may have a rash similar to the exanthem seen in typhus; hepatosplenomegaly and an atypical lymphocytosis may also develop.

Congenital infection in the United States occurs in 1 in 500 to 1 in 3000 deliveries, depending on the geographic region. It should be emphasized that in certain areas of the country, there has been an influx of immigrants from tropical areas where the disease is more prevalent; therefore, special attention should be given to ensure that these patients are properly evaluated. The incidence of congenital infection varies, depending on the trimester during which the infection is acquired. Maternal infection acquired during the 1st trimester is associated with the lowest incidence of fetal infection but is likely to result in spontaneous abortion if the fetus contracts the illness. The highest risk of congenital infection occurs with maternal infection in the 3rd trimester; as noted earlier, however, most newborns infected in the 3rd trimester are asymptomatic and may suffer no sequelae. Others may develop retinochoroiditis, strabismus, blindness, epilepsy, and/or psychomotor or mental retardation months or years later. Infants born with clinical infection may present with retinochoroiditis, hydrocephaly or microcephaly, cerebral calcifications, convulsions, psychomotor retardation, fever, hepatosplenomegaly, jaundice, lymphadenopathy, and rash.

Diagnosis

The diagnosis of toxoplasmosis may be established by isolation of *T. gondii* from body fluids and tissue specimens. This is not a practical method, however, since most institutions do not have the facilities for inoculating mice or tissue cultures. A second method is based on demonstration of trophozoites in tissue sections or smears. This is a difficult procedure in that trophozoites are not easily recognized. Fluorescent antibody techniques have been developed that facilitate the diagnosis and are easier to perform.

Serologic methods have been used most frequently to establish the diagnosis of toxoplasmosis. The Sabin-Feldman dye test, the indirect fluorescent antibody (IFAT) test, and the indirect hemagglutination test (IHAT) are the most frequently used serologic tests. The IFAT and IHAT detect IgG antibodies. The Sabin-Feldman dye test serves as the standard to which all other tests are compared. The IFAT is the most widely used serologic test, and the IFAT and Sabin-Feldman dye test become positive 1 to 2 weeks after acute infection. In 6 to 8 weeks titers of 1:1000 are reached that will decline in several months to titers of 1:4 to 1:64—with these low titers persisting for life.

Another useful serologic test is the IgM–fluorescent antibody test, which becomes detectable within 5 days after infection and disappears 3 to 4 months after infection. The presence in the fetus of IgM antibodies specifically directed against *T. gondii* indicates intrauterine infection, since IgM does not cross the placenta. In a patient suspected of acute toxoplasmosis, serum should be obtained for IgM-IFAT and IgG-IFAT antibodies. If the IgM-IFAT is 1:80 or if there is a serial two-tube rise in titer in specimens run in parallel, then the diagnosis of acute toxoplasmosis is established even in the absence of symptoms. The presence of a positive IgM-IFAT and a rising IgG-IFAT also establishes the diagnosis. A negative IgM-IFAT and a fixed IgG-IFAT titer do not indicate acute infection. However, a negative IgM-IFAT in the presence of a rising IgG-IFAT titer does indicate active disease. The IgG-IFAT titer may become fixed at 1:2400 for years.

Treatment

Whether or not to treat a pregnant woman with asymptomatic toxoplasmosis is a question that is confronted by many obstetricians. Originally it was thought that since the prognosis in untreated asymptomatic toxoplasmosis was good and that disease contracted during one pregnancy would confer immunity during subsequent pregnancies, treatment was not necessary. However, congenital toxoplasmosis may be asymptomatic at first, only to produce serious sequelae many years later. In addition, organisms have been isolated from abortuses, stillborns, and neonates who expired following delivery from women with chronic disease. *Toxoplasma* organisms have, on several occasions, also been recovered from the maternal blood in asymptomatic patients. Therefore, although rare, subsequent congenital infection may occur. It is probably best to have these patients practice some form of contraception for a year's duration or, if the patient is already pregnant, to discuss the risks of treatment and treat for fetal indications.

Individuals who contract the disease during the first trimester risk having a severely affected child if the pregnancy goes to term. If these individuals do not elect abortion, treatment of acute maternal toxoplasmosis appears to decrease the incidence of congenital toxoplasmosis. Treatment should be started with sulfadiazine, 1 g given orally 4 times a day for 28 days. Pyrimethamine (Daraprim), a folic acid antagonist, is contraindicated during the first trimester because it is teratogenic. Sulfadiazine should be discontinued at term, in order to prevent neonatal hyperbilirubinemia. In the second and third trimesters sulfadiazine should be administered in conjunction with pyrimethamine, administered orally in a dose of 25 mg daily for 28 days. Since pyrimethamine is a folic acid antagonist, folinic acid should be given concurrently in dosages of 2 to 10 mg per day, to prevent bone marrow suppression in the second and third trimesters.

In an attempt to prevent acquired and congenital toxoplasmosis, patients should be advised to eat meat that has been thoroughly cooked. Uncooked meat should be kept frozen at 20°C for 24 hours to kill cysts. Fruits and vegetables should be thoroughly washed. Pregnant women should avoid contact with cats and should not change the cat litter. This is especially true for cats that go outdoors and occasionally kill and eat wild animals.

Nursing Considerations in Perinatal Infections

Women who have perinatal infections need emotional as well as physical support. Emotional support involves helping the mother and her family to understand her disease and its ramifications, which in some cases may include the need to isolate the mother from her baby. Good education should be part of this support, especially if the mother has been newly diagnosed with herpes. She will need to understand the importance of cesarean section and what herpes means to her and her sexual partner. The mother may also need supportive care for her physical symptoms, as she may not feel well during her labor and delivery.

Generally speaking, when a woman with a perinatal infection is discharged from a room it should have a thorough terminal cleaning. This includes not only antepartum, postpartum, and labor rooms, but also delivery and recovery rooms. If possible, these mothers should be allowed to labor and deliver, and perhaps recover, in the same room.

Specific isolation, such as enteric precautions, may be necessary. Emotional support for the isolated patient is a well-known need, as such patients start to feel separated from their families and even the staff. Furthermore, as noted, it is sometimes necessary to separate mothers from their babies, thus increasing the mother's frustration. However, in some instances the babies can be isolated with the mothers in a "rooming in" setup. If the mother must be isolated from her baby, she should be encouraged to "view" her baby and to have pictures to promote bonding. Other family members should be encouraged to visit and handle the newborn frequently.

Table 5–4. Management of Perinatal Infections

Infection	Antepartum and Intrapartum Recommendations	Postpartum Recommendations	Breast-Feeding*
Herpes—oral and vaginal	(1) Good handwashing (2) Terminal cleaning of antepartum, labor, and delivery rooms	(1) Rooming-in OR (2) Separate mom and baby so baby doesn't take infection back to nursery from mom (3) Good staff handwashing (4) Good maternal handwashing when handling baby (5) Terminal cleaning of recovery room and postpartum room	Yes, with good maternal handwashing
Rubella	(1) Strict isolation during disease (2) Terminal cleaning of antepartum, labor, and delivery rooms	(1) Isolate baby from mom (2) Strict isolation (3) No pregnant women to attend patient	May breast-feed after infectious period Pump breast and discard milk to preserve lactation until that time
Cytomegalovirus (CMV) (if diagnosed as active)	(1) Strict isolation during disease (2) Terminal cleaning of antepartum, labor, and delivery rooms	(1) Isolate baby from mom (2) Strict isolation (3) No pregnant women to attend patient	May breast-feed after infectious period Pump breast and discard milk to preserve lactation until that time
Varicella-zoster	(1) Strict isolation during disease (2) Terminal cleaning of antepartum, labor, and delivery rooms	(1) Isolate baby from mom (2) Strict isolation (3) No pregnant women to attend patient	May breast-feed after infectious period Pump breast and discard milk to preserve lactation until that time
Hepatitis B, A, and non-A, non-B	(1) Enteric precautions (2) Terminal cleaning of antepartum, labor, and delivery rooms	(1) Isolate baby from mom (2) Enteric precautions (3) Terminal cleaning of recovery room and postpartum room	May breast-feed after infectious period Pump breast and discard milk to preserve lactation until that time
Mumps	(1) Strict isolation during disease (2) Terminal cleaning of antepartum, labor, and delivery rooms	(1) Isolate baby from mom (2) Strict isolation (3) No pregnant women to attend patient	May breast-feed after infectious period Pump breast and discard milk to preserve lactation until that time
Condyloma acuminatum	No restrictions	No restrictions	No restrictions

Table continued on following page

Table 5–4. Management of Perinatal Infections *Continued*

Infection	Antepartum and Intrapartum Recommendations	Postpartum Recommendations	Breast-Feeding*
Syphilis	(1) Terminal cleaning only if patient has open lesions (antepartum, labor, and delivery rooms) (2) Good handwashing	(1) Once treatment started, baby can be with mom (2) Good handwashing (3) Terminal cleaning of room only if patient has open lesions (recovery room and postpartum floor) (4) Test baby for syphilis	Yes, once treatment is started
Tuberculosis	(1) Respiratory isolation with active disease (2) Terminal cleaning of antepartum, labor, and delivery rooms with active disease	(1) Once treatment effective, baby can be with mom (2) Respiratory isolation with active disease (3) If active disease *not* treated: mom and baby to be separated	No, because of active disease or medications
Listeria monocytogenes	Terminal cleaning of antepartum, labor, and delivery rooms	Once treatment started, baby can be with mom	May breast-feed; however, this will be dependent on antibiotic treatment, since breast-feeding is contraindicated with some antibiotics May breast-feed after antibiotic therapy is completed; pump breast and discard milk to preserve lactation until that time
Chorioamnionitis	No restrictions	No restrictions once mom is afebrile	May breast-feed once mom is afebrile; however, this will be dependent on antibiotic treatment May breast-feed after antibiotic therapy is completed; pump breast and discard milk to preserve lactation until that time

Genital mycoplasmas	Unknown	Once treatment started, baby can be with mom	May breast-feed; however, this will be dependent on antibiotic treatment May breast-feed after antibiotic therapy is completed; pump breast and discard milk to preserve lactation until that time
Chlamydia spp.	Terminal cleaning of antepartum, labor, and delivery rooms	Once treatment started, baby can be with mom	May breast-feed; however, this will be dependent on antibiotic treatment May breast-feed after antibiotic therapy is completed; pump breast and discard milk to preserve lactation until that time
Gonorrhea	(1) Good handwashing (2) Terminal cleaning of antepartum, labor, and delivery rooms	Once treatment started, baby can be with mom	May breast-feed; however, this will be dependent on antibiotic treatment May breast-feed after antibiotic therapy is completed; pump breast and discard milk to preserve lactation until that time
Postpartum endometritis	No restrictions	Isolate baby from mom until afebrile	May breast-feed; however, this will be dependent on antibiotic treatment May breast-feed after antibiotic therapy is completed; pump breast and discard milk to preserve lactation until that time
Pneumonia	(1) Good handwashing (2) Terminal cleaning of antepartum, labor, and delivery rooms	Isolate baby from mom until afebrile	May breast-feed; however, this will be dependent on antibiotic treatment May breast-feed after antibiotic therapy is completed; pump breast and discard milk to preserve lactation until that time

Table continued on following page

Table 5–4. Management of Perinatal Infections *Continued*

Infection	Antepartum and Intrapartum Recommendations	Postpartum Recommendations	Breast-Feeding*
Urinary tract infection (UTI)	No restrictions	No restrictions	May breast-feed; however, this will be dependent on antibiotic treatment May breast-feed after antibiotic therapy is completed; pump breast and discard milk to preserve lactation until that time
Trichomoniasis	No restrictions	No restrictions	May breast-feed; however, this will be dependent on antibiotic treatment May breast-feed after antibiotic therapy is completed; pump breast and discard milk to preserve lactation until that time
Toxoplasmosis	No restrictions	No restrictions	May breast-feed; however, this will be dependent on antibiotic treatment May breast-feed after antibiotic therapy is completed; pump breast and discard milk to preserve lactation until that time

*Note: For mothers on antibiotic therapy, breast-feeding will depend on the type of antibiotic used, since some are permissible and others are contraindicated during breast-feeding.

When the mother has a perinatal infection, the baby can usually be breast-fed, provided that treatment has been started and the mother is afebrile. Advisability of breast-feeding will also depend on the medication administered for treatment of the mother's infection (see Chapter 6). If breast-feeding is desired by the mother but contraindicated by her treatment, she can pump her breasts and discard the milk while she is receiving treatment. Once the medication is completed the mother can start to breast-feed her infant.

Table 5–4 gives more specific management for mothers with perinatal infections.

UPDATE ON AIDS*

Acquired immune deficiency syndrome (AIDS) is defined as "A disease that is at least moderately predictive of a defect in cell-mediated immunity, and that occurs in the absence of a known cause for diminished resistance of that disease." Although once

*Based on "Progress in AIDS," FDA Drug Bulletin, Vol. 15, No. 3, October 1985, p. 27; special acknowledgment to Abbe Loveman, R. W., M.B.A.-H.A., Miami, Florida.

thought to be restricted to homosexuals, Haitians, and IV drug users, AIDS is now known to be passed through heterosexual contacts as well and therefore may affect pregnant women and their fetuses.

Since AIDS is transmitted by blood and secretions, care of the AIDS patient revolves around the principles of blood and secretion precautions, which should include the following measures:

- A private room, especially in the intrapartum and postpartum periods, or when amniotic fluid or bleeding are present.
- Use of gowns and/or apron and gloves when handling excretions.
- Use of disposable dishes and trays.
- Linen should be double-bagged and marked contaminated; equipment should be marked contaminated when returned to central supply; waste should be marked contaminated.
- A solution of ½ cup sodium hypochlorite diluted in 1 gallon of water should be used for cleaning.
- Specimens taken to the laboratory should be marked contaminated.
- A bulb syringe or gentle mechanical suction (*not* DeLee suction) should be used for resuscitation of the newborn.

- Gloves should be worn during resuscitation/stabilization of the newborn.
- Attachment should be encouraged and supported.
- Newborns should be bathed immediately after delivery.
- Rooming-in can be utilized.
- Use of bottle feeding, since the HTLV III virus is present in breast milk.
- Puncture-resistant "sharps" containers should be used, and used needles should not be recapped after use by the practitioner.
- Patients with respiratory complications such as *Mycobacterium* tuberculosis, should be placed on *respiratory precautions.*

Treatment for patients with the HTLV III virus and positivity for AIDS includes (1) antiviral antibiotics such as suramin, ribaviran, HPA-23, and PFA; (2) immune stimulators such as interleuken-2 and gamma interferon. Additionally, each of the opportunistic infections is treated with appropriate drugs.

REFERENCES

Amstey, M. S.: Current concepts of herpesvirus in women. Am. J. Obstet. Gynecol. 117:717, 1975.

Beasley, R. P., Hwang, L. Y., Lin, C. C., et al.: Hepatitis B immune globulin (HBIG) efficacy in the interruption of perinatal transmission of hepatitis B carrier. Lancet 2:388, 1981.

Benedetti, T. J., Valle, R., and Ledger, W. J.: Antepartum pneumonia in pregnancy. Am. J. Obstet. Gynecol. 144:413, 1982.

Cassell, G. H., and Cole, B. C.: Mycoplasmas as agents of human disease. N. Engl. J. Med. 304:308, 1981.

Chang, T. W.: Tubella reinfection and intrauterine involvement. J. Pediatrics. 84:617, 1974.

Desmonts, G., and Couvreur, J.: Congenital toxoplasmosis: a prospective study of 378 pregnancies. N. Engl. J. Med. 290:1110, 1974.

Faro, S.: Hepatitis A, B and non-A, non-B in pregnancy. In Amstey, M. S. (ed.): Viral Infections in Pregnancy. New York, Grune & Stratton, 1984, pp. 19–33.

Faro, S.: Sexually transmitted diseases. In Hale, R. N., and Knueger, J. A. (eds.): Gynecology. New Hyde Park, New York, Medical Examination Publishing Co., 1983.

Faro, S., Pastorek, J., and Aldridge, K.: Short course parenteral antibiotic therapy for pyelonephritis in pregnancy. South Med. J. 77:455, 1984.

Faro, S., Sanders, C. V., and Aldridge, K.: Use of single-agent antimicrobial therapy in the treatment of polymicrobial female pelvic infections. Obstet. Gynecol. 60:232, 1982.

Gibbs, R. S., Castillo, M. S., and Rodgers, P. J.: Management of acute chorioamnionitis. Am. J. Obstet. Gynecol. 136:709, 1980.

Giles, C., and Brown, J. A.: Urinary infection and anemia in pregnancy. Br. Med. J. 2:10, 1962.

Gilstrap, L. C., and Cunningham, F. G.: The bacterial pathogenesis of infection following cesarean section. Obstet. Gynecol. 53:545, 1979.

Harris, R. E., and Gilstrap, L. C.: Prevention of recurrent pyelonephritis during pregnancy. Obstet. Gynecol. 44:637, 1974.

Heggie, A. D., Lumica, G., Stuart, L. A., et al.: Chlamydia trachomatis infection in mothers and infants. Am. J. Dis. Child. 135:507, 1981.

Martin, D. H., Koutsky, L., Eschenbach, D. A., et al.: Prematurity and perinatal mortality in pregnancies complicated by maternal chlamydia trachomatis infections. JAMA 247:1585, 1982.

Miehinen, M., Saxen, L., and Saxen, E.: Lymph node toxoplasmosis. Acta Med. Scand. 208:431, 1980.

Nahmias, A. J., Josey, W. E., Naib, Z. M., et al.: Perinatal risk associated with maternal genital herpes simplex virus infection. Am. J. Obstet. Gynecol. 110:825, 1971.

Remington, J. S.: Toxoplasmosis in the adult. Bull. NY Acad. Med. 50:211, 1974.

Sargal, S., Lunyk, O., Larkee, R. P. B., et al.: The outcome in children with congenital cytomegalovirus infection. Am. J. Dis. Child. 136:896, 1982.

Sever, J. L.: Infections in pregnancy; highlights from the collaborative perinatal project. Teratology 25:227, 1982.

DRUGS IN PREGNANCY

DONALD E. MARSDEN

Among the most deeply rooted fears of the pregnant woman is the concern that her baby may be malformed. One of the first questions she asks after the birth is usually "Is the baby normal?", and at the earliest opportunity she will generally examine it herself for reassurance. But for at least 3 percent of mothers such fears are realized by the delivery of a child with a major congenital abnormality. When such an event occurs it is natural for the mother, her family, and her attendants to seek a cause or explanation. For untold centuries the only explanations were divine retribution for actual or imagined sins, witchcraft, or the imprint on the fetus of traumatic events affecting the mother during gestation. The recognition that drugs, radiation and other environmental agents are potentially teratogenic is relatively recent, yet it has captured the imagination of the public at large, and the medical and legal professions in particular. Increased awareness of the risks of drug usage in pregnancy raises the prospect of more sensible and controlled patterns of demand and usage. On the other hand it has spawned a flood of chiefly anecdotal reports in the medical and lay press incriminating, on often dubious grounds, a wide range of drugs in the production of an equally wide range of abnormalities. Some authors advocate "therapeutic nihilism" (Golbus, 1982), an attitude that is encouraged by the package inserts in a large proportion of currently available drugs carrying such disclaimers as "the safety of this drug for use in pregnancy has not been established." These statements greatly increase the medicolegal hazards of prescribing drugs without clarifying the medical risks (Brent, 1982). The end result could easily be a situation in which even potentially lifesaving drugs are withheld for

fear of teratogenesis, and the pregnant woman and her child become "therapeutic orphans" (Shirkey, 1968). Attention has also been drawn to a tragic postscript that may follow the birth of a malformed baby, in which distortion or misinterpretation of available information regarding teratogens can lead to "litigation-produced pain, disease and suffering" affecting the whole family, the medical attendants and attorneys (Brent, 1977).

Although teratogenic effects are the most publicized concern related to drug usage in pregnancy, there are a number of other important considerations. The physical and physiologic changes of pregnancy affect the absorption, distribution, metabolism, and excretion of drugs. For example, plasma levels of ampicillin achieved after a given oral or intravenous dose of ampicillin in pregnancy are significantly lower than those in the same women in the nonpregnant state, even when corrected for weight changes (Philipson, 1977). The potential therapeutic connotations of such changes are readily apparent. Drugs that are relatively safe in nonpregnant women may produce serious toxic reactions in pregnancy. An example is the potentially fatal hepatotoxicity reported to occur in some pregnant women with pyelonephritis who receive tetracycline (Whalley et al., 1964). Drugs used during pregnancy and labor may affect parameters used to assess fetal well-being, without necessarily compromising the fetus. For example, betamethasone given to a woman with threatened premature labor can temporarily reduce plasma estriol levels by as much as 70 percent, yet the fall does not represent fetal jeopardy (Maltau et al., 1979). The potential for neonatal depression from opiates and tranquilizers used in labor is well known. Although this list of factors that have a bearing on drug use in pregnancy is far from complete, it highlights the importance of considerations other than teratogenicity in decision making.

It is the aim of this chapter to present the problems in perspective, to summarize the current state of knowledge relating to various commonly used drugs, and to help the reader develop a rational approach to drug usage in pregnancy.

Establishing the appropriate plan of drug management for the pregnant woman requires collaboration among all members of the perinatal team, as well as the cooperation of family members. This collaborative effort involves education and counseling, including genetic counseling, for those patients taking medications for preexisting medical diseases. Education will also be necessary for patients who will be taking medications they have never taken before, including explanations of how to administer the medication, the necessity for taking it, and any adverse effects that may be anticipated. This education should include the entire family, because the medication regime, its usage, including disposal of syringes when used, and side effects may influence the family's lifestyle.

Drugs as Teratogens

(Table 6–1)

HISTORICAL ASPECTS

The ancient belief that a pregnant woman's experiences impressed themselves on the fetus, producing congenital abnormalities, is accepted in varying degrees by segments of contemporary society. As recently as the 18th century, malformed infants (and often their mothers) were burned as "products of witchcraft or bestiary" (Tuchmann-Duplessis, 1975). (The role of drugs in teratogenesis was suggested in the early 18th and 19th centuries by committees of the Royal College of Physicians and British Parliament, which reported that infants of alcoholic women had a "starved, shriveled, and imperfect look" [Woollam, 1980].)

For the first half of this century, congenital defects in humans were believed to be genetic in origin. Environmental teratogens

Table 6–1. The Teratogenic Status of Various Drugs

Proven Teratogens
 Alcohol (as in alcohol abuse)
 Androgenic hormones
 Cytotoxic agents
  High risk: Folate antagonists, e.g., methotrexate; Alkylating agents, e.g., busulfan cyclophosphamide
  Lesser risk: All others
 Diethylstilbestrol
 Radioiodine
 Thalidomide
 Therapeutic radiation
 Warfarin

Probable Teratogens
 Lithium
 Phenytoin
 Quinine
 Trimethadione

Possible Teratogens
 Barbiturates
 Chloroquine
 Estrogens
 Primidone
 Progestagens

Doubtful Teratogens
 Clomiphene
 Diazepam
 Diphenhydramine
 Penicillamine
 Phenothiazines

Modified from Beely, L.: Clin. Obstet. Gynecol. 8:261, 1981.

were thought to be excluded by a "placental barrier." In 1935 it was shown that anophthalmia in pigs was not inherited but was due to deficiency of Vitamin A (Hale, 1935). Transplacental viral teratogenesis was recognized in 1941 with the description of part of the now classic congenital rubella syndrome (Gregg, 1941). Simultaneous reports from Australia (McBride, 1962) and Germany (Lenz, 1961) of thalidomide-induced abnormalities, most notably phocomelia, demonstrated the fallibility of the "placental barrier." That a supposedly harmless sedative left 5000 grossly deformed infants in Germany alone, and thousands more worldwide (Lenz, 1966), led to intense research into teratogenesis, undermined faith in the medical profession and drug industry, and changed our attitudes regarding prescribing medicine in pregnancy. In 1971, transplacental carcinogenesis was described when diethylstilbestrol (DES) was found to be responsible for an "epidemic" of vaginal adenocarcinoma (Herbst et al., 1971), which was subsequently recognized to be only a relatively uncommon part of a syndrome of genital tract abnormalities in both sexes (Herbst, 1981). The effects of DES are not usually recognized before puberty, a reminder that teratogenicity may not become apparent for many years.

Important though animal and laboratory studies are, "reliable predictability of human teratogenic potential . . . is not possible other than by long term assessment . . . in humans" (Stern, 1981). Such studies are difficult to initiate and execute, yet crucial.

INCIDENCE AND CAUSES OF CONGENITAL ANOMALIES

It is generally accepted that at least 3 percent of newborns have birth defects requiring therapy, one third of them life-threatening. With long-term follow-up the overall rate reaches 7 to 10 percent (Shepard and Fantel, 1981), varying according to standards of observation, definitions of "defect," and racial factors.

Wilson (1973) believed 25 percent of birth defects to be due to genetic or chromosomal factors, 10 percent to environmental factors, and 65 percent to unknown factors. More recently, multifactorial inheritance has been blamed for 30 percent of congenital defects, mendelian inheritance or chromosomal disorders for 20 percent, and drugs and environmental agents for 8 percent, with 42 percent being of unknown etiology (Holmes, 1980). It is important to recognize that the proportion of congenital abnormalities resulting from genetic or chromosomal factors is much greater than that arising from drugs. Nevertheless, drugs may play some role in the sizable category of defects of unknown origin (Golbus, 1982). Thalidomide and DES are unusual teratogens, producing, in a high proportion of exposed fetuses, easily recognized abnormalities that rarely occur spontaneously. More subtle agents may produce abnormalities in a small proportion of cases or increase the incidence of relatively common anomalies.

Teratogenic effects can be species-specific: rats, mice, and rabbits are immune to thalidomide, whereas primates and humans are sensitive. Within a species, genetic factors affect susceptibility to various teratogens. Differing genetic strains of mice vary greatly in the incidence of both spontaneous and cortisone-induced cleft palates (Fraser and

Fainstat, 1951). Many genetically controlled factors, such as palatal closure rate, predispose or protect different strains of mice from drug-induced cleft palate (Fraser, 1980). Susceptibility to drug-induced neural tube defects is genetically controlled in mice (Cole and Trasler, 1980). Furthermore, fetal mice within the same uterus have different sensitivities to maternally administered teratogens, related to enzyme production controlled by a single gene (Nebert and Shum, 1980).

DETERMINING THE TERATOGENIC POTENTIAL OF DRUGS

Animal tests are the "first wall of defense against teratogenesis" (Shepard, 1974). One limitation is variations in sensitivity from one species to another. Dosage is an important consideration: The mother must survive, and there may be only a narrow dose range between the safe dosage and fetotoxic dosages that result in teratogenesis. Massive doses of saline or sucrose are teratogenic in animals (Shepard, 1973). "The production of congenital malformations in experimental animals still is an art," and the application of the results to man is complex (Shepard, 1974). As Blake (1982) has stated, "There are so many examples of inconsistency between results of animal teratogenic studies and the human experience that a credibility gap has developed." The future may lie in testing drugs in cell, organ, or even embryo cultures.

Information regarding teratogenicity in humans may be derived from case reports, controlled or uncontrolled retrospective studies, or prospective studies. All are important, but the most valuable are prospective studies of large populations, which monitor drug exposure and include careful follow-up of the infants (Apgar, 1966).

Retrospective studies usually involve taking a group of women delivering infants with congenital abnormalities, matching them with a "control" group delivering normal infants, and comparing drug usage. This allows study of small numbers of patients, whereas a prospective study may involve, for example, following as many as 10,000 pregnancies in order to gain data on 50 neural tube defects. The problem with retrospective studies is memory bias, with "the control mother forgetting and the mother of the malformed child embroidering events that the latter may blame for her misfortune" (Leck, 1978). This can seriously bias the results of retrospective studies and produce spurious associations between birth defects and pregnancy events. An example of recall bias is a Finnish study of congenital central nervous system abnormalities. In this study, several drugs apparently related to the defects when one control group was used were found to bear no significant relationship to the defects when another control group was used (Granroth, 1978). All who have seen the often desperate attempts of parents of children with congenital abnormalities to find a cause for them will understand how easily false assumptions can be made. Most frequently, such false assumptions are made linking the use of commonly used drugs with uncommon anomalies.

It has been suggested that a national register of birth defects be established, which would indicate changing incidence rates and allow prospective studies of etiologic factors (Apgar, 1966). Difficult though such a project would be to initiate and maintain, it holds the greatest hope for satisfactory monitoring of teratogens.

RELATIVE AND ABSOLUTE RISKS

Virtually all congenital abnormalities associated with intrauterine drug exposure also occur spontaneously in the general population. Thalidomide and diethylstilbestrol were unusual in that they affected a very high proportion of exposed fetuses and produced distinctive abnormalities that occur at a very low frequency in the unexposed population. Most suspected teratogens appear to produce small increases in incidence of more common abnormalities; hence the concept of "relative risk."

Heinonen and coworkers define the relative risk of a drug producing an abnormality as "the ratio of the rate of a defect in exposed children to the rate in non-exposed children" (Heinonen et al., 1977). This offers information on the magnitude of the association and allows one to estimate the reduction in risk if a drug is not used. It is important to keep in mind a number of factors when considering teratogenic risks. First, it will be easier to recognize the teratogenic effect of a commonly used drug producing a rare anomaly than the effect of a rarely used drug producing a commonly seen abnormality. Second, the impact of a teratogen depends on *absolute* risk as well as *relative* risk. For example, a drug with a relative risk of 3 will produce a threefold increase in abnormalities in infants of users compared with those of nonusers. But if the incidence of the abnormality in the unexposed population is 1 in 1000, the incidence in the exposed population is still predicted to be only 3 in 1000. Even where *relative* risks are high, *absolute* risks may be low. Few drugs had relative risks higher than 2 in the study of Heinonen et al. (1977). This is not to diminish the significance of the damage done to affected children but rather to emphasize the importance of considering risk-to-benefit ratios when prescribing in pregnancy.

EXTENT OF DRUG USE IN PREGNANCY

Pregnant women consume an amazing number of drugs. The Collaborative Perinatal Project considered drugs taken from the time of conception to 48 hours before labor and excluded vitamins, iron, antacids, and intravenous fluids. The mean number of medications used was 3.8, with less than 6 percent of all the women studied taking no drugs at all. Furthermore, the study extended from 1958 to 1965, a period that included the thalidomide "epidemic"; yet throughout the time of the study, drug use by pregnant women increased, making it clear that "publicity directed to avoiding unnecessary use of drugs during pregnancy was a failure" (Heinonen et al., 1977).

A report in 1963 noted that of 3072 pregnant women only 8 percent took no prescribed drugs, 20 percent took more than five, and 4 percent took more than ten (Peckham and King, 1963). In addition to prescription drugs, many patients consume "over-the-counter" preparations. Hill and coworkers (1977) studied 231 pregnant patients and found that 95 percent used nonprescription medications, with almost 40 percent using more than three. In the antepartum period their patients used a mean number of 9.6 drugs, 6.4 being prescribed (range 0 to 28) and 3.2 being over-the-counter preparations (range 0 to 12). A more recent prospective study of drug use in pregnancy, which included iron, vitamins, and intravenous fluids, showed that 93 percent of women used five or more drugs (Doering and Stewart, 1978). The average number of products used antenatally (some products including several active ingredients) was 11; in the perinatal period women undergoing vaginal delivery received an average of seven medications.

These figures are cited here not to imply that all drug use in pregnancy is unnecessary but to indicate the frequency with which drugs are used by pregnant women. The most commonly used drugs are antipyretic analgesics, antimicrobials, antinauseants, and antihistamines (Heinonen et al., 1977). Pregnant women and the high-risk team must weigh the potential benefits of any medication against possible risks. Our present knowledge makes the risks of most agents difficult to predict; thus, all that can be hoped for is the avoidance of thoughtless or frivolous prescribing in pregnancy.

Problems in Prescribing Drugs in Pregnancy

(Tables 6–2 and 6–3)

It is beyond the scope of this chapter to discuss all prescribing situations that can occur in pregnancy. Rather, the aim will be to discuss principles. For detailed, practical advice regarding the use of most common drugs, suitable for everyday reference, the reader is referred to the excellent handbook of Berkowitz et al. (1981).

DRUG TREATMENT FOR CHRONIC OR PREEXISTING DISEASE

This area is covered in some detail, as many therapeutic problems become apparent in considering the management of these conditions.

Epilepsy

Epilepsy affects 1 in 200 people (Anderson, 1978), and about 0.3 percent of pregnant women are epileptic (American Academy of Pediatrics Committee on Drugs, 1979). Epilepsy is the most common preexisting neurologic disease seen in pregnancy (Stumpf and Frost, 1978). Data from 11 studies showed that epilepsy and its treatment increased the incidence of congenital anomalies; 6 percent of 1461 liveborn infants of epileptics on anticonvulsants had congenital abnormalities, compared with 4 percent of 455 liveborn infants of epileptics not using anticonvulsants. Control groups totaling 117,176 live births showed a 2.5 percent congenital abnormality rate (Janz, 1975). Thus, both genetic factors and drugs used to control epilepsy appear to contribute to the increased malformation rate.

A single convulsion during pregnancy may lead to fetal morbidity or mortality from a placental abruption or hypoxia, and status epilepticus carries a significant risk of both fetal and maternal mortality (Stumpf and Frost, 1978). Between 30 and 60 percent of epileptics have more frequent convulsions

TABLE 6–2. The FDA Categories for Labeling of Prescription Drugs to Indicate the Risks of Their Use in Pregnancy

Category A:	Controlled studies in women fail to demonstrate a risk to the fetus in the first trimester, and the possibility of fetal harm appears to be remote
Category B:	Animal studies do not indicate a risk to the fetus and there are no controlled studies in humans
	OR
	Animal studies do show adverse effects on the fetus but controlled studies in humans have not shown a risk to the fetus
Category C:	Animal studies have shown the drug to be embryocidal or teratogenic but there are no controlled studies in humans
	OR
	No studies are available in animals or humans
Category D:	Definitive evidence of risk to the human fetus exists, but the benefit in certain situations (e.g., life-threatening situations in which safer drugs are unavailable or ineffective) may justify the use of the drug despite the risks
Category X:	Studies in animals or humans have demonstrated fetal abnormalities or there is evidence of fetal risk based on human experience, or both, and the risk clearly outweighs the possible benefits

(From F.D.A. Drug Bulletin, September, 1979.)

Table 6–3. Safety of Commonly Used Drugs for Use in Lactating Women

	Analgesics: Antiinflammatory Agents	Antibiotics; Antibacterials	Anticoagulants; Vasoactive Drugs	Drugs Acting on the CNS	Hormones and Endocrinologically Active Agents	Miscellaneous Agents
DO NOT USE^a	Indomethacin Phenylbutazone	Chloramphenicol Isoniazid Naladixic acid Tetracycline	Phenindione Reserpine	Lithium Meprobamate	Carbimazole Estrogens (over 50 mcg) Iodine salts	Anthroquinones Antineoplastics Atropine Ergot alkaloids Senna derivatives
USE WITH CAUTION^b	Salicylates**	Aminoglycosides Co-trimoxazole Ethambutol Sulfonamides	Beta blockers Thiazide diuretics Warfarin	Barbiturates** Benzodiazepines** Carbamazepine Phenothiazines** Phenytoin Primadone Sodium valproate	Corticosteroids** Oral hypo-glycemics Progestins Thyroxin	Propantheline
APPARENTLY SAFE TO USE^c	Acetaminophen Codeine Demerol Flufenamic acid Mefenamic acid Paracetamol Salicylates*	Cephalosporins Clindamycin Erythromycin Lincomycin Metronidazole Nitrofurantoin Penicillins Rifampicin	Clonidine Digoxin Heparin Methyldopa	Barbiturates* Benzodiazepines* Chloral hydrate MAO inhibitors Tricyclic antidepressants	Corticosteroids*	Antacids Antihistamines Biscodyl Bulk laxatives Folic acid Iron

Key: * = short-term, low-dose
** = long-term, high-dose.
^a Do not use indicates that the drugs may suppress lactation, that toxic effects have been reported, or that toxic effects are predicted on theoretical grounds.
^b Use with caution indicates that the drugs may be excreted in small amounts in the milk, or that there is insufficient information on their safety.
^c Apparently safe to use indicates that the drugs are either not excreted, or only excreted in minute amounts in milk. (From Read, M. D. Prescribing for the breast feeding patient. Practitioner 225:920, 1981.)

during pregnancy (Knight and Rhind, 1975). In a prospective study of 153 pregnancies in 59 patients, seizures occurred more frequently during pregnancy in 45 percent of cases, and less frequently in only 5 percent (Knight and Rhind, 1975).

Virtually all anticonvulsants have been linked with teratogenesis. Trimethadione has, however, been shown to produce fetal deformities and mental retardation in such a high proportion of exposed fetuses that its use is contraindicated in pregnancy (Feldman et al., 1977). Drugs of the hydantoin group have been associated with increased incidences of relatively common anomalies, as well as producing a specific syndrome. Congenital heart disease is 2 to 3 times more common, and cleft palate 5 to 10 times more common in children of epileptics using hydantoins (often in conjunction with other anticonvulsants) than in those of nonepileptics (Annegers et al., 1974). Furthermore, in one study, 16 to 20 percent of patients with cleft lip or palate had a first- or second-degree relative with epilepsy, emphasizing the importance of common genetic factors (Dronamraju, 1970). A "fetal hydantoin syndrome" is seen in 10 percent of infants exposed in utero, and includes such findings as intrauterine growth retardation, microcephaly, mental retardation, dysmorphic facies, and infantile growth retardation (American Academy of Pediatrics Committee on Drugs, 1979). It is likely that barbiturates play a role in retarding intrauterine growth and brain development (Smith, 1977). Recently it has been suggested that infants with the fetal hydantoin syndrome may be predisposed to childhood neoplasia (Cohen, 1981).

The American Academy of Pediatrics, after considering all available data, have formulated guidelines. They state that anticonvulsants should not be used unnecessarily, but caution that if a patient has been convulsion-free for years and cessation of anticonvulsants is considered, it should be done well before a contemplated pregnancy. Epileptics requiring barbiturates or hydantoins should be advised that the chance of a normal child is 90 percent, but that the risk of congenital abnormalities or mental retardation is 2 to 3 times greater than the average because of either the disease or its treatment (American Academy of Pediatrics Committee on Drugs, 1979). Trimethadione should not be used in pregnancy, but carbamaze-

pine, although teratogenic in animals, appears to be safe in humans (Niebyl et al., 1979).

Anticonvulsant drug dosage in pregnancy should be carefully controlled by checking serum levels. Breast-feeding appears safe, although most anticonvulsants appear in low concentrations in breast milk (American Academy of Pediatrics Committee on Drugs, 1979).

Asthma

Asthma affects approximately 1 percent of pregnant women (Schaefer and Silverman, 1961; Gordon et al., 1970). Collected reports of over 1100 pregnancies in asthmatics suggested that symptoms improved in 36 percent of patients during pregnancy and worsened in 23 percent (Gluck and Gluck, 1976). In a prospective study only 14 percent of asthmatic women improved and 43 percent worsened during pregnancy; the more severe asthmatics generally worsened (Gluck and Gluck, 1976). Hence, asthmatics have a high chance of needing drug therapy in pregnancy, and often in greater doses than when they were not pregnant. Hypoxia is dangerous for both mother and fetus.

"Topical, nonabsorbable, and effective" therapy would be safest for both mother and fetus, but it is not available (Mintz, 1976). Aerosols of adrenergic agents are safe if used according to instructions; the dangers of using adrenergic drugs by several routes simultaneously should be kept in mind. Cromolyn sodium inhalations may be used prophylactically, since less than 10 percent of the inhaled dose is absorbed, and even massive doses in animals have not proved to be teratogenic (Dykes, 1974). There is, however, still concern about its safety in human pregnancy (Turner et al., 1980).

Oral theophylline is the systemic drug of choice, having been used widely with no evidence of teratogenicity (Turner et al., 1980). Toxic symptoms have been seen in some infants following use of theophylline in late pregnancy and labor, but these symptoms settled spontaneously and there were no long-term sequelae (Arwood et al., 1979). Combinations of theophylline, ephedrine, and barbiturates offer no therapeutic advantage, and there is some concern about the teratogenicity of ephedrine (Turner et al., 1980). Oral adrenergic drugs appear to be safe in pregnancy but are best used as an adjunct to theophylline or when it fails (Romero and Berkowitz, 1982). Acute or severe asthmatic attacks in pregnancy are best managed with parenteral aminophylline or adrenergic drugs, the latter possibly being preferable because of their tocolytic actions (Romero and Berkowitz, 1982).

Severe asthmatics may require steroids during pregnancy, and prednisone is the drug of choice. Some reports have linked steroid use to cleft palate, but the risk appears minimal (Turner et al., 1980). Estriol levels may be low as a result of adrenal suppression in the fetus, without indicating fetal compromise (Morrison and Kilpatrick, 1969). Labor constitutes a severe stress, and adequate steroid coverage should be given in women who have been on chronic high doses.

Over-the-counter antiasthmatic drugs may contain iodine as an expectorant. This can lead to congenital goiter and hypothyroidism in the infant, and these preparations should be avoided (Turner et al., 1980; Romero and Berkowitz, 1982).

Cardiovascular Disease

It is not uncommon for a woman suffering from essential hypertension to consider or achieve pregnancy. Such patients are at greater risk themselves, and perinatal morbidity and mortality broadly parallel the severity of the hypertension (Berkowitz, 1980). Superimposed preeclampsia is a common and severe problem (Beilin and Redman, 1977). Thiazide diuretics and furosemide are commonly used in essential hypertension, and although there is no evidence that these agents cause teratogenesis, there are sound reasons for avoiding their use in pregnancy (Witter et al., 1981). These include electrolyte disturbances and contraction of the intravascular space, which may compromise the placental circulation and aggravate the reduced plasma volume of preeclampsia (Berkowitz, 1980). Use of thiazide diuretics in pregnancy has been associated with maternal hyperglycemia, hyperuricemia, pancreatitis, fetal growth retardation, neonatal jaundice, hypoglycemia, and thrombocytopenia (Witter et al., 1981). It is probably reasonable to continue diuretic therapy through pregnancy for those essential hypertensives who used them before pregnancy.

Several studies have testified to the safety of methyldopa in pregnancy (Kincaid-Smith et al., 1966; Leather et al., 1968; Redman et al., 1976). Teratogenesis has not been reported, and perinatal mortality was reduced, largely through a reduced incidence of midtrimester fetal loss (Beilin and Redman, 1977). Methyldopa is therefore still the drug of choice for essential hypertension in pregnancy. Beta blockers, such as propranolol, have been advocated by some, but there are concerns that chronic use of these drugs may lead to intrauterine growth retardation and neonatal hypoglycemia and compromise the ability of the fetus to respond to stress (Stirrat and Lieberman, 1977). Thus propranolol is not generally advised for long-term use in pregnancy. Hydralazine is an effective and apparently safe drug for hypertensive crises in pregnancy. However, since little is known of its safety for long-term use in pregnancy, it is generally not recommended (Witter et al., 1981).

Anticoagulants are occasionally required during all or most of pregnancy, principally in patients with prosthetic heart valves and thromboembolic disease. Warfarin is the most common oral anticoagulant drug, but its use in pregnancy carries the risk of teratogenesis as well as serious maternal, fetal, or neonatal hemorrhage (Witter et al., 1981). A "fetal warfarin syndrome" has been described following first trimester usage. Features include nasal hypoplasia, optic atrophy, epiphyseal stippling, and mental retardation (Hall et al., 1980). It seems likely that some parts of the syndrome may occur even if warfarin is used only later in pregnancy (Goldberg, 1982). Because of these facts it is now recommended that subcutaneous heparin, usually self-administered, is the treatment of choice in those requiring long-term anticoagulation during pregnancy (Goldberg, 1982).

Mental Illness

Mental illness affects all age groups, and the use of psychotropic drugs is common in the reproductive age group. Barbiturates have been widely used over many years, with little convincing evidence of teratogenicity. Such suspicions have been raised when barbiturates have been used, often in conjunction with other drugs, for epilepsy (Meadow, 1970), but as already discussed, this is a complex relationship. Following chronic barbiturate usage in pregnancy, the newborn may suffer typical "withdrawal" symptoms, which occasionally require treatment (Desmond et al., 1972). On the other hand, barbiturate therapy induces enzymes in the fetal liver that enhance its ability to conjugate bilirubin, reducing the incidence of jaundice (Trolle, 1968).

The most widely used group of minor tranquilizers consists of the benzodiazepines, such as diazepam and chlordiazepoxide. There have been reports of increased incidences of congenital abnormalities in general (Milkovich and van den Berg, 1974) and of cleft palate in particular (Safra and Oakley, 1978) associated with these drugs, but there is no convincing evidence of a causal relationship (Hartz et al., 1975). Use in the perinatal period may result in withdrawal symptoms in the neonate (Rementeria and Bhatt, 1977), neonatal depression and hypothermia (Owen et al., 1972), and hypotonia (Shannon et al., 1972).

Tricyclic antidepressant drugs have been implicated in the production of limb reduction deformities and other congenital defects, but no causal relationship has been established (Banister et al., 1972; Rachelefsky et al., 1972; McBride, 1972). Withdrawal symptoms (Webster, 1973) and transient urinary retention (Schearer, 1972) have also been reported in infants following maternal use of these drugs in the perinatal period.

Lithium carbonate, used in the treatment of manic depressive psychosis, is best avoided in early pregnancy. It is teratogenic in animals if even transiently raised serum levels occur, and reports indicate an approximately 11 percent chance of congenital abnormalities, mostly involving the heart, in humans (Weinstein and Goldfield, 1975). Infants of mothers receiving lithium immediately prepartum as well as those being breast-fed by a mother using the drug, may exhibit hypotonia, hypothermia, lethargy, and cyanosis (Ananth, 1978).

Major tranquilizers of the phenothiazine group have been widely used over a long period, and although there have been some reports of congenital abnormalities, the risks appear to be small (Ayd, 1963). Transient extrapyramidal dysfunction has been reported in infants born to psychotic women using phenothiazines (Levy and Wisniewski, 1974).

Thyroid Disease

Thyroid disease is often associated with subfertility and spontaneous abortion. Hyper-thyroidism is seen in roughly 1 in 1000 pregnancies, and hypothyroidism much less frequently (Ramsay, 1977). Severely hypothyroid women rarely achieve pregnancy, but women with mild hypothyroidism may conceive. Although normal infants have been reported (Hodges et al., 1952), spontaneous abortion, stillbirth, and mentally and physically abnormal infants are common in these cases (Man et al., 1971). Hence, thyroid hormone substitution with desiccated thyroid, levothyroxine, or levotriiodothyronine should be used: the latter agent may be preferable because of better placental transfer. Dosage is controlled by serum levels.

Patients with mild thyrotoxicosis may conceive. The diagnosis of thyrotoxicosis in pregnancy can be difficult (Ramsay, 1977) and its treatment controversial. Therapy with radioactive iodine is contraindicated, as it accumulates in, and destroys, fetal thyroid tissue. Medical treatment with thiourea compounds such as propylthiouracil or methimazole may be used, usually in the lowest effective doses, controlled by serum T_3 and T_4 levels. There is no evidence of teratogenesis with these agents (Burrows et al., 1968). Some authors advocate higher doses of antithyroid drugs, together with thyroxin, to maintain normal serum levels (Ramsay, 1977). There is no evidence of any advantage to this approach. Propranolol may be used to provide symptomatic relief in hyperthyroidism, but specific, rather than symptomatic, treatment seems better.

Surgery for hyperthyroidism in pregnancy has been advocated, to avoid drug exposure. In the second trimester of pregnancy, complications from thyroid surgery are uncommon (Howe and Francis, 1962). However, over 30 percent of patients become hypothyroid for a period of time after partial thyroidectomy and may require replacement therapy (Toft et al., 1976). Overall, medical treatment is probably preferable.

PRESCRIBING DRUGS FOR CONDITIONS DEVELOPING IN PREGNANCY

Antiemetic Medications

Antiemetics are commonly used in pregnancy for the relatively common "morning sickness" and the less frequent hyperemesis. There has been great concern about the safety of the most widely used drug, Bendectin, a mixture of doxylamine and pyridoxine. Limb reduction defects, oral clefts, and cardiac defects have all been reported, but recent large controlled studies have confirmed many earlier reports of the safety of this drug (Cordero et al., 1981; Mitchell et al., 1981). Nevertheless, in 1984 Bendectin was taken off the market. For hyperemesis, hospitalization, bedrest, intravenous fluids, and parenteral or rectal phenothiazines are usually safe (Levy and Wisniewski, 1974) and effective.

Antipyretic Analgesics

Drugs of this grouping, mainly obtained over-the-counter, are the most commonly used drugs in pregnancy. This reflects both the common occurrence of a variety of minor aches, pains, and illnesses in pregnancy and the willingness of our society to seek a pharmacologic remedy for all discomfort. The most commonly used drugs are the salicylates and acetaminophen. The salicylates are among the oldest synthetic drugs in use today. Animal studies have shown them to be teratogenic, albeit in very high doses (Warkany and Takacs, 1959; Robertson et al., 1979). Information obtained from retrospective studies using infants with congenital abnormalities as a starting point suggests that salicylates may be teratogenic (Richards, 1969; Nelson and Forfar, 1971; Saxen, 1975), but prospective studies do not support this conclusion (Turner and Collins, 1975; Slone et al., 1976). It has been suggested that chronic usage of large doses of aspirin during pregnancy produces low-birth-weight infants (Turner and Collins, 1975), but that study was performed in Australia at a time when that country had a high incidence of analgesic abuse, especially among women. Studies in the United States show no evidence of retarded fetal growth (Shapiro et al., 1976). Used in late pregnancy, salicylates may lead to prolonged gestation (Lewis and Schulman, 1973) and labor (Collins and Turner, 1973), probably because of their antiprostaglandin action. For a similar reason, postpartum hemorrhage is apparently more common in chronic aspirin users (Lewis and Schulman, 1973).

Salicylates cross the placenta and may have particularly disastrous effects on fetal hemostasis, particularly in premature infants. Intracranial hemorrhage has been shown to occur significantly more often in premature infants whose mothers had consumed aspirin in the last week of pregnancy than in controls or in women using aceta-

minophen in that period (Rumack et al., 1981).

Acetaminophen has been used widely in pregnancy with no evidence of untoward effects, and it is probably a safer drug for occasional use in pregnancy than any of the other commonly used antipyretic analgesics (Lietman and Niebyl, 1982).

Antibiotics

The most common reason for antibiotic use during gestation is urinary tract infection. Sulfonamides are useful first-line drugs and do not appear to be teratogenic in humans, although it is probably not wise to use the combination of sulfamethoxazole and trimethoprim in early pregnancy (Schwarz, 1981). Late in pregnancy sulfonamides are contraindicated, because they cross the placenta, achieve high plasma levels in the fetus, and, should delivery occur, compete with bilirubin for albumin binding sites, which increases the risk of kernicterus (Harris et al., 1950).

Penicillin and its derivatives have been widely used in pregnancy and appear to be safe for both mother and fetus (Hamod and Khouzami, 1982). Little data is available on the use of cephalosporins in pregnancy, but it is known that maternal serum levels tend to be markedly lower for a given dose than for women in the nonpregnant state (Hamod and Khouzami, 1982). Erythromycin appears to be safe in pregnancy, although the estolate form may produce hepatotoxicity (McCormack et al., 1977) and should be avoided. Serum levels are lower than in the nonpregnant state (Hamod and Khouzami, 1982).

Aminoglycosides are ototoxic and nephrotoxic to adults, and it is believed that they may have the same effect on the fetus (Schwarz, 1981; Hamod and Khouzami, 1982). Their use should be limited to life-threatening situations or serious infections resistant to other drugs, and their dosage controlled by serum levels. Prolonged use is unwise.

Tetracyclines form a complex with calcium orthophosphate and become incorporated into the bones and teeth undergoing calcification; this complex causes discoloration. The deciduous teeth begin to calcify at about 5 or 6 months in utero. Therefore, use of tetracyclines after this time will cause staining of the infant's teeth.

Tetracyclines also are passed in the breast milk, so breast-feeding should be discouraged in mothers who are receiving tetracyclines. However, once the treatment is completed, breast-feeding can be resumed.

Three antibiotics that are especially useful for anaerobic infections—chloramphenicol, clindamycin, and metronidazole—are generally contraindicated in pregnancy. Chloramphenicol may produce aplastic anemia in adults and the "gray baby syndrome" in neonates. High fetal serum levels are attained following administration of the drug to the mother (Ross et al., 1950), so its use in pregnancy should be considered only in the most extreme situations. Clindamycin has not been widely used, and judgments as to its safety cannot be made (Hamod and Khouzami, 1982). Metronidazole has been widely used for anaerobic infections in Europe, but fears of its teratogenicity and potential carcinogenic effects have led to cautions against its use in pregnancy in the United States (Schwarz, 1981).

Conclusions

This chapter is not comprehensive. The aim is to emphasize principles of drug administration in pregnancy, using specific drugs or diseases as examples of the problems involved. The monograph of Berkowitz and colleagues, mentioned earlier, is the most useful reference for information regarding specific drugs (Berkowitz et al., 1981).

It must be recognized that there can be no final word on the safety of the vast majority of drugs in pregnancy. As already mentioned, the chance of most congenital abnormalities being drug-induced is far less than the chance of a genetic causation. Furthermore, few known teratogens affect more than a small proportion of exposed fetuses. Before ascribing teratogenic potential to a drug already used by a pregnant woman, or a congenital abnormality to a drug she used, physicians and other health personnel should consider the uncertain state of our knowledge and the load of anxiety and guilt that the mother must carry if she believes her actions have adversely affected her baby. In particular, we must not hide the state of our ignorance behind a false cloak of certainty.

Drugs should never be used without good reason, and this is especially true in pregnancy, when the health of both a mother and a fetus are involved. But the health and safety of the mother and her baby are inter-related, and pregnant women must not be denied necessary medications simply because of their pregnancy.

"Ultimately, to deal effectively with the problem of drug effects in pregnancy, [we] must continue to become better informed and alert to the potential dangers of all agents . . . to supply the appropriate medication when needed, and to withhold it when not needed. . . . Only in this way can the risk of fetal drug toxicity be minimized and the optimal health of both mother and fetus ensured." (Barber, 1981)

REFERENCES

American Academy of Pediatrics Committee on Drugs: Anticonvulsants and pregnancy. Pediatrics 63:331, 1979.

Ananth, J.: Side effects in the neonate from psychotropic drugs excreted through breast feeding. Am. J. Psychiatry 135:801, 1978.

Anderson, V. E.: Genetic Counseling for Epilepsy. In Commission for the Control of Epilepsy and its Consequences: Plan for Nationwide Action on Epilepsy, Vol. 2. Washington, D.C., U.S. Dept. Health, Education and Welfare, 1978, p. 141.

Annegers, J. F., Elveback, L. R., Hauser, W. A., et al.: Do anticonvulsants have a teratogenic effect? Arch. Neurol. 31:364, 1974.

Apgar, V.: The drug problem in pregnancy. Clin. Obstet. Gynecol. 9:623, 1966.

Arwood, L. L., Dasta, J. F., and Friedman, C.: Placental transfer of theophylline: two case reports. Pediatrics 63:844, 1979.

Ayd, F. J.: Chlorpromazine: ten years' experience. JAMA 184:51, 1963.

Banister, P., Dafoe, C., Smith, E. S., et al.: Possible teratogenicity of tricyclic antidepressants. Lancet 1:838, 1972.

Barber, H. R. K.: Symposium on drugs in pregnancy: introduction. Obstet. Gynecol. 58:15, 1981.

Beilin, L. J., and Redman, C. W. G.: The use of antihypertensive drugs in pregnancy. In Lewis, P. J. (ed.): Therapeutic Problems in Pregnancy. Baltimore, University Park Press, 1977.

Berkowitz, R. L.: Antihypertensive drugs in the pregnant patient. Obstet. Gynec. Surv. 35:191, 1980.

Berkowitz, R. L., Coustan, D. R., and Mochizuki, T. K.: Handbook for Prescribing Medications During Pregnancy. Boston, Little, Brown & Co., 1981.

Blake, D. A.: Requirements and limitations in reproductive and teratogenic risk assessment. In Niebyl, J. R.: Drug Use in Pregnancy. Philadelphia, Lea & Febiger, 1982.

Brent, R. L.: Drugs and pregnancy: are the insert warnings too dire? Contemp. Obstet. Gynec. 20:42, 1982.

Brent, R. L.: Litigation-produced pain, disease and suffering: an experience with congenital malformation lawsuits. Teratology 16:1, 1977.

Burrows, G. N., Bartsocas, C., Klatskin, E. M., et al.: Children exposed in utero to propylthiouracil: subsequent intellectual and physical development. Am. J. Dis. Child. 116:161, 1968.

Cohen, M. M.: Neoplasia and the fetal alcohol and hydantoin syndromes. Neurobehav. Toxicol. Teratol. 3:161, 1981.

Cole, W. A., and Trasler, D. G.: Gene-teratogen interaction in insulin-induced mouse exencephaly. Teratology 22:125, 1980.

Collins, E., and Turner, G.: Salicylates and pregnancy. Lancet 2:1494, 1973.

Cordero, J. F., Oakley, G. P., Greenberg, F., et al.: Is Bendectin a teratogen? JAMA 245:2307, 1981.

Desmond, M. M., Schwanecke, R. P., Wilson, G. S., et al.: Maternal barbiturate utilization and neonatal withdrawal symptomatology. J Pediatr. 80:190, 1972.

Doering, P. L., and Stewart, R. B.: The extent and character of drug consumption during pregnancy. JAMA 239:843, 1978.

Dronamraju, K. R.: Epilepsy and cleft lip and palate. Lancet 2:876, 1970.

Dykes, M. H. M.: Evaluation of an antiasthmatic agent, cromolyn sodium. JAMA 227:1061, 1974.

Feldman, G. L., Weaver, D. D., and Lovrein, E. W.: The fetal trimethadione syndrome: report of an additional family and further delineation of the syndrome. Am. J. Dis. Child. 131:1389, 1977.

Fraser, F. C.: Animal models for craniofacial disorders. Prog. Clin. Biol. Res. 46:1, 1980.

Fraser, F. C., and Fainstat, T. D.: Production of congenital abnormalities in the offspring of pregnant mice treated with cortisone. Progress report. Pediatrics 8:527, 1951.

Gluck, J. C., and Gluck, P. A.: The effects of pregnancy on asthma: a prospective study. Ann. Allerg. 37:164, 1976.

Golbus, M. S.: Teratology for the obstetrician: current status. Obstet. Gynecol. 55:269, 1982.

Goldberg, E.: Anticoagulants in pregnancy. In Niebyl, J. R.: Drug Use in Pregnancy. Philadelphia, Lea & Febiger, 1982.

Gordon, M., Niswander, K. R., Berendes, H., et al.: Fetal morbidity following potentially anoxigenic obstetric conditions. VII. Bronchial asthma. Am. J. Obstet. Gynecol. 106:421, 1970.

Granroth, G.: Defects of the central nervous system in Finland. III. Diseases and drugs in pregnancy. Early Hum. Dev. 2:147, 1978.

Gregg, N. M.: Congenital cataract following German measles in the mother. Trans. Ophthalmol. Soc. Aust. 3:35, 1941.

Hale, F.: The relation of vitamin A to anophthalmos in pigs. Am. J. Ophthalmol. 18:1087, 1935.

Hall, J. G., Pauli, R. M., and Wilson, K. M.: Maternal and fetal sequelae of anticoagulation during pregnancy. Am. J. Med. 68:122, 1980.

Hamod, K. A., and Khouzami, V. A.: Antibiotics in pregnancy. In Niebyl, J. R. (ed.): Drug Use in Pregnancy. Philadelphia, Lea & Febiger, 1982.

Harris, R. C., Lucey, J. F., and MacLean, J. R.: Kernicterus in premature infants associated with low concentration of bilirubin in the plasma. Pediatrics 21:878, 1950.

Hartz, S. C., Heinonen, O. F., Shapiro, S., et al.: Antenatal exposure to meprobamate and chlordiazepoxide in relation to malformations, mental development, and childhood mortality. N. Engl. J. Med. 292:726, 1975.

Hawe, P., and Francis, H. H.: Pregnancy and thyrotoxicosis. Br. Med. J. 2:817, 1962.

Heinonen, O. P., Slone, D., and Shapiro, S.: Birth Defects and Drugs in Pregnancy. Littleton, MA, Publishing Sciences Group, 1977.

Herbst, A. L.: Diethylstilbestrol and other sex hormones during pregnancy. Obstet. Gynecol. 58:35S, 1981.

Herbst, A. L., Ulfelder, H., and Poskanzer, D. C.: Adenocarcinoma of the vagina. Association of maternal stilbestrol therapy with tumor appearance in young women. N. Engl. J. Med. 284:878, 1971.

Hill, R. M., Craig, J. P., Chaney, M. D., et al.: Utilization of over-the-counter drugs during pregnancy. Clin. Obstet. Gynecol. 20:381, 1977.

Hodges, R. E., Hamilton, H. E., and Keettel, W. C.: Pregnancy in myxedema. Arch. Intern. Med. 90:863, 1952.

Holmes, L. B., quoted by Knuppel, R. A.: Recognizing teratogenic effects of drugs and radiation. Contemp. Obstet. Gynec. 15:171, 1980.

Janz, D.: The teratogenic risk of antiepileptic drugs. Epilepsia 16:159, 1975.

Kincaid-Smith, P., Bullen, H., and Mills, J.: Prolonged use of methyldopa in severe hypertension in pregnancy. Br. Med. J. 1:274, 1966.

Knight, A. H., and Rhind, E. G.: Epilepsy and pregnancy: a study of 153 pregnancies in 59 patients. Epilepsia 16:99, 1975.

Leather, H. M., Humphreys, D. M., Baker, P. B., et al.: A controlled trial of hypotensive agents in hypertension in pregnancy. Lancet 1:488, 1968.

Leck, I.: Backwards and forwards in search of teratogens. Early Hum. Dev. 2:203, 1978.

Lenz, W.: Malformations caused by drugs in pregnancy. Am. J. Dis. Child. 112:99, 1966.

Lenz, W.: Thalidomide and congenital abnormalities. Lancet 2:1358, 1961.

Levy, W., and Wisniewski, K.: Chlorpromazine causing extrapyramidal dysfunction in a newborn infant of a psychotic mother. NY State J. Med. 74:684, 1974.

Lewis, R. B., and Schulman, J. D.: Influence of acetylsalicylic acid, an inhibitor of prostaglandin synthesis, on the duration of human pregnancy and labor. Lancet 2:1159, 1973.

Lietman, P. S., and Niebyl, J. R.: The use of mild analgesics in pregnancy. In Niebyl, J. R. (ed.): Drug Use in Pregnancy. Philadelphia, Lea & Febiger, 1982.

Maltau, J. M., Stokke, K. T., and Moe, N.: Effects of betamethasone on plasma levels of estriol, cortisol, and HCS in late pregnancy. Acta Obstet. Gynecol. Scand. 58:235, 1979.

Man, E. B., Holden, R. M., and Jones, W. S.: Thyroid function in human pregnancy. VII. Development and retardation of 4 year old progeny of euthyroid and hypothyroxinemic women. Am. J. Obstet. Gynecol. 109:12, 1971.

McBride, W. G.: Limb deformities associated with iminodibenzyl hydrochloride. Med. J. Aust. 1:492, 1972.

McBride, W. A.: Thalidomide and congenital abnormalities. Lancet 1:45, 1962.

McCormack, W. M., George, H., Donner, A., et al.: Hepatotoxicity of erythromycin estolate during pregnancy. Antimicrob. Agents Chemother. 12:630, 1977.

Meadow, S. R.: Congenital abnormalities and anticonvulsant drugs. Proc. R. Soc. Med. 63:48, 1970.

Milkovich, L., van den Berg, B. J.: Effects of prenatal meprobamate and chlordiazepoxide hydrochloride on human embryonic and fetal development. N. Engl. J. Med. 291:1268, 1974.

Mintz, S.: Pregnancy and asthma. In Weiss, E. B., and Segal, M. S. (eds.): Bronchial Asthma: Mechanisms and Therapeutics. Boston, Little, Brown & Co., 1976, p. 971.

Mitchell, A. A., Rosenberg, L., Shapiro, S., et al.: Birth

defects related to Bendectin use in pregnancy. I. Oral clefts and cardiac defects. JAMA 245:2311, 1981.

Morrison, J., and Kilpatrick, N.: Low urinary oestriol excretion in pregnancy associated with oral prednisone therapy. J. Obstet. Gynaecol. Br. Commonw. 76:719, 1969.

Nebert, D. W., and Shum, S.: The murine *Ah* locus: genetic differences in birth defects among individuals in the same uterus. Prog. Clin. Biol. Res. 46:173, 1980.

Nelson, M. M., and Forfar, J. O.: Associations between drugs administered during pregnancy and congenital abnormalities of the fetus. Br. Med. J. 1:523, 1971.

Niebyl, J. R., Blake, D. A., Freeman, J. M., et al.: Carbamazepine levels in pregnancy and lactation. Obstet. Gynecol. 53:139, 1979.

Owen, J. R., Irani, S. F., and Blair, A. W.: Effect of diazepam administered to mothers during labor on temperature regulation in the neonate. Arch. Dis. Child. 47:107, 1972.

Peckham, C. M., and King, R. W.: A study of intercurrent conditions observed during pregnancy. Am. J. Obstet. Gynecol. 87:609, 1963.

Philipson, A.: Pharmacokinetics of ampicillin during pregnancy. J. Infect. Dis. 136:370, 1977.

Rachelefsky, G. S., Flynt, J. W., Ebbin, A. J., et al.: Possible teratogenicity of tricyclic antidepressants. Lancet 1:838, 1972.

Ramsay, I. D.: Thyroid therapy in pregnancy. In Lewis, P. J. (ed.): Therapeutic Problems in Pregnancy. Baltimore, University Park Press, 1977, p. 93.

Redman, C. W. G., Beilin, L. J., Bonnar, J., et al.: Fetal outcome in trial of antihypertensive treatment in pregnancy. Lancet 2:783, 1976.

Rementeria, J. L., and Bhatt, K.: Withdrawal symptoms in neonates from intrauterine exposure to diazepam. J. Pediatr. 90:123, 1977.

Richards, I. D. G.: Congenital malformations and environmental influences in pregnancy. Br. J. Prev. Soc. Med. 23:218, 1969.

Robertson, R. T., Allen, M. L., and Bokelman, D. L.: Aspirin: teratogenic evaluation in the dog. Teratology 20:313, 1979.

Romero, R., and Berkowitz, R. L.: The use of antiasthmatic drugs in pregnancy. In Niebyl, J. R.: Drug Use in Pregnancy. Philadelphia, Lea & Febiger, 1982, p. 41.

Ross, S., Burke, R. G., Sites, J., et al.: Placental transmission of chloramphenicol (chloromycetin). JAMA 142:1361, 1950.

Rumack, C. M., Guggenheim, M. A., Rumack, B. H., et al.: Neonatal intracranial hemorrhage and maternal use of aspirin. Obstet. Gynecol. 58:52S, 1981.

Safra, M. J., and Oakley, G. P.: Association between cleft lip with or without cleft palate and prenatal exposure to diazepam. Lancet 1:478, 1978.

Saxen, I.: Associations between oral clefts and drugs taken during pregnancy. Int. J. Epidemiol. 4:37, 1975.

Schaefer, G., and Silverman, F.: Pregnancy complicated by asthma. Am. J. Obstet. Gynecol. 82:182, 1961.

Schearer, W. T., Schreiner, R. L., and Marshall, R. E.: Urinary retention in a neonate secondary to maternal ingestion of nortriptyline. J. Pediatr. 81:570, 1972.

Schwarz, R. H.: Considerations of antibiotic therapy during pregnancy. Obstet. Gynecol. 58:95S, 1981.

Shannon, R. W., Frazer, G. P., Aitken, R. G., et al.: Diazepam in preeclamptic toxemia with special reference to its effect on the newborn infant. Br. J. Clin. Pract. 26:271, 1972.

Shapiro, S., Siskind, V., Monson, R. R., et al.: Perinatal mortality and birth weight in relation to aspirin taking during pregnancy. Lancet 1:1375, 1976.

Shepard, T. H.: A Catalog of Teratogenic Agents. Baltimore, The Johns Hopkins Press, 1973.

Shepard, T. H.: Teratogenicity from drugs—an increasing problem. In Disease-A-Month, June 1974, Chicago, Year Book Medical Pubs., 1974.

Shepard, T. H., and Fantel, A. G.: Teratology of therapeutic agents. In Iffy, L., and Kaminetzky, H. A. (eds.): Principles and Practice of Obstetrics and Perinatology. New York, John Wiley & Sons, 1981, p. 461.

Shirkey, H. C.: Editorial comment: therapeutic orphans. J. Pediatr. 72:119, 1968.

Slone, D., Heinonen, O. P., Kaufman, D. W., et al.: Aspirin and congenital malformations. Lancet 1:1373, 1976.

Smith, D. W.: Teratogenicity of anticonvulsant medications. Am. J. Dis. Child. 131:1337, 1977.

Stern, L.: In vivo assessment of the teratogenic potential of drugs in humans. Obstet. Gynecol. 58:3S, 1981.

Stirrat, G. M., and Lieberman, B. A.: Fetal outcome in pregnancies complicated by severe hypertension treated with propranolol. In Lewis, P. J. (ed.): Therapeutic Problems in Pregnancy. Baltimore, University Park Press, 1977.

Stumpf, D. A., and Frost, M.: Seizures, anticonvulsants and pregnancy. Am. J. Dis. Child. 132:746, 1978.

Toft, A. D., Irvine, W. J., McIntosh, D. et al.: Temporary hypothyroidism after surgical treatment of thyrotoxicosis. Lancet 2:817, 1976.

Trolle, D.: Decrease of serum total bilirubin concentration in newborn infants after phenobarbitone treatment. Lancet 2:705, 1968.

Tuchmann-Duplessis, H.: Drug effects on the fetus. Sydney, Adis Press, 1975, p. 6.

Turner, E. S., Greenberger, P. A., and Patterson, R.: Management of the pregnant asthmatic patient. Ann. Intern. Med. 93:905, 1980.

Turner, G., and Collins, E.: Fetal effects of regular salicylate ingestion in pregnancy. Lancet 2:338, 1975.

Warkany, J., and Takacs, E.: Experimental production of congenital malformations in rat by salicylate poisoning. Am. J. Pathol. 35:315, 1959.

Webster, P. A. C.: Withdrawal symptoms in neonates associated with maternal antidepressant therapy. Lancet 2:318, 1973.

Weinstein, M. R., and Goldfield, M. D.: Administration of lithium during pregnancy. In Johnson, F. N.: Lithium Research and Therapy. New York, Academic Press, 1975, p. 237.

Whalley, P. J., Adams, R. H., and Combe, B.: Tetracycline toxicity in pregnancy. JAMA 189:103, 1964.

Wilson, J. G.: Environment and Birth Defects. New York, Academic Press, 1973.

Witter, F. R., King, T. M., and Blake, D. A.: Adverse effects of cardiovascular drug therapy on the fetus and neonate. Obstet. Gynecol. 58:100S, 1981.

Woollam, D. H. M.: Teratogens in everyday life. The Milroy Lecture, 1980. J. Roy. Coll. Phys. London 14:213, 1980.

7

NUTRITION IN PREGNANCY

WILLIAM N. P. HERBERT
MILDRED KAUFMAN
ROBERT C. CEFALO

The importance of proper nutrition during pregnancy is receiving increased attention as perinatal care shifts from "crisis" to "preventive" care. All members of the health care team require current scientific information to adequately assess the patient's nutritional status and to encourage her to eat a nutritionally adequate diet. Many patients are unaware of the importance of good food selection practices during pregnancy and often follow fad weight control schemes or substitute multivitamin/mineral supplements for a nutritionally adequate diet. They may also not be aware of the increased tendency for ketosis with overnight or daytime fasting during pregnancy. Preferably, education on nutrition should begin prior to pregnancy, since a woman with good nutritional habits and normal body weight prior to conception has distinct advantages during the course of pregnancy.

This chapter discusses nutritional considerations relating to obstetric care. It provides (1) a review of nutritional requirements during pregnancy; (2) a discussion of obstetric complications that have important nutritional interrelationships; (3) a section on "special situations," e.g., multiple gestation, that require nutritional adjustments; (4) techniques for the assessment of nutritional status; and (5) methods for intervention when nutritional guidance is required.

Nutritional Requirements During Pregnancy

MATERNAL GROWTH AND ENERGY NEEDS

The total energy requirement of pregnancy is estimated to be 75,000 to 80,000 kcal, or an average of an additional 300 kcal daily (Hytten and Leitch, 1971). These calories must be added to the number of calories needed to fulfill the nutritional requirements of the woman that are unrelated to her pregnancy, which vary with her age and physical activity. Table 7–1 contains the recommended dietary allowances (RDA) for calories, protein, vitamins, and minerals during gestation, as proposed by the Food and Nutrition Board, National Academy of Sciences, in 1980.

The actual increase in energy needs varies through the course of pregnancy, with a greater demand in the second and third trimesters than in the first. The Food and Agriculture Organization, a division of the World Health Organization, recommends that the caloric intake be increased by 150 kcal/day during the first trimester and 350 kcal/day thereafter. These are general recommendations and do not reflect individual variation with physical activity.

FETAL GROWTH AND ENERGY NEEDS

Glucose has traditionally been considered the sole energy source for the fetus, but, as noted in the recent review by Moghissi (1978), amino acids may be important for fetal aerobic metabolism. In general, amino acid concentrations are higher in fetal plasma than in maternal plasma (Ghadimi and Pecora, 1964). The capacity of the pla-

Much of the material in this chapter has been developed for presentation at the Intensive Course in Maternal Nutrition supported by the March of Dimes Birth Defects Foundation, White Plains, New York. The authors have served as directors of this course.

Table 7–1. Recommended Dietary Allowances

Females		Nonpregnant				Pregnant
	Years	11–14	15–18	19–22	23–50	
WEIGHT	Pounds	101	120	120	120	
HEIGHT	Inches	62	64	64	64	
ENERGY	Calories	2200	2100	2100	2000	+300
PROTEIN	(g)	46	46	44	44	+ 30
Fat-Soluble Vitamins						
Vitamin A	(RE)[1]	800	800	800	800	+200
Vitamin D	(mcg)[2]	10	10	7.5	5	+ 5
Vitamin E	(mg)	8	8	8	8	+ 2
Water-Soluble Vitamins						
Ascorbic acid	(mg)	50	60	60	60	+ 20
Folacin	(mcg)	400	400	400	400	+400
Niacin	(mg)	15	14	14	13	+ 2
Riboflavin	(mg)	1.3	1.3	1.3	1.2	+ 0.3
Thiamin	(mg)	1.1	1.1	1.3	1.0	+ 0.4
Vitamin B$_6$	(mg)	1.8	2.0	2.0	2.0	+ 0.6
Vitamin B$_{12}$	(mcg)	3.0	3.0	3.0	3.0	+ 1.0
Minerals						
Calcium	(mg)	1200	1200	800	800	+400
Phosphorus	(mg)	1200	1200	800	800	+400
Iodine	(mcg)	150	150	150	150	+ 25
Iron	(mg)	18	18	18	18	18+[3]
Magnesium	(mg)	300	300	300	300	+150
Zinc	(mg)	15	15	15	15	+ 5

[1] Retinol Equivalent (RE) = 5 International Units (IU).
[2] 1 mcg = 40 IU.
[3] The use of an oral iron supplement is recommended.
Data from Recommended Dietary Allowances, 9th ed., 1980. Food and Nutrition Board, National Academy of Sciences, National Research Council, Washington, D.C.

centa to transfer both glucose and amino acids increases throughout pregnancy.

The maternal contribution of protein to the fetus is not limited to placental transfer. Passage of proteins from the mother into the amniotic fluid enables the fetus to swallow, hydrolyze, absorb, and utilize certain amino acids (Gitlin, 1974).

MATERNAL WEIGHT GAIN

Prepregnancy Weight

Next to gestational age, a woman's weight prior to pregnancy and the amount of weight gained through pregnancy are the two strongest determinants of the infant's birth weight. A comprehensive review of weight relationships in pregnancy showed that less than 5 percent of women whose prepregnant weight was 64 kg (140 lb) or greater delivered an infant at term weighing less than 2500 grams, regardless of the amount of weight gained during pregnancy (Eastman and Jackson, 1968). Moreover, less than 2 percent of women whose weight gain during

pregnancy exceeded 14 kg (30 lb) delivered term infants weighing less than 2500 grams, regardless of prepregnant weight. Maternal height does not appear to be a significant factor in regard to birth weight.

Amount of Weight Gain During Pregnancy

While the optimal amount of weight gain during pregnancy is not known, the amount of weight added through pregnancy has been studied repeatedly. Quite consistently, an average gain of 10 to 12 kg (22 to 26 lb) has been found to be associated with the best reproductive outcome. The Committee on Maternal Nutrition of the National Research Council recommends that 11 kg (24 lb) be gained, and the Committee on Nutrition of the American College of Obstetricians and Gynecologists recommends a weight gain of 10 to 12 kg (22 to 26 lb).

The unfounded notion that limiting weight gain prevents toxemia of pregnancy has taken many years for practitioners to abandon. Also, many weight-conscious women fear permanent obesity following pregnancy. It is important that health care providers help women, who are often highly motivated to keep in good health during pregnancy, to understand the importance of adequate weight gain.

Pattern of Weight Gain

Possibly more important than the actual amount of weight added during pregnancy is the rate at which the additional increase in weight occurs. During the first trimester, a total gain of 1.4 kg (3 lb) is recommended. Thereafter, a steady gain of about 0.34 kg (¾ lb) per week or 1.4 kg (3 lb) between 4-week prenatal care visits is suggested.

Although weight gain beyond the first trimester is essentially linear, the utilization of the additional weight changes as pregnancy advances. During the second trimester, the majority of additional weight is used in expansion of the maternal components (uterus, breasts, blood volume, fat deposition). In the third trimester, the products of conception (fetus, placenta, and amniotic fluid volume) predominantly account for the increase in weight (Hytten and Leitch, 1971).

Use of a weight gain grid (Fig. 7–1) as a part of the prenatal health care record emphasizes the recommended pattern of weight gain to the patient and helps health care providers monitor her continuing weight gain status as pregnancy advances.

Components of Weight Gain

The products of conception and the maternal response to gestation share fairly equally in the distribution of total weight gain. At term, products of conception account for approximately 5 kg (11 lb), and the maternal compensatory changes represent approximately 4 kg (9 lb) (Table 7–2).

Therefore, on the average, only weight gain in excess of 9 kg (20 lb) is "additional" weight gain, a portion of which represents fat deposition in preparation for lactation.

Postpartum Weight Change

During the first week following delivery, the average overall decrease in weight is approximately 9 kg (20 lbs), reflecting the weight gain just outlined. During the second to the twelfth postpartum weeks, an additional 3 to 4 kg (6 to 8 lb) is generally lost. The majority of women lose all of the weight gained during pregnancy, especially if they breast-feed. Parity alone has very little influence on maternal weight (Billewicz and Thomson, 1970).

SPECIFIC NUTRIENTS

Protein, Carbohydrates, and Fats

The pregnant woman must increase her dietary intake of *protein* to provide for enlargement of her blood volume, uterus, breasts, and placenta. Fetal protein synthesis requires adequate placental transfer of amino acids. Based upon protein accumulation, as estimated from the nitrogen content of the fetal and maternal compartments, approximately 1 kg of protein is needed through the course of pregnancy. To provide this amount, approximately 10 g of additional protein must be consumed daily. Based on nitrogen balance studies, however, the estimated additional need in pregnancy is 20 to 30 g of protein daily, or a total of about 75 g daily. Because of the uncertainty of these laboratory determinations, this higher figure is used as the recommendation. Adolescents who are still growing them-

Table 7–2. Components of Weight Gain During Pregnancy

Products of Conception		Maternal Response to Gestation	
Fetus	7.5 lb	Enlarged uterus	2.5 lb
Placenta and membranes	1.5 lb	Increased blood volume	3.5 lb
Amniotic fluid	2.0 lb	Increased breast size	1.0 lb
Subtotal	11.0 lb	Increased extracellular fluid	2.0 lb
		Subtotal	9.0 lb
	Total: 20 lb		

Data from Pritchard and MacDonald, 1980.

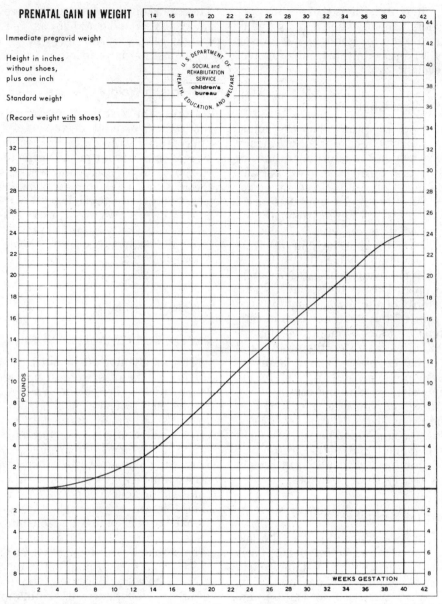

Figure 7–1. Record sheet for prenatal weight gain. (Reprinted with permission from *Clinical Obstetrics*. Copyright © 1953, J. B. Lippincott Co.)

selves have a greater requirement than do adult women.

Although it has been stated that a large nitrogen storage, in excess of the requirements of the fetal and maternal compartments, occurs during pregnancy, recent evidence indicates that the degree of nitrogen storage meets but does not exceed metabolic demands (Johnstone et al., 1981).

Regardless of the amount of maternal protein intake, total serum protein levels decline during pregnancy. After a steady decrease during the first two trimesters, the concentrations approach the nonpregnant levels as late pregnancy is reached. This decline in serum proteins is selective—alpha globulins and beta globulins increase, whereas gamma globulins and albumin decrease.

Carbohydrates are also a primary energy source, both for the mother and for the fetus. As long as total caloric needs are met, pregnancy does not impose any specific requirements for additional carbohydrates. Adequate energy intake from a combination of carbohydrate and fat food sources is necessary for protein utilization and to spare use of protein as an energy source.

For both mother and fetus, glucose and fatty acids provide the main sources of energy, with additional supply from deaminated amino acids. Glucose is the prime fuel on which the fetus heavily depends in order to achieve adequate tissue protein synthesis and conversion of fat to glycogen. Near term the fetal glucose utilization rate is estimated to be 7 mg/kg/min (30 g of glucose a day), as compared with the adult consumption of 2 to 3 mg/kg/min.

Fat storage accounts for one half of the total energy costs of pregnancy and occurs primarily between the 20th and 30th weeks of gestation (Hytten and Leitch, 1971). Fat in the diet is a concentrated source of needed calories. Fat also is a carrier of the essential fat-soluble vitamins A, D, and E, all of which have an increased requirement during pregnancy.

Vitamins

A nutritionally adequate diet meets essentially all of the recommended daily allowances for vitamins listed in Table 7–1. Unfortunately, dietary sources of nutrients are often not adequately stressed and are replaced with the widespread prescription of multivitamin supplementation during gestation. It is important that pregnant women be made aware that multivitamin supplementation cannot substitute for a nutritionally adequate daily diet offering the array of nutrients that interact with the essential macronutrients and micronutrients.

Water-Soluble Vitamins

Folate is important for the growth of maternal, fetal, and placental tissues because of its role in DNA synthesis. Fetal demands, impaired maternal absorption, and defective utilization are related to the increased folate requirements during pregnancy (Kitay, 1969).

Frank megaloblastic anemia is quite uncommon, despite the fact that one fourth of gravidas are "deficient" by nonpregnant standards. Folate deficiency has been associated with a number of abnormalities of pregnancy, including abruptio placentae, congenital malformations, abortion, and pregnancy-induced hypertension. A number of investigators have refuted these claims, however, and at the present time, folate

deficiency seems associated only with megaloblastic anemia (Pritchard and MacDonald, 1980). The offspring of mothers with megaloblastic anemia have normal hemoglobin levels (Pitkin, 1976).

The recommended daily increase of folate is from 400 mcg to 800 mcg. Green leafy vegetables, liver, kidney, and other meats, eggs, and nuts are good dietary sources.

The value of "routine" supplementation of folate is unclear, but the administration of folic acid is necessary for certain patients who are at special risk of developing folate deficiency. Patients with multiple fetuses, hemoglobinopathies and other chronic hemolytic anemias, and those taking diphenylhydantoin (Dilantin) should be supplemented with 1 mg of folate daily throughout pregnancy.

Vitamin B-12 deficiency during pregnancy is rare, since fetal needs total 50 mcg, a small fraction of the maternal store of 3000 mcg. However, patients who are vegans, eating no animal protein foods, do require supplementation during gestation (Leader et al., 1981).

Vitamin B-6 (pyridoxine) concentrations decrease in both plasma and cellular elements of the blood during pregnancy. However, adverse effects are difficult to demonstrate clinically (Pitkin, 1976). Because of its important role in the metabolism of proteins, the need for vitamin B-6 increases during pregnancy to accommodate the greater protein intake. A daily intake of 2.6 mg, which is 0.6 mg above the nonpregnant intake, is suggested to meet this increased demand. Liver, meats, fish, eggs, cabbage, bananas, corn, whole wheat, and rolled oats are good dietary sources.

Vitamin C (ascorbic acid) is essential for normal cell integrity and growth. The RDA for Vitamin C during pregnancy is 80 mg, which represents an increase of 20 mg over the nonpregnant recommendation. Citrus fruits, strawberries, cantaloupe, dark green leafy vegetables, raw cabbage, and green peppers are among the best dietary sources. Paradoxically, intake exceeding 1 g daily has been reported to lead to neonatal scurvy, apparently as a result of conditioning the fetus to an elevated level of vitamin C (Cochrane, 1965).

Fat-Soluble Vitamins

Vitamin A is necessary for normal cellular growth, especially for epithelial cells. To provide adequate Vitamin A for fetal storage, the recommended daily requirement during pregnancy is 5000 retinol equivalents (RE) as compared with 4000 RE for the nonpregnant female. Well-nourished adults maintain hepatic stores of Vitamin A sufficient to meet requirements for several months. Dietary sources of vitamin A are liver, milk (whole or fortified low-fat or nonfat), dark green leafy and deep yellow vegetables, and yellow fruits. Excessive intake of vitamin A in megavitamin supplements has been associated with increased intracranial pressure and congenital malformations in offspring (Rosso, 1980).

Vitamin D is important in regulating the metabolism of calcium and phosphorus. As the need for these minerals increases through pregnancy, vitamin D requirements also rise. The recommended daily allowance during pregnancy is 12.5 mcg daily, compared with 7.5 mcg daily in the nonpregnant state. Exposure to sunshine can provide adequate vitamin D; milk fortified with vitamin D is a good food source. Excessive intake through high-potency supplements has been associated with adverse fetal effects, including aortic stenosis, hyperparathyroidism, and other congenital anomalies (Leader et al., 1981).

Vitamin E is evidently found in sufficient quantities in most diets, since deficiency in humans is rare. Specific functions for vitamin E are unclear, but it is believed to have a significant role in fatty acid metabolism. Neonatal hemoglobinopathies have been reported with vitamin E deficiency in the newborn. The RDA for vitamin E during pregnancy is 12 mg tocopherol equivalents, an increase of 2 mg over the nonpregnant daily recommendation.

Minerals

Pregnancy increases the demand for most minerals, but the need for routine supplementation of multiple minerals, widely practiced by the public and many health care providers, lacks substantiation. With the exception of iron, a nutritionally adequate diet should amply supply the needs of pregnancy for most women.

Iron

Although the primary function of iron is in hemoglobin synthesis and function, iron is involved in many enzyme systems relating to a variety of metabolic processes.

The total iron need during pregnancy has been determined to be between 800 and 1000 g, depending upon whether or not maternal excretion, which through pregnancy totals about 200 mg, is calculated in the amount. Approximately 500 mg of this total iron requirement is necessary to accommodate the expanded maternal blood volume, which occurs in varying degrees in all pregnant women. Another 300 mg is necessary to supply fetal needs.

The blood volume increases by about 50 per cent in pregnancy, with the increase being disproportionate between red cells and plasma. About three fourths of the 1500- to 2000-ml increase in blood volume is due to an elevation in plasma volume, whereas the red cell mass increases by about one third. The hematocrit, which represents the proportion of the total blood composed of cells, decreases as a reflection of these changes.

Whether or not a woman receives iron supplementation, the hematocrit declines slightly through pregnancy, reaching a nadir at about 32 weeks. Thereafter, it increases to approach the prepregnant level. This fact has clinical value—for routine patients whose initial hematologic evaluation does not suggest iron deficiency, the most appropriate time to reassess the iron status is at about 32 weeks, when the hematocrit is expected to be at its lowest point. Largely because of blood loss with menses, the average iron store in young adult women has been estimated to be 270 mg. It is of interest to note that, in a group of apparently healthy young adult nursing students, about one fourth were found to have no stainable iron in their bone marrow (Pritchard and Scott, 1970).

Besides stored iron, the other source of iron is through the diet. The average daily adult diet contains 10 to 12 mg of iron, considerably less than the 18 mg recommended for women of childbearing age. Pregnancy imposes an additional demand of 2 to 4 mg daily. The best dietary sources of iron are liver, red meats, seafood, nuts, legumes, green leafy vegetables, and whole grain and iron-fortified cereals. Iron in the heme form, as in animal foods, and adequate vitamin C (ascorbic acid) in the diet facilitate iron absorption.

Because of the difficulty in obtaining sufficient iron from the diet, iron is the one nutrient supplement usually prescribed for women during pregnancy. It is important to understand that it is the amount of *elemental iron*, not the *iron salt*, that is important. Various salt forms will yield different amounts of elemental iron—a 300-mg tablet of ferrous sulfate and a 300-mg tablet of ferrous fumarate each provides approximately 65 mg of elemental iron; the same dosage of ferrous gluconate provides approximately half this amount.

Side effects of iron supplements are common and troublesome. Nausea and epigastric pain (indigestion) occur in up to 20 per cent of patients, constipation in 10 per cent, and diarrhea in 5 per cent. These effects are primarily the result of iron absorption rather than the type of preparation. Therefore, total lack of side effects may indicate insufficient absorption. Although absorption is maximal when an iron supplement is taken on an empty stomach, ingestion of the iron supplements with meals tends to decrease the side effects described.

Iron toxicity in adults is rare, but infants and young children are particularly prone to its toxic effects, and ingestion of as few as 3 to 5 iron tablets can have catastrophic results. It may be difficult for the mother to have iron tablets readily available for her use, yet away from small children. Child-proof safety caps are strongly recommended.

Oral iron supplements make the stool dark green or almost black in color. Determining a patient's recent compliance concerning intake of the iron supplement includes inquiring as to stool color and performing a simple rectal examination.

Although the fetus has long been thought to be an effective parasite in terms of meeting its iron needs, more recent evidence suggests that iron stores of offspring of iron-deficient mothers are lower than those of offspring whose mothers had adequate iron intake throughout gestation (Fenton et al., 1977). Neonatal serum iron levels are not decreased with maternal iron deficiency.

The majority of iron transferred to the fetus occurs in the last trimester, and it is during this time that fetal iron stores are developed. For this reason, premature infants have diminished stores of iron. Two thirds of the iron transported to the fetus is incorporated into hemoglobin and the remainder is stored as ferritin in the fetal liver for use in the first year of life (McFee, 1979).

Calcium

Calcium is necessary for the development of bones and teeth, and is also important in maintenance of cell membrane permeability, the coagulation process, and neuromuscular excitability (Pitkin, 1975). During pregnancy, the maternal serum concentration of calcium decreases slightly because of a decline in albumin concentration, to which about half of the blood calcium is bound. Calcium absorption is actually increased and excretion decreased during gestation (Heaney and Skillman, 1971).

The total fetal demand for calcium is estimated to be 30 g, mostly required in the later stages of pregnancy (Hytten and Leitch, 1971). Since the total calcium content of an adult is estimated to be 1100 to 1200 g, the fetal need represents a small fraction of that available, and deficiency is extremely rare in developed countries.

Because of the increased calcium need during pregnancy, it is recommended that the daily calcium intake be increased from 800 mg in the nonpregnant state to 1200 mg daily during pregnancy. One quart of milk contains this amount of calcium, along with 400 units of vitamin D. Cheese, other dairy products, and calcium supplements are other sources.

Other Minerals

Phosphorus is primarily combined with calcium in bone formation. The total fetal need of approximately 20 g represents about 3 per cent of the total maternal content of phosphorus (Hytten and Leitch, 1971). The RDA for phosphorus is 1200 mg daily during pregnancy. Its widespread availability makes deficiency unlikely.

Sodium metabolism is strongly influenced by pregnancy, as a result of significantly increased glomerular filtration and increased renal tubular reabsorption. To provide the estimated 750 mEq of sodium to compensate for an average weight gain of 11 kg (24 lb) during pregnancy, a daily increase of 3 mEq is recommended. As the average adult diet contains 100 to 300 mEq, this additional sodium need presents no difficulty. The previous practice of restricting sodium during pregnancy is now discouraged.

Zinc is essential for growth of all tissues, as it is involved in many major metabolic pathways. Short stature, hypogonadism, roughened skin, hepatosplenomegaly, and iron deficiency anemia have been reported with zinc deficiency (Moghissi, 1978).

Iodine requirements are increased during pregnancy to provide sufficient iodine to the fetus and to compensate for the increased renal loss that occurs during pregnancy. A balanced diet plus use of iodized salt is recommended to avoid neonatal cretinism. Conversely, excessive iodine intake may suppress fetal thyroid function.

Potassium concentration does not change substantially during pregnancy, and no disorders peculiar to pregnancy are related to its metabolism.

Obstetric Complications with Nutritional Interrelationships

CONDITIONS COMMON IN PREGNANCY

Anemia

Iron Deficiency Anemia. As noted in the discussion of iron utilization during pregnancy, the plasma volume increases to a greater extent than does the red blood cell mass, resulting in a decline in the hematocrit. This dilutional effect, most marked in the early third trimester, may be compounded by the nutritional deficiencies of iron and folic acid. Anemia is defined as a hematocrit of less than 30 percent or a hemoglobin concentration of less than 10 g/dl at any time during pregnancy (Pritchard and MacDonald, 1980). The majority of cases of anemia in pregnancy are due to iron deficiency, but folate deficiency is also seen. Infection (most commonly pyelonephritis), acute blood loss, hemoglobinopathies and other hereditary hemolytic anemias, thalassemia, and hypoplastic anemia are other causes.

With iron deficiency, a stained smear of the peripheral blood may show the characteristic microcytic and hypochromic appearance of the red blood cells, but these findings are often absent. Likewise, the mean cell volume (MCV), typically decreased with iron deficiency, may be within the normal range. Determination of serum iron and total iron-binding capacity, with a ratio of less than 15 percent being indicative of iron deficiency, has been used to assess iron status. However, very recent iron intake will elevate the serum iron and lead to erroneous conclusions. More recently, serum ferritin has been used to measure iron status. Small amounts of this storage form of iron in serum reflect total iron stores. A level of less than 12 ng/ml suggests deficiency. A bone marrow examination to detect stainable iron is rarely needed during pregnancy.

The objectives of treatment of anemia are to correct the anemia and to replenish stores. Treatment of iron deficiency anemia consists of prescribing a diet high in food sources of iron, protein, and vitamin C, along with approximately 180 mg of elemental iron taken orally daily. This is provided by three tablets of ferrous sulfate or ferrous fumarate, as each tablet of these iron salts contains approximately 60 mg of elemental iron. Ferrous gluconate may be used, but the number of tablets may need to be increased to provide the necessary iron. Doses in excess of 180 to 200 mg daily do not result in more rapid blood cell production and may cause significant side effects. Parenteral iron is seldom necessary and is reserved for the patient with true intolerance to oral iron or who refuses to take the medication as prescribed. Correction of anemia does not occur faster with parenteral than with oral iron.

Response to treatment is quite rapid, but is less than the response seen in the non-pregnant state. Larger basophilic, polychromatophilic red blood cells can be seen in a stained smear of peripheral blood 10 to 14 days after initiation of treatment. The hematocrit rises slowly thereafter at a rate of 1 to 2 percentage points per week. Once the anemia is corrected, continued supplemental iron—e.g., 120 mg daily—is recommended throughout the remainder of pregnancy and for 4 to 6 weeks thereafter.

When there is an apparent lack of response to prescribed iron, patient compliance should be thoroughly determined. As noted earlier, iron ingestion should cause the stool to become dark green or almost black, and therefore stool color is helpful information in determining the patient's iron intake.

Megaloblastic Anemia. Folic acid deficiency is almost always responsible for megaloblastic anemia during pregnancy, as the increasing demand for this vitamin may exceed dietary intake and stores are consumed. The sequence of events following folate deficiency has been evaluated (Table 7–3) (Herbert, 1962). Characteristic megaloblastic

Table 7–3. Sequence of Alterations Following Experimental Folate Deprivation

Event	Weeks After Onset Of Folate Deprivation
Low concentration of serum folate	3
Hypersegmentation of neutrophil nuclei in peripheral blood	7
Elevated urinary FIGLU excretion	14
Low folate in erythrocytes	16
Macro-ovalocytosis	18
Megaloblastic marrow (florid)	19
Anemia	19

Data from Herbert, 1962.

changes in bone marrow occur relatively late in the process. An erythrocyte folate level of less than 150 ng/ml indicates deficiency of this vitamin. A serum folate value of less than 4 ng/ml also suggests folate deficiency, but the increasing plasma volume with pregnancy may make this test less diagnostic during this time (Kitay, 1980).

Treatment of folate deficiency is with oral folate at a dose of 1 mg daily. Response is rapid and first noted as an increase in the reticulocyte count several-fold over the reticulocyte level of 1.5 to 2.5 percent seen in normal pregnancy. In the absence of other factors, the rise in hematocrit is approximately 1 percentage point per day after 1 week.

It is important to remember that folate and iron deficiencies may frequently coexist in pregnancy. Therefore, characteristic hematologic indices may be lacking. For example, the macrocytic changes of folate deficiency may be offset by the microcytic cells indicative of iron deficiency. Other indices may also be misleading—serum iron may be elevated in patients who are both iron and folate deficient because of inefficient erythropoiesis. With folate therapy, however, the serum iron may decrease dramatically as proper iron utilization occurs.

Most cases of anemia during pregnancy can be prevented by stressing good nutrition. Supplementation with iron and possibly folate will ensure adequate intake of these substances. If anemia is identified, attention to diet and simple iron and folate treatment should precede extensive hematologic evaluation, since the vast majority of cases of anemia are due to inadequate intake of these two important nutrients.

Hyperemesis Gravidarum

Nausea and occasional vomiting during the first trimester usually do not interfere with nutrition. Simple treatment includes the taking of small, frequent meals, emphasizing easily tolerated carbohydrates (crackers, baked potato), and taking liquids between meals rather than with food. However, persistent hyperemesis can result in severe physiologic disturbance leading to dehydration, electrolyte imbalance, ketoacidosis, nutritional depletion, and hypovitaminosis. These complications may require hospitalization for sedation, antiemetics, and replacement of fluids, electrolytes, and vitamins. In severe cases total parenteral nutrition may be necessary.

Underweight and Poor Weight Gain

Women who enter pregnancy at a weight that is 10 percent or more below the standard for height (Table 7–4) or women who gain less than 6 kg (13 lb) risk increased rates of prematurity, low-birth-weight infants, and infants with low Apgar scores. The presence of anemia, a history of maternal smoking, and/or poor weight gain in the low-prepregnancy-weight patient markedly increases the incidence of low-birth-weight infants.

The objective of a nutrition and weight gain program in pregnancy is to help ensure the most favorable outcome for both the mother and her infant. The patient should be guided toward a planned goal, beginning with an estimate of her desirable weight, an assessment of her nutritional status, and an estimate of what would constitute an adequate weight gain for her. For an underweight patient this plan may include added calories to gain more than the usual 11 to 12 kg (24 to 26 lb) and to compensate for the degree of underweight.

Optimal fetal growth is dependent on the nutritional status of the mother not only during pregnancy but for many years prior to conception. Ideally, underweight women should obtain their appropriate weight prior to pregnancy.

Pica

As early as the sixth century AD there were accounts of peculiar food and nonfood cravings, or pica. The variety of nonfood sub-

Table 7–4. Table of Standard Weight for Height

Height (with shoes, with 1 inch heels)		Weight (in lb)
4'–10"	=	115
4'–11"	=	117
5'– 0"	=	120
5'– 1"	=	122
5'– 2"	=	125
5'– 3"	=	128
5'– 4"	=	131
5'– 5"	=	134
5'– 6"	=	137
5'– 7"	=	140
5'– 8"	=	143
5'– 9"	=	146
5'–10"	=	149
5'–11"	=	152
6'– 0"	=	155

Height is in inches plus 1 inch to establish a standard for heels. Patients should be weighed with shoes as normally worn. The table above is for medium body build, and except for extreme body build deviations, these figures should be used.

For example, a patient whose height, measured without shoes, is 5 feet 4 inches would have 1 inch added; therefore, her standard weight for height would be 134 pounds.

Ranges are not acceptable in estimating standard weight, since this is an objective observation and represents the midpoint. This midpoint must be used for recording purposes.

For patients under age 25, 1 pound should be deducted for each year.

Adapted from Metropolitan Life Insurance Company: 1983 Height and Weight Tables. Society of Actuaries and Association of Life Insurance Medical Directors of America, 1983.

stances consumed includes laundry starch, clay, ashes, and ice. The propensity of pregnant women for this condition has been singled out as particularly strong, yet research has failed to reveal the underlying etiology (Luke, 1979). A strong and persistent link between this nutritional problem and iron deficiency has been demonstrated, but the exact relation of the two remains unclear. Some suggest that the anemia is a result of the pica; others suggest that it is the cause.

One way in which pica is thought to cause iron deficiency anemia is through the binding of dietary iron, rendering it unusable for the body. In particular, clay with high cation exchange capacity is found to be effective in blocking iron absorption. Magnesium oxide also has been found to be extremely effective in preventing iron absorption in this way. Since cravings have been reported for antacids, some of which contain magnesium,

the cation exchange capacities may have some clinical significance in relation to iron absorption.

Unusual cravings in some women have been eliminated by the treatment of iron deficiency anemia. With serum iron values above 70 mcg percent, the unusual cravings may disappear.

Culture and tradition seem to play a significant role in the condition of pica. Women take clay and other substances such as corn starch, flour, and baking soda in order to relieve nausea, prevent vomiting, relieve dizziness, cure swollen legs, and relieve headaches. In some cultures it is even believed that ingestion of these substances will result in a beautiful child, while failure to have the cravings satisfied is popularly thought by some to cause birthmarks. Others have hypothesized that pica represents an unconscious endeavor to compensate for certain nutritional deficiencies.

Diet counseling should include an open discussion about pica and food cravings. Discussion of a nutritionally adequate diet can include suggestions for foods to substitute for nonfoods. Nonfat dry milk powder has been found to be an acceptable alternative to laundry starch for some women.

ASSOCIATED MEDICAL DISORDERS

Diabetes

Diabetes Mellitus. Changes in maternal glucose level and other metabolites are due not only to drainage by the fetus but also to the action of placental hormones on carbohydrate metabolism. Estrogen, progesterone, and lactogen antagonize the effects of insulin at the cell wall. In addition, placental lactogen is lipolytic, which increases the circulating levels of fatty acids.

As pregnancy progresses, despite the anti-insulin hormonal setting, carbohydrate homeostasis and normal glucose tolerance are maintained in most patients. This is accomplished by an increased maternal secretion of insulin. Hyperinsulinemia has been observed in response to an intake of both glucose and certain amino acids. Although there is an increase in immediate postprandial insulin levels, the fasting level of insulin is reduced because of the fasting hypoglycemic tendency that persists throughout pregnancy.

Caring for a woman with diabetes during pregnancy represents a great challenge. Close teamwork among several health care providers is necessary for the greatest likelihood of a successful outcome. It is clear that perinatal outcome is greatly improved when optimal care is given.

Diabetes and pregnancy may interact in two ways. Evidence of glucose intolerance may appear in a pregnant woman not previously known to be diabetic, or a known diabetic may become pregnant. The patient diagnosed as having diabetes during pregnancy must be counseled carefully and promptly about the management of this disorder and its impact on pregnancy. The previously diagnosed diabetic who becomes pregnant must adjust to the metabolic changes of pregnancy described above. The importance of preconceptional counseling and optimal control of the diabetes cannot be overemphasized, since recent evidence suggests that the incidence of congenital anomalies in the offspring of diabetics may be increased in women whose diabetes is poorly controlled near the time of conception (Miller et al., 1981).

Gestational Diabetes. Gestational diabetes is defined as carbohydrate intolerance that is diagnosed during pregnancy and managed with diet, and that disappears after delivery. It occurs in approximately 5 percent of pregnancies. Perinatal mortality rates are approximately doubled in pregnancies complicated by *undiagnosed* gestational diabetes; these rates may be significantly reduced by identification and close monitoring of such pregnancies. Usually the diagnosis of gestational diabetes is made by screening a high-risk population. All pregnant women who are age 25 years or more or who have persisting glycosuria, a family history of diabetes mellitus, or a history of a previous large baby (greater than 4 kg [9 lb]), previous stillborn, or neonatal death should be tested by a diabetes screening method. Testing should be at the initial visit and repeated at 26 to 28 weeks. An O'Sullivan screening test utilizing a 50-mg oral glucose load should normally yield a plasma glucose level 1 hour later of less than 150 mg/dl. (O'Sullivan et al., 1973). The patient need not be fasting. If the screening result is ≥ 150 mg/dl, a 3-hour oral glucose tolerance test (OGTT) is recommended. Other screening methods are available. A 2-hour postprandial plasma glucose of 140 mg/dl or less is normal; however, a value exceeding 200 mg/dl requires an oral glucose tolerance test. A nonfasting plasma glucose over 200 mg/dl or a fasting greater than 140 mg/dl is indicative of diabetes mellitus and requires an OGTT.

The preferred administration of the glucose tolerance test is by the oral route. It is rarely given by the intravenous route, for the following reasons: (1) the oral route is more physiologic than the IV route; (2) gastrointestinal factors that influence insulin secretion are bypassed in the IV test; (3) tests in high-risk groups have indicated that the oral test is a more sensitive indicator of deterioration in glucose tolerance; (4) the correlation between the oral test and other parameters of carbohydrate metabolism is better than that observed with the IV test; and (5) there is a better standardization for the oral test. The disadvantage of the oral test is that there is a greater variability in the rate of glucose absorption from the gut. However, this has not proved to be a practical problem. There is a practical problem, though, in that the nausea and vomiting of pregnancy may cause some women to have a difficult time ingesting the "Glucola." Foods containing an equal calorie count have been suggested to make the test more palatable.

To be defined as gestational diabetes, the fasting plasma level of glucose should be normal and two of the three glucose tolerance levels should be abnormal. Table 7–5 outlines the accepted plasma glucose levels during pregnancy. Approximately 15 to 20 percent of gestational diabetics will develop overt diabetes mellitus with abnormal fasting and postprandial glucose values.

Table 7–5. Standards for Oral Glucose Tolerance Test in Pregnancy

	Plasma mg/dl	Whole Blood mg/dl
Fasting	105	90
1 hr*	190	165
2 hr*	165	145
3 hr*	140	125

*Post glucose ingestion.
Plasma values are approximately 14 percent higher than corresponding whole blood values.
Glucose load is 100 grams.
For proper interpretation, carbohydrate intake for each of the 3 days preceding the test should exceed 300 g. One candy bar each day helps to ensure that this requirement is met.
Data from O'Sullivan and Mahan, 1964.

Dietary Management of Diabetes. The cornerstone of the management of all types of diabetes mellitus is a meal plan providing consistent dietary intake to control blood glucose. The principles of diet management are based on three general concepts of balance:

1. *Energy Balance*—consistent intake of calories providing the energy needed to maintain ideal maternal and fetal weight gain.

2. *Nutrient Balance*—the proper ratio of macronutrients (carbohydrate, protein, fat) to meet energy needs, and micronutrients (vitamins and minerals) to meet nutritional needs.

3. *Distribution Balance*—consistent distribution of the macronutrients throughout the day, to balance with activity levels, and insulin when prescribed, in order to avoid hypoglycemia and yet provide a sustained availability of glucose.

Energy Balance. During pregnancy the total daily energy requirement is governed by the maternal and fetal metabolic needs, which on the average will require 2000 to 2400 kcal or approximately 30 to 35 kcal/kg of actual body weight. Some authorities suggest 30 kcal/kg of ideal body weight plus 300 kcal/day added during pregnancy (Williams, 1981, and Couston et al., 1980).

Nutrient Balance
CARBOHYDRATE. Contrary to what some formerly believed, carbohydrate should not be disproportionately reduced in a diet prescribed for managing diabetes. However, the carbohydrate should be provided in complex forms (e.g., starches) that are digested and absorbed slowly. Large intakes of concentrated sweets that are quickly digested and absorbed result in greater increments of blood glucose. Approximately 50 percent of the total number of calories, with a minimum intake of 250 g daily, should be provided by carbohydrates. The greater proportion of the carbohydrate calories should be obtained from complex carbohydrate foods, such as starchy vegetables and cereals, with the lesser amounts coming from the simple sugars, as in fruits.

PROTEIN. Proteins are important in controlling diabetes. The diet of a pregnant woman with diabetes should contain approximately 1.5 to 2.0 grams of protein per kilogram of body weight per day, or approximately 100 to 125 g/day. Approximately 25 percent of the total calories should be derived from protein foods.

FAT. Fat needs of the diabetic woman during pregnancy are not primary, so the amount of fat should be kept at moderate levels. Thus, 60 to 80 grams of fat, or approximately 30 percent of the total calories consumed, may come from fat. An effort should be made to keep a 1:1 ratio between saturated and polyunsaturated fats.

FIBER. A diet high in soluble fibers may be useful in the management of diabetes mellitus. Dietary fiber has been defined as the portion of plant material taken in the diet that is resistant to digestion by the secretions of the gastrointestinal tract. As such, fiber remains in the stomach and the small bowel for longer periods of time than does the digestable fraction of food. Fiber increases the volume of bowel contents and might also simultaneously influence general metabolism by altering the rate of absorption from the stomach; this may decrease glucose levels, reduce postprandial hypoglycemia, and diminish insulin requirements (Anderson, 1981).

Fibers may be water-soluble or water-insoluble. The substances that are generally thought of as being fibrous are most often high in cellulose content and predominantly insoluble. The soluble fibers are generally categorized biologically as gums, mucilages, and storage polysaccharides. Soluble fibers are the substances with the greatest likelihood of altering the absorption of nutrients. The fiber content of the diet can be increased by using greater quantities of whole grain breads and cereals, raw fruits, vegetables, and legumes (Anderson and Ward, 1975).

Distribution Balance. The most important aspect of diet for a pregnant diabetic is consistency of mealtimes and time between meals, as well as caloric content of the diet. It is usually desirable to find the patient's preferred eating and exercising patterns and try to adjust insulin to them. To tailor an appropriate insulin schedule, meals should be eaten at the same time each day and be consistent in calories, protein, and carbohydrates. The caloric intake may be divided into three meals and one bedtime snack, using approximately 2/7 of the total calories for each meal and 1/7 for the snack. Some diabetics, especially those who are overweight, may require one to two additional snacks in order to maintain euglycemia. The carbohydrate calories (50 percent of the total calories) are divided about equally for each meal, with an allowance of about 10 percent for snacks. If urinary acetone spillage occurs, then 100 calories in the form of carbohydrate is added to the next meal or snack. If morning fasting acetonuria persists despite increasing the evening snack by 100 calories, then a snack such as 8 ounces of skim milk is added at about 3:00 AM. Alternative snacks containing a combination of protein and complex carbohydrate are also appropriate (Couston et al., 1980; Gabbe, 1981; Williams, 1981). If the patient's insulin is adjusted in the hospital, allowances should be made concerning her exercise when she returns to her usual schedule at home.

The patient should be seen approximately every 2 weeks during her prenatal course. At each visit a fasting and a 2-hour postprandial plasma glucose is obtained, and appropriate adjustments are made.

Insulin Therapy in Diabetes. Insulin is required if the fasting plasma glucose exceeds 105 mg/dl or the 2-hour postprandial value is greater than 140 mg/dl despite the patient's adherence to her prescribed diet. Patients requiring insulin prior to pregnancy often need frequent adjustment throughout gestation. In the pregnant insulin-dependent diabetic, the goal of therapy is to maintain a fasting plasma glucose level of 80 to 100 mg/dl and a 2-hour postprandial level of 120 to 140 mg/dl, which are levels associated with the least perinatal mortality and morbidity. In practical terms, insulin dosage is readjusted if the fasting plasma glucose is more than 100 mg/dl, or if any 2-hour postprandial value is more than 140 mg/dl. Efforts are made to avoid large fluctuations of plasma glucose during the day (Jovanovic and Peterson, 1980).

After 20 weeks' gestation, most pregnant diabetics are treated with combinations of intermediate- and short-acting insulins, with dosages split between morning and evening. Patients take insulin prior to breakfast and dinner each day, using a mixture of intermediate-acting (NPH or Lente) and short-acting (regular) insulin. The fasting plasma glucose reflects the intermediate-acting insulin given at dinnertime on the preceding day, the 2-hour postprandial morning plasma glucose reflects the regular insulin given that morning, and the late afternoon plasma glucose value reflects the morning intermediate acting insulin dose. If an evening glucose can be obtained, it reflects the pre-dinnertime short-acting insulin. In this manner the various components of the day's insulin doses can be adjusted to maintain optimal goals of glucose control.

The detailed management of the pregnant diabetic patient is covered in Chapter 21.

Essential Hypertension and Chronic Renal Disease

In about 30 percent of patients with hypertension during pregnancy, elevated blood pressure will persist after pregnancy and is characterized as hypertension of unknown etiology. When chronic renal disease and hypertension coexist, urinary protein loss may be as high as 5 g/day. If the losses become massive, serum proteins could fall to levels at which their reduced osmotic pressure will allow water to move into extravascular spaces and cause generalized edema. Usually, though, dietary protein supplements are not necessary, because the urinary losses constitute only 5 to 7 percent of the total protein intake.

The general dietary recommendations for essential hypertension with chronic renal disease include a well-balanced diet containing a mixture of essential nutrients (Luke, 1979). Sodium restriction to about 5 g/day may be indicated in patients with essential hypertension. If diuretics are used, it should be acknowledged that potassium as well as sodium may be lost, and the patient should be counseled as to good dietary sources of potassium. These include bananas, orange or grapefruit juice, prunes, potatoes, raisins, and peanuts. It should be remembered that excessive protein intake by patients with impaired glomerular filtration may be hazardous, in that the blood urea level may become elevated.

Cardiac Disease

The two important factors in the nutritional support of pregnancy complicated by heart disease are (1) energy balance in relation to weight control, and (2) careful control of sodium intake. The usual pattern of weight gain should be encouraged. Although sodium is a necessary mineral for the health of the pregnant woman, a woman with heart disease is vulnerable to cardiac failure and should restrict her sodium intake to 5 g/day (Luke, 1979). A diet providing much less than this amount is unpalatable and is associated with a very low rate of patient compliance. This general level of sodium intake can be achieved by (1) omitting salty foods such as salt-cured meats or fish, salted snacks and crackers, pickles, relishes, and condiments, and (2) light use of salt in cooking and none added to food at the table. The nutritionist can assist the patient in planning meals, selecting suitable food, reading food package labels for sodium content, and seasoning food with lemon juice, herbs, and spices rather than with salt.

Maternal Phenylketonuria

Because of the success of past treatment of this disorder, many women with phenylketonuria (PKU) are intellectually normal and are entering into the reproductive age. Since 1957 concern has increased over children born to women with PKU (Dent, 1957). The "maternal PKU syndrome," consisting of offspring with microcephaly, severe mental retardation, congenital heart disease, and intrauterine growth retardation, has been described. It is important that guidelines be established for counseling these young women about diet during their reproductive life. However, uncertainty still exists about the relationship between maternal PKU, diet adequacy, hyperphenylalaninemia, and developmental problems in the fetus. Some believe that the low phenylalanine diet must begin prior to the onset of pregnancy.

Recently the outcome of 34 pregnancies in which dietary therapy was aimed at lowering maternal phenylalanine concentration in an attempt to avoid fetal damage was reported (Lenke and Levy, 1982). The data indicated that most women with PKU have pretreatment phenylalanine blood levels of 20 mg/dl or greater. During dietary treatment in pregnancy, the levels of phenylalanine were generally maintained between 4 and 12 mg/dl, with some values below 1 mg/dl and some above 16 mg/dl. Infant outcome varied from mental normality without other gross fetal effects to neonatal death due to congenital heart disease. There was some relation between protection of the fetus and how early in pregnancy treatment was begun, as well as how effectively the blood level of phenylalanine was controlled. When good dietary control was achieved before conception, 2 of 2 offspring had normal test results for intelligence and no congenital defects were noted. When the diet was started in the first trimester, only 36 percent (4 of 11) of the infants appeared to be normal. The percentage of normal infants when treatment was begun in the second or third trimester was 13 percent (2 of 16) and 50 percent (2 of 4), respectively. The available data tend to support initiation of dietary therapy *prior to conception* for best results, but the number of cases followed in this study is small and points to the need for further research.

The low-phenylalanine diet for maternal PKU is similar to that administered to children who are treated for this disorder. It consists of a specifically designed dietary supplement containing protein free of the amino acid phenylalanine, plus vegetables, fruits, and some specially prepared bread or dessert products. Routine recommendation of prenatal vitamins *should be avoided*, since vitamins are supplied in the dietary preparations. As noted earlier, an excess of vitamins could be harmful to the fetus.

Specifically, the dietary management of maternal PKU should (1) provide sufficient, but not excessive, phenylalanine (250 to 500 mg/day) (the specific prescription of patients' individual tolerances is estimated through monitoring of serum phenylalanine levels for maintenance of target concentration); (2) provide 50 g/day of protein during the first half of pregnancy and 100 g/day during the second half; (3) meet the appropriate caloric needs of both mother and fetus, with needs for the former determined by age, prepregnancy weight, and physical activity.

Gastrointestinal Bypass Procedures

Even though jejunoileal bypass operations are not commonly performed today, pregnancy still occurs in patients who have had the procedure. Usually the alterations in electrolytes and malabsorption of lipids, carbohydrates, and proteins were related to the immediate postoperative weight loss period. Most reports show some degree of stabilization and improvement in all of these parameters occurring within 12 to 36 months. However, some studies have indicated a low serum albumin level (less than 3 mg/dl) in patients following jejunoileal bypass and a persistently diminished level of most essential and nonessential amino acids (Ingardia and Fischer, 1978). A study of the consequences of low maternal protein levels on mean infant weight in relationship to maternal serum albumin found that 76 percent of mothers who were hypoalbuminemic had small-for-gestational-age infants, compared with a rate of 44 percent for mothers whose serum albumin levels were normal (Wong et al., 1981).

Absorption of fat is reduced to 30 to 80 percent in these patients, compared with nearly 100 percent absorption in the normal patient. Likewise, serum cholesterol and triglyceride levels are reduced to 50 percent of normal. Loose stools or frank diarrhea may occur. Following intestinal bypass surgery, increased fecal fat may result in precipitation of insoluble calcium salts, thereby inhibiting calcium absorption. Plasma magnesium levels have also been observed to decrease following intestinal bypass procedures, through a similar mechanism of malabsorption. Marked impairment of liver function may be observed during the initial period of weight loss. In most cases, repeat studies done 1 to 3 years postoperatively, when weight is stabilized, indicate a return to normal liver function and normal amino acid concentrations by most criteria. Carbohydrate absorption abnormalities have also been observed following intestinal bypass procedures. A flat or seemingly unresponsive oral glucose tolerance test is not uncommon. It appears that a rapid transit time may reduce glucose absorption.

Pregnancy during the period of maximum weight loss and malabsorption affects the nutrition of both mother and fetus and increases the likelihood of complications of both. Maternal complications include hypertension, hypocalcemia, hypomagnesemia, hypoalbuminemia, and anemia. Infants of such pregnancies are small for gestational age.

Specific guidelines for the bypass patient during pregnancy are not available and depend upon the time elapsed from the procedure. In general, however, minimal dietary restrictions have been imposed, and progressive weight gain in the absence of ketonuria

has been taken to reflect an adequate diet. Some patients have lost weight during pregnancy but present no evidence of starvation ketosis. No consistency in food tolerance has been noted—milk products are upsetting to some individuals, whereas others are able to consume large quantities of milk and milk products. Some experience severe diarrhea and indigestion from fresh fruits. Most agree that they consume fewer calories after undergoing bypass surgery. A high-protein diet, along with supplementation with iron and other minerals and vitamins, should be encouraged during pregnancy. Vitamin B_{12} levels should be determined periodically, as supplemental administration of this vitamin may be necessary.

Gastrojejunostomy and gastroplasty are alternative procedures for treating morbid obesity, but the effects on the outcome of pregnancy have not been thoroughly studied. As the bypassed duodenum is the site of most iron absorption, women who undergo gastric bypass may have iron deficiency anemia during pregnancy. Therefore, additional oral administration of iron is necessary. If a short jejunoileal loop is not used in the gastrojejunostomy, absorption of calcium and folate may be impaired, since they are absorbed in the upper small bowel. With the gastric stapling partition operation, the normal intestinal continuity is not interrupted. Patients learn to eat small meals and obtain sufficient nutrition without vomiting.

Inflammatory Bowel Disease

Regional enteritis is associated with infertility in one third of patients. However, it may have no significant adverse effects on pregnancy once achieved. In one study, only about 10 percent of the patients with inflammatory bowel disease had an exacerbation during pregnancy (those patients with colonic involvement may be more prone to flare-ups in pregnancy). On the other hand, 24 percent of pregnancies were associated with relapses post partum, which were attributed to the sudden decrease in hormone concentration (Wong et al., 1981).

Also, *ulcerative colitis* is associated with infertility in 10 percent of patients. The majority of pregnancies in women with ulcerative colitis result in live births; however, 20 percent of these patients show an exacerbation of the disease during pregnancy. As in patients with regional enteritis, there is a significant risk of exacerbation post partum.

In pregnant women the management of inflammatory bowel disease is essentially the same as it is in nonpregnant women. The aims are to maintain good nutrition and to correct anemia or electrolyte imbalances. The diet of pregnant women with inflammatory bowel disease should be supplemented by oral administration of iron, folic acid, other vitamins, and by intramuscular administration of vitamin B_{12}. Nutritional support may involve total parenteral nutrition (TPN) in severe episodes, and evidence is accumulating that perinatal outcome is generally successful when TPN has been used (Herbert et al., 1985; Martin et al., 1985).

Special Situations

MULTIPLE PREGNANCY

Theoretically, the nutritional needs of the woman with more than one fetus should increase, as she has both a larger volume and a greater fetoplacental mass. However, there are no published studies to document that the needed requirements for protein, iron, or folic acid should be greater than for the normal pregnant woman with a single fetus.

ADOLESCENT PREGNANCY

Nutritional studies of pregnant adolescents indicate that the nutritional needs of those who conceive before their longitudinal growth is completed are greater than for girls who are 4 or more years postmenarchal. For pregnant adolescents between the ages of 15 and 18, the recommended allowance is 1.5 mg protein/kg/day; for younger girls, 1.7 mg/kg/day is suggested (see Table 7–1). The adolescent's needs for some vitamins and minerals are also increased. There are no differences in the recommended intake for adults and adolescents of vitamins A, E, B_{12}, and folic acid, and of the minerals magnesium, iron, iodine, and zinc.

Assessment of Nutritional Status

Ideally a nutritional assessment prior to conception should be performed. This would identify any weight problems, other nutritional inadequacies, or metabolic alterations that require treatment or correction. In addition, the importance of adequate food intake and weight gain to a successful pregnancy outcome could be stressed.

During pregnancy, the additional and changing nutritive demands require that nutritional assessment be an integral part of all prenatal care. Each prenatal patient should have an assessment at her first prenatal visit, with subsequent reviews at 20, 32, and 38 weeks (ACOG, 1978).

A more meticulous assessment should be made for those women who, because of age, health condition, education, or socioeconomic status, are at greater risk of nutritional deficiency. These include:

- Adolescents who are less than 4 years postmenarchal, who are still undergoing their own linear growth, and who therefore are superimposing these nutrient requirements on the nutrient demands of pregnancy.
- Women who are underweight at the onset of pregnancy, with underweight being defined as below 90 percent of the standard weight for height (see Table 7–4).
- Women with a history of frequent conceptions—i.e., more than two conceptions within the past 2 years.
- Women with a history of low-birth-weight infants (weighing under 2500 g).
- Women with a history of anemia.
- Women with a poor reproductive history, e.g., those who have experienced spontaneous abortions or perinatal loss.
- Women with chronic or infectious diseases that can negatively influence their nutritional status, such as diabetes, hypertension, gastrointestinal disorders (nausea, vomiting, diarrhea, intestinal bypass), allergies, cardiovascular disease, kidney disease, liver disease, and tuberculosis.
- Women with a history of substance abuse, such as habitual smoking, excessive alcohol intake, or other drug abuse.
- Women with a history of unusual dietary practices, including pica, macrobiotic diet, strict vegetarianism (vegans), anorexia nervosa, and bulemia.
- Women in families with insufficient income to purchase a nutritionally adequate diet and/or those who are living in housing without adequate facilities to store and prepare a varied diet.

HISTORY

Much of the data needed for nutritional assessment are found in the patient's medical, family, and social history, which should be included in the prenatal health care record. Pertinent information includes:

- Present age
- Age at menarche
- Previous obstetric history
  —Parity and outcome
  —Weight gain in previous pregnancies
  —Length of interconceptional period
- Weight history
- Diagnosed illnesses, including chronic diseases and infections (including parasitic infections)

DIETARY EVALUATION

Dietary information must be collected in order to assess nutrient intake. This includes data on the variety of environmental, psychosocial, and economic factors that influence food choices, as well as a pattern of usual or current food choices. One should also note the kinds and amounts of foods consumed, how these foods are prepared, and the timing of meals and snacks. Some of the influencing factors that must be investigated are as follows:

- Usual appetite, as well as any problems with nausea and vomiting during pregnancy.
- Regular or irregular eating habits and patterns of meals and snacks.
- Which family member is responsible for planning meals and buying and preparing food, including this person's knowledge of nutrition and attitude regarding meeting individualized nutritional needs.
- Usual food budget and expenditures for food and how many people are fed. Other sources of food, such as available food from a garden, meals provided at employment site, food gifts, or meals provided by parents, etc., should also be taken into account.
- Whether housing and available equipment are in working order to store, refrigerate, and prepare a variety of foods.
- Use of vitamin or mineral supplements, weight-control medications, diuretics, laxatives, antacids, etc.
- Food dislikes, intolerances, or allergies.
- Food or nonfood cravings (pica) during pregnancy.
- Cultural, ethnic, or religious practices that influence food choices.

Current food intake information must be obtained both in order to evaluate the nutritional adequacy of the patient's diet and for use as a starting point in counseling the patient on proper nutrition and diet. The simplest method for obtaining this information is a 24-hour recall, in which the patient is asked to list all the foods she has eaten during the last 24 hours. Questions should be open-ended. Probing questions are used to determine methods of food preparation, amounts of food, and whether added food items such as salad dressings, spreads on breads, toppings, sauces, gravies, sweeteners, etc., were used. Questions also need to be asked to be sure all beverages taken with and between meals are listed.

The patient's eating pattern may vary on weekends or holidays or at different times of the month depending on social activities, changes in schedule, availability of paycheck, welfare allowance, or food stamps. It is advisable to ask the patient to provide a "usual" eating pattern if it is felt the intake during the preceding 24 hours is not typical. A sample form for eliciting, summarizing, and evaluating a day's dietary intake is shown in Figure 7–2.

There are limitations to the validity of dietary intake information, owing to time constraints, variations in the skills of interviewers, variations in the memory and motivation of patients, and difficulty in accurately interpreting information concerning the variety of food eaten by any individual. The greatest value of dietary assessment is to identify gross inadequacies in major food sources of nutrients and to use the patient's own dietary pattern as the basis for remedial diet counseling.

Another commonly employed dietary assessment tool, used to supplement the 24-hour or usual dietary intake listing, is a Food Frequency checklist (Fig. 7–3), which provides insight into the range of foods the patient eats and gives some indication of how often a particular food is consumed. Similar foods are usually grouped together according to the commonly used Daily Food Guide or Four Food Groups. The Food Frequency checklist generally differentiates

24-HOUR TYPICAL FOOD INTAKE   SUMMARY

Name: _____ Interviewer: _____

Date: _____

TIME	PLACE	FOOD EATEN	PREPARATION	AMOUNT	Protein-Rich Foods	Milk and Milk Products	Cereal Products	Vitamin C–Rich Foods	Leafy Green and Yellow Vegetables	Other Fruits & Vegetables
				ASSESSMENT:						
				Servings eaten						
RECOMMENDATIONS AND FOLLOW-UP:				Servings needed	4	4	3	1	2	1
				Addition suggested						

Figure 7–2. Typical food intake (per 24-hour period). (Adapted from Nutrition During Pregnancy and Lactation, California Department of Health, 1975.)

FOOD FREQUENCY CHECKLIST

Name: _____   Date: _____

For each food checked EATEN, write the appropriate number of times eaten in a week (e.g., if eaten daily, number would be 7 — if a food is eaten once a month, put 1/4). A space is provided at the end to add other foods eaten regularly. Any food not eaten regularly should be checked in the DO NOT EAT column.

FOOD	TIMES EATEN PER WEEK	DO NOT EAT
PROTEIN RICH FOODS		
Eggs		
Chicken, Turkey		
Beef, Veal, Lamb		
Pork, Ham		
Liver		
Fish, Shellfish		
Luncheon Meat		
Hot Dogs, Sausage		
Dried Beans, Peas		
Soybeans, Tofu		
Peanut Butter, Nuts		
MILK & MILK PRODUCTS		
Milk (fluid, dried, canned)		
Yogurt		
Cheese (cottage, etc.)		
Ice Cream, Pudding, Custard		
CEREAL PRODUCTS		
Wholegrain Bread		
Enriched White Bread		
Rolls, Biscuits, Muffins, Bagels		
Crackers, Pretzels		
Pancakes, Waffles		
Pasta, Spaghetti, Noodles		
Rice, Grits		
Cereal, cooked		
Cereal, ready-to-eat		
Tortillas		

FOOD	TIMES EATEN PER WEEK	DO NOT EAT
VITAMIN C RICH FOODS		
Orange, Grapefruit, Tangerine or Juice		
Tomato (sauce or juice)		
Cantaloupe		
Strawberries		
DARK GREEN OR YELLOW FRUITS & VEGETABLES		
Greens (beef, collard, kale, turnip, mustard)		
Broccoli		
Peppers (green or red)		
Spinach		
Salad Greens (dark green)		
Carrots		
Sweet Potato		
Winter Squash		
Apricots		
Other Fruits & Vegetables		
Potatoes		
Green/Wax Beans		
Corn		
Peas		
Apples		
Bananas		
Pears		
FATS		
Bacon, Salt Pork		
Butter, Margarine		
Cooking Fat, Oil		
Salad Dressing		

FOOD	TIMES EATEN PER WEEK	DO NOT EAT
MISCELLANEOUS		
Cakes, Cookies, Pies		
Sweet Rolls, Doughnuts		
Candy		
Soft Drinks, Koolade		
Coffee, Tea, Cocoa		
Wine, Beer, Cocktails		
Sugar, Honey, Syrup		
Jam, Jelly		
Chips (potato or corn)		
ANY OTHER FOODS EATEN REGULARLY		

Figure 7–3. Food frequency checklist.

foods that are habitual in the patient's diet from those rarely or never eaten. For example, if the patient rarely or never consumes milk or milk products, a suboptimal intake of calcium, riboflavin, and vitamin D might be assumed. The Food Frequency checklist does not provide information on amounts or time of eating. Although it is a rather subjective assessment, it is useful as a basis for nutrition education.

PHYSICAL EXAMINATION

Indicators of nutritional deficiencies may be observed in the hair, face and neck, eyes, lips, gums, teeth, arms, hands, and lower extremities. Some examples of physical signs of nutrient deficiencies that might be observed in a malnourished, pregnant, or lactating woman are listed in Table 7–6.

It should be recognized that clear-cut physical signs of malnutrition are not frequently observed in the United States; therefore, subclinical signs may be easily confused with conditions unrelated to nutrition. Any signs that might be clues to malnutrition should be incorporated into the routine physical examination and analyzed by the several health professionals involved in the patient's nutritional assessment.

LABORATORY TESTS

Biochemical tests are useful in assessing nutritional status in that they provide objective and precise measurements of nutrient concentrations in tissues, blood, or urine. Some problems in interpretation occur in pregnancy because of the alterations in physiology and the lack of established norms for specific time periods throughout pregnancy. However, the laboratory tests provide baseline data for monitoring nutritional status.

It is generally recommended that hematocrit or hemoglobin and possibly serum folic acid be monitored for all pregnant women initially and in each trimester. Monitoring of serum vitamin B_{12} is desirable for women who are total vegans and who do not eat any animal protein foods. Serum albumin and total serum protein are suggested when a patient's diet appears to be consistently low in protein, calories, or both. According to individual needs, tests of other vitamin levels may also be performed.

Routine testing for blood glucose and urine glucose and ketones is recommended for women with either preexisting or gestational diabetes. Guidelines for criteria for laboratory evaluation of nutritional status are shown in Table 7–7.

ANTHROPOMETRIC ASSESSMENT

The simplest and most common measure of growth during pregnancy is weight gain. The rate of weight gain should be monitored as carefully as the total weight gain. The Prenatal Weight Gain Grid, shown in Figure 7–1, provides a visual reference for the health care professionals to compare each patient's weight gain with the currently recommended pattern. An excessive or sudden weight gain that greatly exceeds this rate is usually due to fluid retention. Sudden or continuous weight loss should trigger concern about severe nutritional or other health problems, and should prompt an assessment for intrauterine growth retardation. The grid is also useful for patient education, to point out any weight loss or inappropriate weight gain.

For the woman who is underweight at conception, with underweight defined as less than 90 percent of standard weight for height (see Table 7–4), the initial weight is plotted to indicate the deficit, and a greater

Table 7–6. Physical Signs of Nutritional Deficiencies

Site	Finding	Deficiency
Generalized	Significant nondependent edema	Protein
Tongue	Filiform papillary atrophy	Iron/folate
Thyroid gland	Diffusely enlarged and visible	Iodine
Skin (upper arms)	Follicular hyperkeratosis	Vitamin A
Gums	Diffusely swollen, red, interdental papillae in a clean mouth	Vitamin C
Lips	Angular fissures and cheilosis	Riboflavin

Data from Assessment of Maternal Nutrition, ACOG, 1978.

Table 7–7. Guidelines for Criteria for Laboratory Evaluation of Nutritional Status in Pregnancy

Test	Acceptable For Pregnancy	Deficient For Pregnancy
Hemoglobin	11.0+ g/100 ml after 6 months	< 9.5 g/100 ml
Hematocrit (packed cell volume)	33%	< 30%
Serum folic acid	6 ng/ml	< 3 ng/ml
Serum albumin	3.5 g/100 ml	< 3 g/100 ml
Total serum protein	6.5 g/100 ml	< 2.5 g/ml
Serum vitamin B_{12}	200 pg/ml	< 80 pg/ml
Thiamine in urine	50 mcg/g creatinine	< 21 mg/g creatinine
Riboflavin in urine	90 mcg/g creatinine	< 30 mcg/g creatinine

Adapted from Christakis, 1973, from Ten-State Survey.

weight gain is recommended. For women who are grossly obese at the onset of pregnancy, a weight gain of about 7 kg (15 to 16 lb) is recommended (Naeye, 1978).

Nutritional Intervention

Nutritional assessment identifies and specifies each woman's need for nutrition education and diet counseling. The Recommended Dietary Allowances of the Food and Nutrition Board of the National Research Council, National Academy of Sciences, provides the frame of reference (see Table 7–1). For pregnant women with adequate income and low-risk pregnancies, nutrition education should focus on providing most of the recommended nutrients through food. Since it is difficult for most American women to consume sufficient iron and folic acid in food, the use of daily supplements of iron (60 to 120 mg) and folic acid (400 to 800 mcg) may be recommended as a routine part of prenatal care. Women who are allergic to milk or who cannot tolerate milk or milk products may also require a calcium supplement, and diet counseling for these women should ensure that adequate calories, protein, and riboflavin are obtained from sources other than dairy products. The focus of individual and/or group nutrition education is on the basic diet for normal pregnancy and recommendations for desirable weight gain. Pregnant women should be advised regarding their nutritional needs for breast-feeding and given information to make an informed choice regarding methods of infant feeding.

Federal, state, and local officials, as well as nongovernmental health agencies, have developed food guides to interpret recommended dietary allowances into practical food groups. Selecting recommended amounts of servings from a given food group is easier and more realistic for most women than calculating amounts of nutrients in foods.

A daily food guide suggested for the pregnant woman is shown in Table 7–8. This is the basic food guide suggested to evaluate the nutritional adequacy of the pregnant woman's diet and to help her develop a meal plan that will meet her nutritional needs for pregnancy.

While the Daily Food Guide, adapted for pregnancy, provides a useful teaching tool, dietary counseling should also involve an exchange between the health professional and the patient, so that the patient can achieve the recommended diet within the constraints of her own individual lifestyle, food preferences, meal patterns, and socioeconomic situation.

Health professionals who conduct nutrition assessment should identify patients with more complex nutritional problems who require more individualized, in-depth counseling, follow-up, and referral. Women with severe nutritional deficiencies or weight problems, with concomitant medical conditions requiring dietary modifications,

Table 7–8. Daily Food Guide*

Food Group	Minimum Number of Servings Recommended During Pregnancy
Milk and milk products	4
Meat, fish, poultry, eggs, dried beans, peas and lentils	4
Leafy green vegetables	1–2
Vitamin C source	1
Other fruits and/or vegetables	1–2
Whole grain or enriched breads and cereals	3

*The Recommended Dietary Allowance (RDA) for calories is not meant to be achieved by this food guide.

with unusual eating patterns, or with emotional problems that affect their eating behavior should be referred to a registered dietitian. The dietitian can provide detailed diet counseling and follow-up with continued monitoring of the woman's nutritional status at each prenatal visit. Registered dietitians are generally available in Level III perinatal centers, major medical centers, community hospitals, local or state public health departments, and private practice.

For women who are unable to afford the recommended diet, all nutrition counseling must include assistance with obtaining adequate food. Most health agencies now participate in the Special Supplemental Food Program for Women, Infants and Children (WIC). Pregnant and lactating women, certified by health professionals as meeting nutritional risk and low-income criteria, receive supplemental foods to assure availability of a quart of milk, an egg, a serving of iron-fortified cereal, and a serving of vitamin C–rich fruit juice each day. These foods provide useful nutrient-dense foods supplemental to a basic nutritious diet, but assume the woman has access to the other components of a nutritionally adequate diet, including needed sources of calories and protein. Women in need of basic food and financial assistance must be referred to the official social services or human service agency administering public assistance (e.g., Aid to Families with Dependent Children) and advised on how to apply for food stamps. For emergency food, many communities now have food banks. Private agencies, such as the Salvation Army and many churches and missions, also provide emergency food or meals.

Another useful community resource is the Expanded Food and Nutrition Education Program of the Cooperative Extension Service. Trained program aides, supervised by a professional home economist, assist young mothers in their homes in learning more about meal planning, food purchasing and preparation, and management of their food budget and food stamps.

The nutritional assessment identifies malnutrition and nutritional risk factors and provides the data for ongoing nutritional care and monitoring during pregnancy and lactation. Nutritional intervention should be provided as indicated. Follow-up, support, and evaluation of the outcome of nutritional care must be provided by the physician and nurse and should include referral to the registered dietitian or public health nutritionist and appropriate community resources. To be effective, nutrition services must accommodate the patient's financial and general living situation, as well as be accessible and individualized. For middle- and upper-income women, the emphasis is on nutritional assessment and nutrition education, with in-depth diet counseling for those identified as at high nutritional risk because of complicating medical or emotional problems or lack of knowledge. For low-income women an added risk is inability to purchase recommended foods. For these women assistance in obtaining nutritious food and providing money for food is an urgent component of nutritional intervention.

REFERENCES AND RECOMMENDED READING

ACOG (American College of Obstetricians and Gynecologists): Nutrition in Maternal Health Care. Chicago, 1974.

ACOG (American College of Obstetricians and Gynecologists) and The American Dietetic Association: Assessment of Maternal Nutrition. Chicago, The American College of Obstetricians and Gynecologists, 1978.

Anderson, J. W.: Fiber, carbohydrates, and diabetes. Nutrition and the M.D. 7:1, 1981.

Anderson, J. W., and Ward, K: High carbohydrate, high fiber diets for insulin-treated men with diabetes mellitus. Am. J. Clin. Nutr. 32:2312, 1975.

Barnes, F. E. F. (ed.): Ambulatory Maternal Health Care and Family Planning Services, Policies, Principles, Practices. Washington, D.C., American Public Health Association, 1978.

Billewicz, W. Z., and Thomson, A. M.: Body weight in parous women. Br. J. Prev. Soc. Med. 24:97, 1970.

Burrow, G. N., and Ferris, T. F.: Medical Complications During Pregnancy, 2nd ed. Philadelphia, W. B. Saunders Co., 1982.

California Department of Health: Nutrition During Pregnancy and Lactation. Sacramento, CA, California State Department of Public Health, 1975.

Christakis, G. (ed.): Nutritional Assessment in Health Programs. Washington, D. C., American Public Health Association, 1973.

Cochrane, W. A.: Symposium on Nutrition: Overnutrition in Prenatal and Neonatal Life: A Problem? Can. Med. Assoc. J. 93:893, 1965.

Committee on Nutrition of the Mother and Preschool Child: Nutrition Services in Perinatal Care. Washington, D.C., Food and Nutrition Board, National Research Council, National Academy Press, 1981.

Couston, D. R., Berkowitz, R. L., and Hobbins, J. L.: Higher metabolic control of overt diabetes mellitus in pregnancy. Am. J. Med. 68:895, 1980.

Davies, N. T., and Williams, R. B.: Zinc balance during pregnancy and lactation. Am. J. Clin. Nutr. 30:300, 1977.

Dent, C. E.: Relationship of biochemical abnormality to development of mental defect in PKU. Report of 23rd Ross Conference, Columbus, OH, 1957.

Eastman, N. J., and Jackson, E.: Weight relationships in pregnancy. Obstet. Gynecol. Surv. 23:1003, 1968.

Fenton, V., Cavill, I., and Fisher, J.: Iron stores in pregnancy. Br. J. Haematol. 37:145, 1977.

Gabbe, S. G.: Optional diabetes control. Contemp. Obstet. Gynecol. 18:105, 1981.

Garden, A. N.: Nutritional Management of High Risk Pregnancy. Reference Manual, Berkeley, CA, Society for Nutrition Education, 1981.

Ghadimi, H., and Pecora, P.: Free amino acids of cord plasma as compared with maternal plasma during pregnancy. Pediatrics 33:500, 1964.

Gitlin, D.: Protein transport across the placenta and protein turnover between amniotic fluid and maternal and fetal circulations. In Moghissi, K. S., and Hafez, E. S. E. (eds.): The Placenta: Biological and Clinical Aspects. Springfield, IL, Charles C Thomas, 1974, pp. 151–191.

Heaney, R. P., and Skillman, T. G.: Calcium metabolism in normal human pregnancy. J. Clin. Endocrinol. Metab. 33:661, 1971.

Herbert, W. P., Seeds, J. W., Bower, W. A., et al.: Fetal growth response to total parenteral nutrition in pregnancy. J. Reprod. Med. (in press).

Herbert, V.: Experimental nutritional folate deficiency in man. Trans. Assoc. Am. Phys. 75:307, 1962.

Hytten, R. E., and Leitch, I.: The Physiology of Human Pregnancy, 2nd ed. Oxford, Blackwell Scientific, 1971.

Ingardia, R. J., and Fischer, J. R.: Pregnancy after jejunoileal bypass and the SGA infant. Obstet. Gynecol. 52:215, 1978.

Johnstone, F. D., Campbell, D. M., and MacGillivray, I.: Nitrogen balance studies in human pregnancy. J. Nutr. III:1884, 1981.

Joint FAO/WHO Ad Hoc Expert Committee: Energy and Protein Requirements. Geneva, WHO, 1973.

Jovanovic, L., and Peterson, C. M.: Management of pregnancy, insulin-dependent diabetic woman. Diabetes Care 3:63, 1980.

Kelly, A. M., MacDonald, D. J., and McDougall, A. N.: Observations on maternal and fetal ferritin concentrations at term. Br. J. Obstet. Gynaecol. 85:338, 1978.

Kitay, D. Z.: Folic acid deficiency in pregnancy. Am. J. Obstet. Gynecol. 104:1067, 1969.

Kitay, D. Z.: Anemia. In Queenan, J. T. (ed.): Management of High Risk Pregnancy. Oradell, NJ, Medical Economics Co., 1980, Chapter 28.

Leader, A., Wong, K. H., and Deitel, M.: Maternal nutrition in pregnancy. Part I: A review. CMA Journal 125:545, 1981.

Lenke, R. R., and Levy, H. L.: Maternal phenylketonuria—result of dietary therapy. Am. J. Obstet. Gynecol. 142:548, 1982.

Luke, B.: Maternal Nutrition. Boston, Little, Brown & Co., 1979.

Mandel, H. G.: Fat-soluble vitamins. In Goodman, L. S., and Gilman, A. (eds.): The Pharmacological Basis of Therapeutics, 5th ed. New York, Macmillan, 1975, p. 1574.

Martin, R., Trubow, M., Bistrian, B. R., et al.: Hyperalimentation during pregnancy: a case report. JPEN 9:212, 1985.

McFee, J. G.: Iron metabolism and iron deficiency during pregnancy. Clin. Obstet. Gynecol. 22:800, 1979.

Miller, E., Hare, J. W., Cloherty, J. P., et al.: Elevated maternal hemoglobin A_{1c} early in pregnancy and major congenital anomalies in infants of diabetic mothers. N. Engl. J. Med. 304:1331, 1981.

Moghissi, K. S.: Maternal nutrition in pregnancy. Clin. Obstet. Gynecol. 21:297, 1978.

Naeye, R. L.: Weight gain and the outcome of pregnancy. Am. J. Obstet. Gynecol. 121:724, 1978.

National Academy of Sciences: Recommended Dietary Allowances, 9th ed. Washington, D.C., 1980.

O'Sullivan, J. B., and Mahan, C. M.: Criteria for the oral glucose tolerance test in pregnancy. Diabetes 13:278, 1964.

O'Sullivan, J. B., Mahan, C. M., Charles, D., et al.: Screening criteria for high-risk gestational diabetic patients. Am. J. Obstet. Gynecol. 116:895, 1973.

Pitkin, R. M.: Calcium metabolism in pregnancy: a review. Obstet. Gynecol. 121:724, 1975.

Pitkin, R. M.: Nutritional support in obstetrics and gynecology. Clin. Obstet. Gynecol. 19:489, 1976.

Pritchard, J. A., and MacDonald, P. C. (eds.): Williams Obstetrics, 16th ed. New York, Appleton-Century-Crofts, 1980.

Pritchard, J. A., and Scott, D. E.: Iron demands during pregnancy. Iron deficiency—pathogenesis—clinical aspects—therapy. New York, Academic Press, 1970, p. 173.

Rosso, P.: Nutritional factors affecting intrauterine growth and development. In American Society for Parenteral and Enteral Nutrition: Syllabus: Nutrition for Growth and Development. Chicago, 1980, pp. 61–66.

Williams, S. R.: Nutritional therapy in special conditions of pregnancy. In Worthington-Roberts, B. S., Vermeersch, J., and Williams, S. R. (eds.): Nutrition in Pregnancy and Lactation. St. Louis, C. V. Mosby Co., 1981, p. 105.

Vong, K. H., Leader, A., and Dutel, M.: Maternal nutrition in pregnancy. Part II: Previous gastrointestinal operation and bowel disorder. CMA Journal 125:550, 1981.

Worthington-Roberts, B. S., Vermeersch, J., and Williams, S. R. (eds.): Nutrition in Pregnancy and Lactation. St. Louis, C. V. Mosby Co., 1981.

PHYSIOLOGIC ADAPTATIONS TO PREGNANCY

KENT UELAND
FREDERICK R. UELAND

Many physiologic changes accompany pregnancy, labor and delivery, and the postpartum period. This chapter focuses on some of these changes. Some may influence the high-risk status of the patient, and others may simply be normal physiologic changes associated with discomfort for her. Table 8–1 summarizes the normal physiologic changes of pregnancy. An awareness of the physiologic changes that occur during pregnancy is necessary for the members of the high-risk team in understanding and caring for the high-risk obstetric patient.

Of the many physiologic alterations that accompany pregnancy, labor, and delivery, those pertaining to the circulation are the most profound. It seems logical, therefore, to begin this chapter with a description of the major hemodynamic changes that take place.

Cardiovascular Adaptations

CARDIAC OUTPUT

The increment in cardiac output at rest is 40 percent during pregnancy (Ueland et al., 1979). As early as 1915 Lindhard reported a 50 percent increase in cardiac output using a nitrous oxide technique (Lindhard, 1915). These values have not changed through the years in spite of the use of much more refined and sophisticated techniques, including echocardiography (Rubler et al.,

1977). Nearly all of the increase is achieved by the end of the second trimester of pregnancy, from which level it is maintained until term when measured in lateral recumbency (Lees et al., 1967; Rubler et al., 1977) or falls slightly (Ueland et al., 1979). When cardiac output is measured in supine recumbency, there is a significant fall in late pregnancy, reaching nonpregnant values (Ueland et al., 1979). The increment in cardiac output, which is the arithmetic product of heart rate and stroke volume, is achieved through two mechanisms during pregnancy. In early pregnancy the increase is due mainly to an augmented stroke volume, whereas late in pregnancy it is due to an increase in heart rate (Ueland et al., 1979). The exact mechanism underlying these changes is unclear, but there is echocardiographic evidence of increased left ventricular dimension in both systole and diastole early in pregnancy (Katz et al., 1978).

The decline in cardiac output in supine recumbency late in pregnancy is due to inferior vena caval occlusion and interference with venous return to the heart, a phenomenon that was eloquently demonstrated by Kerr (Kerr, 1965). When there is inadequate collateral circulation the vena caval occlusion can result in maternal hypotension and bradycardia, the so called "supine hypotensive syndrome" (Howard et al., 1953).

During labor, maternal hemodynamics are again altered, and, as might be expected, the response is influenced considerably by maternal posture, type of anesthesia, and type

Text continued on page 165

Table 8–1. Normal Physiological Changes and Discomforts of Pregnancy

Normal Change or Discomfort	Basis for Change or Discomfort	Time Period	Preventive and Relief Measures (Medical and Nursing Management and Rationale)	Indication of Pathology
		Skin		
1. Pigmentation changes a. Striae	1. Mechanical stretching of skin over abdomen and breasts 2. Increased levels of estrogen and progesterone	Lasts 2nd through 3rd trimester and into postpartum period. Usually remain permanently with some change in color	1. Gradual weight gain; increased stretching 2. Provide moisture to skin, i.e., lanolin, cocoa butter creams, and massage; increase elasticity by increasing surface tension and health of skin. May or may not be effective 3. Support to abdomen decreases sag and stretch. 4. Recognize that striae may occur regardless of counter measures. Body image changes during pregnancy may create alterations in emotional adjustment for women or partners	
b. Vascular spider nevi; palmar erythema c. Chloasma Linea nigra Areola and nipple darkening	High levels of estrogen and progesterone produced by placenta have a melanocyte-stimulating effect Melanocyte-stimulating hormone, a polypeptide similar to ACTH, is remarkably elevated from the end of 2nd month of pregnancy until term	2nd month through postpartum period; may continue permanently. Most begin at 5 to 6 months' gestation.	1. Explain, recognize that changes may happen, discuss feelings and self-image. 2. Stay out of direct sun, use screening agents.	

Table continued on following page

Table 8–1. Normal Physiological Changes and Discomforts of Pregnancy *Continued*

Normal Change or Discomfort	Basis for Change or Discomfort	Time Period	Preventive and Relief Measures (Medical and Nursing Management and Rationale)	Indication of Pathology
		Skin (Continued)		
2. Pruritus a. Vulva	1. Increased blood supply and metabolic rate cause perspiration, which may lead to itching. 2. Leukorrhea—increase in pH favors proliferation of organisms and thus itching (e.g., Döderlein's bacilli)	Throughout pregnancy, increasing in 3rd trimester	1. Cotton underwear 2. Bathe daily to decrease bacteria and remove leukorrhea. 3. Avoid douching—may alter pH 4. Loose clothing to decrease perspiration. 5. Avoid prolonged sitting—this prevents drying of perspiration. 6. Cornstarch or bath powder may prevent intertrigo and increase drying. 7. Avoid scatching and excoriation.	Rule out: 1. Monilia (may be associated with diabetes mellitus) 2. *Corynebacterium vaginalis* 3. Trichomonas 4. Gonorrhea 5. Herpes II 6. Hair follicle cyst (folliculitis) 7. Urinary tract infection
b. Skin	1. Possibly due to retention of bile salts induced by estrogens 2. Increased perspiration and sebaceous gland activity. 3. Possibly related to slightly elevated bilirubin level or other liver function alterations in pregnancy		Cleaniness; avoid drying soaps, perfumed lotions Lotions are of little value, but some get temporary relief from calamine lotion Nonperfumed bath oil may help	1. Scratching may lead to infected excoriations. 2. Intertrigo—red, scaly, irritated rash 3. Gestational herpes manifest by erythematous spots, urticaria, papules, vesicles (on side of extremities, scapular and sacral regions) 4. Jaundice—indication of gallbladder disease, liver pathology, or hyperbilirubinemia.
		Head and Neck		
1. Dental Caries a. Pain	1. Alteration in food choices and variations in salivary pH lead to dental caries. 2. Pain due to increased hyperemia from increased blood volume	Throughout pregnancy	1. Reassurance regarding normality of condition. Dental check-up and removal of plaque when necessary.	Increased incidence of endometritis and postpartum infection

Discomfort	Physiology	Occurrence	Interventions	Complications
			2. Dental repair under local anesthesia when necessary. 3. Dental x-ray and extensive dental work should wait until after pregnancy unless absolutely necessary 4. Regular flossing and tooth brushing 5. Use soft brush; brush gums also 6. If abscessed, follow-up with antibiotics prior to delivery	
b. Gums—sore, bleeding, hyperplasia	Hyperemia from increased blood volume during pregnancy	Midpregnancy	1. Dental check-up to remove plaque early in pregnancy 2. Soft-bristle toothbrush; brush gums gently 3. Rinse mouth with warm saline several times per day 4. Explain normalcy of this happening	1. Gingivitis 2. Epulis (gingival lesion) 3. Oral cancers
2. Headaches	1. In most cases, no cause can usually be found. Possibly hormonal, ocular strain, sinusitis, emotional factors 2. Vasoconstriction with low CO_2 levels 3. Cerebral edema from increased fluid levels	Beginning to middle of pregnancy (headaches usually frontal and mild)	1. Tylenol, if severe 2. If wearing contact lens, may need eye exam	1. Eye problems 2. Preeclampsia (after 20 weeks) 3. Neurologic complications
3. Nasal stuffiness, nosebleeds	1. Vasomotor response to local disturbance of the autonomic nervous system; increased engorgement 2. Nosebleeds due to increased blood flow to the nasal mucous membranes		1. Increase fluids; use saline nose drops 2. Vaporizer to produce moist air 3. Avoid blowing nose vigorously 4. Elevate position of trunk and compress soft outer portion of nose against midline septum for 5–10 minutes.	1. Hypertension can result in severe nosebleeds 2. Trauma 3. Acute sinusitis 4. DIC 5. Drug addiction

Table continued on following page

Table 8–1. Normal Physiological Changes and Discomforts of Pregnancy *Continued*

Normal Change or Discomfort	Basis for Change or Discomfort	Time Period	Preventive and Relief Measures (Medical and Nursing Management and Rationale)	Indication of Pathology
		Head and Neck (Continued)		
4. Ptyalism	Theories vary: 1. May be related to increased dietary starch, which itself may be related to nausea and vomiting 2. Hysterical inability to swallow the normal amount of saliva produced daily (2–3 pints). Nausea may play a part in inability to swallow.	1st trimester or until about time of quickening	1. Relieve nausea and anxieties and therefore causes of condition 2. Mouthwash may help foul taste that may accompany symptoms 3. Decrease dietary starch. 4. Carry Kleenex and container for expectoration 5. Tincture of belladonna may aid by blocking secretion of saliva	1. Observe for parotitis 2. Excess nausea and vomiting can lead to electrolyte imbalance and weight loss 3. Pica for starch can be related to anemia
5. Taste or olfactory distractions	1. Ptyalism caused by increased acidity may affect taste and smell 2. Pyrosis and regurgitation may affect sensory system 3. Nasal stuffiness may be due to increased estrogen 4. More acute sense of smell in pregnancy	Throughout pregnancy	1. Reassure regarding normality; tell partner 2. Correct pyrosis 3. Correct nasal stuffiness	Tumors
		Respiratory System		
1. Dyspnea	1. Increased progesterone affects the respiratory center, lowering levels of CO_2 and raising O_2, often causing a feeling of hyperventilation 2. Pressure of growing uterus on diaphragm 3. Increased engorgement of nasal mucosa 4. Elevation of diaphragm approximately 4 cm	1st to 2nd trimesters 3rd trimester	Good posture 1. Reassure regarding normality of occurrence 2. Do "reaching" exercise to expand the thoracic cavity to its maximum and allow fullest expansion of lungs	Possibility of bronchitis, pneumonia, embolus

Cardiovascular, Peripheral Vascular, and Cerebrovascular Systems

3. Sleep in semisitting position, propped with pillows or blocks under bed, if necessary
4. Eat small, frequent meals to avoid crowding lungs with full (too full) stomach
5. Good posture
6. Inform woman that neither her life nor baby's life is threatened; relief will occur when baby "drops"
7. Saline drops if necessary

1. Dizziness	Early in pregnancy primarily	1. Vasomotor instability associated with hypotension results in transient cerebral oligemia with pooling of blood in legs and in visceral and pelvic areas, especially after prolonged sitting or standing in warm room 2. Hypoglycemia before or between meals can cause light-headedness	1. Avoid sudden changes in position 2. Employ slow, deep breathing, vigorous leg motions, elastic stockings 3. Eat frequently, carry food in purse for periods of hunger between meals 4. Stimulants such as coffee or tea, as well as spirits of ammonia, may be helpful 5. Avoid constricting garments	Be alert for: 1. Anemia 2. Blood pressure problems 3. Hypoglycemia 4. Preeclampsia
2. Edema	2nd to 3rd trimesters	1. Increased blood volume and decreased circulation due to pressure on vessels from growing uterus 2. Sodium and water retention due to ovarian, placental, and adrenal steroid hormones	1. Elevate feet and legs several times a day. Sleep in slight Trendelenburg position 2. Get proper rest 3. Avoid binding clothing—garters, tight slacks, knee socks 4. Position self on left side when lying down 5. Increase protein intake and encourage fluids, especially water 6. Assess blood pressure; assess urine for protein	1. Swelling of face and fingers may be a sign of preeclampsia 2. Kidney, cardiac problems

Table continued on following page

Table 8–1. Normal Physiological Changes and Discomforts of Pregnancy *Continued*

Cardiovascular, Peripheral Vascular, and Cerebrovascular Systems (Continued)

Normal Change or Discomfort	Basis for Change or Discomfort	Time Period	Preventive and Relief Measures (Medical and Nursing Management and Rationale)	Indication of Pathology

3. Hemorrhoids	1. Pressure from enlarging uterus, specifically in the hemorrhoidal veins
	2. Tendency toward constipation in pregnancy
		3rd trimester	1. Avoid constipation:
			  a. Adequate fluid intake
			  b. Warm liquids on rising
			  c. Food containing roughage
			  d. Establishment of good bowel habits
			2. Sitz baths—heat of the water gives comfort and increases circulation
			3. Witch hazel compresses for reduction
			4. Ice packs for pain and reduction
			5. Epsom salt compresses for reduction
			6. Reinsertion of hemorrhoids into rectum in conjunction with Kegel exercises.
			7. Bedrest with hips and lower extremities elevated
			8. Analgesic ointments or topical anesthetics
			9. Topical hemorrhoid preparation
			10. Stool softeners (e.g., Colace)
			11. When trying to have bowel movement place feet on stool (10–12 inches high), take two deep cleansing breaths, and exhale as if pushing
				Thrombosed vein leads to severe pain, considerable bleeding

Discomfort	Cause	Time of Occurrence	Self-Care Measures	Complications to Report

4. Leg cramps (shooting pain in thighs, buttocks)	1. Enlarged uterus exerts pressure on pelvic blood vessels, impairing circulation, or on nerves supplying lower extremities
	2. Imbalance of calcium/phosphorus/magnesium ratio in the body
		Late months of pregnancy	1. Have the woman straighten affected leg and dorsiflex foot
			2. General exercise and good body mechanics
			3. Legs should be elevated periodically throughout the day
			4. Avoid lying in prone position and pointing the toes
			5. Increasing the amount of calcium in the diet while decreasing phosphorus may help
			  a. Decrease milk and take calcium lactate to elevate ionized calcium level of plasma
			  b. Continue to drink 1 quart of milk daily and take aluminum hydroxide, which will trap the dietary phosphorus in the intestinal tract	

5. Perspiration, hot flashes, increased feelings of warmth	Increased levels of progesterone and vasodilatation lead to increased warmth and increased metabolic rate	Throughout pregnancy and postpartum period	1. Wear appropriate clothing—layers that can be removed 2. Frequent baths or showers 3. Adjust temperature of home 4. Inform of normality; explain to pregnant woman and significant others	
6. Supine hypotensive syndrome	1. Compression of the vena cava by large uterus when woman is in supine position 2. Increased progesterone levels 3. Vasodilatation	2nd and 3rd trimesters	1. Turn on to left side from supine position 2. If in supine position, maintain 45-degree angle	1. If accompanied by fever—infection may be present 2. If accompanied by fainting—safety of woman should be discussed

Table continued on following page

Table 8–1. Normal Physiological Changes and Discomforts of Pregnancy *Continued*

Cardiovascular, Peripheral Vascular, and Cerebrovascular Systems (Continued)

Normal Change or Discomfort	Basis for Change or Discomfort	Time Period	Preventive and Relief Measures (Medical and Nursing Management and Rationale)	Indication of Pathology
7. Varicosities—leg and vulvar	1. Increased vascularity of the pelvic organs leads to turgescence of tributary veins of pelvis. Vessels in pelvis and legs relax and dilate in response to progesterone 2. Later in pregnancy, the enlarging uterus may occlude some venous return in inferior vena cava when standing 3. Gravity causes some stasis 4. Familial tendency may predispose to development of varicosities	As early as 4th week and throughout pregnancy Last trimester	1. Full-length support stockings should be put on before arising, keeping leg elevated 2. Lie flat on bed or floor and prop legs on wall vertically for 15 minutes 3. Avoid restrictive clothing, stockings, or garters 4. Avoid prolonged standing or sitting 5. Do not cross legs. When sitting, elevate legs 6. Avoid constipation (see constipation and hemorrhoids) 7. A supportive foam pad may be worn to support vulvar varicosities 8. Elevate hips on a pillow or use knee-chest position. Varicosed vessels may need to be drained 9. Thrombosed vessels may or may not require surgical intervention 10. Do not rub legs because this may dislodge a thrombus	1. Severe calf, vulvar, or femoral pain indicates thrombosis (positive Homan's sign, localized warmth, redness) 2. Dyspnea, pallor, sweating, rales, rhonchi, anxiety, cardiac arrest may indicate pulmonary embolus

Breasts

Change	Timing	Cause	Intervention	Watch for
Breast enlargement: tingling and tenderness	1st and 3rd trimesters	1. Occurs as a result of increased sex hormones: progesterone, estrogen, and human chorionic somatomammotropin 2. Venous stasis	1. Well-fitted bra should be worn 24 hours a day 2. Ice packs and cold compresses may help 3. In late pregnancy, express colostrum to relieve engorgement (*if* planning to breast-feed). Do not express colostrum if there is a history of premature labor	1. Check for palpable mass 2. Check for fever or other signs of infection

Gastrointestinal System

Change	Timing	Cause	Intervention	Watch for
1. Constipation	Throughout pregnancy; increases as uterine size and pressure increase	1. Suppression of smooth muscle motility by increased progesterone and by pressure upon and displacement of intestines by enlarging uterus 2. Nausea and vomiting may cause diet changes (such as eating bland foods)	1. Stress good bowel habits; attempt bowel movement at same time each day 2. Diet: bulk foods, roughage, fruits, liberal fluid intake 3. Encourage exercise 4. Stool softeners or bulk laxatives that are not absorbed and are not irritating to bowel may be used. *Avoid* mineral oil—interferes with absorption of fat-soluble vitamins 5. Avoid strong purgatives that might initiate labor 6. Drink warm liquids in morning	Possibility of intestinal obstruction or impaction
2. Flatulence	Throughout pregnancy but increased in 3rd trimester	1. GI motility is decreased owing to increased progesterone. 2. Uterus displaces and compresses bowel mechanically.	1. Dietary modifications: avoid large meals, fats, gas-forming foods, and chilled beverages 2. Exercise and frequent change of position may help 3. Regular bowel function important	1. Milk intolerance 2. Gallbladder problem

Table continued on following page

Table 8–1. Normal Physiological Changes and Discomforts of Pregnancy *Continued*

Normal Change or Discomfort	Basis for Change or Discomfort	Time Period	Preventive and Relief Measures (Medical and Nursing Management and Rationale)	Indication of Pathology
Gastrointestinal System (Continued)				
3. Heartburn (pyrosis)	Regurgitation of acidic gastric contents into lower esophagus to reverse peristalsis is caused in pregnancy by: 1. Relaxation of the cardiac sphincter of the stomach due to effects of increased amounts of progesterone 2. Decreased gastrointestinal motility leading to delayed gastric emptying results from smooth muscle relaxation—which is caused by increased amounts of progesterone 3. There is lack of room for stomach because of its upward displacement and compression by enlarging uterus	Begins toward end of 2nd trimester and extends through 3rd trimester	1. Small, frequent meals are helpful to avoid overloading the stomach 2. Avoid fats with meals since fat depresses both motility of stomach and secretion of gastric juices 3. Decrease amount of beverages with meals since they tend to inhibit gastric juices 4. Avoid very cold foods with meals because they inhibit gastric juices 5. Drink cultured milk (e.g., buttermilk) rather than sweet milk, drink milk between meals 6. Good posture gives stomach more room to function 7. Avoid specific foods that are identified as causing heartburn 8. Remain upright for 3–4 hours following a meal; avoid bending over immediately after mealtime 9. Low sodium antacids may be taken as ordered 10. No preparations containing sodium bicarbonate should be taken	1. If heartburn persists and becomes severe with pain radiating into neck and is increased in supine position, hiatal hernia may be present 2. Differentiate from epigastric pain, which precedes eclampsia 3. Ulcers

4. Nausea and vomiting	5–13 weeks' gestation	Not known; several theories have been proposed:
		1. Hormonal changes of pregnancy:
		  a. High levels of circulating steroids such as estrogen
		  b. High level of HCG present during 1st trimester
			1. Small, frequent meals instead of three large meals
			2. Dry crackers before getting up in the morning, since emptying stomach seems to precipitate the condition
			3. Eat or drink something sweet (e.g., fruit, fruit juices) before getting up in the morning
			4. Avoid foods with strong or offensive odors
			5. Restrict fats in diet; fat slows peristalsis
			6. Separate liquid and solid intake by ½ hour
			7. Medication: controversy exists because of unknown possible teratogenetic effects of drug on fetus
			8. Reassure mother that it will usually end during the 4th month
				Persistent nausea and vomiting beyond first trimester may indicate:
				  a. Severe emotional problem
				  b. Hyperemesis gravidarum
				  c. Hydatidiform mole

5. Pica and food cravings	Throughout pregnancy	1. Increased appetite may be stimulated by estrogen and progesterone.
		2. Etiology unknown; may be related to
		  a. Psychologic factors
		  b. Social factors
		  c. Iron deficiency
			1. Maintain adequate diet to ensure appropriate nutrition
			2. Check as needed for anemia and decreased intake
			3. Reassure that occurrence is not uncommon
			4. Indulge reasonable cravings
			5. Increase psychologic well-being
			6. Validate intake
				1. Anemia
				2. Intrauterine growth retardation

Table continued on following page

Table 8–1. Normal Physiological Changes and Discomforts of Pregnancy *Continued*

Normal Change or Discomfort	Basis for Change or Discomfort	Time Period	Preventive and Relief Measures (Medical and Nursing Management and Rationale)	Indication of Pathology
Urinary System				
1. Urinary frequency	1. Pressure of the growing uterus on bladder compresses it against pubic bone	1st trimester	1. Avoid drinking large amounts of liquid within 2–3 hours of bedtime	Burning, hematuria, fever, pyuria, CVA tenderness, lower abdominal pain may indicate UTI
	2. Presenting part presses bladder after engagement	3rd trimester, especially after engagement occurs	2. Ingest required intake of liquid earlier in the day	
			3. Instruct woman about signs and symptoms of UTI and tell her to report these to care providers	
			4. Reassure her about normality and causative factors	
2. Nocturia	1. Supine position at night causes better renal perfusion	Throughout pregnancy	As above	As above
	2. Mobilization of dependent edema			
	3. Increased renal filtration			
Reproductive System				
1. Braxton Hicks contractions	Rhythmic tightenings of uterus; occur as part of preparatory changes for labor	Occur approximately every 5–20 minutes throughout pregnancy; most noticeable in last 6 weeks for primipara, last 3–4 months for multipara	1. Reassure woman about normality—the uterus is "getting ready" for labor and birth	Possibly associated with:
			2. Advise mother to try slow deep breathing to enhance relaxation; if active, stop and rest; massage the abdomen lightly	1. Leg cramps due to low calcium levels
			3. Differentiate between true and "false" labor	2. Abruptio placentae
				3. Appendicitis
				4. UTI
				5. Gallbladder problem
				6. Other abdominal problems

2. Dyspareunia	1st and 3rd trimesters depending on cause
	
	Postpartum, especially if breast-feeding
		1. Physiologic:
		  a. Pelvic/vaginal congestion due to pressure and impaired circulation
		  b. Related to enlarging uterus and pressure of presenting part
		2. Physical alterations:
		  a. Enlarged abdomen in way
		  b. Engagement
		3. Psychologic alterations:
		  a. Misconceptions and fears (hurting baby)
		  b. Alterations in libido
		4. Postpartum: decreased vaginal secretions due to decreased estrogens
			1. Positional changes for sexual expression
			2. Alternate sexual expressions; avoid cunnilingus
			3. Accessible congestion may be reduced with ice
			4. Provide explanation and discussion of misconceptions and fears, substituting facts and knowledge; this can be helpful and reassuring
			5. Education of both partners needed; encourage communication
			6. Lubrication if necessary.
			7. Anticipatory guidance with breast-feeding
				Excessive pain

3. Leukorrhea	Begins 1st trimester and occurs again in 3rd trimester	1. Increased vascularity of the cervix and increased mucus formation by the cervical glands due to increased levels of estrogen
		2. Increased desquamation from the cervix and increased transudation through the vaginal walls
		3. Secretions are acidic because of the conversion of an increased amount of glycogen in the vaginal epithelial cells by Döderlein's bacilli into lactic acid
			1. Good hygiene necessary
			2. Frequent change of soft cotton-crotch panties
			3. Use bath powder sparingly
			4. In extreme cases use vinegar douche (2 quarts warm water to 3 T vinegar)
			  a. Never use hand bulb syringes
			  b. Never allow bag to hang higher than about 2 feet above level of hips
			  c. Nozzle is inserted no further than 2 inches into vagina
				Acidic secretions foster growth of organisms responsible for vaginitis
				1. *Trichomonas*
				2. *Candida*
				3. *Gonorrhea*
				4. *Hemophilus*

Table continued on following page

Table 8–1. Normal Physiological Changes and Discomforts of Pregnancy *Continued*

Normal Change or Discomfort	Basis for Change or Discomfort	Time Period	Preventive and Relief Measures (Medical and Nursing Management and Rationale)	Indication of Pathology
Reproductive System (Continued)				
4. Perineal pressure pain	1. Pressure of fetal presenting part 2. Vascular engorgement of tissues due to estrogen and stasis of blood 3. Constipation 4. Bulging membranes if woman is in labor 5. Imminent delivery	3rd trimester	1. Side-lying position to relieve stasis 2. Some practitioners disagree about knee-chest position 3. Elevate hips on pillows	1. Constipation 2. Late stages of labor
5. Pubic pain	1. Progesterone and relaxin cause softening of cartilage of pubic symphasis 2. Increased joint motility can lead to muscle and ligament strain, and thus pain	32–40 weeks	1. Girdle or maternity corset decreases mobility and lends support 2. Correct posture relieves excess strain 3. Avoid activities that require balance and coordination	1. Rule out lower abdominal pain, urinary tract infection, contractions 2. Severe pain 3. Inability to walk 4. Complete separation of symphysis on x-ray
6. Round ligament pain	Round ligaments stretching as uterus enlarges	Sometimes occurs in latter part of 1st trimester but most commonly at 16–32 weeks	1. Pelvic rock and pelvic tilt relieve stretch 2. Avoid prolonged sitting; pain can occur on standing after sitting 3. Use heat—hot pad, warm moist soak 4. Use rest, side-lying position to relieve stretch	Rule out 1. Urinary tract infection 2. Labor 3. Appendicitis 4. Other abdominal infections 5. Constipation
Musculoskeletal, Neurologic Symptoms				
1. Backache (high)	Increase in size and discomfort of breasts	Throughout pregnancy	1. Reassure woman about normality during pregnancy 2. Wear well-fitting and supportive bra 3. Maintain good posture; attempt to hold shoulders back instead of giving in to weight of breasts 4. Stretch arms over head to exercise muscles of upper back	1. CVA tenderness 2. Cervical disk problems 3. Gallbladder problem 4. Predisposition to flu 5. Pleurisy

2. Backache (low)	Muscular fatigue and strain ... due to changes in body balance is caused by growing uterus.	...increases as pregnancy progresses, especially in 3rd trimester	...normality during pregnancy	...knee or ankle, internal
	2. Pressure on nerve roots causes muscle spasm.		2. Improve posture; stress "tall" posture with pelvis tilted forward, buttocks "tucked under"	2. Nerve compression or intervertebral disk syndrome
	3. Pelvic joints are relaxed owing to sex hormones.		3. Instruct about good body mechanics—squatting (to avoid bending and stress on lower back); rolling to side before sitting up from prone or supine position; tailor-sitting	3. Possible sign of premature labor
			4. Perform moderate daily exercise to "tone" and maintain muscle strength—pelvic rock or alternative positions	
			5. Heels of shoes should be medium, not high, to avoid increasing the spinal curvature	
			6. A firm mattress or bed board under mattress can be used to aid support	
			7. Maternity girdle or alteration in regular girdle may be indicated for patient with extreme lordosis or kyphoscoliosis, obesity, or multiple pregnancy	
			8. Local heat or light massage helps	
			9. Assume side-lying position with upper leg supported on pillow(s) for sleep and rest	
			10. Proper arrangement of household appliances at good working level avoids undue stooping or stretching	
			11. Analgesics such as Tylenol can be used for pain relief	
			12. Pelvic tilt stretches and tones side and back muscles	
			13. Rest with legs bent and elevated in chair or on bed	

Table continued on following page

Table 8–1. Normal Physiological Changes and Discomforts of Pregnancy *Continued*

Normal Change or Discomfort	Basis for Change or Discomfort	Time Period	Preventive and Relief Measures (Medical and Nursing Management and Rationale)	Indication of Pathology
		Musculoskeletal, Neurologic Symptoms (Continued)		
3. Gait alterations	1. Increased endocrine hormone relaxin affects sacroiliac joints and pubis 2. Increased motility of joints is characterized by "waddle" gait	Late in 3rd trimester	1. Maintain good body mechanics and good posture 2. Wear low-heeled shoes 3. Watch safety factors 4. Use girdle for stabilization	
4. Paresthesias (numbness and tingling of fingers and toes)	Various theories are suggested: 1. Fingers and upper extremities are affected if lordotic posture is extreme; the head and neck are flexed, putting strain on the brachial nerves and causing tingling of hands and arms 2. Toes and lower extremities are affected if gravid uterus presses on femoral veins and nerves supplying lower extremities, thus interfering with circulation and causing paresthesias 3. Edema may cause pressure and tingling of hands or feet, especially in hands when rising in morning 4. Carpal tunnel syndrome (edema causes pressure on nerves and ligaments within the carpal tunnel) 5. Vitamin B deficiency 6. Hypocalcemia (see Leg cramps, above) 7. Hyperventilation leads to decreased CO_2 normally in pregnancy. This can cause systemic vasoconstriction, which causes tingling	3rd trimester	1. Prevent or relieve edema (see Edema, above) 2. Remove rings and constricting jewelry 3. Exercise hands to relieve edema 4. Correct lordotic posture (see Backache, above) 5. Correct vitamin deficiency with diet and prenatal vitamins 6. Inform patient that she may have to tolerate a certain amount of numbness or tingling 7. Discuss safety measures to prevent dropping objects or skin injury 8. Avoid hyperventilation 9. Maintain adequate but not excessive calcium intake (milk and dairy products) 10. Maintain good bra support 11. Try vitamin B₆ (pyridoxine) supplement with orange juice or banana 12. Wrist splint while sleeping may reduce pain	1. Edema in hands may indicate onset of preeclampsia 2. If lower extremity numbness and weakness are present, rule out herniated disk (this can also occur higher, producing upper extremity symptoms) 3. Generalized tingling and hypertonus of muscles may indicate severe calcium-phosphorus imbalance

From Moore, M. L.: Realities in childbearing, 2nd ed. Philadelphia, W. B. Saunders Co., 1983, pp. 265–279.

of delivery. When the patient is supine, uterine contractions cause a 25 percent increase in cardiac output, a 15 percent decrease in heart rate, and an augmented stroke volume of 33 percent (Ueland and Hansen, 1969a). In lateral recumbency there are no significant changes in hemodynamics induced by uterine contractions. These differences are attributable to inferior vena caval obstruction in supine recumbency along with occlusion of the distal aorta during a contraction. The net effect is an exaggerated hemodynamic response to contractions both from the increased venous return and the fact that the blood is distributed mainly to the upper body.

Caudal anesthesia modifies the progressive rise in cardiac output as labor advances. In women given caudal anesthesia, cardiac output during the first stage of labor remains relatively stable compared with that of women receiving only paracervical block analgesia during labor and pudendal block anesthesia for delivery (Ueland and Hansen, 1969b). The peak increment in cardiac output for women given caudal anesthesia was 60 percent above supine prelabor values, as opposed to an 80 percent increase in women given local anesthesia. The differences are attributed to pain, because in both groups the anesthesia itself does not alter the profound changes in cardiac output accompanying delivery (35 to 40 percent). Cesarean section delivery circumvents the repetitive hemodynamic changes encountered in labor; however, the cardiac output increment at delivery can only be *modified* by anesthesia—it cannot be prevented (Ueland et al., 1972; Ueland et al. (in preparation); Ueland et al., 1968; Ueland et al., 1970). Hemodynamic stability is best maintained with epidural anesthesia *without* epinephrine added to the local anesthetic solution. Balanced general anesthesia (pentothal, N_2O-O_2, succinylcholine) is nearly as effective, whereas spinal anesthesia and epidural anesthesia (with epinephine) cause similar profound changes in maternal hemodynamics.

Blood Volume

PLASMA VOLUME

Changes in plasma volume can be detected as early in pregnancy as the end of the first trimester. Plasma volume increases most rapidly during the first two trimesters and rises slowly during the last trimester (Pritchard, 1965). The rise in plasma volume approximates 50 percent, but there is a wide individual variation (Hytten and Paintin, 1963). There seems to be a correlation between the total increment in plasma volume and the birth weight of the infant in women delivering their first child (Hytten and Paintin, 1963). There also appears to be a relationship between plasma volume expansion and the number of fetuses: In single pregnancies the increment was 48 percent, whereas in twins it was 67 percent and triplets 96 percent (Rovinsky and Jaffin, 1965).

The increase in plasma volume that accompanies pregnancy is the result of major changes in fluid balance, and the underlying mechanisms are complex. Estrogens and progesterone increase plasma renin activity and aldosterone levels and, as a result, promote sodium retention and an increase in total body water (Lipsett et al., 1971; MacGillivray and Buchanan, 1958; Seitchick, 1967). Tubular sodium reabsorption rises, and during a normal pregnancy 500 to 900 mEq of sodium are retained along with an increment of 6 to 8 liters of total body water, two thirds of which is extracellular (Lindheimer and Katz, 1973).

The accumulation of plasma volume and body water is made possible because of progesterone and its relaxant effect on the veins (Wood, 1972). This results in a substantial increase in vascular capacitance, which is further increased by the growth of the venous plexus surrounding the uterus. The altered venous capacity is, therefore, important in the expansion of total blood volume. The fact that the expanded volume is appropriate for the vascular space available is attested to by the fact that aldosterone secretion and excretion responds in a manner similar to that of a nonpregnant individual (Lindheimer and Katz, 1973).

RED CELL VOLUME

The rise in red cell volume in pregnancy is different from that of plasma volume in several ways. The total increment is only 20 to 30 percent. Red cell volume increases progressively throughout pregnancy but much more slowly than plasma volume, and it appears to accelerate slightly in the third trimester (Pritchard, 1965; Scott, 1972). The mechanisms underlying these changes are unclear. However, the differences in timing as well as the disproportionate expansion of plasma volume result in significant changes in hematocrit and hemoglobin values during pregnancy. In one serial study of women with proven iron stores and adequate folate, the hemoglobin decrement reached its lowest point between 16 and 22 weeks of gestation, whereas the values rose toward term (Scott, 1972). In women taking prophylactic iron in the last trimester of pregnancy, compared with a control group taking placebo, there was a significant rise in hemoglobin concentration (Chisolm, 1966). Thus, current evidence supports the fact that iron supplementation significantly improves the oxygen-carrying capacity of maternal blood during pregnancy.

Blood volume loss at vaginal delivery reaches 500 cc and that at cesarean section 1000 cc (Pritchard, 1965; Ueland, 1976). By 3 days post partum the decrement totals 1 liter regardless of mode of delivery (Ueland, 1976). This constitutes 50 percent of the blood volume gained during pregnancy. In those delivering vaginally, half the blood is lost at delivery and the subsequent decline is attributable to diuresis, as the hematocrit rises. In those women delivered surgically, the blood loss is doubled at delivery and the entire decrement is in whole blood; hence the hematocrit falls slightly. Blood values normal for the nonpregnant state are generally reached by 6 weeks post partum (Ueland, 1976).

Respiratory Adaptations

In the broad sense, respiration includes both the transfer of oxygen from air to the blood in the pulmonary capillaries and the consumption of oxygen by the peripheral tissues. The information available in the literature regarding maternal respiratory physiology is incomplete, and much of the data are based on small series of patients reported many years ago. Only the known changes will be discussed in this review.

ANATOMIC CHANGES

Mucosal edema and hyperemia secondary to capillary engorgement are common find-ings in the nasopharynx and the tracheobronchial tract. In fact, the majority of pregnant women have redness and swelling of the larynx that at times can produce changes in the voice. The hyperemia and increased secretion that occurs makes nasal breathing more difficult and is commonly associated with nosebleeds (Gee et al., 1967).

Changes also occur in chest circumference (6 to 7 cm), vertical diameter (4 to 5 cm), and the substernal angle (70° to 105°) (Hellman and Pritchard, 1971; Marx and Orkin, 1958; Thomson, 1938). The increase in chest circumference compensates for the elevation of the diaphragm, so that essentially there is no change in the overall volume of the thoracic cavity.

PULMONARY VENTILATION

During pregnancy a state of hyperventilation exists, i.e. arterial $PaCO_2$ declines. This also has been shown to occur during the postovulatory phase of the menstrual cycle (Goodland and Pommerenke, 1952). The relative hyperventilation increases as pregnancy progresses (Pernoll et al., 1975a). This is accomplished by an increase in tidal volume, not respiratory rate (Pernoll et al., 1975b; Plass and Oberst, 1938). Maternal arterial blood pH does not change appreciably during pregnancy, because of a compensatory increase in renal excretion of bicarbonate. This results in a decrease in standard bicarbonate in the blood from 27 mEq/L to 21 mEq/L (Lucius et al., 1970).

The hyperventilation of pregnancy appears to be related to the direct action of progesterone on the respiratory center (Loescheecke, 1953). One study has shown that when normal male volunteers are given progesterone, hyperventilation is induced (Doring et al., 1947). There also appears to be an increase in sensitivity of the respiratory center to inhaled CO_2 following progesterone administration (Lyons and Antonio, 1959). This response mimics that encountered during pregnancy.

The lowering of $PaCO_2$ in the blood, through maternal hyperventilation, produces a gradient across the placenta. This facilitates removal of CO_2 from fetal cells and produces a CO_2 tension in the fetus similar to what will be found in the newborn.

During labor, ventilation can reach peak values as high as 40 L/min, compared with the average value of 12 L/min seen prior to labor (Wulf et al., 1972). Arterial CO_2 tension also falls progressively during labor, reaching the lowest levels during a contraction in late labor. There is also an associated rise in arterial pH and PaO_2 during contractions (Andersen and Walker, 1970). All these alterations are attributed to the spontaneous hyperventilation produced by painful uterine contractions.

OXYGEN CONSUMPTION

There is a gradual increase in resting oxygen consumption as pregnancy advances (Pernoll et al., 1975b). This increase represents the sum of the increments of many maternal tissues, including the heart, kidneys, muscles of respiration, and reproductive tissues (breasts, uterine muscle, placenta), plus the amount of oxygen consumed by the fetus. The total increment in basal oxygen consumption has been estimated at approximately 50 ml/min, of which half is attributed to maternal reproductive tissues and the fetus. As might be predicted, the oxygen consumption in multiple gestations is even greater (Metcalfe, 1982).

In labor, oxygen consumption rises during each uterine contraction from about 250 ml/min to 750 ml/min, a threefold increase. The average oxygen consumption, which includes that during and between contractions, increases progressively, and in the second stage approaches twice that of the term pregnant woman before the onset of labor.

During pregnancy the affinity of maternal hemoglobin for oxygen decreases. This was shown in a recent study in which there was a statistically significant shift to the right of the oxyhemoglobin dissociation curve (Kambam et al., 1983). This is advantageous for the fetus, since at any given PaO_2 more oxygen is released to the tissues.

LUNG VOLUME PROFILE

During pregnancy the functional residual capacity (FRC) of the lungs is decreased. This represents the volume of air that remains in the lung at the end of quiet expiration. The reduction has been attributed to the elevation of the diaphragm from the enlarging uterus (Novy and Edwards, 1967). Interestingly, this reduction is not accompanied by an increase in airway resistance, even though the lungs are less distended, a condition that would ordinarily result in a decrease in outward traction on the bronchioles. A smaller luminal size would mean an increase in resistance to airflow. However, during pregnancy there is a fall in airway resistance, a phenomenon that must be the result of hormonal (progesterone) relaxation of bronchiole smooth muscle (Gee et al., 1967). The work of breathing is, therefore, reduced in pregnancy.

The mean decrease of 25 percent in functional residual capacity is counterbalanced by a similar increase in inspiratory capacity (IC). This represents the maximum volume of air that can be inspired from the resting expiratory level. The net result is that vital capacity (VC) remains unchanged during pregnancy (Cugell et al., 1953). VC measures the maximum volume of air that can be expelled from the lungs by forceful effort following maximum inspiration. Thus, even in pregnancy, a decrease in vital capacity measured serially could be useful in the early detection of pulmonary congestion or of deterioration in intrinsic lung disease.

Lung compliance does not change during pregnancy, despite the fact that there is evidence of an increase in pulmonary blood volume. This was determined by direct measurements using an esophageal balloon (Gee et al., 1967).

There are some clinical implications from the changes in pulmonary function during pregnancy. The decreased FRC and airway resistance both affect the speed of induction and recovery from inhalation anesthesia (Bonica, 1974). Teleologically speaking, the maternal respiratory as well as cardiovascular adaptations favor the fetal environment. More oxygen-rich blood is delivered to the placental bed, especially early in pregnancy (during embryogenesis and early fetal development), and the oxygen is given up more readily and waste products such as CO_2 are more easily removed because of the gradient created across the placenta. The maternal peripheral vasodilatation allows the metabolically active fetus to dissipate heat, and the vasodilatation and hypervolemia provides the fetus with a generous and constant flow of blood.

Renal Adaptations

The changes in renal function during pregnancy are profound and are surpassed only by those of the cardiovascular system. Major anatomic as well as functional changes are apparent. The following paragraphs will address these adaptations.

ANATOMIC CHANGES

The structural changes of the urinary tract that accompany pregnancy include a slight increase in the size of the kidney (Bailey and Rolleston, 1971). However, the more striking structural changes are those of the ureters, calyces, and renal pelvis. These changes are readily seen as early as the third month of gestation and remain until approximately the 4th month post partum (Lindheimer and Katz, 1975). Since these changes appear long before the gravid uterus is large enough to cause mechanical compression of the ureters, a hormonal effect is postulated. Progesterone, a smooth muscle relaxant, is produced in large concentrations even early in pregnancy, and is most likely the cause of the dilatation and decrease in peristaltic activity (Fainstat, 1963). Later in pregnancy, mechanical compression must certainly play a role. There is no question that the large gravid uterus compresses the bladder and also obstructs the ureters to a varying degree, most likely at the pelvic brim (Dure-Smith, 1968). This results in further dilatation and decreased peristalsis. Interestingly, the dilatation of the upper urinary tract is greater on the right than on the left. The explanation given by some for this phenomenon is that the colon acts as a cushion to protect the left ureter, whereas the right ureter is more exposed.

FUNCTIONAL CHANGES

Of the major functional changes that accompany pregnancy, the most striking is that of glomerular filtration (GFR), which increases by approximately 50 percent (Sims and Krantz, 1958). Renal plasma flow (RPF), on the other hand, increases by approximately 25 percent (Sims and Krantz, 1958). Both begin to change early in the second trimester of pregnancy and in lateral recumbency are maintained at these elevated levels to term. The factors responsible for these changes remain conjectural, but the following have been suggested: (1) the growth hormone–like effect of the hormone human placental lactogen, (2) the increased production and plasma concentration of free cortisol, (3) the increase in blood volume, and (4) the hemodilution and hydremia resulting in decreased colloid osmotic pressure. Regardless of etiology, these functional alterations force us to redefine normal values of renal function during pregnancy.

There is a decrease in serum values of those substances filtered by the glomerulus. The normal serum creatinine in pregnancy is 0.46 mg%, as compared with the nonpregnant value of 0.67 mg%. The BUN decreases to 8.2 mg% from a nonpregnant value of 13 mg% (Sims and Krantz, 1958). Uric acid also declines to a value of 3.1 mg% from approximately 4.5 mg%. Creatinine clearance values increase to 150 to 200 ml/min, as compared with values of 65 to 145 ml/min in the nonpregnant patient.

Although a glomerular-tubular balance exists for sodium during pregnancy, this is not the case for glucose or amino acids. Because of the increased glomerular filtration rate, the filtered load of glucose is so great that it frequently saturates the tubular reabsorptive capacity, resulting in "physiologic" glucosuria. Unlike the increased capacity for sodium reabsorption seen in pregnant women, the tubular maximum for glucose reabsorption (TMG) does not change in pregnancy and hence any excess glucose is excreted in the urine (Christensen, 1958). A similar circumstance prevails with amino acids; hence, aminoaciduria is frequently seen in pregnancy as well. The amino acids alanine, glycine histidine, serine, and threonine are commonly excreted in the urine, leading to lower plasma levels (Hytten and Cheyne, 1972). Like the glucosuria, the aminoaciduria disappears in the early puerperium.

In compensation for the hyperventilation and hypocarbia that occur with pregnancy, there is an increase in bicarbonate excretion by the kidney. This results in an elevation of urine pH.

In addition to the excretion of glucose and most amino acids, there is also an increased excretion of several water-soluble vitamins. There is controversy as to whether or not there is an increase in protein excretion, but regardless of this, it would seem appropriate to consider proteinuria in pregnancy abnormal only if it exceeds 300 mg in 24 hours. The increase in urinary nutrients may be responsible for the increased susceptibility to urinary tract infections during pregnancy. The relative alkalinity of the urine as well as the decreased urine flow may also contribute to this problem.

During pregnancy there is a reversal of the usual nonpregnant diurnal pattern of urinary flow. Hence, urine concentration tests may yield misleading results. During the day, when upright, pregnant women retain an inordinate amount of fluid, mostly in the form of dependent edema. At night, with the woman in a lateral recumbent position, this fluid is mobilized and excreted. Thus, nocturia in pregnancy is a normal event, and failure to excrete a concentrated early morning urine specimen during pregnancy does *not* imply impaired tubular function. In the pregnant woman, urine concentration tests should be conducted by collecting an evening specimen (rather than a morning sample) in order to best determine tubular function.

POSTURE AND RENAL FUNCTION IN PREGNANCY

In nonpregnant individuals the upright posture causes extracellular fluid shifts to the legs, resulting in a relative decrease in central blood volume. The probable reflex response to this phenonenon is the release of renin by the kidney, with a resultant increase in angiotensin production, which stimulates aldosterone secretion. This enhances renal tubular reabsorption of sodium, thus reducing urinary excretion of sodium and water.

In pregnancy this response is exaggerated (Assali et al., 1959), and a similar response also occurs when the supine position is assumed (Pritchard et al., 1955). The extent of the change is a 50 to 60 percent decrease in urine flow and sodium excretion in supine recumbency versus lateral recumbency, accompanied by a 20 percent decrease in renal plasma flow and glomerular filtration. The underlying pathophysiology is likely inferior vena caval obstruction, resulting in pooling of blood in the dilated veins of the lower extremities, dependent edema, decreased venous return, decreased central blood volume, increased aldosterone production, and ultimately decreased urinary excretion of sodium and water. This phenomenon must be considered when performing renal function studies in the latter part

of pregnancy, as the results during this time may be misleading.

It bears repeating that the normal values of renal function are altered appreciably and that values normal to the nonpregnant could indicate substantial renal impairment in the parturient.

Gastrointestinal Adaptations

Compared with the renal and cardiovascular systems, the gastrointestinal system undergoes few significant changes during pregnancy. Gastrointestinal secretion and absorption are slightly affected (Bynum, 1977). More major changes occur in relation to motility or motor function; with these changes likely resulting from the increased production of female sex hormones and, perhaps to a lesser extent, the increased size of the gravid uterus. As with ureteral peristalsis, progesterone appears to affect intestinal peristalsis as well. This decreased motility may lead to *constipation*, a condition frequently encountered during pregnancy. Pressure on the rectosigmoid colon by the large uterus may also be responsible for constipation, especially late in gestation. As in the nonpregnant patient, this constipation is best managed by increased fluid intake, change in dietary habits, and use of bulk agents and stool softeners.

Hemorrhoids are another common problem during pregnancy (Earnest, 1973). Several factors are probably responsible. The major contributing factor must be the partial or complete obstruction of the inferior vena cava and interference with venous drainage, resulting in venous engorgement and increase in hemorrhoidal vein pressure. Hormonally induced venodilation and increased straining at stool because of constipation probably also play a role in the development of this irritating problem. Hemorrhoids can become especially severe in the early puerperium, more commonly in the susceptible patient who experienced a long second stage of labor with repeated bearing-down efforts. Treatment of hemorrhoids during pregnancy should, with rare exceptions, be nonsurgical. Following pregnancy the condition frequently improves dramatically. On occasion, because of severe symptoms, a thrombosed hemorrhoid may need to be evacuated under local anesthesia. However, a hemorrhoidectomy should be avoided. Medical management includes that already recommended for constipation. In addition, hot sitz baths will help alleviate pain, as will local anesthetic ointments, astringent solutions and lubricating suppositories prior to defecation. Correcting constipation frequently improves the problem.

Heartburn is also a frequent accompaniment to pregnancy. Again, there are likely several contributing factors: (a) increased progesterone may cause a relaxation of the lower esophageal sphincter; (b) stomach emptying time is delayed, especially late in pregnancy; and (c) the enlarged uterus exerts upward pressure on the stomach and distal esophagus, so that the intraabdominal portion of the esophagus is lost. The latter, when associated with increased intraabdominal pressure, may compound the problem. Management includes use of postprandial antacids, taking of smaller and more frequent bland meals, avoidance of food for at least 2 hours before bedtime, and elevation of the head of the bed at night.

Nausea (with or without vomiting) is another common gastrointestinal problem encountered during pregnancy. It is most common during the first trimester of pregnancy, is usually self-limiting, and ends spontaneously by the 12th to 14th week. Frequent solid feedings and a mild antinauseant are generally sufficient for relief of symptoms, and most women can function reasonably normally with this approach to management. However, extreme bouts of nausea and vomiting, known as *hyperemesis gravidarum*, represent an ominous sign and can be life-threatening to both mother and fetus. Luckily, hyperemesis gravidarum occurs only rarely. This condition may be associated with an increased level of chorionic gonadotropins, creating an endocrine imbalance, disturbances of the metabolic changes of pregnancy, decreased gastric motility, or psychologic maladjustments to pregnancy (American Association of Critical-Care Nurses, 1983).

In the majority of individuals, few significant changes take place in the liver during pregnancy. There are no major alterations in gross or microscopic hepatic morphology. However, values for several *liver function tests* are outside the normal range. The total serum protein concentration begins to fall in the first trimester, reaching a lowest level by midpregnancy of approximately 1 g% below nonpregnant levels (Alber, 1974; Hytten and Leitch, 1971). The hydremia associated with a substantial increase in plasma volume produces a relative decrease in total protein, yet the absolute mass of intravascular protein is increased. The same pertains to albumin, and there is an associated decline in colloid-osmotic pressure as well during normal pregnancy. In contrast, most globulin fractions rise progressively during pregnancy. The net result is a decrease in the albumin/globulin ratio. Serum alkaline phosphatase rises markedly during pregnancy (Sadovsky and Zuckerman, 1965; Thorling, 1955). The entire rise is attributed to the presence of heat-stable alkaline phosphatase, which is produced in the placenta. It appears in the first trimester and progressively rises to term, at which time it constitutes approximately 50 percent of the total serum alkaline phosphatase activity. In twins the levels are even higher, and in women with preeclampsia they are raised considerably (Bagga et al., 1979). Results from serum copper, alpha fetoprotein serum transaminase, and other laboratory tests that may be indicative of liver disease can also be elevated during pregnancy.

The sex steroids, namely the estrogens, appear responsible for the *cholestasis* that frequently accompanies pregnancy. In its mildest form this results in only a slight decrease in Bromsulphalein (BSP) excretion and possibly a slight elevation in serum bile salts. At its extreme, cholestasis may present as acute hepatic failure in the third trimester of pregnancy or in the early puerperium. This so called acute yellow atrophy is an ill-defined fulminant disease with a maternal mortality estimated as high as 75 percent. It is difficult to characterize because it is associated with a major coagulopathy that precludes a liver biopsy. Much more common is the *cholestatic pruritus* that frequently presents as a nonicteric clinical entity. It is likely secondary to the deposition of bile salts in the skin. At times, it is associated with clinically detectable jaundice, but the most distressing symptom is the persistent pruritus. The disorder is self limiting and usually disappears within 2 weeks of delivery.

As can be seen from the foregoing paragraphs, the usual gastrointestinal changes accompanying pregnancy are rather mild and self limiting, and in the majority of cases are readily treatable by simple measures.

Summary

It is imperative to fully understand the altered physiology of pregnancy, because it affects many of the function studies and laboratory values that are commonly used to diagnose disease. Thus, one has to reset what one perceives as normal. For example, a serum creatinine of 0.9 mg% and a creatinine clearance of 80 ml/min during pregnancy may be indicative of renal compromise. A serum albumin of 3 g% is within the normal range for pregnancy but may well be indicative of hepatic compromise in the nonpregnant state. The reader is referred to the classic work of Hytten and Leitch entitled *The Physiology of Pregnancy* for a complete and detailed review of the physiologic adaptations of pregnancy (Hytten and Leitch, 1971).

REFERENCES

Alber, C. A.: Plasma protein measurements as a diagnostic aid. N. Engl. J. Med. 291:287, 1974.

American Association of Critical-Care Nurses: High Risk Perinatal Nursing. *In* Vestal, K. W., and McKenzie, C. A. M., (eds.) Philadelphia, W. B. Saunders Co., 1983.

Andersen, G. J., and Walker, J.: The effect of labour on the maternal blood gas and acid-base status. J. Obstet. Gynaecol. Br. Commonw. 77:289, 1970.

Assali, N. S., Dignam, W. J., and Dasgupta, K.: Renal function in human pregnancy. II. Effects of venous pooling on renal hemodynamics and water, electrolyte, and aldosterone excretion during normal gestation. J. Lab. Clin. Med. 54:394, 1959.

Bagga, O. P., Mullick, V. D., Madan, P., et al.: Total serum alkaline phosphate and its isoenzymes in normal and toxemic pregnancies. Am. .J. Obstet. Gynecol. 104:850, 1969.

Bailey, R. R., and Rolleston, G. L.: Kidney length and ureteric dilatation in the puerperium. J. Obstet. Gynaecol. Br. Commonw. 78:13, 1971.

Bonica, J. J.: Maternal physiological changes during pregnancy and anesthesia. *In* Shnider, S. M., and Moya, F. (eds.): The Anesthesiologists, Mother, and Newborn. Baltimore, Williams & Wilkins, 1974, p. 3.

Bynum, T. E.: Hepatic and gastrointestinal disorders of pregnancy. Med. Clin. North Am. 61:129, 1977.

Chisolm, M.: A controlled clinical trial of prophylactic folic acid and iron in pregnancy. J. Obstet. Gynaecol. Br. Commonw. 73:191, 1966.

Christensen, P. J.: Tubular reabsorption of glucose during pregnancy. Scand. J. Clin. Lab. Invest. 10:364, 1958.

Cugell, D. W., Frank, N. R., Gaensler, E. A., et al.: Pulmonary function in pregnancy. I. Serial observations in normal women. Ann. Rev. Tuberc. 67:568, 1953.

Döring, G. K., Loeschcke, H. H., and Ochwadt, B.: Weitere Untersuchungen über die Wirkung der Sexualhormone auf die Atmung. Pflügers Arch ges Physiol 252:216, 1950.

Dure-Smith, P.: Ureteric dilatation: its anatomical basis, and relation to sex and pregnancy. *In* O'Grady, F. and Brumfitt, W. (eds.): Urinary Tract Infection. London, Oxford University Press, 1968, p. 172.

Earnest, D. C.: Diseases of the anus. *In* Sleisenger, M. H., and Fordtran, J. S. (eds.): Gastrointestinal Disease. Philadelphia, W. B. Saunders Co., 1973.

Fainstat, T.: Ureteral dilatation in pregnancy: a review. Obstet. Gynecol. Surv. 18:845, 1963.

Gee, J. B. L., Packer, B. S., Millen, J. E., et al.: Pulmonary mechanics during pregnancy. J. Clin. Invest. 46:945, 1967.

Goodland, R. L., and Pommerenke, W. T.: Cyclic fluctuations of the alveolar carbon dioxide tension during the normal menstrual cycle. Fertil. Steril. 3:394, 1952.

Hellman, L. M., and Pritchard, J. A.: Williams Obstetrics, 14th ed. New York, Appleton-Century-Crofts, 1971, p. 260.

Howard, B. K., Goodson, J. H., and Mengert, W. F.: Supine hypotensive syndrome in late pregnancy. Obstet. Gynecol. 1:371, 1953.

Hytten, F. E., and Cheyne, G. A.: The aminoaciduria of pregnancy. J. Obstet. Gynaecol. Br. Commonw. 79:424, 1972.

Hytten, F. E., and Leitch, I.: The Physiology of Human Pregnancy, 2nd ed. Oxford, Blackwell Scientific Publications, 1971, p. 41.

Hytten, F. E., and Paintin, D. B.: Increase in plasma volume during normal pregnancy. J. Obstet. Gynaecol. Br. Commonw. 70:402, 1963.

Kambam, J. R., Handte, R. E., Brown, W. R., et al.: Effect of pregnancy on oxygen dissociation. Abstr. Soc. Obstet. Anesthesiol. Perinatol. 20, 1983.

Katz, R., Karliner, J. S., and Resnik, R.: Effects of a natural volume overload state (pregnancy) on left ventricular performance in normal human subjects. Circulation 58:434, 1978.

Kerr, M. G.: The mechanical effects of the gravid uterus in late pregnancy. J. Obstet. Gynaecol. Br. Commonw. 72:513, 1965.

Lees, M. M., Taylor, S. H., Scott, D. B., et al.: A study of cardiac output at rest throughout pregnancy. J. Obstet. Gynaecol. Br. Commonw. 74:319, 1967.

Lindhard, J.: Über das Minutenvolum des Herzens bei Ruhe und bei Muskelarbeit. Pflügers Arch. ges Physiol. 161:233, 1915.

Lindheimer, M. D., and Katz, A. I.: Renal changes during pregnancy: their relevance to volume homeostasis. Clin. Obstet. Gynecol. 2:345, 1975.

Lindheimer, M. D., and Katz, A. I.: Sodium and diuretics in pregnancy. N. Engl. J. Med. 288:891, 1973.

Lipsett, M. B., Combs, J. W., Jr., Catt, K., et al.: Problems in contraception. Ann. Intern. Med. 74:251, 1971.

Loescheecke, G. C.: Spielen fur die Ruheatmung des Menschen vom O₂-Druck abhangige Erregungen der Chemoreceptoren eine Rolle? Pflugers Arch ges Physiol 257:349, 1953.

Lucius, H., Gahlenbeck, H., Klein, H. O., et al.: Respiratory functions, buffer systems, and electrolyte concentrations of blood during human pregnancy. Respir. Physiol. 9:311, 1970.

Lyons, H. A., and Antonio, R.: The sensitivity of the respiratory center in pregnancy and after the administration of progesterone. Trans. Assoc. Am. Physicians 72:173, 1959.

MacGillivray, I., and Buchanan, T. J.: Total exchangeable sodium and potassium in nonpregnant women and in normal and preeclamptic pregnancy. Lancet 2:1090, 1958.

Marx, G. F., and Orkin, L. R.: Physiological changes during pregnancy: a review. Anesthesiology 19:258, 1958.

Metcalfe, J.: Unpublished data, 1982.

Metcalfe, J., and Ueland, K.: Maternal cardiovascular adjustments to pregnancy. Progr. Cardiovasc. Dis. 16:363, 1974.

Novy, M. J., and Edwards, M. J.: Respiratory problems in pregnancy. Am. J. Obstet. Gynecol. 99:1024, 1967.

Pernoll, M. L., Metcalfe, J., Kovach, P. A., et al.: Ventilation during rest and exercise during pregnancy and postpartum. Respir. Physiol. 25:295, 1975a.

Pernoll, M. L., Metcalfe, J., Schlenker, T. L., et al.: Oxygen consumption at rest and during exercise in pregnancy. Respir. Physiol. 25:285, 1975b.

Plass, E. D., and Oberst, F. W.: Respiration and pulmonary ventilation in normal nonpregnant, pregnant and puerperal women: with an interpretation of the acid-base balance during normal pregnancy. Am. J. Obstet. Gynecol. 35:441, 1938.

Pritchard, J. A.: Changes in the blood volume during pregnancy and delivery. Anesthesiology 26:393, 1965.

Pritchard, J. A., Barnes, C. A., and Bright, R. H.: The effect of supine position on renal function in the near-term pregnant woman. J. Clin. Invest. 34:777, 1955.

Rovinsky, J. J., and Jaffin, H.: Cardiovascular hemodynamics in pregnancy. I. Blood and plasma volumes in multiple pregnancy. Am. J. Obstet. Gynecol. 93:1, 1965.

Rubler, S., Damani, P. M., and Pinto, E. R.: Cardiac size and performance during pregnancy estimated with echocardiography. Am. J. Cardiol. 40:534, 1977.

Sadovsky, E., and Zuckerman, H.: An alkaline phosphatase specific to normal pregnancy. Obstet. Gynecol.: 26:211, 1965.

Scott, D. E.: Anemia in pregnancy. In Wynn, R. M. (ed.): Obstetrics and Gynecology Annual: 1972. New York, Appleton-Century-Crofts, 1972, p. 219.

Seitchick, J.: Total body water and total body density of pregnant women. Obstet. Gynecol. 29:155, 1967.

Sims, E. A. H., and Krantz, K. E.: Serial studies of renal function during pregnancy and the puerperium in normal women. J. Clin. Invest. 37:1764, 1958.

Thomson, K. J., and Cohen, M. E.: Studies on the circulation in pregnancy: vital capacity observations in normal pregnant women. Surg. Gynecol. Obstet. 66:591, 1938.

Thorling, L.: Jaundice in pregnancy: clinical study. Acta Med Scand. 151 (Suppl. 302):1, 1955.

Ueland, K.: Maternal cardiovascular dynamics. VII. Intrapartum blood volume changes. Am. J. Obstet. Gynecol. 126:671, 1976.

Ueland, K., Akamatsu, T. J., Eng, M., et al.: Maternal cardiovascular dynamics. VI. Cesarean section under epidural anesthesia without epinephrine. Am. J. Obstet. Gynecol. 114:775, 1972.

Ueland, K., Akamatsu, T. J., and Der Yuen, D.: Maternal cardiovascular dynamics. VIII. Cesarean section under epidural anesthesia incorporating epinephrine. (In preparation.)

Ueland, K., Gills, R. E., and Hansen, J. Maternal cardiovascular dynamics. I. Cesarean section under subarachnoid block anesthesia. Am. J. Obstet. Gynecol. 100:42, 1968.

Ueland, K., and Hansen, J. M.: Maternal cardiovascular dynamics. II. Posture and uterine contractions. Am. J. Obstet. Gynecol. 103:1, 1969a.

Ueland, K., and Hansen, J. M.: Maternal cardiovascular dynamics. III. Labor and delivery under local and caudal analgesia. Am. J. Obstet. Gynecol. 103:8, 1969b.

Ueland, K., Hansen, J., Eng, M., et al.: Maternal cardiovascular dynamics. V. Cesarean section under thiopental, nitrous oxide and succinylcholine anesthesia. Am. J. Obstet. Gynecol. 108:615, 1970.

Ueland, K., Novy, M. J., Peterson, E. N., et al.: Maternal cardiovascular dynamics. IV. The influence of gestational age on the maternal cardiovascular response to posture and exercise. Am. J. Obstet. Gynecol. 104:856, 1969.

Wood, J. E.: The cardiovascular effects of oral contraceptives. Mod. Concepts Cardiovasc. Dis. 41:37, 1972.

Wulf, K. H., Kunzel, W., and Lehmann, V.: Clinical aspects of placental gas exchange. In Longo, L. D., and Barterls, H. (eds.): Respiratory gas exchange and blood flow in the placenta. Bethesda, MD, U.S. Department of Health, Education, and Welfare, DHEW publication no. (NIH) 73-361, 1972, p. 505.

9

PSYCHOSOCIAL IMPLICATIONS OF HIGH-RISK PREGNANCY

THOMAS M. JOHNSON
JANE M. MURPHY

Pregnancy presents profound social and psychological adaptive challenges to women and their families. Even an uncomplicated pregnancy has been described as a psychobiologic crisis in which the individual physiologic and psychological equilibrium is disrupted, family and work roles are altered, and important interaction patterns between mother and baby are established. There is now considerable freedom of choice regarding pregnancy and the interpretation of the meaning of pregnancy in the light of the currently changing roles of women in society. In the current climate, the social and psychological implications of high-risk pregnancy take on even greater significance because pregnancy and parturition are increasingly viewed as requiring less medical intervention. Indeed, if pregnancy, per se, is an adaptive challenge, the high-risk pregnancy presents even greater social and psychological problems for both patients and practitioners.

The woman who has been diagnosed to be at risk during pregnancy experiences a wide variety of emotions, and the normal emotional changes of pregnancy may be intensified. The patient must deal with realistic fears for her own safety as well as for the life of her unborn child. Because expectations for pregnancy may not have included medical complications, the patient may be confused about what is actually happening to her body, may fear having an abnormal child, and may feel a loss of control over the pregnancy because her choices regarding

pregnancy and childbirth have been limited by her medical condition. Such psychological features of high-risk patients may affect the level of satisfaction and positive involvement in medical care. It is also clear that negative attitudes toward pregnancy leading to increased anxiety contribute to problems with delivery, and later problems with the maternal-infant relationship (McDonald, 1968).

Thus, although specialized, intensive perinatal care has been shown to result in improved fetal and neonatal outcomes (Merkatz et al., 1978), it is equally clear that there must be attention to the psychological as well as physical aspects of care for mothers who are particularly at risk for poor pregnancy outcomes. The long-term hospitalization of pregnant women, for example, may lead to successful parturition and postnatal course but may also prove to be a hardship for other children in the family, place stress on the marriage, and lead to depression for the patient (Smith, 1979).

In short, although maternal and fetal mortality rates have declined as a result of specialized high-risk obstetric care, it has been suggested that morbidity rates for psychological and social factors that affect both mothers and children have increased for iatrogenic reasons and that high-risk obstetric care may be a two-edged sword in which procedures designed to protect mothers and infants from physical damage may simultaneously create profound psychosocial problems (Cohen, 1979).

173

Clearly, if practitioners responsible for the complex management of high-risk pregnancies do not actively consider the psychologic and social implications of intensive testing, lengthy hospitalization, and illness or disability superimposed on pregnancy, the results may be antithetical to the goal of care, which is physically and emotionally healthy mothers and children (Merkatz et al., 1978). It is to a better understanding of the problems of psychosocial adaptation by high-risk patients that this chapter is dedicated.

Adaptations In Pregnancy

Although pregnancy is usually regarded as a period of great joy and anticipation, it is actually a time of complex interrelated changes in physiologic equilibrium and interpersonal associations. Contrary to popular folklore, even when pregnancies are planned, only slightly over one half of primagravidas feel positive about being pregnant and taking on the role of motherhood; many are told primarily negative anecdotes about labor and delivery; over half report decreases in social contacts, and all report negative feelings about body image brought about by physical changes. Clearly, pregnancy is a time of marked emotional upheaval (Deutsch, 1945; Bibring, 1959; Caplan, 1960; Merkatz et al., 1978). Pregnancy demands that a woman redefine herself in terms of her social roles, that she accept the pregnancy and the psychological stresses attendant to it, that she develop an attachment to the fetus, and that she develop and adapt to a relationship with the neonate after parturition.

The decision to become pregnant or the actual fact of pregnancy marks the beginning of an elaborate transition. Adaptations to pregnancy extend far beyond the acceptance of altered energy levels, the tendency toward decrements in social interaction, and in many cases the adjustment to the expectation of future financial difficulties. For the first time, in some cases, a pregnant person must define herself as a "woman" rather than as a "girl." Relationships with parents, spouse, and friends, which have evolved slowly over time and which provide both social support and psychologic equilibrium, are suddenly altered. Changes in sexuality and sexual activity and increased introversion and passivity characteristically occur

from the middle of the second trimester onward, reaching a peak between the 30th and 35th weeks. These factors, coupled with physiologic/hormonal changes that may cause alterations in energy level and mood, may significantly disrupt the family unit and its traditional patterns of activity. Such disruptions cause anxiety, not only for the pregnant woman but also for those with whom she interacts.

Pregnancy has been termed a "life crisis," which implies that the changes that occur pervade all facets of a woman's life, including the somatic, psychological, and social. The importance of psychological variables in life crises is that changes are of such magnitude that an individual's coping style or basic personality may no longer be adaptive. The multilevel disequilibrium of a first pregnancy is a stress for which most women have no personal precedent and which results in anxiety. Despite outward appearances of adaptation, anxiety occurs with all expectant mothers regardless of other aspects of physical or emotional health. Patients, particularly those pregnant for the first time, often present to the physician or nurse with symptoms of overt, repressed, or displaced emotional conflicts.

Pregnant women experience a myriad of psychological symptoms, including introversion, passivity, mood swings, mixed feelings, restlessness, nervousness, irritability, preoccupations, and depression. These appear with such frequency and intensity that there is a statistically higher-than-normal incidence of psychiatric problems diagnosed in pregnant women (Bibring, 1959). Paradoxically, as the pregnant woman strives to develop a degree of comfort with the many changes in social context and psychologic equilibrium, there often occurs a surfacing of old conflicts that were never adequately resolved in earlier developmental periods. For example, pregnant patients may experience conflicts of autonomy with their mothers, renewed rivalry with siblings, or active uncertainty about sexuality, and disturbing fantasies about past relationships, each of which had been adequately dealt with prior to pregnancy but which now result in troubling family interactions or marital discord. Manifest problems in adjustment prior to pregnancy, such as marital discord, economic difficulties, poor self-concept, and neuroticism may be exacerbated by pregnancy.

In short, even in the most well-adjusted patients, life-crisis disturbances can create the clinical impression of more severe decompensation. In general, such disturbances prove to be transient, situational conflicts rather than serious long-term psychiatric problems, but anxiety allowed to go unallayed may lead to maladaptive mother-child interaction, which is of increasing concern because of the deleterious effects maladaptations are purported to have on the child's emotional and cognitive development (Klaus and Kennell, 1976).

To summarize, the pregnant woman must adapt to:
• Altered physiology with associated changes in energy level and mood
• Changes in somatic configuration and body image
• Changing expectations and interactions with parents, spouse, and other significant individuals
• Conflicting overt and covert messages about motherhood, the mechanics of labor and delivery, etc.
• Personal fears, uncertainties, ambivalent feelings, preoccupations
• Feelings of vulnerability, loss of autonomy, lack of precedents, dependency

Maladaptations In Pregnancy

Although most psychosocial adaptation to pregnancy is characterized by some degree of stress, severe psychopathology is seldom seen. Although behaviors and thoughts of maladaptation may occur, they are usually transient in nature. It is important, nonetheless, that health practitioners be able to distinguish those psychosocial features of pregnancy that may be troublesome but occur with great frequency and those that are indicative of more severe pathology. In one sense, pregnancy can be viewed as a testing ground for mental health. Because of the great reorientation demanded by pregnancy, women with preexisting psychiatric problems may well show evidence of acute decompensation for which psychiatric collaboration is essential.

Many women, however, simply have difficulty achieving the "developmental milestones" of adaptation to pregnancy and the neonatal period. There are many signs and symptoms of psychosocial maladaptation to pregnancy. Many women express early ambivalence about being pregnant, but in some cases denial of pregnancy persists well into the second trimester. Such problems with acceptance of pregnancy may be manifested by a denial of body or appearance changes or, conversely, overreaction to such changes. Clinically, the woman who persists in wearing regular fashions that hide pregnancy changes or who wears maternity clothes prior to physical need may be having some difficulty accepting the fact of pregnancy. Other signs of early ambivalence about pregnancy are frequent complaints about or preoccupations with vague personal, physical, or emotional problems during prenatal visits, often to the exclusion of normal concerns about the developing fetus.

Failure to develop a meaningful emotional affiliation with the growing fetus is a psychosocial maladaptation that is occasionally seen in obstetric practice. In this situation, mothers present with either a subnormal or a supernormal response to the first fetal movements and later may express no interest in fetal heart tones, position of the fetus in utero, etc. These women may also show symptoms of regressive behavior, such as being demanding, uncooperative, provocative, hostile, passive, controlling, or disinterested in care. The clinician may get the impression that the mother is in competition with the fetus for attention and that she has strong needs to be "cared for" or "treated" because of multiple problems unrelated to the baby. Paradoxically, women who are having difficulty accepting pregnancy and developing a relationship with the growing fetus may present with extreme anxiety about the condition of the baby and will be hypervigilant in looking for signs that "something is wrong" with the pregnancy. Ambivalence about names for the baby or the baby's sex, or absence of speculation or fantasies about the baby's physical characteristics, when persisting well into pregnancy, may be similarly indicative of problems in adaptation.

An additional psychosocial maladaptation of pregnancy is failure to make adequate, concrete plans for postnatal care of the baby. The absence of family members or friends to help care for the baby or, at the other extreme, passivity and overreliance on family members are signs of difficulty in adapting to pregnancy, as is unrealistic planning or inadequate preparation for managing the baby at home.

To summarize, obstetric practitioners are cautioned to be alert to the following conditions in their patients, and should screen for them during office visits (Cohen, 1979):

- Deficiency or lack of maternal figure in the patient's life
- Chronic conflict with mother or other female relatives
- Previous birth of a damaged child or the presence of another child with emotional disturbances or behavioral disorders
- Chronic marital discord or acute discord if the conflict is in the area of childbearing or childrearing
- Little or no preparation for sexual experience, childrearing, or childbearing
- Reports of experiences that it is feared will have damaged the baby
- Third-trimester behavior indicative of overt or disguised rejection of the pregnant state
- Absence of plans for care of the baby after birth

Psychosocial Problems in High-Risk Pregnancy

In general, there are two major types of high-risk patients: those who have chronic conditions that predispose them to problems in pregnancy, and those who become pregnant and only subsequently develop conditions that demand special care or hospitalization. In either case, however, consideration must be given to important psychological factors that affect total obstetric care. In the former case, when the pregnant patient has a preexisting condition such as diabetes or past obstetric complications, there will be a history of adaptation to chronic disease that is of utmost importance. In the latter case, in which a woman becomes pregnant and only later develops complications, the unexpected superimposition of problems on pregnancy can be especially stressful.

HIGH-RISK PATIENTS WITH PREEXISTING MEDICAL CONDITIONS

Patients with longstanding medical complications that place them at risk during pregnancy (such as diabetes mellitus, chronic hypertension, sickle cell disease, or systemic lupus erythematosus) deserve special attention from the psychosocial perspective. For women with preexisting problems, the best predictor of adaptation to high-risk pregnancy is their adaptation to the previous health problems. In patients whose chronic conditions result in a persistent negative self-image, there can be an exaggeration of the expected body image disturbances or a persistence of negative fantasies and fears about the unborn baby.

Some women who have preexisting conditions to which they have not adapted psychologically (for example, an adolescent with juvenile-onset diabetes who denies or minimizes the significance of her illness) may view pregnancy and having a baby as evidence of their "normalcy" (Merkatz et al., 1978). High-risk obstetric care for such a patient reinforces feelings of abnormality, but now for reasons of both diabetes *and* pregnancy. In younger patients who are grappling with issues of self-image, the pregnancy that they thought would be liberating in terms of the ambiguity of adolescence becomes instead an albatross that perpetuates normal feelings of inadequacy and typically leads either to dangerous denial of medical problems or to a regression to even greater dependency.

Such patients deserve the opportunity for counseling, not only to help them deal with their high-risk pregnancy but also to enable them to come to terms with their preexisting medical conditions. Practitioners must strive to help these patients overcome their denial of their medical problems, so that they will be more likely to endorse medical measures necessary to ensure both their health and the health of the fetus. In doing so, however, the physician must be careful not to impose an overprotectiveness that will result in total rejection of physician recommendations or, at the other extreme, in dependency difficulties during hospitalization.

PATIENTS WITH PREGNANCY-INDUCED COMPLICATIONS

Unlike women with prediagnosed conditions who tend to have psychological adaptations to high-risk pregnancy that mirror their adaptations to their chronic conditions, women with high-risk conditions discovered as a result of pregnancy characteristically exhibit signs of a classic grief reaction (Lindemann, 1944). Women in this situation must adapt to two stresses, the pregnancy *and* the newly diagnosed complication. Women who are unexpectedly confronted with the possibility of hospitalization for complications during a pregnancy that was previously "normal" may react with symptoms of anger, disbelief, anxiety, fear, and depression, all of which may be misinterpreted by health care professionals. A period of time in which the patient tries to come to terms with an additional health problem is essentially a time of grieving for the loss of a formerly healthy self and for hopes of a "normal" pregnancy. There may be anger, particularly if the physiologic changes of pregnancy precipitated the emergent problem, coupled with guilt for having feelings of regret about having become pregnant or for wishing that pregnancy had not occurred.

Many women whose pregnancies precipitate medical problems go through phases similar to the grieving process associated with the death of a child. Davidson (1979) describes four stages of grief: (1) shock and disbelief, (2) searching and yearning, (3) disorganization and despair, (4) resolution and reorganization. In the case of the high-risk patient, the grief reaction results from the "death" of the idealized, trouble-free pregnancy that the patient had expected to have. Although classified into "stages," the psychological reactions of these patients are seldom so mechanistic: stages may be skipped entirely, superimposed on one another, or experienced with varying intensity.

When a woman finds that she is at risk, she may feel stunned and in a state similar to shock. The high-risk patient may actually be unaware of or unable to remember what she is told during this phase. Often, the shock phase is the patient's way of protecting herself against the news she has heard. In providing patient education, practitioners should be alert to this problem and be prepared to give explanations more than once without becoming frustrated. Rather than providing unsolicited information, it is more appropriate for practitioners to answer the patient's questions, thereby proceeding at the patient's own pace.

Expectant parents often feel helpless and may not want to believe what they are told in regard to medical problems. Women have reported feeling nothing, being overwhelmed by a feeling of numbness. As a symptom of the need for denying the existence of complications, patients may fail to keep medical appointments, may leave the hospital against medical advice, or may avoid discussion of their medical complication.

During the searching and yearning phase, the patient may ask, "Why me?" She may feel she has "failed" in her role as a mother because she has developed a complication. Many women feel guilty, believing that something they did early in pregnancy caused their problems; they will search through their entire pregnancy and their past personal and family medical history trying to establish causal explanations. Usually their complications are unrelated to the variables they feel are the cause. Women sometimes feel that they are being punished for some act they may have committed years ago, or they may blame their problems on dietary indiscretions, arguments with their spouse, etc. Patients need to find reasons and need something or someone to blame for their predicaments. Most often a patient blames herself, feeling guilty about normal ambivalent feelings she might have had early in pregnancy.

During the disorganization and despair stage, women are characteristically insecure about decisions that have to be made. Patients become confused and disorganized at a time when much medical information regarding treatment decisions must be comprehended. Patients often feel isolated from friends and family who do not understand what they are going through. Helplessness and isolation breed feelings of anger, which are often directed toward health care professionals. Ultimately, most patients achieve some level of resolution as they begin to come to terms with the problems and to reorganize their plans for the pregnancy. The intense emotions experienced at first will begin to lessen, and patients will be better able to make informed decisions, but only if practitioners are able to understand the dynamics of grief reactions and can help the patient avoid maladaptive countertransference reactions. The insensitive clinician who reacts to the patient's emotionality as a personal affront rather than as a symptom of adaptation may permanently compromise the therapeutic relationship.

Finally, couples often deal with their feelings independent of one another, which can cause increased emotional stress. Families should be encouraged to communicate their feelings so that they better understand how all members feel. Practitioners must recognize when parents react differently and fail to communicate, and must learn to treat the couple as the "patient."

Medical Care for the High-Risk Pregnant Woman

The nature of the diagnosis and the stage of pregnancy in which it is made will affect the mode of treatment in high-risk obstetrics. Depending on the diagnosis and the time it is made, one of the following may occur: (1) the patient may be referred early in pregnancy to a Regional Perinatal Intensive Care Center (RPICC) for outpatient care by perinatologists who specialize in high-risk obstetrics; (2) the patient may be determined to be at high risk in a hospital that has inadequate facilities to care for a critically ill mother or premature or sick infant and may be transported to an RPICC; or (3) the patient may unexpectedly deliver a sick or premature infant, with the baby then transported to a regional center.

This chapter is primarily concerned with the woman who has been transferred to a regional center for high-risk obstetric care. Patients may be transported in critical condition with an imminent delivery of a premature infant, or they may be referred to face an extended hospital stay and/or extensive outpatient care. In either situation, the expectant parents face a time of emotional turmoil and confusion.

PATIENT-PRACTITIONER RELATIONSHIPS

Because the patient-physician relationship is very special in obstetrics, it is common for a patient to have invested a great deal of time and emotion in choosing her personal obstetrician. When a pregnant woman has been referred to a regional center and to a set of new, specialized practitioners, a mutually satisfying relationship with her former physician may be seen as being lost, and she may even feel abandoned by her original obstetrician (Souma, 1979). Practitioners specializing in high-risk pregnancies and the relative inflexibility of high-risk care

will often be compared unfavorably by patients with original and more familiar nurses and physicians.

If referred to a regional center, the patient will likely be cared for by several physicians and other health care professionals working as a team (Freeman, 1982). Teams typically include several physicians, nurses, social workers, dietitians, and other health care professionals. Team members have specialized areas of expertise and responsibility relating to the patient, and although the team concept is crucial to high-risk care, it can confuse the patient. It is important that each team member be introduced to the patient and that different responsibilities are clarified so that the patient understands each team member's role. Once the patient feels comfortable with the team concept, she can utilize the diversity of its members to her best advantage. Often patients develop a special relationship with one team member and may feel more comfortable dealing with this person on a one-to-one basis. The team member closest to the patient may be better able to communicate her needs by acting as her advocate or "case manager" in the team setting.

DIAGNOSTIC TESTS AND PROCEDURES

High-risk care usually involves many diagnostic procedures with which patients may have little familiarity. Tests such as amniocentesis, ultrasonography, the nonstress test, or the GTT (glucose tolerance test) can confuse and frighten a patient who does not understand their purposes. It is essential that patients be made familiar with the procedures so that they will feel more comfortable. A particular problem occurs when symptoms are ominous to the obstetrician and demand special testing (such as elevated blood sugar, elevated blood pressure, or intrauterine growth retardation) but are unrecognized or are not considered significant by the patient. In such cases patients do not feel ill, and it is quite common for friends and family members to minimize signs such as edema or high blood pressure by telling patients, "That's exactly what happened to me during my pregnancy and everything was fine!" Such patients, particularly if confronted with the additional burden of young children at home or the need to continue to work to support the family, may be reluctant to undergo diagnostic procedures or to enter the hospital for a long period of antenatal care, and may even be resistant to the prescription of a special diet or medication.

High-risk obstetric care also runs counter to current cultural trends that increasingly promote pregnancy and childbirth as "natural" and condemn the "technologization" of the birth process. For this reason, as well, there is resistance to high-risk care on the part of some women, and care should be taken to negotiate mutual understandings and expectations between patient and practitioner (Johnson, 1981). This involves careful elicitation by the clinician of the patient's "explanatory model" of her special condition and of her pregnancy in general, including possible cause of the problem, onset of symptoms, pathophysiology, likely course of illness (chronicity, severity, outcome), and treatment. Although it is possible to alter the wording, the following are examples of questions designed to elicit patient explanatory models (Kleinman et al., 1978):

1. What do you think has caused your problem?
2. Why do you think it started when it did?
3. What do you think your sickness does to you and your baby?
4. How does it work?
5. What kind of treatment do you think you should receive?
6. What are the most important results you have to receive from this treatment?
7. What problems have been (or will be) caused by your condition?
8. What do you fear most about your sickness?

Persistence and patience in such questioning, even in the face of patient hesitancy, will provide bases for comparing physician and patient expectations, identifying discrepancies that may cause clinical management problems, and planning patient education activities.

ADAPTATIONS TO HOSPITALIZATION

Hospitalization, a major feature of high-risk obstetric care, is inherently stressful and represents an adaptive challenge to both the pregnant woman and her family (Wu, 1973; Volicer, 1974; Williams, 1974). Women who are at special risk during pregnancy may be hospitalized for extended periods to allow close medical supervision. Such antepartum patients face the difficult situation of being placed in the hospital when they are actually feeling well. For example, a diabetic patient who is pregnant may have to be hospitalized for monitoring and control of blood sugar, even though she is feeling normal. Similarly, a woman who has been confined to bed owing to premature labor may not feel ill. Under such circumstances, both the patient and the medical staff face unusual circumstances in that the medical staff may not be accustomed to caring for someone who feels so well, and the patient may not understand why she must stay in the hospital. "Hospitals are for sick people, and I'm not sick," is often heard on the antepartum floor.

Patients who see themselves as being healthy usually have problems adapting to hospitalization (Rosen, 1975), particularly because of boredom, restlessness, and irritation caused by having to adhere to the rules and regulations of the hospital. Again, extensive negotiation and explanation is needed to educate the patient and her family so that they will better understand the reasons for hospitalization and will be able to make a better informed and more willing decision. From their end, practitioners must make an effort to make the patient's hospital stay more bearable by modifying traditional hospital procedures—e.g., by discontinuing the taking of vital signs in the middle of the night, relaxing strict visiting hours, and allowing for "passes" out of the hospital.

Hospitalization results in a loss of autonomy and of decision-making responsibility in pregnant patients. Moreover, it has been demonstrated that hospitalization does not become easier with the passage of time but that patients who are hospitalized for periods greater than 2 weeks show increased distress as the hospital stay becomes extended (Merkatz, 1976). Indeed, hospitalization may heighten a sense of dependency, and regressive adaptations in pregnancy may become even more profound as a result of prolonged periods in the hospital setting.

Hospitalization also involves a loss of familiar territory, personal identity, privacy, and control, which can result in patients responding with overassertiveness or anger displaced toward hospital personnel, hospital routine, family members, etc. At any time, physicians, nurses, medical technicians, social workers, dietitians, food service personnel, and housekeepers may revolve through the patient's room without warning or explanation. When patients are in semi-private rooms, twice the usual number of interruptions occur.

Many patients may be afraid of being in a hospital. Even today, hospitals are often viewed as places to die. Such fears may be especially acute for the patient who is referred from another hospital or community. Tertiary centers frequently have reputations for being depersonalizing (Boehm et al., 1979), a factor that may increase the patient's anxiety and influence her relationship with the health care team. Community education and close coordination with the referral source may help to alleviate some of these fears (Boehm et al., 1979; Oh et al., 1977; and Souma, 1979). Many patients feel reassured if RPICC staff maintain contact with their own physician during the course of their hospitalizations.

Perhaps because of lengthy hospitalization, with its inherent isolation from family and friends, but also as a result of proximity and shared perspectives, a powerful patient "subculture" exists on many high-risk wards that influences patient adaptation to hospitalization. Patients commonly compare treatment recommendations, special orders, and other features of care, so that exceptions to rules or general routine for one patient will quickly lead to similar requests from others. Poor outcome of delivery or diagnostic tests for one patient will also be known to all patients fairly quickly, as will other administrative problems on the ward. Both may lower satisfaction with care or raise new fears about being pregnant. Some accounts of adverse effects of hospitalization or diagnostic tests on patients may reach mythologic proportions and be passed along from patient to patient until long after the woman who originally encountered the difficulties has been discharged from the hospital. It is not uncommon for patients to threaten to leave the hospital against medical advice on the basis of unrealistic fears generated by other patients. On the other hand, patients often are tremendously insightful about the concerns of other patients and can be valuable therapeutic allies. Practitioners should listen to patients, not just for what they are saying about themselves, but for what they reveal about the social milieu of the hospital unit.

The responses of patients and family members to long-term hospitalization are highly variable. Many patients become active participants in their own care, becoming quite self-reliant in the hospital, whereas others become extremely dependent and/or rebellious. Difficulties can arise between the patient and the father if the latter resents the coming baby, whether on a conscious or subconscious level. In such cases, the resentment may be made worse by the woman's hospitalization, since the father blames the pregnancy for causing their separation. In other instances, the father may not resent the situation at all, but the patient nevertheless fears that such resentment exists. It is not uncommon for patients to become acutely agitated, demanding to be discharged immediately, because of fears that their partners are becoming permanently alienated by their absence. In any case, wide fluctuations in affect can be expected to occur in patients during hospitalization, but the absence of lability of affect, including depression, should be more alarming than its presence.

High-risk patients have been shown to express characteristic areas of distress during antenatal hospitalizations (Merkatz et al., 1978). The most frequently mentioned concerns are about the baby, personal health, children at home, outcome of pregnancy for the baby, and concern about spouse or mate. Less frequently verbalized areas of distress include being bothered by hospital regulations or routine, depression, concern about receiving inadequate information about plans for care, loneliness, unhappiness with the performance of health personnel, and dissatisfaction with food. Events usually thought of by health professionals as stressful during hospitalization, such as sleeping in a strange bed, disruption of eating habits, wearing hospital gowns, having to stay in bed all day, or using bedpans are actually considered least stressful by patients. On the other hand, patients are most frequently and severely stressed by such unfortunately common problems in hospitals as not being told their diagnosis, not knowing what illness they have, not getting pain medications when needed, and not knowing the reasons for or the results of diagnostic procedures.

Patients frequently complain about those things that are not actually very stressful, such as quality of food or the hospital routine, when they are actually concerned about the more stressful aspects of high-risk care. The astute clinician will be alert for these displaced expressions of anxiety, which are much more likely to be reflections of uncertainty about diagnosis, treatment, personal health, family functioning, and so on. On the other hand, it is not uncommon for patients to have so many personal problems that the hospital represents a refuge to which they cling. One should interpret a certain level of patient complaining as a healthy symptom of adaptation.

EFFECTS ON FAMILY LIFE

One of the most difficult aspects of hospitalization is the separation of the patient from her family. She may be forced to leave her partner and children and be unexpectedly admitted to the hospital for an indeterminate period of time. The patient who has children at home often feels guilty because she is no longer able to fulfill her maternal responsibilities. Finding alternative caretakers for children may be difficult, and other adult family members may be forced to alter their daily routines to stay home and take care of children. Hospitalization of young primagravidas who have been living at home with their parents will also be a source of worry and disruption. Hospitalization may be inherently stressful for young patients because it is their first time away from home and family.

Family members often feel "left out" in the medical setting. Bedside rounds are typically made when relatives are not in the hospital, and physicians and nurses who have primary responsibility for patients may not be available during visiting hours. Thus, family members who are concerned about the decisions that are being made are not always given needed information or included in the decision-making process and may have difficulty relating to the health care team. Their sense of isolation is often expressed in terms of resentment of the medical system and hostility toward high-risk practitioners. It is also not uncommon in such situations for family members to exert emotional pressure on patients to resist treatment. Working at cross-purposes with family members is best avoided by keeping them apprised of the issues and of progress in treatment.

FINANCIAL CONSIDERATIONS

Finances are a common but often overlooked concern for most high-risk patients and their families. Practitioners are often naive about the subtleties of health care financing and may not realize that increased visits to the physician, numerous diagnostic procedures, and potentially lengthy hospitalizations for mother and baby often force patients and family members to quit jobs or seek additional employment. Financial burden and economic uncertainty increase anxiety about pregnancy and high-risk care. Although many regional perinatal centers have special funding that may assist the patient in paying her bills, in any case the family should be advised to consult hospital social workers or financial counselors to ensure that every possibility for assistance is explored. All members of the health care team should be aware of what financial assistance is available, so that the social worker, physician, and financial counselors are not giving the patient mixed messages about available assistance. Also, the patient can make more rational decisions about health care options based on the real need to consider finances. Such consultation has the secondary function of helping family members feel useful and needed, which reduces their frustration with hospitalization.

PATIENT EDUCATION

Childbirth education classes have become an accepted practice in modern obstetric care, and have been demonstrated to reduce anxiety in patients (Browne and Dixon, 1978). Unfortunately, many women are hospitalized in specialized high-risk programs precisely at the time when they would ordinarily be starting such classes. Because of the association between high-risk hospitalization and increased chance of prematurity, need for care of newborns in a specialized neonatal intensive care unit, and increased incidence of neonatal abnormalities, educational programs should be an integral part of comprehensive high-risk care.

Routine tours of the neonatal intensive care unit (NICU), during which parents can receive detailed explanations in response to questions they may have, as well as an opportunity to become familiar with the staff, are recommended. Indeed, many parents have fears about giving birth to a deformed or partially formed fetus and, although visiting the NICU can be a frightening experience, reality is seldom as frightening as patient fantasy. A formalized NICU visitation program will help allay anxiety prior to the birth, will make postnatal visitation by parents less traumatic, and may improve the collaboration of patients and staff in the care of babies in the NICU.

High-risk patients are also at increased risk for cesarean delivery, and they and their partners deserve specialized counseling and patient education to prepare them for this possibility. Although this is not always possible (as in cases of unforeseen emergency cesarean deliveries), it is known that patients who have received special counseling are better able to feel a part of the decision-making process. Some hospitals also allow fathers who have undergone prenatal classes to be in the delivery room during cesarean sections, an arrangement that can be of real benefit to both the patient and her partner.

MATERNAL-INFANT INTERACTION

A most important problem is that high-risk mothers are at a greater risk of being separated from their newborn children. It is crucial that some way to compensate for this be found, given evidence that the amount of contact between mother and infant following birth and the first days of life will influence her attachment to and relationship with the baby (Brown, 1979; Klaus and Kennell, 1970, 1976; Seashore et al., 1973).

Lynch (1975) suggests that failure for the mother and infant to bond relates to the pregnancy perinatal experience and early ill-health of the infant, and he identifies the following six factors that were over-represented in the history of abused children when compared with their nonabused siblings: (1) abnormal pregnancy, (2) abnormal labor or delivery, (3) other separations, (4) illness in the mother in the first year of life, (5) illness in the first year of life in the infant. Lynch concludes that "episodes of ill-health in vulnerable families during pregnancy, delivery, and early childhood put the parent/child bond at risk."

Barnet and co-workers (1969) suggest that mothers who have a longer period of interactional deprivation experience differences in commitment to their infants, have less self-confidence in their ability to mother appropriately, and behave differently toward their infants than do mothers who have not been separated from their babies. They question whether separation might also produce effects upon the infant to the extent that stimulation of the infant at home may be affected by the prior separation experience in the hospital.

Stern (1973) suggests that in trying to understand how parents can develop negative feelings resulting in child abuse or neglect, one must include the possibility that anticipatory grief, guilt over a child's condition at birth, or prolonged separation for intensive medical care may prevent positive emotions from developing and growing. When mothers have to be hospitalized for long periods of time, the mothers and their families may have negative feelings toward the baby for "keeping her in the hospital." Sometimes mothers will say that it is more important to be at home with their children than to stay in the hospital for the child that is not yet born. These feelings certainly can interfere with bonding.

In short, the responsibility not only for the health of women but also of future families lies with the obstetric staff in collaboration with those in pediatrics to develop and change hospital policies regarding childbirth and early separation of mother and infant. Klaus and Kennell (1976) found that visitation in the nursery posed no increased medical hazard. Weekly bacteriologic infectious disease surveillance showed that when more lenient visitation was allowed, there was no increase in the occurrence of infection; in fact, the number of cultures with potentially pathogenic organisms declined.

Mothers should be encouraged to see and touch their infants as much as possible after birth. It has been shown that mothers have difficulty forming an attachment when they are separated from their babies during the first hours of delivery. Kennell suggests that many factors influence the behavior of the mother (Klaus and Kennell, 1976). It is important that the influence of hospital practices and the behavior of the health care team be a positive one in terms of providing as much interaction as possible between mothers and their infants and between them and the rest of the family members.

Summary and Recommendations

From the preceding discussion of psychosocial adaptations in high-risk pregnancy, a series of recommendations can be derived. If these are followed, care of high-risk pregnant women should be more effective and mutually satisfying.

1. Conduct early psychosocial screening for factors such as conflict with maternal figures, poor outcome in previous pregnancies, marital discord, inadequate sexual or childbearing experience, persistent ambivalence or fears about pregnancy, or absence of realistic plans for the baby.

2. Because patients who are at risk are stressed more by uncertainty than by almost any other factor, elicit patient perceptions of their problem and share with patients the rationale for therapy, what she can expect regarding hospitalization, the nature and results of diagnostic procedures, and the probabilities for a successful outcome to the pregnancy.

3. Because pregnancy is something that happens to the family, not just to the patient, focus intervention strategies on all members of the family. Assess family functioning and include family members in the decision-making process and in activities such as financial planning. Anticipate potential problems and assist family members in dealing with patient frustration, depression, and displaced anger. Be alert to the problem of family members' exerting pressure on patients to resist treatment.

4. Recognize that pregnancy in general, and high-risk pregnancy in particular, may be associated with psychological disequilibrium. Differentiate those psychological problems that are situational reactions (such as a grief reaction) from those that are manifestations of a chronic personality style. Request early mental health consultation in either case.

5. Modify hospital routines that are designed for acutely ill patients to better suit women who are basically feeling well but must be hospitalized for problems related to their pregnancy. For example, patients may be more comfortable wearing their own clothes, visiting privileges can be modified, passes out of the hospital can be arranged, and so forth. It is also advisable to encourage patients with extended antepartum hospitalization to decorate their rooms with familiar, personal items. Staff should regard these rooms as "belonging" to the patients and be respectful of this territory.

6. Arrange for early psychosocial assessment and have a member of the care team who listens to patients visit regularly but for brief periods. Such a person (sometimes referred to as a "no needle" person in pediatric settings) should not be directly involved in obstetric care. It is easier for patients to express their full range of feelings about treatment to such a person than to those who are figures of authority and upon whom the patient feels dependent and vulnerable. It is also possible to use hospitalization as a catalyst for long-term psychotherapy, if indicated.

7. If in a tertiary care center, recognize potential negative patient stereotypes about such facilities and possible prior emotional attachment to primary care obstetric practitioners. Consult effectively and regularly with such sources of referral to ensure continuity of nursing and medical care from inpatient-outpatient and from regular high-risk care. Keep patients informed of this consultation and collaboration.

8. Provide childbirth education programs for high-risk patients in the hospital, including tours of neonatal intensive care units and delivery rooms. Encourage participation of family members and include educational preparation about both normal and cesarean deliveries. Also educate patients about the team approach to high-risk care, and arrange for team members with special rapport to advocate for the patient in team meetings.

9. Because high-risk patients are in a compromised psychologic position in the hospital, in that their sense of control and expectations for pregnancy have been changed, afford patients as much control over care as possible. This can involve active decision-making, self-monitoring (such as blood glucose; see Fig. 9–1 for an example), etc.

10. In order to anticipate psychosocial reactions of high-risk patients, differentiate those who have a past medical history of a condition that places them at risk during pregnancy from those who only after conception have developed complications demanding specialized high-risk care. In the former patients, the best predictor of adaptation to high-risk care will be their adaptation to prior conditions; in the latter patients, practitioners should expect the myriad of emotional responses that accompany any grief reaction. Some of these responses may be disconcerting, such as when denial or anger is directed personally toward a member of the hospital staff, but all of them must be dealt with professionally.

HOME BLOOD GLUCOSE MONITORING

WHY: You will learn how to check your blood glucose (sugar) at home in order to determine if it is high or low. The goal is better diabetic control during pregnancy.

WHEN: 1. Do a Chemstrip test when you feel well in order to periodically check glucose levels.
- A. Do this in the morning beore you eat breakfast and before you take your insulin.
- B. Do another test before you eat supper.
2. Do a test when you have symptoms of high or low blood sugar.
3. Do a test if you feel sick (cold, flu).

We want you to keep a record of your blood glucose levels at home during the weeks be-tween each clinic visit. Record them on this graph. BRING A GRAPH OF BLOOD GLUCOSE LEVELS WITH YOU TO EACH CLINIC VISIT. THAT GRAPH SHOULD HAVE THE BLOOD GLUCOSE LEVELS ON IT FROM THE PRECEDING WEEK.

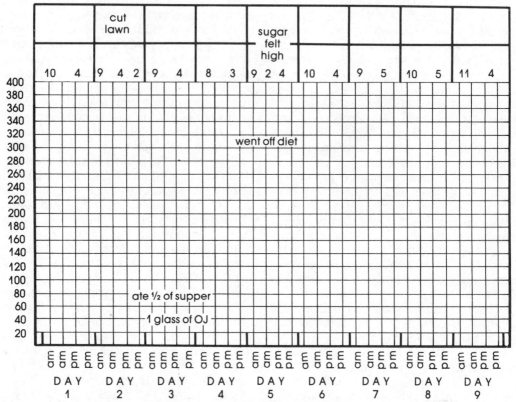

Figure 9–1. Chart and instructions for self-monitoring of blood glucose levels. (Courtesy of Marian Lake and Tom Johnson, University of South Florida, Tampa, FL.)

Illustration continued on opposite page

BLOOD SUGAR LEVEL

Figure 9–1 *Continued.* This portion shows the actual graph for the patient. The gray area indicates where the blood sugars should fall, making it easy for the patient to see if her blood sugars are in control.

11. Establish postnatal practices that maximize maternal-infant interactions. Hospital routines and policies should allow the earliest possible interaction between parents and their infant.

REFERENCES

Barclay, R. L., and Barclay, M. L.: Aspects of the normal psychology of pregnancy: the midtrimester. Am. J. Obstet. Gynecol. 125:207, 1976.

Barnet, C. R., Leiderman, P. H., Grobstein, R., et al.: Neonatal separation, the maternal side of interactional deprivation. Pediatrics 45:197, 1970.

Beckhard, R.: Organizational issues in the team delivery of comprehensive health care. Milbank Memorial Fund Quarterly 50:287, 1972.

Bibring, G.: Some considerations of the psychological processes in pregnancy. Psychoanal. Study Child. 14:113, 1959.

Blum, L.: Psychological Aspects of Pregnancy, Birthing and Bonding. New York, Human Services Press, 1980.

Boehm, F. H., Haire, M. F., Davidson, K., et al.: Maternal-fetal transport: inpatient and outpatient care. J. Tenn. Med. Assoc. November, 1979, pp. 829–833.

Brazelton, T. B.: The early mother-infant adjustment. Pediatrics 32:931, 1963.

Brown, W. A.: Psychological Care During Pregnancy and the Postpartum Period. New York, Raven Press, 1979.

Browne, J. C. M., and Dixon, G.: Browne's Antenatal Care. London, Churchill Livingstone, 1978.

Cagan, J., and Meier, P.: A discharge planning tool for use with families of high risk infants. J.O.G.N. Nurs. 8:146, 1979.

Caplan, G.: Emotional implications of pregnancy and influences on family relationships. In Stuart, H., and Prugh, D. (eds.): The Healthy Child. Cambridge, MA, Harvard University Press, 1960, pp. 72–81.

Chabon, I.: Awake and Aware: Participating in Childbirth Through Psychoprophylaxis. New York, Delacorte Press, 1966.

Cohen, R. L.: Maladaptation to pregnancy. Semin. Perinatol. 3:15, 1979.

Davidson, G. W.: Understanding Death of the Wished-For Child. Springfield, IL, OGR Service Corp., 1979.

Deutsch, H.: The Psychology of Women; Vol. 2: Motherhood. New York, Grune & Stratton, 1945.

Freeman, R. K., and Pescar, S. C.: Safe Delivery: Protecting Your Baby During High Risk Pregnancy. New York, Facts on File, 1982.

Gabbe, S. G., and Quilligan, E. J.: General obstetric management of the diabetic pregnancy. Clin. Obstet. Gynecol. 24:91, 1981.

Gorsuch, R. L., and Key, M. K.: Abnormalities of pregnancy as a function of anxiety and life stress. Psychosom. Med. 36:352, 1974.

Grimm, E. R., and Venet, W. R.: The relationship of emotional adjustment and attitudes to the course and outcome of pregnancy. Psychosom. Med. 28:34, 1966.

Helfer, R. E., and Kempe, C. H.: Child Abuse and Neglect. Cambridge, MA, Ballinger, 1976.

Johnson, T. M.: Interpersonal skill in physical diagnosis. In Burnside, J. (ed.): Physical Diagnosis: An

Introduction to Clinical Medicine. Baltimore, Williams & Wilkins, 1981, pp. 20–21.

Jones, A. C.: Life change and psychological distress as predictors of pregnancy outcome. Psychosom. Med. 40:402, 1978.

Kane, R.: The interprofessional team as a small group. Soc. Work Health Care 1:19, 1975.

Kitzinger, S.: Sex before and after childbirth. Midwife and Health Visitor 8:315, 1972.

Klaus, M. H., and Kennell, J. H.: Mothers separated from their newborn infants. Pediatr. Clin. North Am. 17:1015, 1970.

Klaus, M. H., and Kennell, J. H.: Maternal-Infant Bonding. St. Louis, C. V. Mosby Co., 1976.

Klaus, M. H., and Kennell, J. H.: Parent-Infant Bonding. St. Louis, C. V. Mosby Co., 1982.

Kleinman, A., Eisenberg, L., and Good, B.: Culture, illness, and care: clinical lessons from anthropological and cross-cultural research. Ann. Intern. Med. 88:251, 1978.

Lindemann, E.: Symptomology and management of acute grief. Am. J. Psychiatry 101:141, 1944.

Lynch, M. A.: Ill-health and child abuse. Lancet 2:317, 1975.

McDonald, R. L.: The role of emotional factors in obstetric complications: a review. Psychosom. Med. 30:222, 1968.

Merkatz, R. B.: Behavioral Responses of Hospitalized High Risk Maternity Patients. Unpublished thesis; Case Western Reserve University, Frances Payne Bolton School of Nursing, 1976.

Merkatz, R. B., Budd, K., and Merkatz, I. R.: Psychologic and social implications of scientific care for pregnant diabetic women. Semin. Perinatol. 2:373, 1978.

Oh, W., Cowett, R. M., Clark, S., et al.: Role of an educational program in the regionalization of perinatal health care. Semin. Perinatol. 1:279, 1977.

Parad, H. J.: Crisis Intervention: Selected Readings. New York, Family Service Association of America, 1965.

Plovnik, M., Fry, R., and Rubin, I.: Managing Health Care Delivery: A Training Program for Primary Care Physicians. Cambridge, MA, Ballinger, 1978.

Rosen, E. L.: Concerns of an obstetric patient experiencing long-term hospitalization. J.O.G.N. Nurs. 4:15, 1975.

Rubin, I., Plovinick, M., and Fry, R.: Improving the Coordination of Care: A Program for Health Team Development. Cambridge, MA, Ballinger, 1975.

Schwartz, N. L., and Schwartz, L. H.: Vulnerable Infants. New York, McGraw-Hill, 1977.

Seashore, M. J., Leifer, A. D., Barnett, C. R., et al.: The effects of denial of early mother-infant interaction on maternal self-confidence. J. Pers. Soc. Psychol. 26:367, 1973.

Smith, D. H.: Psychologic aspects of gynecology and obstetrics. Obstet. Gynecol. Ann. 8:457, 1979.

Souma, M. L.: Maternal transport: behind the drama. Am. J. Obstet. Gynecol. 134:1904, 1979.

Stern, D.: The effect of the infant on its care giver. In Lewis, M., and Rosenbloom, L. A.: Origins of Behavior: The Effect of the Infant on Its Care Giver. New York, Wiley, 1974.

Taylor, P. M.: Parent-Infant Relationships. New York, Grune & Stratton, 1980.

Tylden, E.: Psychological problems during pregnancy. Midwife and Health Visitor 8:311, 1972.

Volicer, B. J.: Patients' perception of stressful events associated with hospitalization. Nurs. Res. 23:235, 1974.

Weinberg, J. S.: Body image disturbance as a factor in the crisis situation of pregnancy. J.O.G.N. Nurs. 7:817, 1978.

Williams, F.: The crisis of hospitalization. Nurs. Clin. North Am. 9:37, 1974.

Wolkind, S., and Zajicek, E.: Pregnancy: A Psychological and Social Study. London, Academic Press, 1981.

Wu, R.: Behavior and Illness. Englewood Cliffs, NJ, Prentice-Hall, 1973.

10

SEXUAL INTIMACY IN PREGNANCY

HOWARD J. OSOFSKY
JOAN E. DRUKKER

Pregnancy is a period of time that can be conceptualized as a major developmental phase for the mother and father both as individuals and as a couple. It is an exciting and eagerly anticipated time for most couples, and it commonly results in significant adult growth. Yet, like other important developmental periods in human life, pregnancy involves struggles and upheavals and requires a tremendous amount of adjustment. Adapting to parenthood, especially with a first pregnancy, is a complex task for the individuals and the couple. Considering the stresses and adjustments that the couple must go through, it is not at all surprising that sex during pregnancy can become problematic (Osofsky, 1980; Dameron, 1983; White and Reamy, 1982). In this chapter we will review some of the issues that seem to be of concern for both mothers and fathers, and some of the ways that they may deal with these issues.

The Mother-To-Be

Although there is considerable variability in the reports concerning coital frequency during the first two trimesters of pregnancy, our experience and a number of the reported studies indicate that in general there is some decline in frequency as the pregnancy progresses, with a more apparent decline in the third trimester (Falicov, 1973; Holtzman, 1976; Lumley, 1978; Masters and Johnson, 1966; Solberg, 1973). During the first trimester, the woman may not be aware of her pregnancy and therefore there may be no changes in sexual arousal or activity. Most women experience a considerable decline in interest, frequency of intercourse, and sexual arousal and sexual enjoyment during the last 2 months of pregnancy, and many prefer to forego sex entirely at that point. Some women wish to be held and feel close to their partner although not feeling desirous of intercourse (Hollender, 1974). Varying factors may contribute to these feelings. Suggestions have been made that hormonal fluctuations may influence the reported changes in sexual desire and behavior. However, although Ford and Beach (1951) found that hormonal changes influenced eroticism in animals, they found less of a hormonal influence as one moves up the evolutionary scale to higher mammalian species. Thus, despite hormonal increases during pregnancy, sexual activities seem to decrease, especially in the third trimester. It should be noted that in contrast to these general findings, a fair number of women report an *increased* desire for sex at various times during pregnancy. While these feelings can fluctuate during pregnancy, many women feel increased arousal, especially during the first several months of pregnancy. Several studies have also shown increased arousal in the second trimester (Masters and Johnson, 1966; Falicov, 1973). Ironically, women with increased sexual desires may wonder if they are normal or worry about whether their partner will think they are abnormal. They sometimes feel that pregnant women are not supposed to enjoy sex, that their focus should now be solely on their impending motherhood. On the other hand, many women whose sexual interest increases see pregnancy as a proof of their womanhood and find that in itself to be arousing.

From the degree of variability in the reports that we have heard from many women, it is likely that cultural and psychological factors as well as physical changes determine individual desire and behavior. Many women may decrease their sexual behavior during pregnancy because they see themselves as less attractive, and also because they recognize that they are shifting into the new role of mother as well as wife. The woman who attracted her partner as a young, slender, sexy lover is now uncertain about how he will react to her with the physical and emotional changes that occur during pregnancy. This may cause the woman to feel preoccupied, and her partner may feel isolated and lonely. Both may feel uncertain and insecure, with a pregnancy reawakening old doubts and introducing new pressures. Each may feel cut off from the other. The woman may even become annoyed with her partner if he seems more concerned about himself and his sexual desires and less concerned than she about the baby growing inside her. Sharing feelings and supporting one another can allow for some degree of relief, minimize the difficulties that occur, and improve and strengthen the couple's relationship.

As pregnancy becomes a reality, it may awaken conflicts a woman has about dependency needs, reminding her of rivalries with her mother or siblings, which may influence her relationship with her husband and bring forward her attitudes toward herself as a female. Often women are afraid to have intercourse during pregnancy for fear of hurting the baby. The woman may worry about the infant being traumatized by penile thrusting during intercourse, or she may fear that this will cause premature labor. Although concerns have been raised by some authors (Goodlin et al., 1971; Naeye, 1979), including theories that fetal anoxia during orgasm will result in lower IQs and increased mental retardation in children (Limner, 1969), most reports have not found intercourse or orgasm to be harmful to either the mother or her fetus (Mills, 1981; Perkins, 1979; Wagner, 1976).

In addition, some women may have feelings that a pregnant woman should be a Madonna-like figure for whom sex is dirty and inappropriate. During intercourse, some pregnant women imagine that they are impure and that both they and their partners are doing something that is simply wrong. Psychologically, pregnancy is influenced by how a woman feels about her pregnancy and its representative body changes, how she handles new stress, how she adjusts to changes in her relationship with her partner, and finally, her dependency needs.

Cultural influences also affect the way a woman responds sexually during pregnancy. In the United States, women are frequently advised by friends and medical personnel not to have intercourse in the last 4 to 6 weeks of pregnancy. Ford and Beach (1951) collected sexual data from 60 societies, all of which had an increase of taboos against sex in the last trimester of pregnancy. However, all but two of the societies that prohibit sex during all or most of pregnancy were polygamous, and therefore other sexual outlets were available for the male partner. In contrast to these taboos _against_ sex during pregnancy, in the Liberian culture it is believed that the woman will not have a healthy baby unless sexual activity is continued throughout pregnancy.

Perkins (1979) found that the rate of sexual activity declined at a lesser rate than would be expected by the decline of sexual interest on the woman's part, suggesting her willingness to participate for her partner's sake. This may also be influenced by rumors of infidelity of men during their partners' pregnancy.

Physiologic changes during pregnancy also influence how women feel about sex during pregnancy. Intercourse during pregnancy can feel different for the woman in a number of ways as she undergoes physiologic changes. Her tissues become more swollen and congested, particularly in the breasts and pelvic area. Vasocongestion is increased because of the pregnant woman's increased blood volume, and this may alter her sexual responses. Sometimes women feel vaginal irritation and experience discomfort or even pain during foreplay and the insertion of the penis. During the early part of pregnancy, such normal symptoms as increased breast tenderness due to hormonal and vascular changes and increased fatigue may contribute to a woman's feeling less sexually aroused. The breast tenderness, instead of being erotic, may result in discomfort if the breasts are stimulated during foreplay. The discomfort may decrease the woman's interest in intercourse or may turn her off completely. Furthermore, the tendency to nausea and increased sensitivity to odors may result in decreased sexual interest or pleasure. For example, her partner's normal breath or body odors at the end of the day may turn the woman off or even make her nauseous. With more relaxed communication, care to avoid discomfort, and more attention to hygiene such as showering and brushing the teeth at the end of the day, the couple may enhance their sexual relationship and avoid some of the factors that contribute to less frequent and pleasurable sex during pregnancy.

As the pregnancy progresses, many women become more aware of their uterus and its increasing size; they are distinctly aware of the presence of the baby in the uterus during intercourse. The uterus may contract during coitus, and tonic contractions during orgasm may occur, with a slowing of fetal activity and then a compensatory time of hyperactivity. Transient bradycardia in the fetus has been noted during these episodes with no apparent ill effects (Masters and Johnson, 1966). These changes in fetal activity may make it difficult for the woman to feel sexually relaxed.

The sensation of orgasm sometimes has a painful component during pregnancy that may persist for some time after intercourse, since vasoconstriction is not well relieved, and the residual feeling of fullness may be uncomfortable and persistent (Masters and Johnson, 1966). On the other hand, the pelvic congestion and the intensity of the Braxton-Hicks contractions cause the sexual experience and orgasm to be heightened in some women, and some even find themselves orgasmic for the first time during pregnancy. However, other women may find themselves distracted by the contractions and thus less able to enjoy intercourse. Especially during a first pregnancy, they may worry about whether intercourse and the accompanying contractions will cause them to go into labor prematurely. Sometimes in subsequent pregnancies, when women become more comfortable about the normality of intercourse in pregnancy, they report that the heightened contractions are pleasurable and an enjoyable part of the sexual experience.

During the latter months of pregnancy, other issues may come up. For example, some women feel particularly embarrassed about their appearance. They may feel awkward, obese, bloated, and conscious of additional swelling around the vaginal area. It may be difficult for them to find a position in which intercourse is easy and comfortable. Women who previously felt free in their sexual experiences and in their nudity during intercourse may now feel more inhibited, vulnerable, and exposed. As noted earlier, while many women may not feel much spontaneous enthusiasm for sex, they may still have a need to be held and cuddled.

As pregnancy progresses and the woman's uterus enlarges, some of the sexual techniques that the couple have used and enjoyed in the past may have to be modified to decrease awkwardness and deep penile penetration. For example, most couples usually have intercourse in the so-called "missionary position," i.e., with the man on top of the woman. Late in pregnancy the couple

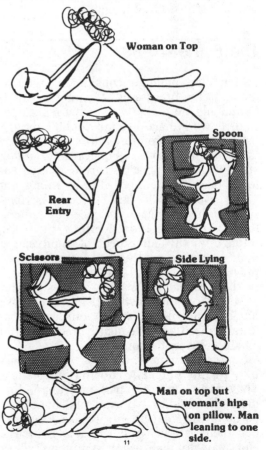

Figure 10–1. Alternative positions for intercourse during pregnancy. (From Hager, Ann: Some things about sex and pregnancy. Publication available through author, 8240 Margaret Lane, Cincinnati, OH 45240, 1981. Illustration by Joel Momberg.)

may find this position awkward. This problem, however, is not universal, and some couples report relatively little difficulty with this position even in late pregnancy. Some couples may find alternative positions helpful (Fig. 10–1). If the couple can be flexible and patient with one another, they can usually find positions that do not seem awkward and that are comfortable for both partners.

In our experience, it is preferable for the pregnant woman to discuss with her partner her feelings concerning her fears and physical changes. The couple should be encouraged to explore and discuss their individual sexual desires and needs during pregnancy and not feel embarrassed to make specific requests of one another or acknowledge temporarily decreased interest in sex. By confiding in each other, they may recognize that they are experiencing similar pressures; they may become more sexually relaxed and/or they may find alternative solutions that are acceptable to both of them.

The Father-To-Be

Men also undergo considerable adjustments in the process of becoming a parent. Commonly the father-to-be experiences periods of worry, anxiety, and doubt, although he may be less comfortable in recognizing them and may have less opportunity to talk about them than does his partner. Stereotypically the man is supposed to be strong and supportive. Duvall (1971) has described some of the feelings experienced by fathers-to-be. These include feelings of being trapped, ambivalence, fear of approaching their partners sexually, guilt for causing the pregnancy, jealousy of the newcomer's place in their partner's life, and depression and anxiety about their own inadequacies. These human concerns and vulnerabilities may go unrecognized and frequently receive little attention by professionals.

Some men treat their pregnant partners like fragile porcelain during pregnancy. They focus on their partners' impending motherhood and have concerns about their partners and their unborn babies. They notice their partners' full and tender breasts and react to their early symptoms. They respond to changes that they perceive, worry about their partners' symptoms and at times discomfort, and fear hurting them. In the area of sexual intimacy, it is important for

professionals to convey to women that having intercourse will not be harmful to either the woman or the baby. It is also helpful for the man to realize that his concerns are shared by many other fathers-to-be. Men may experience greater or lesser sexual arousal during their partners' pregnancies. A study done by Landis and coworkers (1950) showed an increasing decline of sexual interest in both men and women with each successive trimester. This was a retrospective study in which participants were asked to recall data from a period that was sometimes 2½ years previous to the time of the study. It also was carried out 34 years ago, but it is worth mentioning because it included male sexual interest during pregnancy.

Commonly fathers experience more pressures and complex emotions related to the general situation involving the pregnancy and impending fatherhood. They are both aroused by and fearful of the thought of having sex with their pregnant partners, feelings that can be confusing and troubling. As a result of emotional pressures, fathers may experience psychosomatic disorders, mood swings, anxiety, and difficulties in their relationships. Psychosomatic symptoms, such as nausea and abdominal pain, are referred to as the couvade syndrome. The primitive ritual of couvade is when the father goes to bed while his child is being born and submits to fasting and purification (Trethowan, 1972). The couvade ritual can be explained as sympathetic magic practiced by the father to protect his partner and their unborn child as well as to establish his paternity. These symptoms probably are related in varying degrees to ambivalence toward the pregnancy, identification and empathy toward the pregnant partner, and/or "conception envy" and jealousy of the woman's ability to bear a child (Trethowan, 1972).

Many men find the experience of having intercourse with their pregnant partner to be quite different from the way it was when she was in the nonpregnant state. Her body feels different. Her breasts are fuller, and her skin feels tighter. Her vagina is more congested, and the tissues around the vagina sometimes feel swollen. As the pregnancy progresses, her abdomen enlarges. She does not look the same, and the man may feel uncertain about how much foreplay is appropriate and even how to proceed with the sexual act. He is also dealing with feelings about having intercourse not just with his lover but with the woman who is going to be the mother of his child. The feelings may be complex; some men may want to have intercourse but feel that it would be profane to touch a pregnant woman or even think of having sexual relations with her. On the other hand, some men find that they are more sexually aroused when their partners are pregnant.

Obviously, many reasons underlie the increased sexual excitement that men may experience, at least intermittently, during their partners' pregnancies. The man may feel extremely close to the woman who is carrying his child. If the couple had used contraception prior to the conception and found it at all awkward, they no longer have to worry about it. The man may feel a new sense of adulthood and view his partner as more of an adult. He may find it exciting to think of having intercourse with a pregnant woman even with or possibly because of the knowledge of a growing baby in the uterus. He may find the pregnant body to be seductive and attractive. He may enjoy the feel of his partner's larger breasts, find her new fullness appealing, and the vaginal congestion and labial enlargement arousing.

On the other hand, there are also men, and even the same men mentioned above at differing times during the pregnancy, who find the sight of a pregnant woman less sexually appealing, sometimes even unsettling, and they prefer to have intercourse with their partners when they are not pregnant (Osofsky, 1980; Dameron, 1983). Especially later in pregnancy a man may find it awkward to try to maneuver himself into a position in which intercourse is comfortable, so that the enlarged uterus and fetus are not in the way abdominally. Women tend to have more vaginal secretions during pregnancy, which some men find disturbing, especially those for whom oral foreplay is an important part of intercourse. In addition to the awkwardness of position, some men report that the increased size of the labia and the vaginal congestion late in pregnancy are vaguely disturbing.

Feeling afraid is one of the common concerns men have during a pregnancy and is one of the frequent reasons for their diminished sexual advances toward their partners. As the pregnancy progresses and the fetus and uterus enlarge, men become very much aware of the presence of the fetus. They sometimes feel it move or become more active during intercourse. Men frequently report worrying about whether they have hurt the baby during intercourse. They worry about whether they can cause anomalies to the baby as a result of intercourse; some have described specific concerns about injuring the baby's head, especially when they can feel movement of the vertex against the penis late in pregnancy when engagement has occurred. A father obviously has a natural desire to protect his unborn child and to do whatever is necessary to ensure its health. Some of the feelings also appear to stem from his rivalry with the unborn child. When he is having intercourse, he is acutely aware of the presence of this other, growing person. The fetus may seem like a person who is in the way, someone who is competing for his partner's affections.

Because of the Braxton-Hicks contractions that occur during intercourse, men are concerned about causing miscarriage, premature labor, or a stillbirth. The penis, the semen, and the act of intercourse itself can all be felt, on an emotional level, to be harmful. This can be especially true during the first pregnancy. With subsequent pregnancies the couple usually is more relaxed and less concerned about these contractions.

A few men wear condoms during intercourse when their wives are pregnant, because of having heard that prostaglandins in the semen cause uterine contractions that may induce abortions or preterm deliveries. However, the link between prostaglandins in the ejaculate and the initiation of labor appears to be conjecture (White, 1982), and these men are likely to be reacting to their anxieties about being able to set off labor. In any case, it is important to reassure them that intercourse during pregnancy is safe for both women and the babies.

Many men find during the course of their partners' pregnancies that they fantasize about having relationships or affairs with other women. In a study by Masters and Johnson (1966) of 79 men, 12 found sexual release outside of marriage during the pregnancy and 6 during the postpartum period. It would be interesting to see how these statistics might differ in the 1980s as a result of the change in moral climate since 1966.

Often when men have an affair during their partner's pregnancy it is the first affair during their relationship (Osofsky, 1980; Masters and Johnson, 1966). Men have occasionally reported to us that they have had affairs during each of their wives' pregnancies, but not in between. The affairs may begin when their partners start to look pregnant. In some, but not all, cases the extramarital relationship terminates with delivery.

A number of reasons exist for the fantasies, and even for the affairs. As has been noted, some men find their wives physically less appealing during pregnancy and feel a preference for slim, "more attractive" females. The other woman can be exclusively the lover and not the mother. A male does not have to worry about sharing her with a child. He also does not have to deal with his own feelings about having made his partner pregnant and thus having put himself, at times, in the ambivalent position of being both attracted to and repelled by a motherly individual. When a man's partner becomes pregnant and motherly, it may evoke some of his "little boy" feelings about his own mother, feelings that seem foolish and inappropriate to him. These feelings may be repugnant to him, but they do contribute to the fantasies and to the occasional affairs. Although it is hard for the woman and the husband to believe, the husband's fantasies, and even the affairs, may in part be his attempt to protect his partner from his confusing and possibly hurtful feelings. If the man becomes involved in a relationship with another woman he can avoid some of the feelings that he may have and inhibitions that may result from his being involved sexually with his "wife-mother."

Although fantasies about other women are normal, a man's having an affair is often a sign of some significant underlying difficulty. The man and woman are frequently not communicating well, are harassing one another, or are pushing each other away. The stresses of the affair are likely to cause or contribute significantly to marital difficulty. The man may not understand his feelings, and the partner, if she knows about the affair, is likely to feel angry, let down, and rejected, and alternately worthless and the source of the problem. At such times couples may find it helpful to obtain professional counseling, which may help both of them work through the contradictory feelings that pregnancy may exacerbate.

A study in Chicago (Hartman, 1966) showed an increase in deviant sexual behavior in men whose wives were pregnant. These behaviors included exhibitionism, pedophilia, rape, homosexual acts, transvestism, and the making of obscene phone calls (and/or letter writing). When they occur, homosexual attractions and fantasies tend to take place most commonly during the latter part of the pregnancy and may produce some degree of panic in the husbands. They fear that they are becoming homosexual and are afraid to share these feelings with others. The increased attraction toward other males, however, is usually temporary and precipitated by the stresses of pregnancy, especially the changes that are taking place in his partner's body. Unusual stress such as pregnancy at various times in life can arouse temporary homosexual feelings and panic in some men who are usually comfortable in their heterosexual lives. In addition, a man may suffer a negative reaction to the physiologic changes his partner is undergoing. The woman's sexual organs are suddenly becoming much bigger, and as a result, the man's sexual equipment may by comparison seem smaller and less significant. As mentioned, although the feelings can be very frightening to the male and although the panic is very real, the experience is usually temporary and a direct result of the pregnancy-related changes. Following the birth of the baby and the wife's gradual resumption of her prepregnancy figure, the husband usually feels considerably more comfortable, and the disturbing feelings tend to fade with time.

Because of their concerns, a number of men report some degree of sexual difficulty during their partners' pregnancies. A man may lose much or all of his desire for intercourse. He may have difficulty obtaining an erection, lose the erection before achieving orgasm, or become impotent for considerable periods of time. When he is able to achieve orgasm he may be terrified of the results for the baby or the pregnancy. If his partner seems sexually receptive, he may feel angry toward her, afraid that she will encourage him to commit the act that will cause the destruction of the pregnancy. The husband wants to have intercourse and yet he may feel so concerned about hurting the fetus or his partner that he needs to deny those feelings.

It is extremely important for a couple to discuss their sexual inhibitions and pressures during pregnancy, since talking about them can often help relieve tension and allow for more spontaneous sexual activity. If they have medical concerns, it is worthwhile for them to discuss these concerns with their physician. Often their fears can be quickly put to rest. If a physician recommends restrictions to intercourse, the couple, through communication, can decide whether abstinence from all forms of sexual activity makes the most sense for them. Some men may masturbate during their partners' pregnancy, and some couples feel comfortable with the women performing masturbation or fellatio during times when abstinence is recommended medically, having the men achieve orgasm in this manner instead of having no sexual contact. The woman may need cuddling and tenderness during this period of time. However, we have also seen husbands who feel extremely guilty about masturbation and couples who feel that the partners' providing alternate forms of sexual release for their husbands is improper or profane. Some men describe seeing themselves as adults—fathers-to-be— and say that when they engage in masturbation they feel as though they are doing something immature, adolescent, and forbidden. It is important to emphasize that individuals and couples know themselves and their preferences. They should be encouraged to do what they feel comfortable with and not participate in activities in which they do not feel at ease.

How the mother accepts or rejects the father during pregnancy may be a predominant factor in how he accepts or rejects the child. And because the father's actions affect the mother, they also affect the mother's regard for the child. Therefore, providing counseling and education for the parents at the beginning and throughout pregnancy is imperative to prevent miscommunication between the couple during pregnancy.

Complications

Since *Homo sapiens* is the only species known to copulate during pregnancy, some authors have speculated as to the safety of sexual practices during pregnancy. Some have suggested that the decreased interest in coitus during pregnancy is due to a subconscious "holding back" of orgasm to prevent harming the baby. However, most authors are of the opinion that coitus and orgasm are *not* harmful to the normal pregnant woman or her fetus (Falicov, 1973; Bing, 1977; Goodlin, 1969; Mills, 1981; Pugh and Fernandez, 1953; Connell et al., 1981; Perkins, 1979). However, there are some concerns regarding coitus, orgasm, and breast stimulation in cases in which risk situations exist or are likely to develop, for example, bleeding, repeated fetal wastage, premature labor, incompetent cervix, premature rupture of the membranes, infection, and multiple gestation. Traditionally, intercourse is discouraged in cases of threatened abortion, rupture of the membranes, premature labor, and vaginal bleeding, as well as during the last 6 weeks of pregnancy and the first 6 weeks post partum. With these recommendations even normal patients would have to abstain from intercourse for 3 months. These recommendations were based on fears of penile thrusting against the cervix causing labor; contractions of coitus and orgasm inducing labor; intercourse causing rupture of the membranes; and physical discomfort. However, in most pregnancies, sexual activities can be safely maintained throughout pregnancy and resumed about 2 to 4 weeks into the postpartum period. There are cases in which complications may limit sexual behavior, and these are discussed in the remainder of this section.

BLEEDING AND FETAL WASTAGE

In the first trimester, bleeding may occur as a prelude to spontaneous abortion. Couples should refrain from coitus whenever there is active bleeding. If this resolves, the couple can resume their normal sexual activity.

If there have been repeated spontaneous abortions it is imperative that the products of conception be studied for anomalies, genetic abnormalities, infection, or placental defects. If the miscarriages were due to any of the above factors, further gynecologic assessment may be indicated. The conditions that produced the risk may be correctable and/or not likely to cause problems in the current pregnancy. Intercourse will not affect the outcome in most of these situations; the factors should be evaluated and discussed with the patient. A "blighted ovum" miscarriage is a statistical risk in any pregnancy, occurring in 1 out of every 10 pregnancies. Again, coitus and orgasm will not affect this outcome. If, however, factors such as congenital uterine anomalies or fibroid distortions rather than embryonic death are the cause of bleeding and first-trimester abortion, it is best to counsel against intercourse and orgasm (Grover, 1977). Resolution of these problems between pregnancies may be wise.

If couples spontaneously decide not to engage in sexual activities because of previous early losses, they should be supported in their decision. However, as the pregnancy progresses, milestones such as fetal heart tones and fetal movement may encourage the couple to accept the pregnancy and again enjoy sexual activities.

In the second and third trimesters, bleeding can be caused by uterine anomalies, placental abruption, or placenta previa, or it may be of unknown origin. Naeye (1981) studied the association between coitus and antepartum bleeding from placental abruption and antepartum bleeding of unknown origin. He found that there was an association between these two types of bleeding and coitus (orgasm not identified) that was independent of other factors, such as hypertension, smoking, and placental infarcts that cause abruption, although he was unable to show a causal relationship between coitus and antepartum bleeding.

Placenta previa is mentioned in the literature as a reason for avoiding intercourse during pregnancy. It is not clear whether this avoidance is advised only in cases in which there is active bleeding. However, because of the possibility that contact of the penis against the lower uterine segment may cause disruption of the placenta and bleeding, intercourse should probably be avoided by all patients with placenta previa. Contractions during orgasm may also cause bleeding and should be avoided. If the placenta should migrate away from the cervix, intercourse may be resumed; this is dependent on the location of the placenta and the physician's discretion.

PREMATURE LABOR

It has been documented that throughout pregnancy uterine contractions occur with and without orgasm (Perkins, 1979; Goodlin et al., 1972; Fox et al., 1970; Jarvet, 1957; Masters and Johnson, 1966; Goodlin, 1971), especially in the last 2 months of pregnancy, when the uterus is more sensitive to stimuli

of all types. In a study by Goodlin (1969), 55 percent of women who were orgasmic reported painful uterine contractions, pains of the back or pelvis, or pressure or round ligament type of pain after orgasm. Perkins (1979) described varying percentages of women who had contractions during sexual activity. Fox and coworkers (1970) measured uterine contractions during intercourse and orgasm. They found that regular uterine contractions occurred during coitus, irrespective of orgasm, which were interrupted by more irregular, sometimes tonic, contractions during orgasm. The regular contractions returned after orgasm. Perkins (1979) reported that multiparous patients perceived uterine irritability more readily than did nulliparous patients during coitus.

Oxytocin may play a part in initiating these contractions. Fox and coworkers (1970) found that there were small amounts of oxytocin in the peripheral bloodstream within 1 minute after orgasm. A pressure gradient exists between the vagina and uterus after female orgasm, which may also play a part in uterine irritability (Fox et al., 1970). However, most authors agree that these contractions during coitus and orgasm are not strong enough to initiate labor (Rayburn and Wilson, 1980; Perkins, 1979; Masters and Johnson, 1966; Pugh and Fernandez, 1953; Solberg, 1973; Wagner, 1976; Naeye, 1979; Goodlin et al., 1972). Many of these authors recommend that unless intercourse is uncomfortable, it need not be discontinued in the normal pregnancy.

Several studies have been done to try to determine whether there is a relationship between coital or orgasmic contractions and premature labor. Perkins (1979) found no adverse associations between orgasm and onset of labor. As a matter of fact he found that orgasmic patients consistently had a lower percentage of early deliveries. Perkins also reported that the type of stimulation used to achieve orgasm was not important, except that masturbation was consistently associated with a lower risk of prematurity throughout pregnancy. However, Wagner (1976), in a small matched study sample of a larger study group, noted that a higher frequency of mothers of premature infants had, in the first trimester, experienced one or more of the following: (1) a higher frequency of orgasmic coitus; (2) orgasm from noncoital stimulation; (3) multiple orgasm; and (4) a greater frequency of cramps and contractions following coitus than did mothers of nonpremature infants. Wagner questioned whether orgasm in early pregnancy could significantly affect the developing fetus so as to cause preterm birth. It should be noted that when this matched study group of mothers of premature infants was compared with the entire study, there was no statistically significant relationship between orgasm and prematurity.

Rayburn and Wilson (1980) found no relationship of coital activity with orgasm to the delivery of premature infants.

Goodlin (1969) found that there was an increased incidence of orgasm in those women delivering prematurely. However, this group also had a 3-times higher incidence of history of premature labor than did the control group delivering at term. In 1971, Goodlin again found a relationship between increased orgasm and premature delivery. In that study Goodlin asked four women at term to try to initiate labor with orgasm, and three were successful in starting labor shortly after orgasm.

One of the problems with the comparison of frequency of coitus and orgasm in relationship to premature labor is that the frequency of sexual activity is higher in the second than in the third trimester. Thus, although many women have more sexual activity in the second trimester, few go into premature labor at that time. Goodlin (1971) found that many women who abstained from coitus, for fear that penetration would harm the baby, continued to achieve orgasm by other means.

From the information now available, the recommendations of the authors cited in this section seem to be consistent despite differences in outcomes. The recommendations are to advise abstention from coitus and orgasm only in cases of (1) a poor reproductive history; (2) arrested premature labor in the present pregnancy, until the fetus reaches maturity; (3) a prior *unexplained* premature delivery; and (4) incompetent cervix or early ripening of the cervix on vaginal examination (Rayburn and Wilson, 1980; Herbst, 1979; Goodlin, 1971; Perkins, 1979). Grover (1977) agrees with these recommendations, with the exception that he allows his cerclage patients to continue intercourse, although intercourse was occasionally discontinued owing to the discomfort of the band on the penis.

Two other factors—seminal fluid and breast stimulation—should be considered in relation to premature labor. Seminal fluid, rich in prostaglandins and enzymes, has been implicated as a possible initiator of labor. Lavery and Miller (1981) reported that the short-term exposure to the prostaglandins that occurs with ejaculation is not enough to cause premature labor. Breast stimulation has been used to initiate labor at term. At this time no studies have been reported on the possibility that premature labor may be initiated through breast stimulation during sexual activities (Herron et al., 1982; Cheek, 1969).

Creasy describes stress as a component of the initiation of premature labor (Herron et al., 1982). It would seem that sexual proscription would add to the life stress of pregnancy itself and might therefore actually increase the risk of premature labor. Also, many couples who are unable to abstain from their sexual activities become guilty from their lack of abstinence, especially if complications arise, and this creates further stress. Therefore it would behoove practitioners to assess the situation carefully before proscribing sexual activities for the couple. It should be remembered that sexual activities can be resumed when fetal maturity is achieved (as determined by L/S ratio).

As a final note regarding premature labor, it would be interesting to compare cervical changes in those women who have contractions during coitus, those who have contractions during coitus and orgasm, and those who do not have any contractions. This information might be helpful in making recommendations regarding sexual activities.

RUPTURE OF THE MEMBRANES AND INFECTION

There have been several theories on the cause or causes of premature rupture of the membranes (PROM), including poor nutrition, cigarette smoking, coitus, parity, prior surgery to the cervix, and infection (Naeye, 1982). (See also Chapter 16). In regard to coitus, it is believed that the contractions that occur during orgasm are not strong enough to cause PROM. In the laboratory, both normal and prematurely ruptured membranes usually resist pressures generated as high as those of labor (Danforth and Hull, 1958; Embrey, 1954; Al-Zais, 1980; Lavery and Miller, 1979). Most of the strength of the membranes is found in a zone of connective tissue beneath the amnion. No difference has been found between the collagen content of normal membranes and that of membranes ruptured prematurely (Al-Zais, 1980). It has been noted that the membranes may rupture along areas of membrane abnormalities, leaving the normal membrane areas intact. Artal et al. (1979) postulated that damage is caused by enzymatic depolymerization of the collagen fibers. Acute infection releasing proteolytic enzymes or the collagenase-like enzymes in seminal fluid are possible mechanisms for this damage. However, Lavery and Miller (1981) found that seminal fluid acting alone does not appear to weaken the membranes. Naeye (1979) reported finding coitus combined with infection as a mechanism for PROM, although his methods have been criticized because of his definition of infection found in the placenta. Since intercourse is more frequent in the second trimester, this may skew the data toward an association between more frequent coitus and PROM (Herbst, 1979; Perkins, 1983). Mundsley et al. (1966) reported a high incidence of placental inflammation and infection without clinical correlation to PROM. Also, Kappy et al. (1979) found that half of the patients with PROM who were thought to be infected before delivery were found to be free of histologic or bacteriologic evidence of infection; and half of those who were judged prenatally to be without infection had bacterial colonization in the placenta or uterus or had chorioamnionitis. Although many of these patients had prolonged PROM, there is the implication that little is known about this type of bacterial infection.

Naeye's (1982) findings suggested that previous cervical damage may cause harboring of bacteria, which predisposes to PROM; his report included a recommendation for further studies in this area. He also suggested that guidance for sexual activity is not clear, because even though there is an *association* between coitus and PROM, this does not constitute proof of a *causal* relationship. Naeye's recommendations were to counsel patients to abstain only if there is previous cervical damage or cervical change. He suggests fastidious cleaning of the genitalia and the use of condoms to decrease contact with seminal fluid and reduce the risk of infection. However, Herbst (1979) refutes this,

and at present Naeye's suggestions remain unsubstantiated.

OTHER COMPLICATIONS

Some authors have suggested abstinence from sexual activities when *uterine anomalies* (such as fibroids) are present that might cause uterine irritability or decrease uterine capacity (Grover, 1977). If there are recurrent problems, surgery between pregnancies may resolve the situation.

Since *multiple gestation* increases uterine size and may cause uterine irritability, some researchers recommend that coitus and orgasm be avoided (Rayburn and Wilson, 1980; Connell, 1981), although others feel that abstention is necessary only with cervical changes or a poor reproductive history (Perkins, 1979; Herbst, 1979; Goodlin et al., 1971; Grover, 1977).

Another area of concern is whether there is *fetal distress* during orgasm. Grudzinskas (1979) reported that women who were sexually active during the last 4 weeks of pregnancy had an increase of meconium-stained fluid and lower 1-minute Apgar scores. He questions whether there is a temporary compromise in fetal circulation associated with uterine contractions. Limner (1969) in his book *Sex and the Unborn Child* suggests, based upon a review of the literature, that the fetus may become anoxic during orgasmic contractions, and that this may cause mental retardation. And Javerts, cited in Goodlin et al. (1971), reported that couples who refrained from coitus during pregnancy had children with higher IQs. However, to date, most clinical information supports the idea that sexual activity *does not* harm the fetus (Dameron, 1983).

Goodlin and colleagues (1971) measured one patient for uterine pressure and fetal heart tones during female orgasm. They noted decelerations of the fetal heart rate and questioned whether fetal distress was present. (From the tracings in the article, the fetal decelerations appeared to be mild variables). Butler, cited in Connell (1981), stated, "If coitus did play a significant role in fetal loss, the planet would be empty."

There is one notoriously dangerous sexual activity during pregnancy. This is the practice of *insufflating air* into the vagina under pressure during cunnilingus. Sudden maternal deaths have been reported during this activity secondary to air embolism.

Postpartum Sexual Activity

Ford and Beach (1951) found that of the societies they studied, one half had sexual taboos for 2 to 4 months after delivery, while the other half had even longer taboos. Masters and Johnson (1966) found that there was a return to coitus starting at 2 weeks to 3 months in women in the United States. One half of the women studied had resumed sex by the 4th postpartum week; however, only 12 percent of these women felt that it was safe. Masters and Johnson (1966) also found a more prompt return to sexual activity in breast-feeding women. Kenny (1973) reported that desire for coitus returns by about the 4th week post partum. However, this may be influenced by the fact that all but one of the mothers studied were breast-feeding.

Richardson and coworkers (1976) reported that women on the postpartum unit had less pain and resumed sexual activities earlier (2 to 3 weeks post partum) when fine polyglycolic acid suture was used with a fine needle. This finding was also reported by Livingstone et al. (1974), Rogers (1974), and Tompkins (1972).

Kyndely (1978) has suggested that intercourse can be resumed when bleeding has stopped, when there is no perineal discomfort, and when the couple is psychologically ready. Resumption of sexual activity may be hampered by the fatigue and tension caused by the stress of a new baby. Some women still have a decreased sexual interest as late as 7 months post partum. Counseling is important to guide couples through this stressful time, and to help them to feel comfortable in resuming their sexual activities. Couples should be informed that there will be an involuntary leakage of milk with sexual activity and that sexual arousal may occur during breast-feeding, both of which are normal. Teaching and counseling ahead of time can make the transition back to a sexual relationship easier.

Recommendations

Research seems to indicate that sexual activity is normal and safe during pregnancy. However, in the presence of (a) bleeding in general, and specifically with placenta previa, (b) a poor reproductive history secondary to factors that could be influenced by coitus, or (c) cervical changes, discontinuance of coitus, orgasm, and perhaps breast stimulation is recommended. Clinicians should be careful not to interfere with the couple's sexual activities or to give them information that would make them feel guilty or frustrated and angry when this is not necessary. If there have been previous miscarriages or other problems, couples may decide temporarily to discontinue sexual activities. These patients should be supported in their decision. As the pregnancy progresses, they may be encouraged to resume intercourse.

It should also be recommended to counsel patients as to when they can resume intercourse, i.e., when bleeding has stopped or when the fetus reaches maturity (as determined by L/S ratio).

The couple should be counseled together, especially when abstinence is recommended, to avoid conflict and so that appropriate recommendations can be made. Tenderness and cuddling can be advised, and nongenital sexual play and gratification can be discussed. When recommendations are made, they should be very specific: Don't just say, "No sex." The woman may still want to continue pleasuring her partner through oral or manual stimulation when intercourse is proscribed. The couple should be encouraged to explore broader aspects of their physical and emotional relationship during abstinence. Often pamphlets like "Some Things About Sex in Pregnancy," by Ann Hager can help in counseling the couple throughout pregnancy. Taking an initial sexual history can be helpful. This history can be updated as the pregnancy continues, with counseling to the couple on both physical and emotional needs. New parenting is an ideal time for the expression of love. The couple's sexual relationship can help to maintain them as a couple as the new baby, especially in the primipara, changes the family structure.

REFERENCES AND RECOMMENDED READINGS

Al-Zais, N. S., Bov-Resli, M. N., and Goldpink, G.: Bursting pressure and collagen content of fetal membranes and their relation to premature rupture of the membranes. Br. J. Obstet. Gynaecol. 87:227, 1980.

Artal, R., Burgeson, R. E., Hobel, C. J., et al.: An in vitro model for the study of enzymatically mediated biomechanical changes in the chorioamniotic membranes. Am. J. Obstet. Gynecol. 133:656, 1979.

Bing, E., and Colman, L.: Making Love During Pregnancy. New York, Bantam Books, 1977.

Cederqvist, L. L., Francis, L. C., Zervoudakis, I. A., et al: Fetal immune response following prematurely ruptured membranes. Am. J. Obstet. Gynecol. 126: 321, 1972.

Cheek, D. B.: Significance of dreams in initiating premature labor. Am. J. Clin. Hypn. 12:5, 1969.

Connell, E. B., Butler, J., and Goodlin, R.: What do you advise patients concerning the safety of sexual relations during pregnancy? Med. Aspects Human Sex. 15:91, 1981.

Dameron, G.: Helping couples cope with sexual changes pregnancy brings. Contemp. Obstet. Gynecol. 21:23, 1983.

Danforth, D. N., and Hull, R. W.: The microscopic anatomy of the fetal membrane with particular reference to the detailed structure of the amnion. Am. J. Obstet. Gynecol. 75:536, 1958.

Duvall, E. M.: Pregnancy—the premise of parenthood. In Family Development, 4th ed. Philadelphia, J. B. Lippincott Co., 1971.

Ellis, D.: Sexual needs and concerns of expectant parents. JOGN Nurs. 9:306, 1980.

Embrey, M. P.: On the strength of the foetal membranes. Br. J. Obstet. Gynaecol. 61:793, 1954.

Falicov, C. J.: Sexual adjustment during first pregnancy and post partum. Am. J. Obstet. Gynecol. 117:991, 1973.

Ford, C., and Beach, F.: Patterns of Social Behavior. New York, Perennial (div. of Harper & Row), 1951.

Fox, C. A., Wolff, H. S., and Baker, J. A.: Measurement of intra-vaginal and intra-uterine pressures during human coitus by radiotelemetry. J. Reprod. Fertil. 22:243, 1970.

Gnarpe, H., and Friberg, J.: T-microplasmas on spermatozoa and infertility. Nature 245:97, 1973.

Goodlin, R. C.: Orgasm and premature labour. Lancet 2:646, 1969.

Goodlin, R. C., Keller, D., and Raffin, M.: Orgasm during late pregnancy; possible deleterious effects. Obstet. Gynecol. 38:916, 1971.

Goodlin, R. C., Schmidt, W., and Creevy, D. C.: Uterine tension and fetal heart rate during maternal orgasm. Obstet. Gynecol. 39:125, 1972.

Grover, J. W.: Coitus during pregnancy for women with a history of spontaneous abortion. Med Aspects Human Sex. 5:113, 1977.

Grudzinskas, J. G.: Does sexual intercourse cause fetal distress? Lancet 2:692, 1979.

Hager, A.: Some Things About Sex and Pregnancy. Publication available through Ann Hager, 8240 Margaret Lane, Cincinnati, OH 45240, 1981.

Hames, C.: Sexual needs and interests of postpartum couples. JOGN Nurs. 9:313, 1980.

Hartman, A. A., and Nicolay, R. C.: Sexually deviant behavior in expectant fathers. J. Abnormal Psychol. 61:232, 1966.

Herbst, A. L.: Coitus and the fetus. N. Engl. J. Med. 301:1235, 1979.

Herron, M. A., Katz, M., and Creasy, R. K.: Evaluation of a preterm birth prevention program: preliminary report. Obstet. Gynecol. 59:452, 1982.

Hollender, M., and McGehee, A.: The wish to be held during pregnancy. J. Psychosom. Res. 18:193, 1974.

Holtzman, L.: Sexual practices during pregnancy. J. Nurse Midwife 6:21, 1976.

Hott, J. R.: The crisis of expectant fatherhood. Am. J. Nurs. 76:1436, 1976.

Israel, S. L., and Rubin, I.: Sexual Relations During Pregnancy and Post-Delivery Period. New York, Sex Information and Educational Council of the United States, Study Guide Number Six, 1967.

Jarvet, C. T.: Spontaneous and Habitual Abortion. New York, McGraw-Hill, 1957.

Kappy, A., Cetrulo, C. L., Knuppel, R. A., et al.: Premature rupture of the membranes: a conservative approach. Am. J. Obstet. Gynecol. 134:655, 1979.

Karim, S. M., Trussell, R. R., Hillier, K., et al.: Induction of labor with prostaglandin F₂. Obstet. Gynecol. Surv. 25:210, 1970.

Kenny, J. A.: Sexuality of pregnant and breastfeeding women. Arch. Sex. Behav. 2:215, 1973.

Knox, J. C., and Hoerner, J. K.: The role of infection in premature rupture of the membranes. Am. J. Obstet. Gynecol. 59:90, 1950.

Kyndely, K.: The sexuality of women in pregnancy and postpartum: a review. JOGN Nurs. 7:28, 1978.

Landis, J. T., Poffenberger, T., and Poffenberger, S.: Am. Sociol. Rev. 15:766, 1950.

Lavery, J. P., and Miller, C. E.: Deformation and creep in the human chorioamniotic sac. Am. J. Obstet. Gynecol. 134:366, 1979.

Lavery, J. P., and Miller, C. E.: Effect of prostaglandin and seminal fluid on human chorioamniotic membranes. JAMA 245:2425, 1981.

Limner, R. R.: Sex and the Unborn Child. New York, Julian Press, Inc., 1969.

Livingstone, E., Simpson, D., and Naismith, W. C.: A comparison between catgut and polyglycolic acid sutures in episiotomy repair. J. Obstet. Gynaecol. Br. Commonw. 81:245, 1974.

Lumley, J.: Sexual feelings in pregnancy and after childbirth. Aust. New Zeal. J. Obstet. Gynecol. 18:114, 1978.

Lungquist, F., Thorsteinsson, T., and Buus, O.: Purification and properties of some enzymes in human seminal plasma. Biochem. J. 59:69, 1955.

Masters, W. H., and Johnson, V. E.: Human Sexual Response. Boston, Little, Brown & Co., 1966.

Mills, J. L., Harlap, S., and Harley, E. E.: Should coitus late in pregnancy be discouraged? Lancet 2:136, 1981.

Mitchell, M. D.: Plasma concentrations of prostaglandins during late human pregnancy: influence on normal and preterm labor. J. Clin. Endocrinol. Metabol. 46:947, 1978.

Moghissi, K. S.: Sperm migration through cervical mucus. In Sherman, A. I. (ed.): Pathways to Conception: The Role of the Cervix and the Oviduct in Reproduction. Springfield, IL, Charles C. Thomas, 1971, p. 214.

Morris, N. M.: The frequency of sexual intercourse during pregnancy. Arch. Sex. Behav., 4:501, 1975.

Mundsley, R. F., Brix, G. A., Hinton, N. A., et al.: Placental inflammation and infection: a prospective bacteriologic and histologic study. Am. J. Obstet. Gynecol. 95:648, 1966.

Mueller, L. S.: Pregnancy and sexuality. JOGN Nurs. 14:289, 1985.

Naeye, R. L.: Coitus and associated amniotic fluid infection. N. Engl. J. Med. 301:1198, 1979.

Naeye, R. L.: Safety of coitus in pregnancy. Lancet 2:686, 1981.

Naeye, R. L.: Coitus and antepartum haemorrhage. Br. J. Obstet. Gynaecol. 88:765, 1981.

Naeye, R. L.: Factors that predispose to premature rupture of the fetal membranes. Obstet. Gynecol. 60:93, 1982.

Naeye, R. L., and Peters, E. C.: Causes and consequences of premature rupture of fetal membranes. Lancet 1:192, 1980.

Naeye, R. L., and Ross, S.: Coitus and chorioamnionitis: a prospective study. Early Hum. Dev. 6:91, 1982.

Obrzut, L. A.: Expectant fathers' perception of fathering. Am. J. Nurs. 76:1440, 1976.

Osofsky, H. J., and Osofsky, J. O.: Answers for New Parents: Adjusting to Your New Role. New York, Walker Publishers, 1980.

Perkins, R. P.: Sexual behavior and response in relation to complications of pregnancy. Am. J. Obstet. Gynecol. 134:498, 1979.

Perkins, R. P.: Sexuality in pregnancy: What determines behavior? Obstet. Gynecol. 59:189, 1982.

Perkins, R. P.: Adverse pregnancy outcome and coitus. Obstet. Gynecol. 26:399, 1983.

Pugh, W. E.: Coitus and late pregnancy, delivery and the puerperium. Am. J. Obstet. Gynecol. 64:333, 1952.

Pugh, W. E., and Fernandez, F. L.: Coitus in late pregnancy. Obstet. Gynecol. 2:636, 1953.

Rayburn, W. F., and Wilson, E. A.: Coital activity and premature labor. Am. J. Obstet. Gynecol. 137:972, 1980.

Richardson, A. C., Lyon, J., Graham, E., et al.: Decreasing postpartum sexual abstinence time. Am. J. Obstet. Gynecol. 126:416, 1976.

Rogers, R. E.: Evaluation of post-episiorrhapy pain: Polyglycolic acid vs. catgut sutures. Milit. Med. 139:102, 1974.

Semmens, J. P.: Female sexuality and life situations. Obstet. Gynecol. 38:555, 1971.

Shephard, B. D., and Shephard, C. A.: The Complete Guide to Women's Health. (A Plume book). New York, New American Library, 1985.

Sloan, D., and Bing, E.: Sex and pregnancy: will prematurity result? The Female Patient 8:24, 1983.

Solberg, D., Butler, J., and Wagner, N.: Sexual behavior in pregnancy. N. Engl. J. Med. 288:1098, 1973.

Speroff, L., and Ramerell, P. W.: Prostaglandins in reproductive physiology. Am. J. Obstet. Gynecol. 107:111, 1970.

Swanson, J.: The marital sexual relationship during pregnancy. JOGN Nurs. 9:267, 1980.

Tompkins, M. G., and Lea, R. H.: The use of polyglycolic acid sutures in obstetrics and gynecology. Can. Med. Assoc. J. 106:675, 1972.

Trethowan, W. H.: The couvade syndrome. In Howells, J. G. (ed.): Modern Perspectives in Psycho-Obstetrics. New York, Brunner-Mazel, 1972.

VanDenBerg, B. J.: Coitus and amniotic fluid infections. N. Engl. J. Med. 302:632, 1980.

Wagner, N., Butler, J., and Sanders, J.: Prematurity and orgasmic coitus during pregnancy: data on a small sample. Fertil. Steril. 27:911, 1976.

White, S., and Reamy, K.: Sexuality and pregnancy: a review. Arch. Sex. Behav. 11:429, 1982.

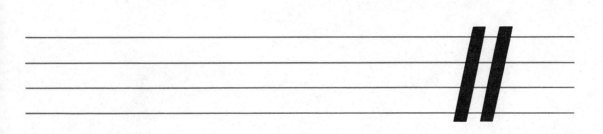

COMPLICATIONS AND DELIVERY

11

LABOR

ROY H. PETRIE
ATHANASIA M. WILLIAMS

Following fertilization, embryogenesis, organogenesis and a period of growth and development, the fetus reaches a point at which a nonconfined and separate life is undertaken. In those animal species in which the developing fetus is carried inside the mother and such a transformation is accomplished by expulsion of the fetus or fetuses from the mother by rhythmic contractions in the muscular portion of the reproductive tract, this transition is known as *labor*. In the human, labor is generally thought of as that interval from the onset of regular rhythmic uterine contractions, initiating the movement of the fetus down the genital tract, until the time when the fetus is expelled from the mother and ends its dependence on her for vital physiologic support, assuming its independent life as a neonate.

The foregoing general description satisfies an overall biologic consideration of labor. In any biologic consideration, reproduction is the ultimate of all biologic functions, and as such occupies a central drive and effort in order to maintain the species. The maintenance of the species by procreation generally requires multiple attempts at procreation by any one member of the species to replace that member. Evaluation of the reproductive process demonstrates that it is a somewhat wasteful process in terms of the numbers of conceptions that take place compared with the numbers that reach maturity with the ability to reproduce. This wastefulness is obvious in the lower species, and upon careful scrutiny it is similarly true in the human. It has been estimated that as few as 50 percent of all human conceptions reach the age of 1 year. The transition from an intrauterine life into an extrauterine existence is

called the birth process, and the mechanism by which it is accomplished is called labor. It is during labor that enormous maternal and fetal/neonatal changes are experienced, and it is during this interval that a major applied evaluation and analysis of this process is necessary. After biologic and other considerations are analyzed, medical management processes are designed to ameliorate and correct steps that previously have yielded damage and loss. Implementation of these prescribed medical processes then results in improved outcome in human reproduction.

The Uterus

EMBRYOLOGY

During the 3rd week of fetal development, the intraembryonic mesoderm is noted to differentiate into three distinct parts: (1) the paraxial portion, which ultimately forms the somites; (2) the lateral plate, which forms the somatic and splanchnic mesoderm, or the layers lining the coelom; and (3) the intermediate mesoderm, which connects the paraxial portion and the lateral plate. The intermediate mesoderm at the cervical region loses contact with the somites and segmentally forms small cell clusters known as nephrotomes. The nephrotomes grow laterally and caudad and develop a lumen. In the thoracic, lumbar, and sacral areas, the intermediate mesoderm loses contact with the coelomic cavity, segmentation disappears, and the nephrogenic cords form excretory tubules. Thus begin the three different and yet slightly overlapping renal systems embryologically noted in the human. Henceforth, the development of the urinary and genital systems is an interconnecting and intertwining saga that explains all of the basic anatomic relationships found in the adult.

The first of the renal systems to develop is the pronephros, which is located in the cervical region. The pronephros is replaced by the mesonephros in the thoracic and lumbar regions, which in turn is replaced by the metanephros in the lower lumbar and sacral regions. During the 4th embryonic week, genital ridges are noted on each side of the midline of the intermediate mesodermal plate between the mesonephros and the dorsal mesentery. By the 6th embryonic week both male and female embryos have two pairs of genital ducts: the wolffian, or mesonephric, duct and the müllerian, or paramesonephric, duct (which runs parallel to the wolffian duct). In the female the müllerian duct subsequently forms the primary skeleton of the internal female genital system: The upper part forms the fallopian tube, or oviduct, and the lower part comes together, fuses, and forms the uterus and upper vagina. While the mesonephric or wolffian duct becomes the primary genital duct in the male, it disappears for all practical purposes in the female (Arey, 1965).

ANATOMY

The uterus is a slightly flattened, pear-shaped muscular organ that lies between the vagina below and the fallopian tubes above. The opening to the uterus from the vagina is through the cervical os. The cervix is attached to the body, or corpus, of the uterus; the fallopian tubes enter the uterus laterally through the cornua, and that area above the cornua is known as the fundus. The cervix and the transitional area between the cervix and the body of the uterus are made up of connective tissue tapering into the muscular tissue as the body of the uterus is approached. The cervix contains connective tissue, which includes elastin (Leppert et al., 1982), and it is that part of the uterus that dilates during the course of labor to allow the fetus to move from the uterine cavity down the vagina to the outside. The uterine wall is made up of muscle tissue that has no singular vectorial orientation, but rather runs in all directions, in order to properly control bleeding from the multiple

vessels supplying blood to this area when delivery is accomplished. The purpose of this is to avoid exsanguination.

The uterus in the very young and very old is quite small, perhaps no larger than an adult large thumb. As the uterus enters the interval during which reproduction takes place, the body and fundus of the uterus enlarge in order to accommodate the implantation of the fertilized ovum (embryo); further enlargement takes place in all aspects, but particularly in the muscular portion, in order to allow for the growth of the fetus during the developmental process. Uterine size and growth are under the control of the hormones. The uterus has a peritoneal covering for that portion found in the peritoneal cavity; the uterus is lined with endometrium. The urinary bladder is anterior to the cervicovaginal junction, and the rectum of the bowel is posterior to the cervical ligaments. The attachments to the uterus include the utero-ovarian or infundibulopelvic ligament, which is attached from the lateral side wall to the upper lateral one third of the uterus, and the cardinal ligaments, which connect the area just at the junction of the body and cervix to the side wall, thus forming the base of the broad ligament. Supporting each side of the uterus is the broad ligament, the superior boundary of which is the round ligament. The uterosacral ligament connects the posterolateral aspect of the cervicouterine junction with the sacral vertebrae (Fig. 11–1). The chief blood supply of the uterus is through the utero-ovarian artery, the uterine artery, and the superior branch or cervical branch of the vaginal artery (Fig. 11–2).

UTERINE ACTIVITY AND THE ONSET OF LABOR

The etiology of the onset of labor is unknown, although a considerable amount of information regarding the onset of labor has been acquired in the past few years. There are a number of theories that deal with the onset of labor and the control of labor. For example, it is known that prior to the onset of labor, the maternal estrogen/progesterone ratio generally shifts in favor of estrogen. It is further known that the predominance of estrogen and the formation of the prostaglandins from arachidonic acid result in an inflammatory reaction similar to that which is

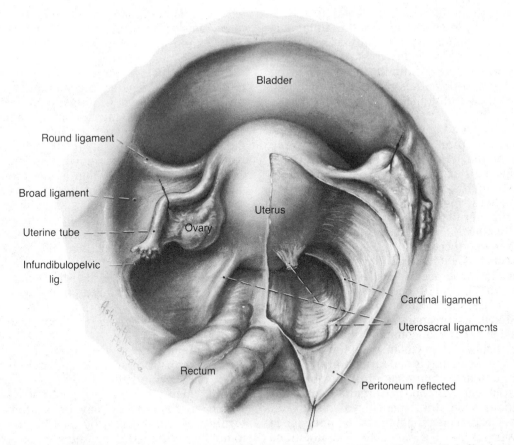

Bladder

Round ligament

Broad ligament

Uterine tube

Infundibulopelvic
lig.

Ovary

Uterus

Cardinal ligament

Uterosacral ligaments

Rectum

Peritoneum reflected

Figure 11–1. Ligaments of the female pelvis. (From Jacob, S. W., Francone, C., and Lossow, W. J.: Structure and Function in Man, 5th ed. Philadelphia, W. B. Saunders Co., 1982.)

Figure 11–2. Blood supply of uterus and ovary. (From Moore, M. L.: Realities in Childbearing, 2nd ed. Philadelphia, W. B. Saunders Co., 1983.)

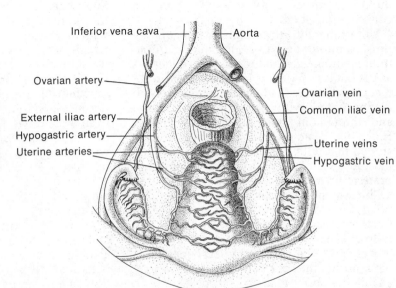

Inferior vena cava

Aorta

Ovarian artery

Ovarian vein

Common iliac vein

External iliac artery

Hypogastric artery

Uterine arteries

Uterine veins

Hypogastric vein

seen with an infection (Mitchell, 1983). It is interesting to speculate that this inflammatory environment (similar to that seen with an infection) provides a biochemical-biophysical source of stimuli that provoke and alter action potentials that may be required to initiate individual muscle cells to contract.

It has been known for some time that the posterior pituitary octapeptide oxytocin causes the term or near-term uterus to respond with contractions, whereas, the nongravid uterus or the uterus early in gestation does not respond to oxytocin (Petrie, 1981). As the uterus grows near to term, and especially after the onset of uterine activity, the uterus may become exquisitely sensitive to oxytocin. Oxytocin receptors in the myometrium have been identified (Soloff, 1973 and 1977), and it has been demonstrated that more functional oxytocin receptors are available as pregnancy and labor progress (Fuchs, 1981). Concomitant with the rise in the number of oxytocin receptor sites that become available is the formation of apparent cellular communication routes or myometrial gap junctions. Garfield (1981) has demonstrated the specialized cell-to-cell contacts that are thought to lower impedence to current flow between cells. Gap junctions are present in increased number as parturition approaches and as labor ensues. The release of arachidonic acid from the fetal membranes and the formation of the prostaglandins, particularly $F_{2\alpha}$ and the E_2 fraction, clearly establish that these compounds are intimately involved as uterine stimuli in the initiation of uterine activity and the continuation of labor.

Unfortunately, the relationship of the prostaglandins and oxytocin in the initiation, maintenance, and regulation of labor is as yet unclear. Myometrial prostaglandin $F_{2\alpha}$ receptors have been identified and have been demonstrated with impending parturition and throughout labor (Hartelendy, 1982). Hall (1957) and Rusu (1966) have demonstrated that with pregnancy, the serum magnesium levels fall. With the onset of either preterm or term labor, a further fall related to the impending onset of labor can be identified. Considering that the myometrial contraction chemically can be expressed by the following equation: actin + myosin + ATP + calcium → a contraction response, it is obvious that the control of calcium flow may enable the obstetrician to control labor. The beta$_2$-sympathomimetic agents are thought to regulate calcium by altering cyclic AMP control, and magnesium probably displaces calcium.

It appears that the uterus as it approaches term is being prepared biochemically and physiologically to perform its function. Hormone levels shift; microscopic anatomic changes occur; hormones are released; hormones are formed; the myometrium is prepared initially to act somewhat independently at a cellular level; and as the process ensues, more and more of the entire myometrium acts in unison as a singular muscular effort. The exact etiology of the onset of spontaneous labor is as yet unknown. However, it is clear that there may be multiple physiologic, biochemical, and pharmacologic avenues by which labor may ensue, and correspondingly, there may be multiple avenues by which the onset of uterine activity leading to labor may be blocked.

For the purposes of discussion, it is interesting to construct an analogy between the onset of labor and the starting of an automobile engine. There are many ways by which an automobile may be started—by turning an ignition key, by pushing the automobile with another engine such as a car, by "cross-wiring" an ignition system, and so on. There are also several conditions that promote the starting of an automobile: the proper fuel being available in the carburetor, sufficient oxygen for the combustion of the fuel, etc. By the same token, it is known that several conditions can cause labor. Labor is more likely to ensue with overdistension of the uterus, as occurs with twin gestations; with a Ferguson reflex (a cervical reflex), which causes the generation of uterine activity; with cervical dilatation; with the rupturing of the membranes if conditions in the myometrium are right, including the correct hormone relationship being present either from a maternal, fetal, or exogenous source; and with infection or an electric stimulus, which may provoke sufficient uterine activity to initiate labor. *Once sufficient uterine activity from whatever source has been generated to initiate labor, the process will usually proceed on its own*, much as the running of the automobile engine continues once it has been started by one of various avenues. The analogy is not complete, but it is sufficiently similar to warrant consideration as a pattern or template when thinking about the biochemistry, physiology, and pharmacology of labor.

Normal Considerations of Labor

Normal considerations of labor should include the "Four P's." Traditionally there have been "Three P's": *Power, Passage,* and *Passenger.* However, recently a fourth P has been added: *Psyche* (Moore, 1980).

POWER (UTERINE ACTIVITY)

In the strict clinical sense labor is defined as rhythmic uterine contractions that result in cervical effacement and dilatation with descent of the presenting fetal part.

In labor, repeated rhythmic uterine contractions provide a setting in which, during the course of each contraction, there is the possibility that the intramyometrial pressure may exceed the intravascular blood pressure; this would partially or completely interrupt blood flow to the placenta and the intervillous space, where maternal red cells unload oxygen and take on a new supply of carbon dioxide from the fetal red cell. Normally the human fetus has sufficient reserve to tolerate this intermittent interruption in carbon dioxide–oxygen exchange. However, in circumstances of reduced placental surface, excess uterine activity, lowered maternal blood pressure, or increased fetal demands, the fetal tolerance may be exceeded and the Krebs cycle can no longer supply all of the fetus's needs for energy in the form of ATP, because of insufficient oxygen. At this point the anaerobic glycolytic pathway must be utilized for the production of ATP. As a result, lactic acid will be formed, which has the potential to cause nervous system damage, which in turn may lead to fetal death. Thus, hypoxia causing acidosis and asphyxia is a potential result of the labor process.

In order to reduce the potential for fetal/neonatal damage or death as a result of labor conditions exceeding a fetus's ability to tolerate them, it became necessary to critically and extensively analyze the labor process and to quantitate the various divisions of labor. Thus, normal limitations and normal fetal tolerances can be established as guidelines for appropriate management. Although this concept of analysis and the establishment of normal ranges appears to be simple, logical, and necessary, it was not until the last quarter to half century that any meaningful consideration of these aspects of labor was undertaken.

Evaluation and Quantitation of Uterine Activity and Labor Progress

Vital to the current analysis and consideration of labor is the concept of force in relation to action. In labor, the force (uterine contraction) is quantitated into a measurement of uterine contraction (activity) and compared with the demonstrated effects of that force in the form of action on the cervix and fetus, as measured by cervical effacement/dilatation and descent of the presenting fetal part (labor).

The uterus differentiates into two parts during labor; the actively contracting upper segment becomes thicker as labor advances; the lower portion (lower uterine segment and cervix) is rather passive and develops into a much thinner-walled muscular passage for the fetus. The upper passage contracts, retracts, and expels the fetus. In response to the force of contractions of the upper segment, the lower uterine segment and cervix dilate and thereby form a greatly expanded, thinned-out muscular and fibromuscular tube through which the fetus can pass.

With each contraction the uterus changes shape. The ovoid uterus becomes elongated simultaneously with a decrease in the horizontal diameter. This produces a straightening of the fetal vertebral column, which presses the upper fetal pole firmly against the uterine fundus, while the lower fetal pole is driven downward into the pelvis. During this lengthening of the uterus, the longitudinal uterine fibers are drawn tight, pulling the lower segment and cervix upward over the lower fetal pole. This effect on the lower uterine segment and cervix is important to cervical dilatation and effacement. Although not essential for successful labor and delivery, the round ligaments can contract and pull the uterus forward.

In the second stage of labor the main force that expels the fetus is intraabdominal pressure created by contraction of the abdominal muscles simultaneous with forced respiratory efforts, i.e., pushing.

Crucial to any analysis of this type is the concept of quantitating and comparing uterine contractions (uterine activity) and progress of labor in the form of cervical effacement/dilatation with the amount of fetal descent by time elapsed. When uterine activity (contractions) is compared with labor progress over an interval of time, normal ranges and expectations for each of these components and for the two integrated together can be established. Therefore, methods of quantitation of both uterine activity (contractions) and labor progress are essential to clinical investigation, analysis, and clinical management decisions.

Methods of Uterine Activity Analysis

There are three currently available methods of evaluating and quantitating uterine contractions (uterine activity): (1) timing and palpation, (2) external tocography, and (3) internal monitoring.

Timing and palpation. It is simple to time the frequency of contractions, and this can be done by measuring from the onset of one contraction to the onset of subsequent contractions; likewise, it is relatively easy to make a crude measurement of a contraction's duration simply by timing the interval from the onset to the end of the contraction. Estimating the intensity of a uterine contraction is somewhat more difficult; however, by placing one's hand on the abdomen overlying the gravid uterus, one can palpate uterine contractions and estimate whether the contraction is mild, moderate, or strong. Once a uterine contraction reaches a point of being palpated and appreciated as being painful by the patient, the intensity of the contraction probably has reached approximately 40 torr (mm Hg). For many clinical applications, particularly when attempting to establish whether true labor has begun, this form of analysis may be sufficient, despite the fact that it is rather subjective.

In order to palpate a contraction properly, it is necessary to leave one's hand on the fundus for a period of time when it is in both the relaxed and contracting states. Since all uteri have some degree of tone all throughout labor, a determination of the intensity of each contraction can be made only by comparing it with that patient's resting tone or with the tone between contractions.

External tocography. A more quantitative form of analysis of uterine activity is the use of external tocography, in which a tocodynamometer transducer (tocotransducer) is placed on the abdomen overlying the gravid uterus in a position so that changes in the curvature of the abdomen that result from uterine contractions can be measured and appropriately recorded on a graph. Thus, the onset of a contraction can be better quantitated, as can the duration of the contraction. However, the exact beginning and end of the contraction may be difficult to define, especially if the patient is moving around in the bed. (Defining the end of the contraction may be crucial to the recognition of deceleration patterns.) The evaluation of intensity of the uterine contraction remains somewhat semiquantitative using this method of evaluation, owing to placement of the transducer and movements of the mother and fetus. This form of analysis of uterine activity is currently used in labor until such time as the fetal membranes are ruptured and the internal pressure form of uterine activity analysis is initiated.

It is important to note that in the placement of the external transducer, it is vital to remain with the patient during a few contractions to ensure that the tocotransducer is situated in the proper position. If the patient complains of pain or one is able to palpate increased tone in the uterus and it is not recording on the graph, it is then necessary to move the transducer in order to properly record contractions and progress of labor. It should be recalled here that external monitoring does not demonstrate the *intensity* of contractions. In an obese patient a mild-appearing contraction can actually be a very strong one, whereas the reverse may be true in a thinner patient. Therefore, manual palpation of the contractions should be done in conjunction with use of the tocotransducer. As an aside, in this era of return to natural childbirth, the practitioner may encounter patients who do not want to be monitored during labor. It is vital to discuss and explain the reasons for monitoring with all monitored patients, ideally during pregnancy rather than when the patient arrives in the delivery suite.

Internal monitoring. The third form of uterine activity analysis is performed with the

MONTEVIDEO UNITS

Average 1 x Frequency / 10 min

ALEXANDRIA UNITS

Average 1 x Frequency / 10 min
x Average duration (min)

ACTIVE PLANIMETER UNITS

Area under active pressure curve
x 10 min

TOTAL PLANIMETER UNITS

Area under entire curve
x 10 min

AVERAGE RATE OF RISE

Intensity / Tr

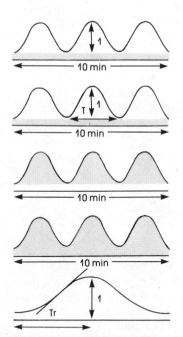

Figure 11–3. Alternative methods for the quantitation of frequency, duration, and intensity of the uterine contractions. (From Miller, F. C., Yeh S.-Y., Schifrin, B. S., et al.: Quantitation of uterine activity in 100 primiparous patients. Am. J. Obstet. Gynecol. 124:308, 1976.)

use of an intrauterine catheter inserted transcervically into the amniotic cavity to measure pressure. By this manner quantitation of frequency, duration, and intensity of the uterine contraction can be accomplished. A number of methods of graphing quantitation of uterine activity (contractions) have been developed (Fig. 11–3) (Miller, 1976). Utiliz-

ing the total area under the uterine pressure curve, Miller and associates (1976) and Huey and associates (1976) have demonstrated the normal amount of uterine activity (contractions) required to achieve delivery in a large number of nulliparous and multiparous patients, as shown in Figures 11–4 and 11–5. By itself, the quantitation of uterine contrac-

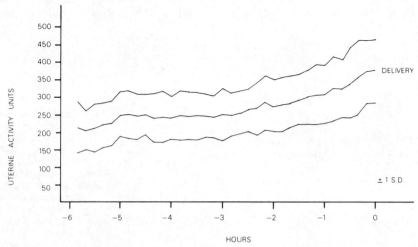

Figure 11–4. Mean uterine activity units for 100 patients (nulliparas) plotted every 10 minutes for 6 hours preceding delivery. (From Miller, F. C., Yeh, S.-Y., Schifrin, B. S., et al.: Quantitation of uterine activity in 100 primiparous patients. Am. J. Obstet. Gynecol. 124:308, 1976.)

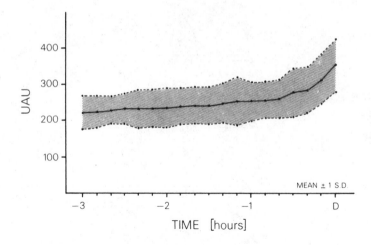

Figure 11–5. Mean uterine activity units for 149 patients (multiparas) plotted every 10 minutes for 3 hours preceding delivery. (From Huey, J. R., Al-Hadjiev, A., and Paul, R. H.: Uterine activity in the multiparous patient. Am. J. Obstet. Gynecol. 126:682, 1976.)

tions (activity) can indicate only whether a normal or an abnormal amount of uterine contractions (uterine activity) is being generated by a given patient, and accordingly this measurement contributes minimally to the overall clinical evaluation of labor. This form of uterine activity analysis is now available on some commercially available fetal monitoring units. When the quantitation of uterine activity is combined with the quantitation of the progress of labor, it can be of considerable benefit in the evaluational process and in the management and decision-making efforts.

If a satisfactory external recording of fetal heart rate and uterine activity has been achieved, internal monitoring may be unnecessary. However, if only a poor tracing is recorded or if oxytocin is being adminis-

tered, it is highly recommended to avail oneself of the additional information that internal monitoring can provide. Since kinking and clogging of a catheter can occur, periodic flushing with sterile water should be performed in order to ensure the patency of the catheter and the accuracy of the information received.

Graphing Labor Progress

Friedman (1954), in the major cornerstone system of labor analysis upon which rest our current concepts of the process of labor and its evaluation and management, introduced the evaluation of labor by graphing cervical dilatation/effacement with descent of the presenting fetal part against the passage of time. Clinically the station of the presenting part (distance above or below the interischial

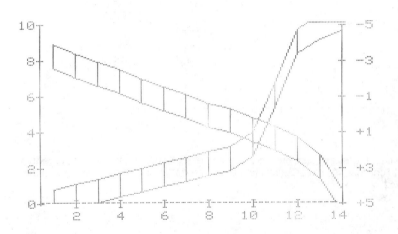

Figure 11–6. The "S"-shape projected nulliparous labor curve (one of 48 computer-generated labor curves available showing standard deviation) appropriately adjusted for parity, medication status, membrane status, and onset of labor for this nullipara. The curve from the upper left downward shows the station descent with standard deviation. (Courtesy of Henry R. Rey and Dr. Roy H. Petrie, Columbia University, New York.)

STANDARD FRIEDMAN CURVES

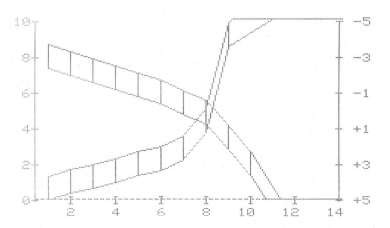

Figure 11–7. The "S"-shape projected multiparous labor curve appropriately adjusted for parity, medication status, membrane status, and onset of labor for this multipara. (The wide band indicates standard deviation.) The curve from the left corner downward indicates the standard deviation. (Courtesy of Henry R. Rey and Dr. Roy H. Petrie, Columbia University, New York.)

spine plane) and the cervical dilatation are graphed on the vertical axis, with subsequent measurements graphed further along on the vertical axis according to the elapsed time. Thus a characteristic S-shaped curve will result for a normal labor. Normal S-shaped labor curves have been established for both the nullipara and multipara, as demonstrated in Figures 11–6 and 11–7. Figures 11–8 and 11–9 demonstrate normal patients meeting labor goals. During the past 20 or 30 years, the use of this graph to record labor progress has enabled the obstetrician to evaluate labor more logically than in the past. As a result, subsequent comparisons between neonatal outcome and the progress

of labor have enabled obstetricians to make advances in neonatal salvage and the quality of neonatal life based on this factor alone. When these evaluations are compared with uterine activity (contractions) and the fetus's tolerance to labor in the form of fetal heart rate data, considerable improvement in fetal/neonatal salvage and quality of life is possible.

Characteristically when labor is analyzed by the comparison of cervical dilatation and descent of the presenting part against elapsed time, three biologic divisions of labor are identified. The first period runs from the onset of contractions and minimal cervical dilatation until the point at which

STANDARD FRIEDMAN CURVES

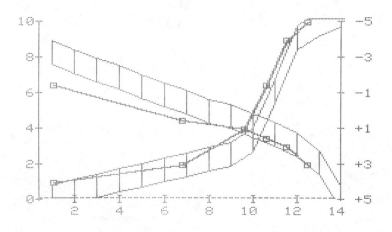

Figure 11–8. The actual labor data for a nullipara who met most of her projected labor guideline goals and experienced a normal nulliparous labor. The lines connecting the boxes represent the patient's actual dilatation and station changes. The wide bands indicate standard deviation for dilatation and station. (Courtesy of Henry R. Rey and Dr. Roy H. Petrie, Columbia University, New York.)

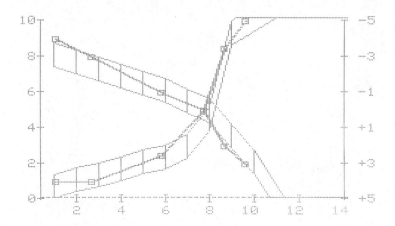

Figure 11–9. The actual labor data for a multipara who met most of her projected labor guideline goals and experienced a normal multiparous labor. The lines connecting the boxes represent the patient's actual dilatation and station changes. The wide bands indicate standard deviation for dilatation and station. (Courtesy of Henry R. Rey and Dr. Roy H. Petrie, Columbia University, New York.)

approximately 3 cm of cervical dilatation are achieved (latent phase) or until a point at which rapid changes should be expected in cervical dilatation, which generally occurs at about 3 to 4 cm of dilatation (active phase). The latent phase may take from a few to many hours. Most conservative obstetricians now consider that the latent phase of labor becomes prolonged after approximately 20 hours. It has been established that a prolonged latent phase is associated with an increased risk of fetal/neonatal damage and death. Once accelerated cervical dilatation begins to occur, usually at about 3 to 4 cm, subsequent cervical dilatation with descent of the presenting part is rapid and usually falls within the 1 to 2 cm/hr range. At approximately 8 cm, rapid cervical dilatation slows down, and the steepness of the cervical dilatation curve is diminished somewhat through delivery. Once complete cervical dilatation is accomplished, the interval to delivery may be short, as is usually seen in the multipara, or it can be longer, up to 1 or 2 hours normally in the nullipara. Many clinicians consider that as long as there is descent of the presenting part and the fetus demonstrates good health by appropriate fetal surveillance, the interval from complete cervical dilatation to delivery may actually reach 2, 3, or more hours (Fig. 11–10) with no harm to the fetus. A number of

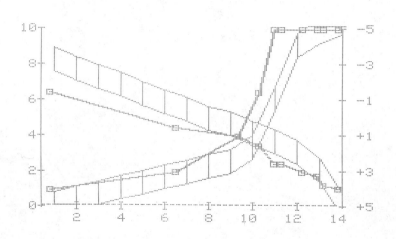

Figure 11–10. A nullipara who reached complete full dilatation of the cervix at approximately 11 hours into the labor with prolonged or slow descent of the head. Note that the second stage of labor is over 3 hours; however, progress in descent is being made and the fetus is tolerating labor well as judged by fetal rate monitoring. A low or outlet forceps type of instrument-assisted delivery was subsequently accomplished. The lines connecting the boxes represent the patient's actual dilatation and station changes. The wide bands indicate standard deviation for dilatation and station. (Courtesy of Henry R. Rey and Dr. Roy H. Petrie, Columbia University, New York.)

factors, including age, parity, position, gestational duration, labor duration, cervical maturity, medication, membrane status, and pelvic size, may affect the duration of the various stages of labor. From clinical analysis of the various stages of labor, it has been demonstrated that a too-rapid or too-slow advancement of cervical dilatation/effacement and descent of the presenting part may have a deleterious effect on fetal/neonatal outcome.

As a patient is being evaluated during labor, she should be informed as to how the labor is progressing and exactly what it means. Not all patients are aware of what the physiologic changes are in labor, and this unawareness can cause fear and anxiety that often are severe enough so as to obstruct the normal course of labor. An informed patient, on the other hand, can relax and therefore optimize the true potential of labor.

Importance of an Integrated Evaluation

In the clinical evaluation and management of the course of labor, it has been demonstrated by several investigators that age, parity, duration of pregnancy, cervical quality, position, and sedation and administration of other medications play an important role in the generation of uterine activity, and that the generation of uterine activity with the passage of time directly influences the "S-shape" labor curve that demonstrates the progress of labor (Burnhill et al., 1962; Miller et al., 1976; Huey et al., 1976). Thus, it is important in managing labor to integrate both methodologies of labor quantitation: evaluation of uterine activity *and* the progress of labor per unit of time. This allows evaluation of centimeters of progress and the amount of uterine activity required to achieve this progress, as depicted in Figures 11–11 and 11–12. Note that with the passage of time, lesser amounts of uterine activity are required to achieve cervical dilatation than were required earlier in the labor process. This is a critical concept to remember for the proper active management of the labor process, especially when aggressive management may be needed. As long as the progress of labor is normal, less attention can be paid to the amount of uterine activity (contractions) generated; however, if normal progress is not occurring, then the analysis of uterine contractions (uterine activity) may become rather important.

Differentiation Between True and False Labor

The consideration of definitions as well as that of the normal parameters of labor is essential to the proper analysis and management processes. For the purpose of this discussion, *prodromal labor* may be defined as the somewhat erratic, nonregular to regular uterine contractions that are present prior to the establishment of the regular, rhythmic contraction pattern that is seen during the true labor process. *False labor* may be defined as the somewhat regular, rhythmic uterine contractions that simulate *true labor* but are not accompanied by either cervical

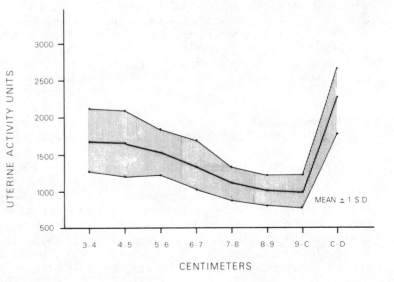

Figure 11–11. The average uterine activity units generated for each centimeter of cervical dilatation during the labors of 100 primiparas, demonstrating a progressive increase in the efficiency of uterine activity as labor advances. (From Miller, F. C., Yeh, S.-Y., Schifrin, B. S., et al.: Quantitation of uterine activity in 100 primiparous patients. Am. J. Obstet. Gynecol. 124:308, 1976.)

MEAN TOTAL UAU AT EACH CM.

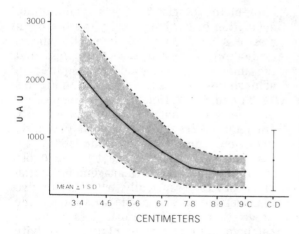

Figure 11-12. The average total uterine activity units generated for each centimeter of cervical dilatation during the labors of 149 multiparas, demonstrating a progressive increase in the efficiency of uterine activity as labor advances. (From Huey, J. R., Al-Hadjiev, A., and Paul, R. H.: Uterine activity in the multiparous patient. Am. J. Obstet. Gynecol. 126:682, 1976.)

dilatation/effacement or descent of the presenting part. In some cases the differentiation between true and false labor requires an interval of observation. During this observation period, after obtaining a brief monitoring strip to ensure the fetus's ability to tolerate the stress of the contractions, it is often helpful if a patient is encouraged to ambulate. Quite often ambulation will diminish or totally eradicate false labor, whereas real labor will continue and increase in intensity. In true labor, ambulation can aid in the descent of the fetal presenting part, thereby making labor more effectual. The *latent phase* of labor is often confused with *prodromal labor;* however, the latent phase of labor is a slow steady effacement and dilatation of the cervix that occurs from the time of the onset of contractions until the start of the active phase of labor. It is somewhat normal for the labor in the primigravida to last between 8 and 12 hours from the onset of contractions through to delivery. Various phases of labor will be dependent upon parity as well as age, gestational duration, cervical ripeness, medications used, and so on.

The Stages of Labor

For clinical consideration, labor is divided into stages; the first, second, and third. The *first stage of labor* represents the interval between the onset of contractions and the point at which full cervical dilatation is achieved. This is a time when a woman needs a great deal of support and encouragement from the intrapartum team as well as her coach. A patient needs to know where she is in the laboring process and how much

more work must be done until delivery. With adequate knowledge and support, the patient can cope more effectively with the progressive intensity of her labor. An analgesic agent may be needed during this stage. The *second stage of labor* lasts from the onset of full cervical dilatation through the delivery of the fetus. This can be the most difficult part of labor. After many hours of laboring, it is now necessary for the potentially exhausted patient to expend the most energy. She needs encouragement to summon up all her strength to push as efficiently and forcefully as possible. Even the most prepared of patients can lose control at this time. It is necessary to relax the patient as much as possible and to reinforce use of the most effective positions and techniques for accomplishing her goal. The *third stage of labor* is the interval from the delivery of the baby through the delivery of the placenta. At this point the fetus and mother are usually bonding. The patient still needs encouragement and help in handling her newborn infant. If the neonate cannot be with the mother, the mother should be made aware of the infant's condition as soon as possible. Some institutions classify a *fourth stage of labor*, defined as the first 1- to 2-hour interval following delivery of the placenta. It is during this interval that the recently delivered mother (parturient) is observed carefully for blood loss, proper uterine contraction, changes in blood pressure, and overall state of well-being. If the mother is in the recovery room with the newborn, this is an excellent opportunity to help the mother to examine her baby, to encourage continuation of bonding, and to allay any fears the mother may have for her baby's well-being.

THE PASSAGE

The type of maternal pelvis may have an effect on labor. The *gynecoid pelvis* is considered the most satisfactory for normal labor. It allows effective uterine contractions and vaginal delivery. The wide pubic arch reduces perineal tears.

In women with an *anthropoid pelvis*, the fetal head is often in an occiput posterior position, and the woman may deliver with the fetus in that position. Labor and delivery are usually without difficulty.

The *android pelvis* usually causes the fetal head to engage in a transverse or posterior position, and it may not rotate, which often results in the need to use forceps for rotation and delivery. Such a delivery may be difficult, causing stress to the fetus. Perineal tears are common because of the narrow pubic arch.

In a *platypelloid pelvis* the baby may never be able to enter the pelvis inlet, because of the short anteroposterior, posterior sagittal, and anterior sagittal diameters. The outlook for the fetus is poor unless this pelvis shape is recognized and the fetus is delivered by cesarean delivery.

THE PASSENGER

Fetal Attitude

It is important to consider the concept of the anatomic relationship of the fetus to the mother. *Attitude* is the relationship of the fetal limbs and head to its trunk and should be one of flexion. Therefore, the fetus forms a compact, ovoid mass that accommodates itself well to the uterine cavity. To help determine this relationship, Leopold's maneuvers (examination of the gravid uterus) (Fig. 11–13) can be helpful. However, in some instances it is difficult to determine the relationship of the fetus to the mother, and the use of an additional evaluation technique, such as real-time ultrasound, can be immediately illuminating.

Fetal Lie (Fig. 11–13)

The fetus's vertebral column in relation to the maternal vertebral column is referred to as the *lie*. There is a longitudinal lie when the fetus's vertebral column is parallel to the maternal vertebral column. With a transverse lie, a fetus's vertebral column is at an approximately 90-degree angle to the maternal vertebral column. In cases of transverse lie, the extremities may be cephalad (extremities up) or caudad (extremities down). With an oblique lie, the fetus's vertebral column is neither at right angles nor parallel to the maternal vertebral column, but at some angle in between.

Fetal Presentation (Fig. 11–13)

It is also important to know and evaluate the type of *presentation*, or that part of the fetus that is being applied to the cervix and will be delivered first. The most common is the cephalic presentation. The cephalic presentation may be in varying degrees of flexion or extension. The most common cephalic presentation is the vertex, which represents the back of the head or the extreme form of flexion. The sinciput presentation is neither flexed nor extended. The brow presentation shows some degree of extension, and a face presentation is the extreme form of hyperextension.

The second most common presentation is the breech, which may be of three types: frank—the feet extended fully toward the head; complete—the knees bent; or footling—the feet presenting first. On occasion there may be an acromial or shoulder presentation, and in rare instances there may be a compound presentation such as an arm and leg, arm and head, or some other combination.

Fetal-Maternal Position (Fig. 11–14)

Likewise it is important to know the position of the presenting part in relationship to the maternal anatomy. *Position* is the relationship of the presenting part to one of the four quadrants of the maternal pelvis. The four quadrants would be anterior, posterior, and lateral (right and left). In giving fetal position, the maternal symphysis is referred to as anterior and the sacrum as posterior, with the right maternal femur referred to as right and the left maternal femur, left. The same applies to breech presentations. A right sacrum posterior indicates that the fetal sacrum is directed to the right of the maternal vertebral column and pointed in the direction of the maternal sacrum.

With a face presentation the position is determined by the fetal mentum. For example, a mentum posterior position indicates that the fetal mentum is directed toward the maternal sacrum.

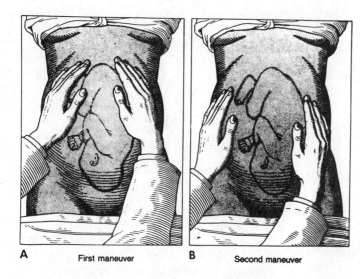

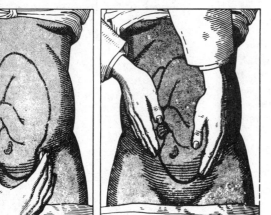

| A | First maneuver | B | Second maneuver |

| C | Third maneuver | D | Fourth maneuver |

Figure 11–13. Leopold's maneuvers for determining (A) lie, attitude, and presentation of fetus; (B) position; (C) engagement; and (D) position and flexion. (From Pritchard, J. A., and MacDonald, P. C.: Williams Obstetrics, 16th ed. New York, Appleton-Century-Crofts, 1980.)

These relationships are important in determining whether or not labor will progress normally. When the fetus is askew, dysfunctional labor can ensue.

THE PSYCHE

Some studies have suggested the possibility of an interrelationship between difficulties during labor and delivery and sociocultural or psychologic factors. There has been shown to be a relationship between anxiety and uterine dysfunction, in that women who reported more than average symptoms of muscle tension during pregnancy, and who demonstrated at the beginning of labor more than average physiologic and behavioral signs associated with anxiety, are more likely to develop physiologic disturbances related to uterine dysfunction.

Rosengren (1961) noted the relationship between the tendency to take the sick role during pregnancy and subsequent difficulty during labor and delivery. His findings suggested that "the more a woman regarded herself as 'ill' during pregnancy, the greater was the likelihood of a longer period of active labor."

There is also a relationship between anxiety and pain. Several physiologic changes are initiated by anxiety. A major response is the production of epinephrine and norepinephrine: Epinephrine stimulates both alpha and beta receptors, whereas norepinephrine stimulates primarily alpha receptors. Alpha-

Left Occipito-Anterior   Left Occipito-Transverse   Left Occipito-Posterior

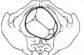
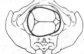

Right Occipito-Anterior   Right Occipito-Transverse   Right Occipito-Posterior

Left Mento-Anterior   Right Mento-Anterior   Right Mento-Posterior

Left Sacro-Anterior   Right Sacro-Anterior   Right Sacro-Posterior

Figure 11–14. Positions in relation to various presentations, with fetus viewed from below. (From Pritchard, J. A., and MacDonald, P. C.: Williams Obstetrics, 16th ed. New York, Appleton-Century-Crofts, 1980.)

adrenergic receptor stimulation causes uterine vasoconstriction (as well as generalized vasoconstriction) and an increase in uterine muscle tone, leading to both a decrease in uterine blood supply and an increase in maternal blood supply and maternal blood pressure. Beta-adrenergic receptor stimulation causes vasodilatation and relaxation of uterine muscle. Since the uterine vessels are already fully dilated, the dilatation of other vessels reduces the flow of blood to the uterus. Decreased uterine blood flow may produce fetal bradycardia. Morishima et al. (1978) and Meyers and Meyers (1979), in animal studies, were able to produce fetal bradycardia by frightening monkey mothers.

Lederman et al. (1977) found that high epinephrine levels correlated with maternal anxiety and led to decreased uterine activity and longer labors. Newborn Apgar scores tend to be lower in those mothers demonstrating a high degree of anxiety.

Therefore, it would seem that anxiety may sometimes play a role in dysfunctional labor. It is very important, therefore, to assist mothers psychologically during their labor. This can be done by providing support, ensuring that her coach is present, encouraging the timid coach to participate more, and providing information to reduce anxiety.

Exceptional Labor Circumstances

DYSFUNCTIONAL LABOR

Labor does not always proceed as expected, nor does it fall within normal limits for all individuals in a given population. Many terms have been applied to this situation, such as "failure to progress," "clinical cephalopelvic disproportion," and various classifications of "dystocia." It would perhaps be simpler and more appropriate to list all of these disorders of nonprogressive labor under the term *dysfunctional labor*, which could then be further defined as existing with excessive, normal, or subnormal amounts of uterine activity.

Evaluation

Frequently a review of the patient's history and/or a reevaluation of the pelvis is needed in these cases, since the primary causes of a dysfunctional labor include inadequate uterine activity, pharmacologic agents that reduce uterine activity, and even perhaps cephalopelvic disproportion. The effects of drugs on uterine activity are reasonably well known, and many of the sedative and narcotic drugs used during labor may reduce uterine activity to such a degree that inadequate progress of labor will occur. The use of oxytocin to augment labor by increasing uterine activity will be discussed in the chapter on the medical control of labor. Potential bony disproportion between the fetus and the mother is always a consideration with dysfunctional labor, and therefore it requires appropriate evaluation. A careful physical examination to evaluate and estimate fetal size in relation to pelvic size and space must be performed; *clinical pelvimetry* is considered the appropriate method of evaluation of potential cephalopelvic disproportion. (X-ray pelvimetry is still used at some centers, but has fallen to disfavor in recent years; see Delivery Considerations, next section.)

There is little reason to suspect that the generation of additional uterine activity will promote additional progress in labor in patients in whom the contraction pattern is essentially normal (contractions occurring every 2 to 3 minutes and lasting approximately 40 to 90 seconds, with an intensity of 40 to 90 mm Hg and a resting tone of 5 to 20 mm Hg) during the active phase of labor. If the fetus is tolerating the labor well, as evidenced by a normal fetal heart rate tracing, and uterine activity (i.e., contractions) has not reached this "normal" level, then perhaps an augmentation of the labor with oxytocin should be considered. In many cases of inadequate progress of labor, the condition may correct itself within 2 to 3 hours, and simply waiting and observing the patient for this period of time may be sufficient; however, many clinicians prefer a more aggressive form of labor management, with the use of oxytocin in the active phase. In some instances when there is lack of progress of labor with otherwise normal-appearing uterine contractions, or when the patient is excessively tired, especially during the latent phase (very early first stage) of labor, the use of sedatives to rest the patient for a few hours may be deemed appropriate.

Delivery Considerations

Some institutions rely upon the use of x-ray pelvimetry to assess the potential of disproportion between the fetal vertex and the maternal pelvis. This form of fetal surveillance, however, has generally fallen into disfavor in many places, and most obstetricians today prefer to make a clinical evaluation of the pelvis, based on whether there is adequate uterine activity and normal progression of labor. In the presence of an abnormal lie or presentation, such as a breech or transverse lie, the use of ultrasound scanning is considered the primary diagnostic tool, although x-ray pelvimetry is still considered an acceptable approach. Any abnormal presentation, whether a breech, transverse lie, oblique lie, or an aberrant form of the cephalic presentation, can be of major concern. Today it has become almost axiomatic that all large breech presentations (greater than 4000 grams) should be subjected to cesarean section, and in many institutions all small breech presentations (less than ± 1750 grams) are also subjected to cesarean section (Gimovsky and Petrie, 1982) in order to avoid the obvious problems of prolapsed cord and traumatic delivery. In some institutions *all* breech presentations are delivered by cesarean section; however, other institutions still maintain that it is unsafe to deliver term breech presentations of normal size (2 to 4 kg) from below (Gimovsky et al., 1981), especially with primipara women with untested pelves. In cases of an oblique lie (with the fetal vertebral column crossing the maternal vertebral column at less than right angles), many institutions will allow labor to continue with a cephalic presentation, with the expectation that the oblique lie will convert to a longitudinal lie. The oblique lie that may convert to a breech presentation is more likely to be considered an indication for cesarean section, especially by those institutions favoring this mode of delivery for breech presentations.

With the cephalic presentation, the head may be fully flexed, as with a vertex (occiput) presentation, or fully extended, with the face (mentum) presenting. Fetuses in all variants of cephalic presentation with or without asynclitism (lateral deflexion of the head) to a more anterior, posterior position in the pelvis can be delivered vaginally from any position except for one: the mentum posterior. This means that the fetal chin presents directly into the maternal sacral hollow with the fetal forehead coming under the symphysis pubis. Should the delivery occur from the mentum posterior position, insufficient room exists, and sufficient trauma will occur to a term-size fetus to bring about damage or death. In order to deliver the fetus with this type of presentation, rotation of the head must be achieved, either spontaneously, manually, or by forceps, so as not to deliver the baby in the direct mentum posterior position. In general, labor with presentations other than the vertex tends to proceed at a slightly slower rate, and descent is often somewhat retarded. Because with breech presentations the largest part of the fetal body (the head) is delivered last, thus leaving no time to mold the fetal head, some investigators mandate that during the active phase of labor, in order to allow a breech to continue labor, the cervix must dilate at least 1 cm/hr in the nullipara and 1 to 1½ cm/hr in the multipara (Gimovsky et al., 1981). The breech presentation, the second most common presentation, constitutes only 2 to 4 percent of all term deliveries. Thus the transverse lie, oblique lie, and the compound presentations are extremely uncommon, and there is a general trend toward delivery of all abnormal or uncommon presentations by cesarean section in order to avoid a prolonged labor and a traumatic delivery process.

PREMATURITY AND POSTMATURITY

Prematurity represents the single largest cause of perinatal mortality (Nochimson et al., 1980) and morbidity, and suspected postmaturity or postdatism is the single largest indication for antepartum fetal surveillance, because of the inexactness of data regarding true gestational age (Yeh and Read, 1982). Both of these conditions require special management of the labor process, as do cases of intrauterine growth retardation (IUGR), diabetes, and preeclampsia.

Prematurity, postmaturity, intrauterine growth retardation, and a fetus of a severe preeclamptic or diabetic mother appear to be a divergent group of conditions. Nevertheless, the same physiologic considerations exist in each of these disorders to warrant special consideration during the process of labor. The underlying principle is that each of these fetuses has the potential to be remarkably sensitive to hypoxia, stress, and trauma. The premature fetus has minimal reserves in the form of glycogen and body mass; the postmature may be large and marginally oxygenated owing to a deteriorating biologic function of the placenta; the intrauterine growth retarded (IUGR) infant may be small, poorly oxygenated, and with minimal amniotic fluid to cushion the stresses of labor. The diabetic infant likewise may be macrosomic or growth-retarded, with marginal oxygenation and a high degree of sensitivity to the stresses of hypoxia and trauma. The fetus of a preeclamptic mother may have uteroplacental insufficiency as a result of the poor vascularization of the placental bed caused by the hypertension. This may cause a decrease of oxygenation and consequent stress or distress to the fetus.

Because of the potential for respiratory distress syndrome, cord problems, and reduced biologic reserves, many centers tend to be very protective of these infants and observe fetal response to labor very carefully, with the aim of not allowing significant hypoxia or stress during labor. Generally speaking, a short, uncomplicated labor and delivery process is desired, and if this cannot be reasonably expected or achieved, an atraumatic cesarean section, in which hypoxia and asphyxia would not be factors, should be elected.

The Delivery Process

Parturition, or delivery of the fetus, can occur from almost any maternal anatomic position. Depending on the culture and society, deliveries may take place from a squatting, sitting, reclining, or lounging position. In Western cultures and societies, two maternal delivery positions are most common: (1) the reclining position or its variant, the dorsolithotomy position, which allows greater anatomic access to the perineal area, and (2) the lateral Sims position, in which the patient is lying on her side with her dependent leg slightly flexed and the superior leg elevated above the obstetrician's/midwife's neck. The lateral Sims position is frequently used when a spontaneous delivery is expected and additional perineal elasticity may be needed.

There are three delivery process techniques: spontaneous vaginal delivery, instrument-assisted vaginal delivery, and cesarean section delivery. In spontaneous delivery the presenting part is simply guided over the perineum with or without an episiotomy (incision into the perineum either obliquely or vertically) to allow additional delivery space. Instrument-assisted deliveries are of two types: (1) by the application of obstetric forceps around the face and head of the fetus, with downward traction to assist in the delivery process, and (2) by the application of a vacuum extractor device, in which negative pressure is exerted on the fetal head with downward traction to assist in the delivery process. The decision as to which of these two types should be used is based on the relative position of the presenting part (usually the vertex) in the pelvic cavity: i.e., the mid-cavity versus the outlet delivery. Engagement of the presenting part (vertex) occurs when the greatest diameter of the fetal vertex has successfully traversed the inlet of the pelvis, and generally this has occurred when the leading part of the vertex has reached the level of the interischial spinal plane. This is called *station zero*. For further reference, the point at which the fetal head is sufficiently low in the vagina to begin to distend the vulva in preparation for delivery, and the scalp is easily visible (as a 4- to 5-cm circle), is called *crowning*. When the fetal vertex is sufficiently low (usually 4 to 5 cm below the level of the ischial spine) so as to allow the easy application of forceps or a vacuum extractor, this is called an *outlet* or *low forceps* delivery. Application of the vacuum extraction apparatus or the obstetric forceps at a level between station zero and station four (4 cm below the interischial spine plane) is known as a mid-cavity forceps or mid-forceps delivery.

Deliveries that necessitate the application of the instrument at a level above station zero (floating) are *not* performed. In the past such deliveries *were* performed and were termed "high forceps." However, analysis of experience with instrument-assisted deliveries has demonstrated that the perinatal and maternal morbidity and mortality associated with high forceps deliveries is simply too great for them to be used, and a cesarean section should be performed instead. If an instrument-assisted delivery should be necessary, analysis of cumulative experience with instrument-assisted delivery of the mid-forceps and low-forceps varieties has demonstrated that there is no significant difference between the spontaneous vaginal delivery and the outlet type of instrument-assisted delivery. However, there *is* a significant increase in perinatal morbidity, mortality, and maternal morbidity with the use of mid-forceps–assisted deliveries (Friedman, 1983). It is the opinion of many skilled obstetricians that the major portion of fetal morbidity and mortality associated with the mid-forceps delivery is found in those deliveries that require considerable manipulation and, in particular, rotation of the fetal vertex and delivery from some position other than one in which a direct application of the forceps to an occiput anterior or posterior is possible.

An instrument-assisted delivery of the outlet or low type may be elected in order to shorten the second stage of labor, or it may be indicated for one of several other reasons, including inability of the mother to adequately push the baby out, fetal distress, or perhaps excessive bleeding. The decision of whether to use forceps or the vacuum extraction method to assist delivery is often based upon the obstetrician's background, training, and experience. The vacuum extractor functions by applying suction to the fetal scalp. The suction is formed under a latex or metal cup that is applied over the posterior fontanelle, with the sagittal suture pointing to the center of the cup. If the fetal occiput remains posterior or transverse, traction from the vacuum will usually allow the fetus to rotate on its own; the fetal head should *not* be rotated manually. In some cases in which there is minimal room for the application of forceps, a vacuum extraction device for delivery may be warranted. This also decreases injury to the vagina, bladder, uterus, and bowel. Since the vacuum extraction does not press on the mother, it is less painful; however, inclusion of these tissues into the cup can cause maternal trauma. This should not happen with proper application of the device.

The major disadvantage of the vacuum extractor is the development of the chignon, an edematous, occasional ecchymotic area beneath the vacuum cup. In the majority of cases, this regresses in 2 to 3 days. Small abrasions are sometimes seen around the rim of this area.

The use of the vacuum extractor has not been as popular in the United States as it has been in Europe. However, with the development of the latex cups, it has increased in popularity.

Philosophy of Labor Management

Once it has been established that a labor process is under way, the goal of the health care professional managing the labor should be to have the labor and delivery proceed as normally as possible with regard to duration, intensity, maternal and fetal responsiveness, and, of course, outcome. In other words, as long as all aspects of the labor process are normal, the health care professional managing labor simply observes and waits for delivery to occur. It is the obligation and duty of the health care professional managing the labor and delivery process to constantly evaluate and observe the labor process for abnormalities. This requires analysis, measurement, timing, and emotional and psychologic support of the parents. To provide this

Table 11–1. Patient Care Summary for Labor*

	First Stage	Second Stage	Third Stage	Fourth Stage (Postpartum)
BP, P, R	On admission; then q 1 hr	q 30 min	q 15 min	On admission; then q 15 min × 4; then q 30 min × 2; then q 1 hr until stable; then on discharge to postpartum floor
T	On admission; then q 4 hr	q 4 hr	—	On admission; then q 4 hr; then on discharge to postpartum floor
Urinalysis for protein	On admission; then with each void			
Fetal heart rate	Continuous during labor, preferably with internal monitor Without monitor, q 30 min to 1 hr, listening through 2 to 3 contractions	Continuous during labor, preferably with internal monitor Without monitor, q 5 to 10 min		
Contractions —Frequency —Duration —Quality —Resting tone	Continuous during labor, preferably with internal monitor Without monitor, q 1 hr	Continuous during labor, preferably with internal monitor Without monitor, q 15 min		
Sonogram	On admission			
Chemistry	On admission			
I&O	Each shift	Each shift	Each shift	While in recovery, note first void
Lochia				On admission; then q 15 min × 4; then q 30 min × 2; then q 1 hr until stable; on discharge to postpartum floor; then q 4–8 hr
Fundus				On admission; then q 15 min × 4; then q 30 min × 2; then q 1 hr until stable; on discharge to postpartum floor; then q 4–8 hr
H&H	On admission			Morning following delivery

*Nurse–patient ratio = 1:2.

supervision, the nurse–patient ratio should be 1:2, or 2:3 to allow for adequate labor and delivery management.

Unfortunately, not all labor processes are normal, and it is the responsibility of the health care professional to recognize when an abnormality is present and to take the appropriate medical, psychologic, pharmacologic, and if necessary, surgical measures to ensure that a healthy mother and a healthy neonate emerge from the labor process. In the past two to three decades, the significant advances made in maternal and fetal surveillance, blood banking, pharmacology (particularly antibiotics administration), and labor management have resulted in a significant decline in both maternal and fe-

tal/neonatal morbidity and mortality (Shamsi et al., 1979). There remains room for significant additional reductions in morbidity and mortality rates; however, these will be achieved only through considerable additional hard work, evaluation, and critical analysis in order to promote further refinements of management protocol that will result in improved care. As the population at large becomes more educated about health care, health professionals must strive to do even more teaching, including educating patients as much as possible in areas involving their own health care. Only by so doing can we hope to achieve the highest quality of medical care. Table 11–1 summarizes the management of the labor patient.

REFERENCES

Arey, L. B.: Developmental Anatomy, rev. 7th ed. Philadelphia, W. B. Saunders Co., 1974.

Burnhill, M. S., Danezis, J. D., and Cohen, J.: Uterine contractility during labor studies by intraamniotic fluid pressure recordings. Am. J. Obstet. Gynecol. 83:561, 1962.

Friedman, E. A.: The graphic analyses of labor. Am. J. Obstet. Gynecol. 68:1568, 1954.

Friedman, E. A.: Effects of labor and delivery procedures on the fetus. *In* Cohen, W. R., and Friedman, E. A. (eds.): Management of Labor, Baltimore, University Park Press, 1983.

Fuchs, A. R., Fuchs, F., Husslein, P., et al.: Oxytocin receptors in human parturition. Scientific Abstract #231, 28th Annual Meeting of Society for Gynecologic Investigation, San Antonio, 1981.

Garfield, R. E., and Hayashi, R. H.: A review of formation and regulation of gap junctions of myometrium during labor. Scientific Abstract #10, Society of Perinatal Obstetricians, San Antonio, 1981.

Gimovsky, M. L., Petrie, R. H., and Todd, W. D.: The neonatal performance of the term vaginal breech delivery. Obstet. Gynecol. 56:687, 1981.

Gimovsky, M. L., and Petrie, R. H.: The neonatal performance of the low birth weight vaginal breech delivery. J. Reprod. Med. 27:45, 1982.

Hall, D. G.: Serum magnesium in pregnancy. Obstet. Gynecol. 9:158, 1957.

Hartelendy, F., and Linter, F.: Myometrial $F_{2\alpha}$ receptors during pregnancy and parturition. Scientific Abstract #293, 29th Annual Meeting of Society for Gynecologic Investigation, Denver, 1982.

Huey, J. R., Jr., Al-Hadjiev, A., and Paul, R. H.: Uterine activity in the multiparous patient. Am. J. Obstet. Gynecol. 126:682, 1976.

Lederman, R. P., McCann, D. S., Work, B., Jr., et al.: Endogenous plasma epinephrine and norepinephrine in last trimester pregnancy and labor. Am. J. Obstet. Gyncol. 129:5, 1977.

Leppert, P. C., Keller, S., Cerreta, J., et al.: Elastin in the uterine cervix, its role in dilation. Dallas, Society for Gynecologic Investigation, Scientific Abstract #104, 1982.

Meyers, R. E., and Meyers, S. E.: Use of sedative, analgesic, and anesthetic drugs during labor and delivery: bane or boon? Am. J. Obstet. Gynecol. 133:83, 1979.

Miller, F. C., Yeh, S.-Y., Schifrin, B. S., et al.: Quantitation of uterine activity in 100 primiparous patients. Am. J. Obstet. Gynecol. 124:398, 1976.

Mitchell, M. D., Strickland, D. M., Brennecke, S. P., et al.: New aspects of arachidonic acid metabolism and human parturition in initiation of parturition: prevention of prematurity. Report of the Fourth Ross Conference on Obstetric Research, Columbus, OH, 1983, p. 145.

Moore, M. L.: Realities in Childbearing, 2nd ed. Philadelphia, W. B. Saunders Co., 1980.

Morishima, H. O., Pederson, H., and Fenster, M.: The influence of maternal psychological stress on the fetus. Am. J. Obstet. Gynecol. 131:899, 1978.

Nochimson, D. J., Petrie, R. H., Shah, B. L., et al.: Comparison of conservative and dynamic management of premature rupture of membranes/premature labor syndrome. Clin. Perinatol. 7:17, 1980.

Petrie, R. H.: The pharmacology and use of oxytocin. Clin. Perinatol. 8:35, 1981.

Rosengren, W. R.: Some social psychological aspects of delivery room difficulties. J. Nerv. Ment. Dis. 132:515, 1961.

Rusu, O., Lupan, C., Baltescu, V., et al.: Magneziul seric in sarcina normala la termen si nasterea permatura: rolul magneziterapiei in combatera nasterii permature. Obstetrica Si Ginecologia 14:215, 1966.

Shamsi, H. H., Petrie, R. H., and Steer, C. M.: Changing obstetrical practices and amelioration of perinatal outcome in a university hospital. Am. J. Obstet. Gynecol. 133:855, 1979.

Soloff, M. S., Schroeder, J., Chakraborty, J., et al.: Characterization of oxytocin receptors in the uterus and mammary gland. Fed. Proc. 36:1861, 1977.

Soloff, M. S., and Swartz, T. L.: Characterization of a proposed oxytocin receptor in rat mammary gland. J. Biol. Chem. 248:6471, 1973.

Yeh, S.-Y., and Read, J. A.: Management of post-term pregnancy in a large obstetric population. Obstet. Gynecol. 60:282, 1982.

12

INDUCTION OF LABOR

ROY H. PETRIE
ATHANASIA M. WILLIAMS

Until the past few years there was no scientifically valid manner of influencing the onset, the stimulation, or the suppression of labor; therefore, all gestations continued until spontaneous labor occurred and the fetus was delivered. Maternal morbidity and mortality was commonplace, and perinatal morbidity and mortality, even in the most advanced countries, was unacceptably high. Today maternal mortality has become somewhat unusual, and perinatal morbidity and mortality has generally been restricted to the very low birth-weight infant. Analyses of the obstetric practices that have produced these improvements in outcome reveal that the improvements in large part consist of a few philosophical, diagnostic, and therapeutic innovations. One of these is the ability to medically control uterine activity in order to cause the uterus either to contract and expel the fetus and/or the products of conception or to suppress uterine contractions in order to achieve an improved outcome. Thus in some instances of labor it has become medically desirable to inhibit uterine contractions, whereas in other cases it is desirable to evoke and promote uterine activity in order to affect delivery. Although there are a number of nonpharmacologic approaches to the control of uterine activity (labor), in the majority of cases control of labor is of pharmacologic origin.

Definitions

Induction of labor may be defined as the nonspontaneous initiation of uterine activity in order to provoke the onset of uterine contractions that will result in progressive cervical effacement and dilatation with de-

scent of the presenting part. Generally speaking, induction of labor is carried out near term and when there is a *medical indication* for the termination of a given gestation.

Augmentation of labor is the medical stimulation, once labor has already begun, of *additional* uterine activity in order to bring about more progressive cervical dilatation/effacement and descent of the presenting part. Almost uniformly, augmentation of labor today is of pharmacologic origin. Generally augmentation is required when there is a dysfunctional (nonprogressive) form of labor or less than the normal amount of uterine activity that is required to promote progressive cervical effacement/dilatation and descent of the presenting part.

The Physiology of Labor

A number of outstanding investigators, including Csapo, Liggins, Turnbull, MacDonald, du Vigneaud, and Karim, along with a host of other individuals who have done outstanding work, have advanced our concepts relating to the physiology and origin of labor. A great body of research has been done and is being currently performed that deals with these concepts; nevertheless, the exact origin of the onset of spontaneous labor and its exact physiology are as yet unknown. For discussion purposes, in Chapter 11 an analogy was drawn between the starting of an automobile engine and the initiation of labor. Analogies of this sort serve the purpose of clinical consideration and thinking only; however, clinical expression must be buttressed by biologic facts and concepts.

There are a number of theories, supported by a considerable body of evidence, that deal with the onset and control of labor. For example, it is known that prior to the onset of labor the maternal estrogen/progesterone ratio generally shifts in favor of estrogen. It is further known that the predominance of estrogen and the formation of the prostaglandins from arachidonic acid results in an inflammatory reaction similar to that seen with an infection (Mitchell, 1983). It is interesting to speculate that this inflammatory environment provides a biochemical-biophysical stimulus that provokes and alters action potentials that may be required to initiate the contraction of individual muscle cells.

It has been known for some time that the posterior pituitary octapeptide oxytocin causes the term or near-term uterus to respond with contractions; however, the nongravid uterus or the uterus early in gestation does not respond well at all to oxytocin administration (Petrie, 1981). The uterus growing near to term, and especially after the onset of uterine activity, becomes exquisitely sensitive to oxytocin. Oxytocin receptors in the myometrium have been identified (Soloff and Swartz, 1973; Soloff et al., 1977), and it has been demonstrated that more functional oxytocin receptors are available as pregnancy and labor progress (Fuchs et al., 1981). Concomitant with the rise in the number of oxytocin receptor sites that become available is the formation of apparent cellular communication routes or myometrial gap junctions. Garfield and Hayashi (1981) have demonstrated the specialized cell-to-cell contacts that are thought to lower impedence to current flow between cells. Gap junctions are present in increased number as parturition approaches and as labor ensues. The release of arachidonic acid from the fetal membranes and the formation of the prostaglandins, particularly the $F_{2\alpha}$ and the E_2 fractions, clearly establishes that these compounds are intimately involved as uterine stimuli in the initiation of uterine activity and the continuation of labor. Unfortunately the information dealing with the relationship of the prostaglandins and oxytocin in the initiation, maintenance, and regulation of labor is as yet unclear. Myometrial prostaglandin $F_{2\alpha}$ receptors have been identified and have been demonstrated to increase with impending parturition and with the duration of labor (Hartelendy and Linter, 1982).

It has also been demonstrated that as pregnancy progresses, serum magnesium levels fall (Hall, 1957; Rusu et al., 1966). With the onset of either preterm or term labor, a further fall in serum magnesium can be identified. Considering that the myometrial contraction can be expressed chemically in the following equation: actin + myosin + ATP + calcium yields an actin − myosin − ATP − calcium complex, or a contraction response, it is obvious that controlling calcium flow probably will enable the obstetrician to control labor. The beta$_2$-sympathomimetic agents are thought to regulate calcium by altering cyclic AMP control, and magnesium probably acts by displacing calcium.

It appears that the uterus approaching term is being prepared biochemically and physiologically to perform its contractile function. Hormone levels shift, microscopic anatomic changes occur, hormones are released, hormones are formed, the myometrium is prepared initially to act somewhat independently from a cellular level, and, as the labor process ensues, the various elements of the myometrium increasingly function in unison to produce a singular muscular effort. The exact etiology of the onset of spontaneous labor is as yet unknown; however, it is clear that there may be multiple physiologic, biochemical, and pharmacologic avenues by which labor may ensue, and accordingly, there may be multiple avenues by which the onset of uterine activity leading to labor may be blocked.

Considering the changes required to achieve active labor, it is accordingly much easier to appreciate the importance of the lesser amounts of uterine activity that are required to bring about progress of labor (see Figs. 11–11 and 11–12). The same applies to the oxytocin augmentation/induction schedules, which utilize a reduction in dosage and a lengthening in the temporal interval between the increases in doses that are subsequently recommended in this chapter. To summarize, it takes lesser amounts of uterine activity, and therefore lesser amounts of pharmacologic stimulation, to achieve the amount of cervical dilatation between 7 and 8 centimeters than it does to achieve the same amount at the earlier stage between 2 and 3 centimeters of cervical dilatation.

From a more philosophical standpoint, to what degree does the clinician really need to alter or control uterine activity or labor? Obviously the ability to provoke normal labor may be desirable in certain clinical situations. Likewise, the inhibition of labor is also desirable in some circumstances, although the true indications for the latter may be far fewer than initially suspected. An overall cost-benefit analysis with regard to the control of labor is needed each time its use is entertained.

Methods and Techniques of Labor Induction and Augmentation

Historically, four medical techniques have been used to induce or augment labor: electrical stimulation, surgical intervention, mechanical intervention, and pharmacologic administration. However, although electrical stimulation of the uterus has been used in the past to stimulate uterine activity (Waltner and Hassimi, 1966), it is seldom used in the United States today, and thus we will limit our discussion to the three methodologies currently in common use: surgical, mechanical, and pharmacologic.

SURGICAL METHODS

Surgical induction of labor is perhaps the most easy to perform of all the artificial forms of induction. When it has been established in the term gestation that there is pulmonary maturity or that the gestation should be medically terminated, the surgical rupture of membranes is followed by spontaneous uterine activity that leads to productive labor in the vast majority of instances within the first 12 to 24 hours. It is uncommon in the multiparous patient at term that this form of induction will be unsuccessful; however, in a few instances this form of labor induction may have to be supplemented by the pharmacologic approach. Generally speaking, with a favorable (ripe) cervix, the membranes are ruptured by inserting an instrument through the cervix or through an endoscope placed through the cervix. Care must be taken that a prolapsed cord does not occur; for this reason many clinicians will not rupture membranes in the presence of an unengaged presenting part. Although the success rate using the surgical induction of uterine activity to promote labor in the nulliparous patient is slightly less than for the multiparous patient, it is nonetheless frequently used because the

resultant labor is of a spontaneous nature and type (Turnbull and Anderson, 1967). The underlying theory is that with rupture of the membranes, arachidonic acid is converted into prostaglandins, which then initiate uterine activity, and once the uterine activity is initiated, it is further regulated and augmented with the release of endogenous oxytocin. Once labor is initiated, of course, no further stimulation is required. Because surgical induction of labor is an irreversible process—i.e., the rupturing of the fetal membranes, which mandates the delivery of the fetus—many clinicians are afraid to take this step, although it is a very legitimate form of labor induction.

MECHANICAL METHODS

Mechanical induction of uterine activity and labor can be achieved in several ways: (a) by mechanical stimulation of the uterus by *manual palpation*; (b) by *artificial dilatation of the cervix* with the use of laminaria or a cervical vibrator (Beard et al., 1973); and (c) by the digital separation of the membranes overlying the lower uterine segment through a process known as *digital stripping of the membranes* (Swann, 1958). Mechanical measures to induce labor have not been used extensively in the United States, because of the risk of damaging the cervix or introducing an infectious agent.

It is most likely that the digital separation of the membranes from the underlying cervix/uterus works in a manner similar to that of surgical induction of labor. It is also less successful than are other forms of induction, and it has the potential of introducing an infectious process at a time when it is not desirable or in the best interest of the patient; therefore, experienced clinicians tend to use stripping of the membranes only in those instances in which the cervix is very ripe and a short induction is anticipated (Muldoon, 1968).

The insertion of desiccated seaweed (laminaria) into the cervical canal is gaining favor in this country after reports of successful outcomes with this method from around the world (Darney, 1983). The desiccated material is packed into the cervical canal, where it absorbs fluid and slowly and progressively dilates the cervix, thereby promoting uterine activity over several hours, probably through the same mechanism as stripping of the membranes and the surgical induction of labor. Many clinicians will insert laminaria the evening before an anticipated induction the next day, in order to "prime" the cervix for rupture of the membranes and/or the infusion of a pharmacologic uterine stimulant. It must be noted, however, that there is minimal but real potential for the introduction of an unwanted infection with this method.

PHARMACOLOGIC METHODS

Whenever a pharmacologic preparation for the induction or augmentation of labor is to be used, it is necessary that a careful delivery system be employed. This requires use of a primary intravenous infusion, with all pharmacologic preparations administered as a secondary intravenous system into the first, using the "piggyback" method. This secondary IV should be inserted as close to the needle site as possible. A "Y" type insertion well above the site should not be used, as the fluid between the "Y" and the needle site contains oxytocin and would give the patient a bolus of fluid if the patient's primary IV is increased, as in the case of fetal distress. Most institutions now consider that the technique of administration of these pharmacologic preparations is of such importance that a regulated infusion system is necessary. Regulated infusion systems come in two types: a regulated drip system and a constant infusion system. The two systems are similar, but their implementation requires the use of different administrative protocols.

Before one decides which technique—surgical, mechanical, or pharmacologic—should be used to alter or control labor, it is vitally important that the condition of both the mother and the fetus be known and that both the mother and the fetus be medically able to safely undergo the proposed therapy for labor control. For every agent used, there are maternal and fetal complications and side effects. As an example, the chief side effects for both mother and fetus for oxytocin are listed in Table 12–1.

Pharmacologic uterine stimulants include the estrogens, the $F_{2\alpha}$ fraction of prostaglandins, the E_2 fraction of prostaglandins and oxytocin. The ergot alkaloids and the alkaloid tocosamine (sparteine) are such potent stimulants of the uterus that they are no longer used if a living fetus/neonate is the expected product from the labor. Intravenous infusion of large doses of estrogen to simulate the fall of progesterone will induce some uterine activity and contractions, but this infrequently provokes labor unless the cervix is very ripe, and for this reason estrogen infusions are rarely used. Other agents, such as quinine, that promote some uterine activity by stimulating surrounding organs are no longer in the medical arsenal.

The $F_{2\alpha}$ fraction of the prostaglandins has been used intravenously to promote uterine activity and labor; however, it has not received approval by the Food and Drug Administration for use for this purpose at term, because of associated side effects that include nausea, vomiting, hyperthermia, and an elevated baseline uterine pressure tone. Using a low-dose approach, some investigators have found an intravenous infusion of $F_{2\alpha}$ (Baxi et al., 1980) to be most effective. The E_2 fraction of prostaglandins has been used in a number of clinics, either administered orally (Yip et al., 1973) or applied as a local, extraamniotic cervical vaginal gel used to "prime" or pretreat for a routine induction process (Calder et al., 1974; Clarke et al., 1980).

The only agent currently approved for the induction of term labor is oxytocin. It has been known since the first decade of this century that extracts of the posterior pituitary gland had uterine stimulant properties. By the 1930s it was confirmed that there were *two* substances in the posterior pituitary extract, and subsequently these were separated. In the 1950s both vasopressin (also called antidiuretic hormone, or ADH) and oxytocin were synthesized de novo in the laboratory (du Vigneaud et al., 1953; du Vigneaud, 1956). For this work the Nobel Prize was awarded. A pure preparation of oxytocin enabled the obstetrician to use oxytocin for the augmentation or induction of uterine activity without the side effects that the original Pitressin carried as an extract of the posterior pituitary. Oxytocin is destroyed in the stomach by trypsin, and accordingly it is given as a nasal spray, a

Table 12–1. Side Effects of Oxytocin

Fetal Effects	Maternal Effects
Hyperbilirubinemia	Allergy
Hypoxia	Uterine hypertonus
Asphyxia	Uterine rupture
Death	Water intoxication
	Hypertension
	Hypotension

buccal tablet (Chalmers and Prakash, 1971), or as an intramuscular (Rysso and Kosar, 1967) or intravenous injection. Because of an erratic and unpredictable uptake and absorption, *only the intravenous infusion of oxytocin is now considered to be appropriate for the induction of term labor.* The half-life of synthetic oxytocin has been determined to be between 1 and 6 minutes in early pregnancy and between 1 and 3 minutes in late pregnancy and during lactation. The liver, kidneys, and functional mammary glands remove oxytocin from the plasma. Oxytocinase has been found in plasma, and it inactivates oxytocin by breaking the cystine-tyrosine bond in oxytocin (Petrie, 1981).

Table 12–2 provides an oxytocin infusion schedule for augmentation and induction of labor utilizing a Harvard pump. For convenience, the infusion rates using milliunits per minute and the approximate equivalent number of drops per minute and cc per hour are included. Note that two different standard solutions—10 international units (IU) per 250 milliters of intravenous solution and 15 IU per 250 milliliters of intravenous solution—are used; this is in order to obtain flexibility of doses delivered at the greater dosage schedule. For those using an infusion pump such as the Sigma 5000, oxytocin protocols are given in Table 12–3. Once again, in order to provide flexibility of infusion rates, two different stock solutions are used and two schedules are provided. Note that the 1:4 diluted stock solution gives the greatest flexibility of doses delivered in the lower dosage ranges. The clinical goal with oxytocin induction/augmentation is to simulate a normal labor pattern—i.e., contractions every 2 to 3 minutes, lasting 40 to 90 seconds at an intensity of 40 to 90 mm Hg (torr)—and provide adequate progress of

labor. It is relatively easy to exceed the optimal oxytocin dose range. A summary of the factors involved in oxytocin administration is given in Table 12–4.

Based on the recent work of a number of investigators (Baxi et al., 1980; Seitchik and Castillo, 1983), a schedule of increasing the dose of oxytocin delivered that employs an interval between the increasing dose rate of between 45 minutes and 1 hour is provided (see Table 12–3). Studies on the use of such a schedule have shown that most patients undergoing oxytocin induction or augmentation of labor will generate sufficient uterine activity to bring about progress of labor with use of a mean dose of 4 to 5 mU/min, and that the majority of patients will respond appropriately to doses of 8 mU/min or less. Using this slower temporal and low-dose approach for augmentation and induction of labor, minimal cervical change may be noted during the first few hours of induction; however, quite frequently the active phase of labor will be reached after a few hours and then proceed at a normal to slightly accelerated pace. Quite frequently during an induction of labor, once the patient has reached 4 to 5 cm of cervical dilatation, the oxytocin infusion can be reduced or eliminated, and labor will proceed without further pharmacologic stimulation; likewise, frequently augmentation of labor with oxytocin will proceed well with the use of very minimal (less than 2 mU/min) doses of oxytocin. Frequently when an adequate labor has been established, an augmentation infusion can be discontinued altogether. It should be noted that in some cases when the uterus is not properly prepared for labor by whatever unknown mechanisms may be involved, doses of oxytocin of 10 to 20 mU/min (or even higher) may be

Table 12–2. Administration Using an Oxytocin Infusion Pump (Harvard) for Augmentation and Induction (30-ml Syringe Only)

10 IU Oxytocin/250 ml IV Solution		Setting Number	15 IU Oxytocin/250 ml IV Solution	
Milliunits	Approximate Equivalent in Drops/Minute		Milliunits	Approximate Equivalent Drops/Minute (and cc/hour)
0.2 mU/min	—	12	0.35 mU/min	— (0.35 cc/hr)
0.5 mU/min	—	11	0.75 mU/min	1.5 gtt/min (0.75 cc/hr)
1.0 mU/min	2 gtt/min	10	1.50 mU/min	3.0 gtt/min (1.50 cc/hr)
2.0 mU/min	4 gtt/min	9	3.50 mU/min	6.0 gtt/min (3.50 cc/hr)
5.0 mU/min	8 gtt/min	8	7.50 mU/min	12.0 gtt/min (7.50 cc/hr)
10.0 mU/min	16 gtt/min	7	15.00 mU/min	24.0 gtt/min (15.00 cc/hr)
20.0 mU/min	32 gtt/min	6	35.00 mU/min	56.0 gtt/min (35.00 cc/hr)
50.0 mU/min	80 gtt/min	5	75.00 mU/min	120.0 gtt/min (75.00 cc/hr)

Table 12–3. Sigma 5000 Oxytocin Infusion Protocols for Augmentation or Induction of Labor Using Measured-Volume Burette Sets

I. Preparation of Undiluted Stock Solution
   A. Add 30 IU of oxytocin (3 vials) to 500 cc of D5W or RL
      This is the stock solution—60 mU/ml.
   B. Carefully label as "Stock Solution Oxytocin 60 mU/ml."

II. Dilution of Stock Solution 1:4
   A. Make a label "Diluted Oxytocin 1:4 (15 mU/ml)" and place it on the burette.
   B. Run 10 ml of stock solution into the burette. *Do not fill IV tubing with the original undiluted stock solution.*
   C. Add 30 ml of fresh D5W or RL to the burette to make a total volume of 40 ml. This is the stock solution diluted 1:4 (15 mU/ml).

Infusion Schedule #1—Diluted 1:4 stock solution of oxytocin (15 mU/ml)
A. Fill the IV tubing with the diluted 1:4 stock solution.
B. Insert the IV tubing into the Sigma 5000, following the instructions printed on the pump.
C. Insert the IV tubing into the main infusion line as a "piggyback" at the infusion site nearest the needle insertion.

To Administer:

Milliunits	*Approximate Equivalent in Drops/Minute* (10 IU/1000 ml)	*Toggle in this Flow Rate:*
0.25 mU/min	—	1 ml/hr
0.50 mU/min	1 gtt/min	2 ml/hr
1.00 mU/min	2 gtt/min	4 ml/hr
2.00 mU/min	4 gtt/min	8 ml/hr
2.50 mU/min	5 gtt/min	10 ml/hr
3.50 mU/min	6 gtt/min	14 ml/hr
5.00 mU/min	8 gtt/min	20 ml/hr
7.50 mU/min	12 gtt/min	30 ml/hr
10.00 mU/min	16 gtt/min	40 ml/hr
15.00 mU/min	24 gtt/min	60 ml/hr
20.00 mU/min	32 gtt/min	80 ml/hr
25.00 mU/min	40 gtt/min	100 ml/hr

After toggling in the correct infusion rate on the Sigma 5000 pump, set the total volume to be infused, press the reset total volume button, and start the pump.

Infusion Schedule #2—Undiluted Stock Solution of Oxytocin (60 mU/ml)
The undiluted stock solution may be used for infusion rates of 1.0 mU/min or greater.
A. Disconnect the "piggyback" IV tubing from the patient.
B. Empty the burette and tubing of any remaining diluted stock solution 1:4. Remove the "Diluted Stock Solution" label from the burette.
C. Make a new label "Stock Solution Oxytocin 60 mU/ml" and place it on the burette.
D. Fill the burette and IV tubing with the undiluted stock solution (60 mU/ml).
E. Connect the IV tubing to the patient's main infusion line as a "piggyback" at the site nearest the needle insertion point.

To Administer:

Milliunits	*Approximate Equivalent in Drops/Minute* (10 IU/1000 ml)	*Toggle in this Flow Rate:*
1.0 mU/min	2 gtt/min	1 ml/hr
2.0 mU/min	4 gtt/min	2 ml/hr
3.0 mU/min	6 gtt/min	3 ml/hr
5.0 mU/min	8 gtt/min	5 ml/hr
7.0 mU/min	12 gtt/min	7 ml/hr
10.0 mU/min	16 gtt/min	10 ml/hr
15.0 mU/min	24 gtt/min	15 ml/hr
20.0 mU/min	32 gtt/min	20 ml/hr
25.0 mU/min	40 gtt/min	25 ml/hr
30.0 mU/min	48 gtt/min	30 ml/hr
35.0 mU/min	56 gtt/min	35 ml/hr
40.0 mU/min	64 gtt/min	40 ml/hr
45.0 mU/min	72 gtt/min	45 ml/hr
50.0 mU/min	80 gtt/min	50 ml/hr

After toggling in appropriate infusion rate on the Sigma 5000 Pump, set the total volume to be infused, press the reset total volume button, and start the pump.

Table 12–4. Medication Summary for Induction of Labor*

Medication	Action	Route	Dose	Pregnancy Precautions	Maternal Side Effects	Nursing Considerations	Fetal/Neonatal Considerations	Breast-Feeding
Oxytocin	Appears to act primarily on uterine myofibril activity by increasing the permeability of the cell membrane to sodium ions, therefore increasing uterine contractility	IV with constant infusion pump	0.25 mU/min Double dose q 45–60 min (after 8 mU, increase at 1 mU q 45 min) until adequate contraction pattern is established (q 2–3 min lasting 45–90 sec with 50–80 torr amplitude & ≤20 torr resting tone) Be prepared to reduce dosage or discontinue in active phase labor Discontinue with fetal distress or hyperstimulation	Contraindications: 1. Significant cephalopelvic disproportion 2. Unfavorable fetal positions or presentations that are undeliverable without conversion prior to delivery. 3. When the benefit-to-risk ratio for either the fetus or mother favors surgical intervention 4. Fetal distress when delivery not imminent 5. Hypertonic uterine patterns	Uterine hyper-stimulation Uterine rupture Water intoxication	Oxytocin should not be given simultaneously by more than one route. Incompatible with: fibrolysis; levarterenol bitartrate; prochlorperazine edisylate; protein hydrolysate; warfarin sodium. Compatibility with other IV fluids may be influenced by drug concentration, pH, and other factors. Monitor maternal vital signs every 15 to 30 min; monitor fetal heart rate and uterine activity q 15 min, preferably with internal monitoring. Do not freeze. Hourly I & O. Discontinue if contractions (1) occur less than 2 minutes apart, or (2) last longer than 90 seconds. May cause severe hypertension if given within 3–4 hours of vasoconstriction in patients receiving caudal anesthetic	Prematurity Fetal distress	No known contra-indications

*Nurse–patient ratio = 1:2

required to effectively stimulate adequate labor. It should also be noted that any time a labor is being induced or augmented by *any* means, including pharmacologic uterine stimulants such as oxytocin, great attention must be paid to how well the fetus is tolerating the stresses of labor. Primarily this is accomplished by external or preferably internal fetal heart rate and uterine activity monitoring and by appropriate backup fetal surveillance based on acid-base determinations whenever fetal heart rate data do not completely reassure the obstetrician of fetal well-being.

Before the induction of labor is begun, it is essential to check the working condition of the infusion pump. Once this is done, the induction may proceed by slowly increasing the amount of medication administered. Careful observation of the patient is necessary in order to ascertain whether the medication should be increased or kept at the present dosage. Since every individual has different responses to drugs, no fixed dose of medication can be given. It is important to administer the oxytocin by secondary infusion, so that if one creates a hypertonic response in the uterus or if fetal bradycardia or decelerations occur, the infusion can very simply and quickly be discontinued. One should always have magnesium sulfate and/or other tocolytic agents readily available during an induction of labor in case hypertonicity occurs.

Oxytocin has a weak antidiuretic effect. This could cause water intoxication in the mother if a large volume of fluid is given during oxytocin administration. Therefore, unnecessary fluids should not be given, and a careful intake and output assessment should be made. The patient's fluid intake should be kept to 1000 ml per 8-hour shift, unless the patient is dehydrated.

In an induction of labor, it is of utmost importance to allay the fears of the patient. Many patients feel that induced labor is "unnatural" and have been told by other women that induction causes a much more severe labor than would occur naturally. It should be explained to any patient who expresses these fears that induced labor is not really stronger than "natural" labor, it is only the way in which labor progresses that is different. In spontaneous labor the uterus slowly contracts in an irregular mild pattern, building up to strong regular contractions, thereby allowing the patient to gradually get used to and cope with the intensity and duration of the contractions. However, in induced labor, this prodromal, early form of labor does not exist with many induction techniques, and the patient may progress from complete absence of discomfort to strong active labor. This sudden sensation of pain tends to frighten a patient and cause her a great deal of difficulty in managing to control herself during the labor process. If a patient is aware that this will occur, she can better prepare herself for the onset of the active phase of labor.

It is important to keep the patient assessed of all progress being made during labor, so that she will be encouraged to continue dealing with the contractions, thereby facilitating the advancement of the fetus. The patient should be made aware that natural childbirth is still possible in induced labor; however, as in spontaneous labor, once a regular active pattern of contractions is achieved, the option of analgesia or anesthesia should be offered.

The necessity for the medical induction or augmentation of labor does not terminate with the delivery of the fetus/neonate. During the so-called fourth stage of labor, which includes 1 or 2 hours following delivery, the use of pharmacologic preparations to bring about sufficient uterine contractions to close the uterine sinuses and inhibit excessive blood loss from the uterus is almost essential for the proper management of some patients. Almost routinely, in order to promote effective uterine contractions, intramuscular or intravenous oxytocin is administered just as the fetus is delivered or immediately following the delivery of the placenta. When the intravenous form of oxytocin is administered, great care must be taken to avoid the direct administration of large doses of oxytocin, because of the potential for hypotension and shock (Hendricks and Brenner, 1970). Generally 10 to 30 IU of oxytocin are added to 1000 ml of an electrolyte-containing solution, and the infusion is administered at 100 to 150 ml/hr. More oxytocin may be added to the intravenous solution as needed, or it may be given intramuscularly.

In cases in which the uterus does not contract appropriately (atony), more potent uterine stimulants may be required. Ergonovine and methylergonovine maleate may be administered intramuscularly or on occasion intravenously. The dosage is generally 0.2 mg, and this dosage may be repeated one or two times as necessary. Because of the potential of these alkaloids to provoke hypertensive states, they are not commonly used in patients with elevated blood pressure. In extreme instances of postpartum hemorrage, the use of prostaglandin preparations for injection directly into the myometrium is suggested by some authors (Tropper and Petrie, 1983). A summary of patient treatment is given in Table 12–5.

Failure of a Pharmacologic Agent to Induce or Augment Labor

When oxytocin fails to adequately induce or augment labor, several questions must be addressed. If the induction has not involved rupture of the membranes, is it wise to wait and attempt the induction the following day, or is it better to proceed with surgical rupture of the membranes in order to determine if this will augment the induction effort? With ruptured membranes and an attempt to induce labor, most obstetricians will consider the presence of good contractions (i.e., 40 to 80 mm Hg in intensity, lasting 40 to 90 seconds every 2 to 3 minutes) for a period of 8 to 12 hours as an adequate trial of labor before resorting to cesarean section.

The concept of attempting to shorten the latent phase of labor by either amniotomy or the use of oxytocin is a controversial one; however, some authorities feel that neither may be very effective, whereas others feel that oxytocin is of some benefit. Once the latent phase of labor has reached approximately 20 hours, many clinicians feel that an attempt should be made to achieve active-phase labor by means of intravenous oxyto-cin augmentation. Although the concept and ideas regarding latent-phase labor may vary from physician to physician, from institution to institution, and from patient to patient, most clinicians feel that an attempt of between 6 and 12 hours of adequate uterine activity augmentation is needed before resorting to delivery by cesarean section.

Although some variation of opinion may exist, most clinicians feel that arrest of labor of 4 hours' duration in the midst of the active phase of labor, with the membranes ruptured and adequate uterine activity that would normally bring about progress of labor, is sufficient indication for a cesarean section to be performed. Some variation is allowed with regard to the patient's parity, with 3 to 4 hours of lack of progress in the active phase considered an indication for cesarean delivery in the multipara, while 4 to 5 hours may be allowed in the nullipara before proceeding to cesarean section. Figure 12–1 shows the labor curve of a multipara who has experienced an arrest of labor in the active phase. The patient has intact membranes, and evaluation of uterine activity demonstrates that a subnormal amount of uterine activity has been generated. After appropriate evaluation, augmentation of the labor was begun with intravenous oxytocin. Figure 12–2 is the labor curve of a multipara undergoing induction of labor for prolonged rupturing of the membranes. Although a normal amount of uterine activity has been generated, there is an arrest of labor in the active phase, and delivery will be accomplished by cesarean section in this patient,

Table 12–5. Patient Care Summary for Induction of Labor*

	Intrapartum	Postpartum
BP, P, R	On admission; then q 15 min while increasing dose q 30 min on maintenance dose	On admission to RR; then q 15 min × 4; then q 30 min × 2; then q 1 hr until stable; on discharge to PP floor; then follow normal PP routine
T	On admission; then q 4 hr; q hr with ROM	On admission to RR; then q 4 hr; then on discharge to PP floor
Fetal monitoring	Continuous during labor, preferably internal Without monitor, q 10 to 15 min, listening through 2 to 3 contractions	—
Contractions Duration Frequency Quality Resting tone	Continuous during labor, preferably internal monitoring Without monitoring, q 10 to 15 min	—
I & O	q 8 hr (observed for water intoxication)	—

*Nurse–patient ratio = 1:2

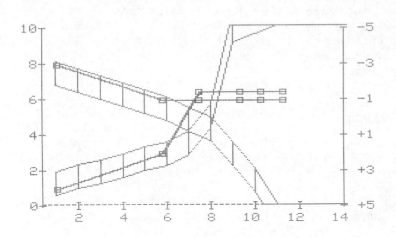

STANDARD FRIEDMAN CURVES

Figure 12–1. Labor curve for a multipara with inadequate uterine activity to effect progress of labor. If an evaluation of the patient warrants it, oxytocin will be used to achieve sufficient uterine activity to produce progress of labor. Should an amniotomy be performed or oxytocin be used, the computer will then select a different projected labor curve for the expected progress of labor. The lines connecting the boxes represent the patient's actual dilatation and station changes. The wide bands are the new projected labor and station curves using standard deviation. (Courtesy of Henry R. Rey and Dr. Roy H. Petrie, Columbia University, New York.)

for whom a clinical diagnosis of cephalopelvic disproportion has been made.

Effects of Other Pharmacologic Agents on Uterine Activity and Labor

The principles of the primary pharmacologic agents that are currently used to control uterine activity have been discussed; however, almost any pharmacologic agent used in labor has the potential for affecting uterine activity and labor. Some agents, such as the local anesthetics, may either increase or decrease uterine activity depending on the patient's gravidity, the dosage and mode of administration of the agent, and the timing of its administration within labor itself.

Many drugs given as an intravenous bolus will provoke a temporary increase in uterine activity. Some drugs, such as Nisentil (alphaprodine HCl), may initially increase uterine activity only to decrease it later from the same injection (Petrie et al., 1976); thus, whenever one is managing or controlling labor, great care must be exercised in administering pharmacologic agents, so that undesirable results are avoided.

In some instances, depending on the pharmacologic agent used and the timing of its administration, one may effectively control uterine activity and yet promote the progress of labor. For example, studies quantitating uterine activity have shown that although meperidine (Demerol) may decrease uterine activity, when the agent is administered in

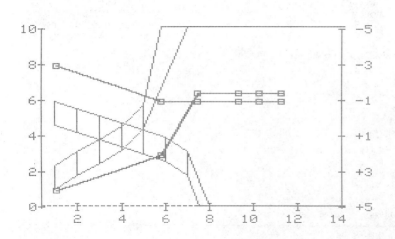

STANDARD FRIEDMAN CURVES

Figure 12–2. Labor curve for a multipara with adequate uterine activity to effect progress of labor, which has been stimulated with oxytocin. There has been an arrest of labor in the active phase for 4 hours. Delivery will be accomplished by cesarean section. The lines connecting the boxes represent the patient's actual dilatation and station changes. The wide bands indicate standard deviation for dilatation and station. (Courtesy of Henry R. Rey and Dr. Roy H. Petrie, Columbia University, New York.)

the early to mid-active phase of labor, sufficient relaxation, through the relief of pain and perhaps the diminution of the release of catecholamines, may actually result in greater *effectiveness* of the uterine activity that is generated, thus providing greater progress in labor as measured by the degree of cervical dilatation/effacement with descent of the presenting part. Recall the concept from Chapter 11 that less uterine activity is required to achieve a centimeter of cervical dilatation later in labor than in the early stages. Generally, tranquilizing agents tend to suppress uterine activity, perhaps by mechanisms that are the same as or similar to alcohol—that is, by decreasing the outflow of oxytocin as well as having a general sedative effect. However, Shepard and coworkers have demonstrated an agent such as Dramamine (dimenhydrinate) as oxytocin-like uterine stimulant properties, especially when given as an intravenous bolus (Shephard et al., 1976). Similarly, some agents that independently have a tendency to decrease uterine activity when given alone, may actually increase uterine activity when administered in combination, particularly as an intravenous bolus injection (Riffel et al., 1973). The use of meperidine and Phenergan (promethazine HCl) as a combination intravenous injection has been demonstrated to do exactly this. Patients who are being treated for preeclampsia with an anticonvulsant such as magnesium sulfate have been noted to have longer labors and require augmentation of labor in a greater than normal percentage of cases (Hall et al., 1959). Patients with asthma who are using a beta$_2$-sympathomimetic agent may also require the use of oxytocin augmentation to bring about effective labor, inasmuch as the beta$_2$ agent may be acting on uterine smooth muscle as well as on the bronchial smooth muscle.

EVALUATION OF THE PATIENT

The obstetrician who is considering using labor control or manipulation must take into account one factor above all others: to wit, a detailed cost-benefit analysis must indicate that the patient and her fetus would be more likely to be benefited than harmed by artificial control of labor. In other words, before attempting to control uterine activity and/or labor there should be a good medical indication for inducing labor. Not only is it a consensus, but it has been mandated by the Food and Drug Administration (Postotnik, 1978) that oxytocin should be utilized for the induction of labor *only* when there is a *medical* indication to induce labor. Accordingly, the same can be said for the use of oxytocin to augment labor.

The practice of obstetrics has seen more changes in the past two decades than in the previous few centuries. Accordingly, the indications for the induction and/or augmentation of labor are not static but dynamic, and are usually relative; nevertheless, there do exist uniformly accepted indications for the induction of labor. Generally speaking, situations in which the mother and/or fetus would be best served from a medical standpoint by accomplishing delivery warrant the induction of labor, provided the uterus is sufficiently receptive to the induction technique to be used and the fetus is sufficiently able to tolerate labor. It must be emphasized that this indication does *not* include the *elective* induction of labor for the convenience of the patient or her physician. A judicious weighing of the pros and cons is necessary in situations that do not represent either absolute medical indications or absolute nonindications. For example, the induction of labor in a multiparous patient who has a history of short labors with well-controlled hypertension and who lives some 2 hours from the hospital may appear to be a convenience type of induction of labor when actually there may be reasonable justification to induce labor, particularly in the presence of favorable physical findings indicating that a labor could be accomplished easily.

Using the same philosophical approach as in determining whether to induce labor, the decision to augment labor should not be undertaken without a good indication. Generally speaking, the medical indication for the augmentation of labor is based on lack of progress in labor in the presence of subnormal amounts of uterine activity. Whenever labor is induced or augmented, careful attention must be paid to the fetal response to the additional potential insult of increased uterine activity.

Once the decision has been reached to induce labor, certain criteria should be met *before* the actual induction is carried out, in order to ensure that everything possible has been done to anticipate and, where possible, avoid problems that may be encountered during the induction of labor. These considerations may vary from one institution to another, but for the most part the following criteria must be met:

- Data supporting fetal pulmonary maturity and/or a medical indication that the benefit of a premature delivery will outweigh the possible risk associated with prematurity
- Absence of fetal distress
- Absence of absolute cephalopelvic disproportion
- Absence of overdistention of the uterus with a multiple gestation or hydramnios
- Absence of vaginal bleeding from placenta previa, abruptio placenta, or vasa previa
- Absence of a uterine scar
- Absence of an unfavorable presentation or position of the fetus
- Absence of grand multiparity
- Absence of uterine trauma and/or past infection
- A fetal weight that is not estimated to be excessive for the maternal pelvis
- An evaluation of the cervix (Bishop's score) (Table 12–6) that is diagnostic of a successful outcome.

Many of the considerations to be met for the induction of labor also apply to the augmentation of labor. The primary consideration in any case in which progress is not being made in the active phase of labor is to determine whether cephalopelvic disproportion is the cause. The belief of many obstetricians that it is prudent to attempt to shorten a prolonged latent phase of labor (20 hours or more) by using intravenous oxytocin before the 20th hour is still open to question; nevertheless, a number of authorities believe that, particularly in the presence of ruptured membranes, oxytocin should be utilized in an attempt to reach the active phase of labor.

Central in any equation to consider induction or augmentation of labor is the concept of cervical ripeness or maturity. While biologic and biochemical considerations are the basic criteria used in determining uterine preparation for labor, clinical evaluation of the cervix adds considerably to the overall concept of labor control, as does any history of the prior performance of a patient in labor. A careful evaluation of the cervix for its general position in relation to the long axis of the vagina, its dilatation, its effacement, its consistency, and the station and position of the presenting parts are all vitally important in making an accurate assessment for the induction and/or augmentation of labor. Inasmuch as many of these factors are somewhat difficult to express scientifically and it is important to communicate accurate information from one individual to the next, a system whereby cervical ripeness may be objectively evaluated has been developed by Bishop (Bishop, 1964) and is shown in Table 12–6.

Philosophical Considerations in the Control of Labor

The techniques to induce or augment uterine activity are tools available to the obstetrician to attempt to improve outcome in terms of morbidity and mortality for both the fetus/neonate and the mother. The old adage of "for every advantage there is a disadvantage" applies to the control of labor. The techniques and pharmacologic agents used to achieve desired results are often potent and accordingly have potential side effects, with which the obstetrician and medical staff involved must be completely familiar, in order to anticipate and avoid problems. Likewise, artificial induction and control of labor requires careful surveillance

Table 12–6. Bishop Score

Component	Points*			
	0	1	2	3
Cervical dilatation (cm)	0	1–2	3–4	5–6
Cervical effacement (%)	0–30	31–50	51–70	>70
Cervical consistency	Firm	Medium	Soft	—
Cervical position	Posterior	Mid	Anterior	—
Station	−5/−3	−2	−1	+1/+2

*Total score of 0–5 points = easy induction; 6–13 = difficult induction.
*Adapted from Bishop, E. H.: Pelvic scoring for elective induction. Obstet. Gynecol. 24:266, 1964.

of both mother and fetus, in order to ensure an optimal outcome.

In all probability our current approach to the control of labor still leaves much room for improvement, and current protocol concepts and techniques will need to be altered as we become more knowledgeable about the labor process itself and additional pharmacologic agents become available. An overall analysis of this medical endeavor indicates that considerable research from both a basic and a clinical standpoint will be needed before the clinician who is involved in controlling labor can be completely comfortable.

REFERENCES

Baxi, L. V., Petrie, R. H., and Caritis, S. N.: Induction of labor with low dose PFG$_{2a}$ and oxytocin. Am. J. Obstet. Gynecol. 136:28, 1980.

Beard, R., Boyd, I., and Holt, E.: A study of cervical vibration in induced labor. J. Obstet. Gynaecol. Br. Commonw. 80:9, 1973.

Bishop, E. H.: Pelvic scoring for elective induction. Obstet. Gynecol. 24:266, 1964.

Calder, A. A., Embray, M. P., and Hillier, K.: Extraamniotic PGE$_2$ for the induction of labour at term. J. Obstet. Gynaecol. Br. Commonw. 81:39, 1974.

Chalmers, J. A., and Prakash, A.: Optimal dosage of buccal oxytocin for the induction of labor. Am. J. Obstet. Gynecol. 111:227, 1971.

Clarke, G. A., Letchworth, A. T., and Noble, A. D.: Comparative trial of extraamniotic and vaginal prostaglandin E$_2$ in tylogel for induction of labor. J. Perin. Med. 8:23, 1980.

Darney, P. D.: What's the status of laminaria and other cervical dilators? Contemp. Obstet. Gynecol. 21: 209, 1983.

du Vigneaud, V., Ressler, C., Swan, J. M., et al.: The synthesis of an octapeptide amide with the hormonal activity of oxytocin:enzymatic cleavage of glycinamide from vasopressin and a proposed structure for the pressor-antidiuretic hormone of the posterior pituitary. J. Am. Chem. Soc. 75:4879, 1953.

du Vigneaud, V.: The isolation and proof of structure of the vasopressins and the synthesis of octapeptide amides with pressor-antidiuretic activity. In Liebecq, C. (ed.): Proceedings of the Third International Congress on Biochemistry, New York, Academic Press, 1956.

Fuchs, A.-R., Fuchs, F. Husslein, P., et al.: Oxytocin receptors in human parturition. Scientific Abstract #231, 28th Annual Meeting of Society for Gynecologic Investigation, San Antonio, 1981.

Garfield, R. E., and Hayashi, R. H.: A review of formation and regulation of gap junctions of myometrium during labor. Scientific Abstract #10, Society of Perinatal Obstetricians, San Antonio, 1981.

Hall, D. G.: Serum magnesium in pregnancy. Obstet. Gynecol. 9:158, 1957.

Hall, D. G., McGaughey, H. S., Corey, E. L., et al.: The effects of magnesium sulfate therapy on the duration of labor. Am. J. Obstet. Gynecol. 78:27, 1959.

Hartelendy, F., and Linter, F.: Myometrial F$_{2\alpha}$ receptors during pregnancy and parturition. Scientific Abstract #293, 29th Annual Meeting of Society of Gynecologic Investigation, Denver, 1982.

Hendricks, C. H., and Brenner, W. E.: Cardiovascular effects of oxytocic drugs used postpartum. Am. J. Obstet. Gynecol. 108:751, 1970.

Mitchell, M. D., Strickland, D. M., Brennecke, S. P., et al.: New aspects of arachidonic acid metabolism and human parturition in initiation of parturition: prevention of prematurity. Report of the Fourth Ross Conference on Obstetric Research, Columbus, OH, 1983, p. 145.

Muldoon, M. J.: A prospective study of intrauterine infection following surgical induction of labor. Journal of Obstetrics and Gynaecology of the British Commonwealth. 75:1144, 1968.

Petrie, R. H., Wu, R., Miller, F. C., et al.: Effects of drugs on uterine activity. Obstet. Gynecol. 48:431, 1976.

Petrie, R. H.: The pharmacology and use of oxytocin. Clin. Perinatol. 8:35, 1981.

Postotnik, P.: Drugs and pregnancy. FDA Consumer 12:7, 1978.

Riffel, H. D., Nochimson, D. J., Paul, R. H., et al.: Effects of meperidine and promethazine during labor. Obstet. Gynecol. 42:738, 1973.

Rusu, O., Lupan, C., Baltescu, V., et al.: Magneziul seric in sarcina normala la termen si nasterea permature: rolul magneziterapiei in combatera nasterii permature. Obstetrica Si Ginecologia 14:215, 1966.

Rysso, J. N., and Kosar, W. P.: The use of intramuscular oxytocin for the elective induction of labor. Am. J. Obstet. Gynecol. 97:203, 1967.

Seitchik, J., and Castillo, M.: Oxytocin augmentation of dysfunctional labor. II. Uterine data. Am. J. Obstet. Gynecol. 145:526, 1983.

Shephard, B., Cruz, A., and Spellacy, N.: The acute effects of dramamine on uterine contractility during labor. J. Reprod. Med. 16:27, 1976.

Soloff, M. S., and Swartz, T. L.: Characterization of a proposed oxytocin receptor in rat mammary gland. J. Biol. Chem. 248:6471, 1973.

Soloff, M. S., Schroeder, J., Chakraborty, J., et al.: Characterization of oxytocin receptors in the uterus and mammary gland. Fed. Proc. 36:1861, 1977.

Swann, R.: Induction of labor by stripping membranes. Obstet. Gynecol. 11:74, 1958.

Tropper, P. J., and Petrie, R. H.: Current management of postpartum hemorrhage. In Quilligan, E. J. (ed.): Current Therapy in Obstetrics and Gynecology, 2nd ed. Philadelphia, W. B. Saunders Co., 1983, pp. 87–89.

Turnbull, A. C., and Anderson, A. B. M.: Induction of labour. I. Amniotomy. J. Obstet. Gynaecol. Br. Commonw. 74:849, 1967.

Waltnar, R., and Hassimi, M.: Electrical current for induction or augmentation of labor. Am. J. Obstet. Gynecol. 105:220, 1966.

Yip, S. K., Ma, H. K., and Ng, K. H.: Induction of labour with oral prostaglandin E$_2$. J. Obstet. Gynaecol. Br. Commonw. 80:442, 1973.

13

FETAL DISTRESS

CYDNEY I. AFRIAT
FRANK C. MILLER

The ability to predict the condition of the fetus prior to birth has been a goal of obstetricians for decades. The traditional methods for detecting fetal distress during labor include the appearance of meconium in the amniotic fluid and auscultation of fetal heart rate. However, during the past 20 years, electronic fetal heart pattern monitoring and analysis of fetal blood pH have become successful tools in the assessment of fetal condition.

Perinatal Mortality and Morbidity

During the past three decades, perinatal mortality and morbidity have steadily declined, although no one factor can be isolated as the reason. Perinatal mortality has fallen from 32.5/1000 in 1950 to 14.6/1000 in 1978 (Table 13–1).

Duration of pregnancy and intrauterine growth are major determinants in infant mortality and morbidity. Both of these factors are reflected in the infant's weight. The lower the birth weight, the greater the chances for death, serious congenital anomalies, or other severe impairments. Despite very little change in birth weight in the United States, the infant mortality rate has decreased. This reduction in mortality may be attributed in large part to major advances in neonatal intensive care and also to more careful intrapartum fetal management.

Methods of Detection of Fetal Distress

The incidence of meconium passage in utero is approximately 3 to 5 percent until term, at which time it increases to approximately 10 to 12 percent. Postterm fetuses (gestational age 42 weeks or greater) pass meconium prior to delivery as frequently as 40 to 44 percent of the time.

The reliability of meconium passage as an indicator of fetal distress has been questioned. Low 5-minute Apgar scores are found in only approximately 10 percent of cases in which meconium has been passed. Indeed, in more than 90 percent of the cases in which meconium is present, the Apgar

Table 13–1. Perinatal Mortality (per 1000 Cases)

| | Neonatal | | | |
	Under 28 Days	Under 7 Days	Late Fetal Mortality Rate	Perinatal Mortality Rate
1950	20.5	17.8	14.9	32.5
1955	19.1	17.0	12.9	29.7
1960	18.7	16.7	12.1	28.6
1965	17.7	15.9	11.9	27.6
1970	15.1	13.6	9.5	23.0
1975	11.6	10.0	7.8	17.7
1978	9.5	8.0	6.6	14.6

Vital Statistics of the United States, Vol. II, 1950–1978. Public Health Service. Government Printing Office, Washington, D.C.

score is greater than or equal to 7. However, meconium passage in association with abnormal heart rate patterns, specifically late decelerations, and/or a pH less than 7.25 does increase the risk of delivering an asphyxiated infant.

Because of this increased incidence of perinatal asphyxia in the presence of meconium, two clinical interventions are recommended. At the first recognition of meconium, a direct fetal heart rate electrode is placed in order to accurately assess fetal heart rate patterns and variability. If the pattern is without periodic changes and the variability is average, labor continues as normal, for such an infant falls in the 90 percent group with good outcome. However, since the risk of meconium aspiration syndrome at birth still exists, a second clinical intervention is advised, as follows: With the delivery of the head, but before the thorax is delivered, the mother is instructed to stop pushing while the clinician suctions the fetal mouth and nose with a DeLee suction catheter. After the birth is complete, careful attention is given to avoid stimulation of the infant. The infant is then handed directly to the waiting pediatrician for visualization of the vocal cords by direct laryngoscopy. If meconium is present at the cords, direct suctioning of the trachea with a DeLee catheter or mouth endotracheal tube is performed (Carson et al., 1976). However, appropriate suctioning of the infant *before* the delivery of the thorax will usually eliminate the need for tracheal suctioning. This procedure of suctioning by the obstetrician (or obstetric assistant) significantly reduces the incidence of meconium aspiration syndrome and effectively prevents severe disease (Carson et al., 1976).

AUSCULTATION

Auscultation of the fetal heart was first described by Mayo in 1818. In 1822, Kergaradec, using a stethoscope, suggested that "perhaps it will be possible to judge the state of health or disease of the fetus from variations that occur in the beat of its heart." In 1893, Von Winckel defined criteria of fetal distress as a fetal heart rate above 160 or below 120.

Clinicians have long been aware that intermittent auscultation of the fetal heart could not reliably diagnose fetal asphyxia.

In 1968 Benson and coworkers studied the utility of auscultation of fetal heart rate in their Collaborative Perinatal Study and concluded that "no reliable single auscultatory indicator of fetal distress exists in terms of fetal heart rate, save in an extreme degree."

One suspected reason for this inaccuracy may be that the auscultation period is usually relatively brief, varying from 15 seconds to 1 minute every 30 minutes to 1 hour during the first stage of labor and every 5 minutes during the second stage of labor. At best, one is listening for 1 out of 5 minutes— i.e., only 20 percent of the time. Additionally, there is a considerable degree of listener bias. There is an unconscious tendency for the listener to perceive the fetal heart rate as "normal" in cases in which it is actually outside the normal range.

Despite these limitations, Haverkamp reported a study of 485 high-risk patients in labor in which the effectiveness of intermittent auscultation of fetal heart rate (FHR) with one-to-one nursing care was compared with that of continuous electronic FHR monitoring (Haverkamp et al., 1979). The outcome, as judged by newborn Apgar scores and cord blood gases, was not different between these two groups. However, there was a higher incidence of *diagnosed* fetal distress and a higher cesarean section rate for fetal distress in the continuously monitored fetuses. Haverkamp has suggested that concepts of fetal heart rate patterns learned from continuous electronic fetal heart rate monitoring have influenced clinical interpretations of auscultated FHR. Instead of simply auscultating an average rate, clinicians are more conscious of subtle changes in rate, perhaps indicating late or variable decelerations. This could explain the divergence of his findings from those of Benson.

ELECTRONIC FETAL HEART RATE MONITORING

It is agreed that the electronic fetal heart rate monitor is only as good as the people interpreting the patterns. It has been suggested that when monitoring is first introduced in an institution, the increase in cesarean section rates that is often seen may be partly due to the staff's lack of confidence or education in pattern interpretation, rather than being a problem with the electronic monitoring itself. Additionally, it has been suggested that the increase in cesarean sections may be due to a failure to provide nonsurgical intervention (i.e., turning off oxytocin and/or changing the patient's position) prior to resorting to surgery.

A prerequisite for providing effective remedies for fetal distress is a thorough understanding of the underlying mechanisms of normal FHR patterns. Only then can a comprehensive understanding of abnormal patterns become possible and specific interventions be applied.

Rhythmic contractions of the fetal heart, as with the adult heart, result from an intrinsic pacemaker function. A normal sinus rhythm is generated from the pacemaker site, the sinus node, which is found in the wall of the right atrium. This pacemaker site provides the electric stimulus to begin cardiac contraction and will continue to do so unless interrupted. The heart muscle may continue pumping even when isolated from the body, as demonstrated in biology classes when the heart of a pithed frog maintains pumping action in a saline bath. Comparably, in the human with brain injury or death, the heart muscle continues mechanical function for an indefinite period of time. However, the loss of central nervous system influences on the heart prevents variation in rate or rhythm. It is the two branches of the autonomic division of the central nervous system (CNS)—the sympathetic and parasympathetic—that control changes in heart rate. An unexpected event (e.g., being startled) may cause the heart rate to speed up (sympathetic response), and a Valsalva maneuver may produce a slowing of rate (parasympathetic). Therefore, heart rate cannot be discussed separately from the CNS.

From one electric stimulation of the heart to the next there is a slight fluctuation in rate produced by the autonomic nervous system. The sympathetic division is constantly attempting to increase the heart rate, and the parasympathetic division is trying to counteract this by slowing the rate. The end result is similar to a tug of war, with a little bit of ground gained and lost with each pull, or in this case, beat of the heart. In the well-oxygenated, nonmedicated human this competition occurs with every beat, causing slight changes in rate that cannot be felt or auscultated, yet may be mechanically recorded by a machine that detects each beat-to-beat variation. These beat-to-beat changes are termed *variability*.

Multiple factors may influence the presence or absence of variability, oxygen deprivation being of primary importance. Inhibition of oxygen flow to the CNS impedes its function, causing a decrease or complete loss of variability and indicating an acid-base shift. It is this correlation of lack of oxygen to loss of variability that has led researchers to determine that fetal distress may be determined by changes in fetal heart rate patterns recorded on electronic fetal monitors.

Baroreceptors and chemoreceptors influence fetal heart rate regulation. Baroreceptors are small stretch receptors located in the arch of the aorta and in the carotid sinus, at the junction of the internal and external carotid arteries. These stretch receptors are sensitive to increases in blood pressure. When the blood pressure rises, impulses are sent from these receptors through the glossopharyngeal or vagus nerve to the midbrain. Further impulses are then sent via the vagus nerve to the heart, which slows cardiac activity. This is a protective mechanism that attempts to lower the blood pressure by decreasing the heart rate and cardiac output when the blood pressure increases (Parer, 1983). Therefore, when the umbilical cord arteries are compressed, causing an increase in the fetal blood pressure, the baroreceptors are stimulated and the fetal heart rate drops, as mediated by the vagus nerve.

The chemoreceptors are affected by chemical changes in the blood, such as decreases in O_2, increases in PO_2, and the presence of H^+. The chemoreceptors are found in both the peripheral and central nervous systems. The peripheral receptors are located in the carotid and aortic bodies, and the central receptors are found in the medulla oblongata. When there is a decrease in arterial oxygen perfusion or an increase in CO_2, there is usually a reflex tachycardia to increase cardiac activity. There is also an increase in the arterial blood pressure. These changes are mediated through the central receptors. Although the interplay between the peripheral and central chemoreceptors is not clearly understood, the end result of asphyxia is fetal bradycardia and hypertension (Parer, 1983).

The parasympathetic nervous system decreases the fetal heart rate. The parasympathetic nervous system originates in the medulla oblongata, extending through the vagus nerve to the SA and AV nodes. Stimulation of the vagus nerve causes a release of acetylcholine at the nerve endings, thereby decreasing the heart rate by lowering the rate of firing of the SA node and decreasing the transmission of impulses from atrium to ventricle (Parer, 1983).

The sympathetic nervous system increases the fetal heart rate. The sympathetic nerves distributed throughout the heart muscle, when stimulated, release norepinephrine at the nerve endings, which increases the rate of cardiac contractions and thus cardiac output (Parer, 1983).

There is normally a tonic sympathetic and parasympathetic influence on the heart to maintain a consistent rate. When this equilibrium is disturbed, accelerations and decelerations occur.

FETAL HEART RATE PATTERNS

Prior to discussing the actual fetal heart rate patterns, specific definitions need to be clarified. Fetal heart rate patterns are divided into two major categories: (a) baseline heart rate and (b) periodic and nonperiodic changes.

Baseline Heart Rate

Baseline heart rate (Table 13–2) is determined by assessing a tracing for a minimum of 10 minutes. Rate changes between contractions or between periodic changes are considered baseline changes. After the con-

Table 13–2. Baseline Heart Rate*

Categories	
Tachycardia	*Bradycardia*
a rate greater than 155 BPM or a sustained rise in rate 30 BPM above the previous baseline rate	a rate less than 110 or a sustained drop in rate 20 BPM from the previous baseline rate
Differential Diagnosis	
Asphyxia (compensatory)	Asphyxia (late)
Maternal fever	Reflex
Infection	Hypothermia
Fetal arrhythmia	Fetal arrhythmia
Drugs	Drugs
Prematurity	

*Definition: The heart rate between contractions or between periodic changes in heart rate. "Normal" is considered to be in the range of 120–160 BPM.

Note: Many normal fetuses have a heart rate below 120 or above 160 BPM.

traction has concluded, it is determined whether the rate is the same, greater, or less than it was following each and every contraction during that period of time. If the rate has slowly risen over this period of time, this increase is called a *rise in rate*. If the rate is persistently 160 beats per minute or more, it is defined as a *tachycardia*. If the rate is slowly dropping during this segment, it is described as a *falling baseline rate*. If the baseline rate is persistently below 120 beats per minute, it is defined as a *bradycardia*.

Three factors must be kept in mind when assessing fetal heart rate patterns. First, although the textbooks define normal fetal heart rate as 120 to 160 beats per minute, each fetus must be assessed individually, as the following example illustrates. If, upon admission, the fetal heart rate is 130 beats per minute, and then 2 hours later the rate is 150 beats per minute, this change represents a fetal tachycardia for this particular fetus, even though the two rates are within the "normal" range. Investigation into the cause of the tachycardia should follow, along with appropriate treatment. It should also be noted that if periodic or nonperiodic decelerations are occurring, the assessment of the baseline rate must be made after the *recovery* of the heart rate following the deceleration pattern. Finally, the assessment of variability is made during this same recovery baseline period, not during the deceleration itself.

Baseline Changes. The causes of baseline changes are many, some potentially harmful to the fetus, others not. It must be kept in mind, however, that a tachycardia or bradycardia alone is not necessarily an indication of fetal distress. Many normal fetuses have heart rates above 160 beats per minute and below 120 beats per minute.

Known causes of fetal tachycardia are maternal fever, maternal dehydration, fetal or maternal infection, maternal anxiety, stimulation of the fetus, fetal cardiac arrhythmias (such as supraventricular tachycardia and paroxysmal atrial tachycardia), and asphyxia. During recovery from an asphyxial episode, tachycardia may be seen as a sympathetic response to stress. Drugs such as the betamimetics (Yutopar) or parasympathetic blockers (atropine, scopolamine) will cause fetal tachycardia when administered to the mother.

Fetal bradycardias may be caused by medications, such as those drugs used for paracervical blocks ("caine" drugs) or beta blockers (propranolol). Bradyarrhythmias, e.g., complete heart block, are another cause of fetal bradycardia. When bradycardia persists, it is associated with a 20 percent incidence of congenital cardiac structural anomalies (Parer, 1983). Bradycardia is also associated with maternal connective tissue disease and fetal hypothermia.

The initial response of the normal fetus to acute hypoxia or asphyxia is always bradycardia (Parer, 1983). When the bradycardia is accompanied by average variability it represents only a stressful incident that is usually well tolerated by the fetus. However, bradycardia accompanied by absent variability usually represents an obstetric emergency.

Baseline Variability. Although the physiologic origin of variability is not clear, there is evidence to show that its presence indicates an intact nervous system. It originates either from the interplay of the sympathetic and parasympathetic divisions or from numerous, sporadic inputs traveling from various areas of the cerebral cortex to the cardiac integratory centers in the medulla oblongata and then transmitted down the vagus nerve (Parer, 1983). This interplay or these impulses cause an irregularity, or jitter, in the heart rate. This jitter is caused by the slight difference that the nervous control causes in the interval between the heart beats. (If all of these beat-to-beat intervals were the same, the heart rate pattern would be smooth.) The jitter is detectable only with internal methods of heart rate counting and is assessed during the baseline heart rate. If there is a discrepancy in the variability during decelerations and the baseline, the correct assessment is made in the baseline period only.

The variability is described as increased, average, decreased, or absent. An increase in the baseline variability usually results from some event that has stimulated the fetal central nervous system. A loose or defective fetal heart rate electrode may also simulate increased variability.

A loss of variability can result from many factors, but the one that most concerns the perinatal team is asphyxia. With fetal hypoxia, central nervous system and heart function will continue, but variability may be diminished or absent. In addition, non-asphyxial factors such as medication administration (including narcotics, alcohol, tranquilizers, barbiturates, and anesthetics) or fetal congenital anomalies can cause a possible loss or decrease in variability. Premature fetuses have less variability than term fetuses, because of immaturity of the autonomic nervous system. In addition, when tachycardia is present at rates over 180 beats per minute, variability decreases because there is less time between each beat, causing fewer fluctuations (Table 13–3).

Figure 13–1 shows a tracing indicating decreased variability secondary to narcotic administration. Note that the last 4 minutes of the tracing show a beginning return of variability as the medication loses its effectiveness. Figure 13–2 is a tracing that shows a loss of variability due to asphyxia.

Periodic and Nonperiodic Heart Rate Changes

The second category of fetal heart rate changes comprises periodic and nonperiodic deviations above or below the baseline. Periodic heart rate changes are those deviations in rate occurring in response or in relation to contractions. Periodic changes are further divided into two subgroups, accelerations and decelerations (not to be confused with tachycardia and bradycardia). Periodic accelerations may be of three types: uniform, variable, or rebound overshoot (Table 13–4). Decelerations are classified as early, late, or variable. Nonperiodic heart rate changes are also divided into two subgroups: accelerations and decelerations. These accelerations and decelerations do not occur repetitively with contractions and therefore do not meet the criteria of periodic changes. These can

Table 13–3. Factors Affecting Variability

Decreased Variability	Increased Variability
Asphyxia	Contractions
Drugs	Second stage of labor
Prematurity	Application of direct electrode
Tachycardia	Vaginal exams
Arrhythmias	pH sampling
Fetal sleep	Fetal movement
Anesthesia	Fetal breathing movement
Cardiac and CNS anomalies	Following moderate and severe variable decelerations

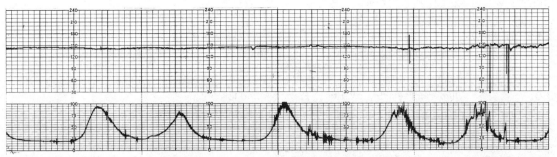

Figure 13–1. Mode: Direct electrode, intrauterine catheter. Baseline stable, periodic changes absent, variability decreased but increasing at end of tracing. Demerol 50 mg IV push 1 hour prior to this portion of tracing. (From Afriat, C. I.: Fetal Heart Rate Monitoring Pattern Assessment, Parts I and II, 4th ed. Monterey, CA, Perinatal Productions, 1985.)

further be defined as undefined or prolonged.

Periodic Accelerations. *Uniform accelerations* begin with the onset of the contractions and end with the termination of contractions. The shape of the acceleration is smooth—it gently rises as the contraction builds and decreases as the contraction subsides. The acceleration also mirrors the size of the contraction—the stronger the contraction, the greater the acceleration. Uniform accelerations are believed to be benign and *not* associated with fetal compromise. Although the exact mechanism is not known, uniform accelerations are believed to be caused by a lack of parasympathetic stimulation during the contraction in the nonvertex presentation. Because the head is not in the pelvis, only the torso of the fetus is being stimulated during the contraction. This causes the sympathetic nervous system to raise the heart rate without the counterbalance of the parasympathetic generally produced by the stimulation of the presenting fetal head. This can also occur in the nonen-

gaged vertex presentation. No treatment of this pattern is indicated, but a vaginal examination is warranted to determine the presenting part.

Variable or *shoulder accelerations* may precede or follow variable decelerations, with the mechanism of this believed to be the result of umbilical vein compression. When only the vein is compressed (as opposed to compression of both the vein and arteries), blood flow to the fetus is impaired, which causes a drop in fetal blood pressure, thus stimulating the baroreceptors to increase the heart rate as a compensatory mechanism. Occasionally a cord compression develops so slowly that, initially, the vein alone is compressed, causing the acceleration. Then, as the compression continues, the arteries are also compressed, causing an abrupt drop in fetal heart rate and thus variable deceleration. The same process may occur during the recovery stage: As the compression is alleviated, first the arteries are no longer compressed, allowing the fetal heart rate to begin to return to the baseline, but the continuance of umbilical *vein*

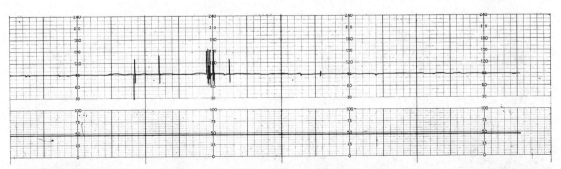

Figure 13–2. Mode: Direct electrode, no uterine activity monitoring. Baseline bradycardia, periodic changes absent, variability absent. No medications given. Diagnosis: chronic fetal asphyxia with poor outcome. (From Afriat, C. I.: Fetal Heart Rate Monitoring Pattern Assessment, Parts I and II, 4th ed. Monterey, CA, Perinatal Productions, 1985.)

Table 13–4. Periodic Changes in Heart Rate: Accelerations

Designation:	*Uniform*	*Variable (Shoulders)*	*Overshoot (Rebound)*
Character:	Mirrors uterine contraction	Abrupt rise and fall	Following variable decelerations
Mechanism:	Nonvertex presentations Umbilical vein compression	Response to fetal movement Precedes and follows variable decelerations	Autonomic imbalance
	Stimulation	Stimulation	

compression creates the acceleration until the point at which compression ceases totally and the heart rate returns to the baseline. These particular accelerations do not require treatment for themselves, but treatment for the variable *decelerations* should be instituted (Fig. 13–3). They are always associated with variable decelerations and good variability.

The last type of periodic acceleration is the *rebound overshoot*, which is the only potentially ominous type of acceleration. The characteristics of overshoots are that they only *follow* variable decelerations with *absent* variability. This pattern is seen either in the premature fetus, because the autonomic nervous system is immature, or in the fetus that has received atropine—a parasympathetic blocker—across the placenta. However, in the term fetus who has received no systemic atropine or atropine-like drug, overshoot is an indication of asphyxia and demands intervention. Overshoots in these cases are probably caused by adrenal activation from asphyxia, resulting in a very unstable heart rate. After the heart rate decelerates, it is so unstable that it overshoots the baseline before it stabilizes at the baseline rate. These accelerations should not be confused with shoulders, variability being

the key for distinguishing between the two types. Therefore, prior to determining whether an acceleration following a variable deceleration is a shoulder or an overshoot, a direct fetal electrode must be placed so that an accurate assessment of the variability may be made (Fig. 13–4).

Periodic Decelerations. Periodic decelerations are classified as early, late, or variable according to their shape and timing in relation to periodic uterine activity. The characteristics of each deceleration pattern should be committed to memory so that error is avoided when making the interpretation. If a deceleration pattern does not fulfill the characteristics stated, then a specific interpretation should be avoided and the pattern classified as undefined (Table 13–5).

Early decelerations begin with the onset of a contraction and end with the termination of the contraction. The drop in rate is very slow and smooth, rarely falling more than 10 to 15 beats per minute below the baseline rate. These decelerations mirror the contraction, so that the stronger and longer the contractions, the longer and deeper the decelerations will be. They tend to occur repetitively, with each contraction. Early decelerations occur more commonly in primi-

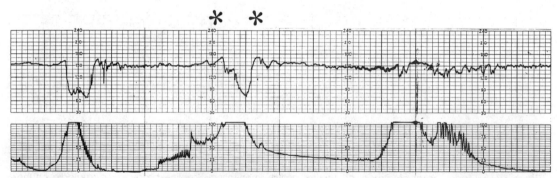

Figure 13–3. Mode: Direct electrode, external tocodynamometer. Baseline rate stable, variable decelerations with shoulders,* average variability. (From Afriat, C. I.: Fetal Heart Rate Monitoring Pattern Assessment, Parts I and II, 4th ed. Monterey, CA, Perinatal Productions, 1985.)

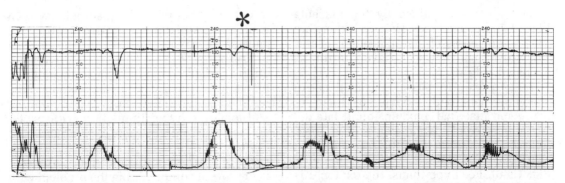

Figure 13–4. Mode: Direct electrode, external tocodynamometer. Baseline tachycardia, variable decelerations with overshoots,* absent variability. (From Afriat, C. I.: Fetal Heart Rate Monitoring Pattern Assessment, Parts I and II, 4th ed. Monterey, CA, Perinatal Productions, 1985.)

gravidas. Regardless of cervical dilatation or stage of labor, the decelerations remain smooth in shape, do not drop abruptly, and are not associated with acidosis. Early decelerations are the result of head compression or parasympathetic stimulation, so that a change in maternal position will not necessarily alleviate the compression. Therefore, no treatment is necessary (Table 13–5).

Late decelerations have all the same characteristics of early decelerations except that the onset of the deceleration occurs *after* the onset of the contraction (frequently at the peak of the contraction). The recovery of the heart rate to the baseline occurs well after the contraction that caused it has ended. Therefore, late decelerations have a late onset and a late offset and are repetitive. Additionally, late decelerations have a gradual drop in rate and return to the baseline rate. The size and depth of the deceleration are not important in its interpretation. Some of the most ominous patterns are depicted by very subtle late decelerations. Remember that the deceleration pattern indicates the

mechanism of the insult, whereas the variability indicates fetal reserve. The underlying mechanism of late decelerations is uteroplacental insufficiency. As the contraction builds, the blood flow through the placenta is diminished, leaving the fetus to rely on reserve oxygen. Without adequate reserve because of chronic placental insufficiency, the fetal heart rate begins to slow as the contraction increases in intensity, to allow for maximum use of this minimal blood flow. After the contraction has ended, blood flow resumes and the fetus generally recovers. However, this repeated insult can lead to fetal hypoxia, and eventually death (Table 13–5).

Uteroplacental insufficiency may be viewed from two perspectives, that which we can control and that which we cannot. In the woman with diabetes or other chronic problems such as hypertension or renal or collagen disease, the placenta may deteriorate very slowly over a long period of time. Certainly, what we do during labor will affect the fetus, but we cannot correct the

Table 13–5. Periodic Changes in Heart Rate: Decelerations*

	Early	Late	Variable
Definition:	Vagally mediated response to fetal head compression	Response to impaired uterine blood flow	Response to umbilical cord compression
Characteristics:	Uniform shape	Uniform shape	Variable shape (abrupt drop)
	Begins at beginning of contraction	Begins at peak of the contraction	Occurs at any time
	Repetitive	Repetitive	May be repetitive
	Reflects amplitude and duration of contractions	Reflects amplitude and duration of contractions	Variable shape
	Ends with the end of the contraction	Ends after the end of the contraction	Variable duration
	Benign	May be associated with acidosis	May be associated with acidosis

*If the deceleration does not have the characteristics as listed above, it is termed "undefined."

damage already sustained by the placenta (Fig. 13–5) in such cases. However, there are some acute causes of uteroplacental insufficiency over which we do have control, as discussed below.

The two main threats to placental perfusion are hyperstimulation from oxytocin infusion and maternal hypotension. If late decelerations result from oxytocin-induced hypertonus or hypotension, recovery will occur once the insult has been eliminated (Fig. 13–6). For hypertonus, the oxytocin is turned off *completely,* and for hypotension, the mother is repositioned to her left side and fluids are increased. Late decelerations caused by these factors may be referred to as *iatrogenic,* since they are being caused by extraneous forces. Iatrogenic late decelerations may be corrected nonsurgically. If these conditions are allowed to persist, however, morbidity and mortality could ensue. However, it must be pointed out that not only can such decelerations be easily corrected, but they can just as easily be avoided altogether. As noted in Chapter 12, oxytocin should be administered only through a "piggyback" line, by constant infusion pump, beginning with a low dose and increasing the dose very slowly. Monitoring should be with a direct electrode and internal intrauterine pressure catheter to provide information about fetal well-being, as well as to quantify the precise intensity of the uterine contractions and baseline resting tone. In addition, all pregnant women should undergo labor in the lateral position, to avoid hypotension and maximize venous return and placental perfusion. Iatrogenic uteroplacental insufficiency can thus be avoided.

The woman whose pregnancy is complicated by a chronic medical problem leading to chronic uteroplacental insufficiency is in a different situation. Late decelerations in such cases may be treatable only by surgical intervention. Prior to labor and delivery, all efforts should be made to maximize uterine blood flow by maintaining the woman in the left lateral position, improving hydration, and avoiding hyperstimulation with oxytocic agents. The fetus should be monitored directly and observed closely, with a minimum of a 1:2 nurse–patient ratio. The goal is to prevent compounding the problem with iatrogenic factors.

Variable decelerations, the third type of periodic deceleration, may occur before, during, or after the contraction, or when no contractions are present. (Variable decelerations can also be considered nonperiodic if they do not occur with contractions.) The key characteristic of variable decelerations is the abrupt drop in heart rate, followed by an equally abrupt return to the baseline (Fig. 13–7). This is commonly caused by cord compression and acute cessation of umbilical blood flow. Variable decelerations may last any length of time, from a few seconds when the cord is briefly compressed, to a prolonged period of time if the cord is trapped. When the cord is trapped, variable decelerations are seen with every contraction for as long as the cord remains trapped. If the fetus accidentally kicks or squeezes the cord, the variable deceleration may be a one-time-only event. Variable decelerations may vary in size, timing, duration, and depth. They may be benign, but they may also be ominous or threatening and require treatment (Table 13–5).

Krebs et al. (1982) described six atypical variable decelerations: loss of initial and secondary acceleration; prolonged secondary acceleration; loss of variability; contin-

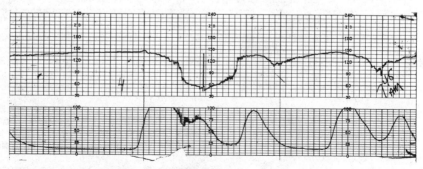

Figure 13–5. Mode: Direct electrode, intrauterine catheter. Baseline rate stable, late decelerations, absent variability. Chronic uteroplacental insufficiency. (From Afriat, C. I.: Fetal Heart Rate Monitoring Pattern Assessment, Parts I and II, 4th ed. Monterey, CA, Perinatal Productions, 1985.)

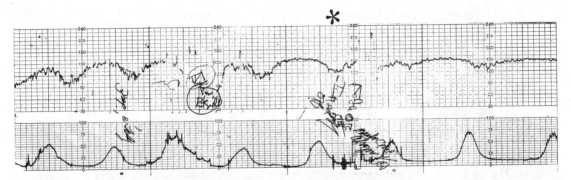

Figure 13–6. Mode: Direct electrode, intrauterine catheter. Baseline rate stable, late decelerations, average variability. Oxytocin turned off.* Late decelerations resolving. Iatrogenic fetal distress. (From Afriat, C. I.: Fetal Heart Rate Monitoring Pattern Assessment, Parts I and II, 4th ed. Monterey, CA, Perinatal Productions, 1985.)

uation of the baseline at a lower level; biphasic deceleration (W-shaped); and slow recovery to the baseline. The authors suggest that the more atypical signs that are demonstrated, the greater the chance of poor fetal outcome. *However,* their study showed that "the number of low Apgar scores in cases of pure or atypical variable decelerations associated with increased variability was not significantly different from pure or atypical variable decelerations with normal variability."

The goal in treating variable decelerations is to alleviate the cord compression. To do this, a variety of maternal position changes may be initiated, such as turning from side to side or assuming the knee-chest position. Another possible measure is elevation of the presenting part; however, this may cause a prolapsed cord and should be performed only in an emergency situation by nurses.

Nonperiodic Accelerations. Nonperiodic accelerations are isolated accelerations in response to fetal movement or stimulation. The basis for the antepartum nonstress test

is observation for fetal heart rate acceleration in response to fetal movement. These accelerations are abrupt in rise and fall. When they are seen in both the antepartum and intrapartum period, good fetal outcome may be anticipated (Fig. 13–8).

Nonperiodic Decelerations. Nonperiodic (prolonged or undefined) decelerations may be caused by either cord compression or uteroplacental insufficiency. The heart rate drops and stays down for several minutes, or an isolated small deceleration may occur that appears to be unrelated to any of the characteristics described thus far. Generally such decelerations are intermittent and do not produce any recognizable pattern. They may be either benign or ominous, and further pattern assessment, especially of variability, is indicated (Fig. 13–9).

Pattern Assessment

Assessment of fetal heart rate patterns should be done in a very organized, systematic fashion, beginning with the determination of the mode of monitoring. Because the

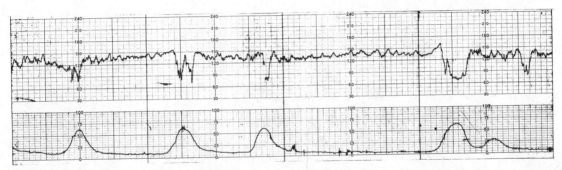

Figure 13–7. Mode: Direct electrode, intrauterine catheter. Baseline stable, variable decelerations with shoulders, average variability. (From Afriat, C. I.: Fetal Heart Rate Monitoring Pattern Assessment, Parts I and II, 4th ed. Monterey, CA, Perinatal Productions, 1985.)

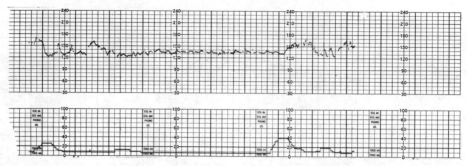

Figure 13–8. Mode: External ultrasound and tocodynamometer. Stable baseline rate, variable accelerations in response to fetal movement—reactive nonstress test. (From Afriat, C. I.: Fetal Heart Rate Monitoring Pattern Assessment, Parts I and II, 4th ed. Monterey, CA, Perinatal Productions, 1985.)

ability to assess variability is limited to tracings obtained with the direct fetal electrode, the precise mode of monitoring must be taken into consideration. With the external ultrasound transducer, information on variability may not be reliable. Precise determination of uterine baseline tone and the intensity of contractions can be obtained only with the intrauterine pressure catheter. After defining the mode of monitoring, the baseline rate is determined, as well as any changes in this rate (rise, fall, tachycardia, bradycardia). The presence or absence of periodic changes (accelerations or decelerations) is noted, and then the baseline variability is assessed as being increased, average, decreased, or absent. Uterine activity is evaluated by determining frequency, duration, and the intensity of the contractions, as well as the tone of the uterus at rest. Once these facts have been collected, the next step is to gather together all of the abnormal factors and formulate a differential diagnosis based on the possible causes of the abnormal factors. Once the differential diagnosis has been made, treatment specific to the possible causes of the problem can be carried out.

Therapy for Abnormal Fetal Heart Rate Patterns

It is clearly a nursing responsibility to assess fetal heart rate tracings and begin treatment, when necessary, with nonsurgical methods. When any pattern appears suspicious or threatening, the physician or nurse midwife should be notified immediately and all information documented in the nursing notes.

The possible causes of tachycardia were cited earlier in the chapter (p. 239). To properly treat tachycardia, it is best to do the easiest, most noninterventional action first, which would be to take the maternal temperature. If the patient is afebrile, infection and dehydration may be ruled out. In the event that she is febrile, an IV line should be started and fluids infused. Further investigation may be necessary to determine the origin of the infection, and appropriate treatment should be initiated.

It should also be kept in mind that premature fetuses have an inherently higher heart rate than that of full-term infants. Therefore, knowledge of gestational age is

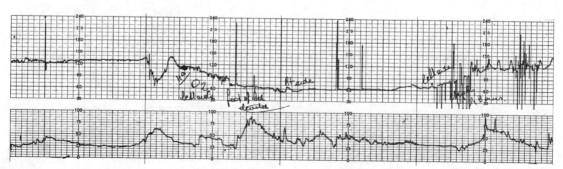

Figure 13–9. Mode: Direct electrode, external tocodynamometer. Baseline rate stable, prolonged deceleration, decreased variability. (From Afriat, C. I.: Fetal Heart Rate Monitoring Pattern Assessment, Parts I and II, 4th ed. Monterey, CA, Perinatal Productions, 1985.)

necessary. In the event that the fetus is at full term, shows no periodic changes, and has average variability, the final possible cause of the tachycardia would be an arrhythmia or hypoxia.

Fetal bradycardia alone with average variability and a stable baseline rate warrants observation but not necessarily intervention. Of primary importance is the need to rule out fetal demise. In the event of a fetal death, the maternal heart rate may be conducted through the dead fetal tissue and trigger the machine so that the maternal heart rate is counted in the absence of the fetal heart rate. It has been reported in the literature that emergency cesarean sections have been done for fetal bradycardia when in fact the fetus had been dead for several hours or days. This situation is easy to avoid by either taking the mother's pulse and comparing the rates or by doing a real-time ultrasound scan to observe fetal heart motion.

Bradycardias are most often seen during the second stage of labor. A distinction must be made between "end-stage" bradycardia and terminal bradycardia. When there has been a previously normal tracing and the bradycardia is accompanied by average variability, the condition is characterized as "end-stage" bradycardia, and vaginal delivery may be anticipated. It is suggested, however, that oxygen be given to the mother, and that the woman be encouraged to push in the left lateral position, or perhaps to push with every other contraction, to allow for maximum placental blood flow.

However, if variability is absent with bradycardia, it is called "terminal" bradycardia and may be cause for immediate abdominal delivery (unless vaginal delivery would be faster), as the fetus may be asphyxiated.

Other causes of fetal bradycardia are reflex action, vagal stimulation, drugs (primarily associated with paracervical blocks), cardiac and central nervous system anomalies, and asphyxia. In the event of a bradycardia, each possible cause must be ruled out systematically. Fetal blood pH sampling may be used to diagnose asphyxia (Table 13–6).

Since variable decelerations result from decreased blood flow through the umbilical cord, treatment begins with altering maternal position to alleviate the cord compression. Oxygen may be given at 7 liters per minute by face mask, and an IV should be started in preparation for surgical intervention. If oxytocin is infusing, it should be terminated immediately. However, if the variability remains average and the variable decelerations are not deep, the oxytocin may continue if the presence of stronger contractions does not increase the fetal stress. A vaginal examination may be performed to palpate for a prolapsed cord. If the physician or nurse midwife is not present, the information must be conveyed as to what has occurred and what treatment measures have been taken.

Since late decelerations indicate decreased blood flow through the placenta, the initial treatment of late decelerations is to turn the woman to her side to correct supine hypotension. Intravenous fluids should be increased at a rapid rate, to expand maternal blood volume and/or alleviate dehydration. Oxygen may be given by mask. Oxytocin, if infusing, should be turned off *immediately* (Table 13–7).

A common concern of perinatal practitioners is deciding on the appropriate time to intervene. Unfortunately, electronic fetal monitoring is not an exact science, and thus it is difficult to set specific time guidelines

Table 13–6. Management of Baseline Changes in Fetal Heart Rate*

Tachycardia	Bradycardia	Decreased Variability
Take maternal temperature (rectal or axillary)	Rule out fetal death (counting maternal heart rate)	Check for possible drug effect (including analgesics and anesthetics)
Rule out fetal arrhythmia (fetal ECG)	Rule out fetal arrhythmia (fetal ECG)	Stimulate fetus (abdominal palpation, vaginal exam)
Average variability and no decelerations, observe	Average variability and no decelerations, observe	Change maternal position
Decreased variability and/or decelerations, see fetal distress	Decreased variability and/or decelerations, see fetal distress	No decelerations, observe
pH sampling (?)	pH sampling (?)	pH sampling (?)

*While asphyxia is the most *important* cause of bradycardia, tachycardia, and decreased variability, it is not the most *common* cause. If decelerations are absent, the cause is usually something other than asphyxia. However, if these baseline changes are associated with late or variable decelerations, asphyxia becomes the most likely explanation.

Table 13–7. Principles of Treatment for Fetal Distress*

Objective: To improve blood flow to the fetus and to increase oxygen transfer		
	FHR Pattern	
	Variable Decelerations	*Late Decelerations*
CHANGE POSITION:	To alleviate cause of cord compression	To improve maternal venous return; correct hypotension
INCREASE IV FLUIDS:	—	To increase effective maternal volume
TURN OFF OXYTOCIN:	To improve uterine blood flow; eliminate potentiating factors	To improve uterine blood flow; eliminate potentiating factors
AVOID MEDICATIONS:	To avoid other causes of fetal depression	To avoid other causes of fetal depression
OXYGEN:	To increase oxygen flow across placenta (questionable effect)	To increase oxygen flow across placenta
OMINOUS CHANGES:	Decreased variability; rebound accelerations	Decreased variability; rising baseline

*If fetus shows no signs of recovery, prepare for a cesarean birth; with fetal distress, all uterine activity is considered "excessive."

that will apply to every case. Each situation of fetal distress is different and requires a thorough assessment of the fetal and maternal conditions before a decision can be made. The basic guideline is to determine what type of periodic change is occurring, which indicates the mechanism of the insult, and to assess baseline recovery and variability as indicators of fetal tolerance or reserve. If after attempting nonsurgical techniques, no positive change is noted indicating recovery, surgical intervention must be considered. For example, Figure 13–10 indicates clearly late decelerations and average varia-

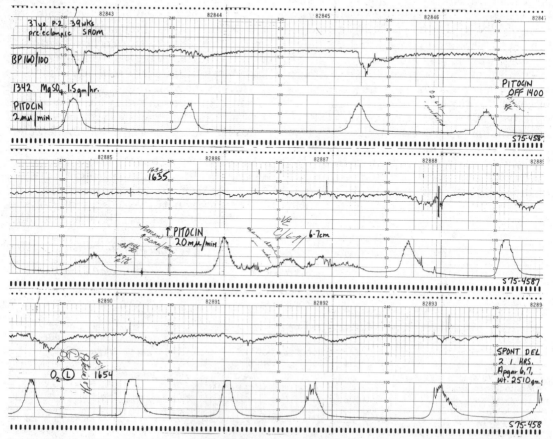

Figure 13–10. Late decelerations with oxytocin infusion. (From Afriat, C. I.: Fetal Heart Rate Monitoring Pattern Assessment, Parts I and II, 4th ed. Monterey, CA, Perinatal Productions, 1985.)

bility. This provides the information that the fetus has a problem with oxygenation because of uteroplacental insufficiency. What may not be clear is that at time 1654 the oxytocin was turned off, and almost immediately the contractions began to space out and the late decelerations began to subside. This indicates fetal distress, but it is remediable by removing the insult to the fetus and placenta. If, for some reason, the oxytocin needs to be restarted, it should be done only under the following conditions: (1) after the baseline heart rate has stabilized at the rate prior to the distress; (2) late decelerations are absent; (3) the variability is average; and (4) the contractions are greater than 2 minutes apart, are lasting less than 90 seconds, and are less than 75 mm Hg in strength. When all four of these criteria are fulfilled, oxytocin can be restarted, but *always* under careful observation, with a 1:1 nurse–patient ratio.

Ominous Signs

The presence of variable decelerations with a normal baseline rate and average variability constitutes a warning pattern that needs to be watched. The patient should be kept on her side to avoid supine hypotension and should have an IV. Signs of this pattern worsening would be a rise in baseline rate, loss of variability, and/or presence of overshoots. Ominous changes in the presence of late decelerations with average variability would be a rise or fall in baseline rate and a decrease in variability. This would indicate that the fetal reserve is decreasing and intervention is warranted. With either late or variable decelerations, the presence of tachycardia or bradycardia would also indicate a worsening situation. In all of the forementioned situations, the use of oxytocin would be contraindicated. With fetal distress, all uterine activity may be "excessive." Also, consideration must be given to the fact that if decelerations are present with average variability, medications will cause a diminishing of variability, thus removing a vital factor in assessing fetal condition.

In the presence of threatening or ominous patterns, additional concrete information regarding fetal condition may be obtained through the use of blood pH sampling to determine the presence or absence of fetal asphyxia. Sampling is also used as a tool for the practitioner who is less experienced with pattern interpretation or in the event of unusual patterns requiring more information.

ACID-BASE ASSESSMENT

The investigation of fetal acid-base balance was pioneered by Yippo, who in 1916 reported that, by adult standards, the cord blood of the fetus was acidotic. The current techniques of fetal blood sampling were introduced by Saling in 1964. Fetal capillary blood pH is of clinical interest because it is directly related to tissue oxygenation. With inadequate oxygenation, the fetus will suffer brain damage and, ultimately, death. The pH is used more frequently with PO_2 because PO_2 is more difficult to measure, is more subject to technical error, and fluctuates more rapidly. The PO_2 reflects the status of the fetus only at the time of sampling and gives no indication of what the preceding levels may have been. The pH of blood is influenced by both respiratory and metabolic factors and, therefore, may reflect rapid (respiratory) and/or prolonged (metabolic) changes.

Base excess is measured from the known values of Ph and carbon dioxide tensions by means of a nanogram. It is a measure of the amount of change of the metabolic acid-base change from normal.

The pH is defined as the negative logarithm to the base 10 of the activity of hydrogen ions in solution. Hydrogen ion activity in pure water is 10^{-7}. By convention, solutions having hydrogen ion activity greater than 10^{-7} are alkaline solutions. The Henderson-Hasselbalch equation demonstrates the metabolic and respiratory components of pH:

$$pH = pK + \log \frac{[Base]\,[HCO_3]}{[Acid]\,[CO_2]}$$

In a simplified way, changes in CO_2 (respiratory) will inversely affect pH. Retention of CO_2 will cause a reduction in pH (respiratory acidosis), while a decrease in CO_2 (respiratory alkalosis) will result in an elevated pH. In metabolic acidosis, bicarbonate (HCO_3) is utilized to buffer the metabolic acids. This reduction in bicarbonate will cause a fall in pH (see above equation). While the respiratory effect on pH is rapid, the metabolic rate is slower to respond and to return to normal.

The fetus is subject to both respiratory and metabolic acidosis. One major function of the placenta is to serve as the fetal lung. Conditions that interrupt the normal blood flow to and from the placenta, such as umbilical cord compression and other intermittent mechanisms, will cause an increase in fetal PCO_2 and a fall in pH. More prolonged or chronic conditions that result in reduced oxygen supply interfere with normal aerobic metabolism, with subsequent development of anaerobic metabolism and metabolic acid production.

Normal Acid-Base Range

The range for so-called normal pH values is considerable. Table 13–8 is a summary of pH values from 14 different studies. The results fell into two different groups.

Modanlou and others have clearly shown that the fetal pH decreases as labor progresses (Modanlou et al., 1973). There is also a correlation between fetal acidosis and progressively severe FHR patterns, as reported by Kubli and coworkers (1969) and by Renou and Wood. Apgar scores correlate in a general way with fetal pH values in late labor, although there is considerable overlap. Hon and colleagues (1969) reported a false-normal rate of 20.1 percent and a false-abnormal rate of 57.7 percent. Bowe and coworkers (1969) reported a false-normal rate of 10.4 percent and a false-abnormal rate of 7.5 percent.

Conditions that may result in a false-normal pH (good pH, low Apgar) include the following:

1. Maternal hyperventilation
2. Drugs
3. Airway obstruction (newborn)
4. Prematurity
5. Infection
6. Congenital anomalies
7. Asphyxia between sampling and delivery

Some causes of false-abnormal pH (low pH, good Apgar) are:

1. Contraction during sampling
2. Stage of labor when sampling done
3. Maternal acidosis
4. Anesthesia and/or analgesia
5. Small amount of bleeding from scalp, causing slow collection

Table 13–8. Normal Acid-Base Range

	Lower Limits	Upper Limits
pH	7.15 to 7.30	7.33 to 7.47
pCO_2 (mm Hg)	22 to 34	50 to 67
pO_2 (mm Hg)	7 to 17	23 to 36
Base excess	−14.1 to −5.3	−4.3 to +3.0

Table 13–9. Indications for Fetal Blood Sampling for pH

- Absent variability on initiation of monitoring without known cause
- Absent variability in the case of potential fetal hypoxia
- Late decelerations with decreasing variability when the problem is not resolved in a reasonable time (30 minutes)
- Unusual tracings, i.e., sinusoidal, arrhythmias

Lesser Considerations for pH
- Late decelerations with good variability that cannot be resolved
- Severe variable decelerations with good variability that cannot be resolved

6. Delay in analyzing the sample
7. Caput succedaneum (?)

There are several sources of evidence that the fetal scalp blood is a reliable index of fetal central circulation. Bowe and coworkers reported a positive correlation between the pH of the scalp blood just prior to delivery and the pH of blood from the umbilical artery and vein.

Adamson and coworkers, working with the rhesus monkey fetus, compared the pH of blood taken simultaneously from the fetal scalp and that from the carotid artery and jugular vein. They reported that capillary blood remained representative even under conditions of extreme asphyxia (Adamson et al., 1970). The capillary blood more closely resembled the jugular venous blood.

Fetal Blood Sampling Technique

Fetal heart rate monitoring should be used as a screening tool to detect abnormal heart rate patterns and fetal blood pH taken after the failure of in utero treatment to correct such a pattern. Indications for fetal blood sampling for measurement of pH are listed in Table 13–9. Withdrawal of blood for a pH should be obtained over the scalp or buttocks—not over the face, brow, or genitals. Other contraindications to this procedure would be: (1) when the fetus has a known or suspected blood dyscrasia, hemophilia, or von Willebrand's disease; (2) when it might cause undesirable rupture of the membranes; (3) when there is vaginal bleeding; and (4) when 10 to 12 previous incisions have been made.

To obtain a fetal blood sample for pH, the patient is placed in the lithotomy position at the end of her bed or in the delivery room.

The presenting part is visualized through an endoscope, and debris is removed with long cotton-tipped applicators. Silicone cream can be placed over the anticipated site to help contain the blood droplet. Increased blood perfusion of the fetal skin may be produced by spraying it with ethyl chloride. However, this is not generally recommended, as it may alter the results of the blood tests. Once the skin is prepared, a single incision is made with a 2 × 1.5 mm blade. The sample of blood should then be collected from free flowing blood into a capillary tube. The sample should be collected between contractions, as values from samples obtained during decelerations may be falsely low. Sampling from the caput succedaneum or air contamination during collection can cause inaccuracy in sampling. Table 13–10 lists considerations for interpretation of values.

After the sample has been collected, pressure should be applied to the incision site to prevent bleeding. Other complications include: (1) potential bleeding from sites during vacuum extraction; (2) fetal death due to exsanguination (rare); (3) scalp infections (usually fewer than 1 per cent require only local treatment); and (4) lacerations, which occasionally require suturing.

In current practice, pH is used primarily in a supportive or complementary role to electronic FHR monitoring. Use of pH has not spread from the academic institutions to the community hospitals, as the majority of physicians have not been trained in the technique, and few hospitals have a micro–blood gas analyzer available 24 hours a day. FHR monitoring has the advantage of providing a record that immediately reflects changes in the fetal condition, and it can be almost universally applied. In situations in which there is some question about the FHR

Table 13–10. Considerations for Interpretation of Fetal Blood Sample

- Relationship to maternal pH and base excess
- Degree of accuracy of sampling and measurement
    - Caput succedaneum?
    - Air contamination?
    - Correct machine calibration?
- Type of acidosis (metabolic or respiratory)
- Stage of labor
- Transient vs. permanent asphyxial insult
- Influence of an in utero treatment
- Relationship of sampling to uterine contractions
- Relationship of pH to FHR patterns and clinical situation

results, a pH determination may help to clarify the problem. When the two tests agree, confidence in diagnosis is increased whether they are both normal or both abnormal. It is difficult to establish exact limits of pH that would indicate when intervention is required. The most reasonable approach is to observe trends. A very low pH not associated with a correctable condition or an acidotic trend in pH with an abnormal FHR pattern would be cause for intervention.

Scalp Stimulation

Scalp stimulation with associated acceleration may reduce the necessity for scalp blood sampling (Clark et al., 1984). One hundred fetuses with tracings judged to be suggestive of fetal asphyxia were entered into the study. Each fetus was stimulated by firm digital pressure on the scalp followed by a pinch with an atraumatic clamp. Following this, scalp blood sampling was carried out in the usual manner. If the fetus demonstrated an acceleration of 15 BPM lasting 15 seconds, the pH was uniformly found to be ≥7.19. Fifty-one of the 100 fetuses responded with acceleration to the stimulation. Clinical application of scalp stimulation could reduce the necessity for scalp pH determination. It may also have application when a vaginal examination may not permit a scalp blood sample or if scalp blood sampling is not available to the patient.

Patient Education and the Team Approach

As is true with all types of medical and nursing care, thorough explanation of the procedure (in this case, fetal heart rate monitoring and fetal blood sampling) and its benefits and risks should be provided prior to the procedure. Since labor itself can be a stressful period for the patient, this information should be given prior to the onset of labor, preferably during the antepartum period. This ensures that the parents will have time to digest the information, have their questions answered, and investigate the procedure more thoroughly, if desired. This encourages the woman (and her partner) to participate more fully in her plan of care.

Written literature is an important supplementary source of information for the patient, so that she does not have to rely on memory from conversation alone. Many hospitals provide a booklet explaining electronic fetal monitoring, along with the hospital policy and procedure. Other information is frequently provided in childbirth education classes or during hospital tours.

After all the information is given and all questions are answered, the parents may decide that they do not wish to have the monitor applied. If an agreement cannot be made during the antepartum period, the parents may have to choose another midwife or physician who shares their opinions on how to deliver the baby.

Open avenues of communication will benefit all health care practitioners. However, it must be remembered that communication does not stop after the patient has consented to be monitored. In the event of fetal distress, when many manipulations and treatments may be carried out in a very harried fashion, one member of the team must take responsibility for explaining what is being done *as it is being done*. Reassurance and comfort must be given continually. The entire perinatal team must work together in support of this mother and fetus. It must be remembered that although many of these events are daily occurrences for the nurses and clinicians, they constitute a new experience for this family. When a decision is made to perform an emergency cesarean section, it must be remembered that the parents are feeling tremendous anxiety for both the mother and the fetus as the mother is rushed down the corridor to the operating room. We, as professionals, often lose sight of this level of anxiety, which may remain with families for many years following this type of event.

Conclusion

Technology in obstetrics has advanced at a rapid rate during the last 30 years and will most likely continue to do so in the years ahead. Obstetricians, nurse midwives, obstetric nurses, and all other members of the health care team have a responsibility to provide optimum care for the pregnant woman and her baby. Since diagnosis of fetal distress based on information provided by blood pH and electronic heart rate mon-

itoring is still relatively new, these techniques and the possibilities they offer for optimum treatment of the fetus and newborn must all be kept in perspective and be open to improvement. Advances are being made and new equipment is being introduced. Outcome predictions based on this information are becoming more accurate, but there is still a long road ahead.

The current state of technology tells us that, in combination, fetal blood pH trends and electronic fetal monitoring improve our ability to predict fetal distress. The years ahead may bring still other alternatives. While trying to absorb and at the same time perfect and improve upon all this, it should be kept in mind that we are using high level technology to assist in one of the most human experiences life holds.

REFERENCES

Adamson, K., Beard, R. W., and Myers, R. E.: Comparison of the composition of arterial, venous and capillary blood of the fetal monkey during labor. Am. J. Obstet. Gynecol. 107:435, 1970.

Afriat, C. I.: The nurse's role in fetal heart rate monitoring. J. Perinatol. Neonatal. March 1983, p. 29.

Afriat, C. I., and Schifrin, B. S.: Sources of error in fetal heart rate monitoring. J.O.G.N. Nurs. 5(Suppl.):5, 1976.

Benson, R. L., Shubeck, F., Deutschberger, J., et al.: Fetal heart rate as a predictor of fetal distress. Obstet. Gynecol. 32:259, 1968.

Bowe, E. T., Beard, R. W., Finster, M., et al.: Reliability of fetal blood sampling. Am. J. Obstet. Gynecol. 107:237, 1969.

Carson, B. S., Losey, R. W., Bowes, W. A., et al.: Combined obstetric and pediatric approach to prevent meconium aspiration syndrome. Am. J. Obstet. Gynecol. 126:712, 1976.

Clark, S., Gimovsky, M., and Miller, F.: The scalp stimulation test: a clinical alternative to fetal scalp blood sampling. Am. J. Obstet. Gynecol. 148:274, 1984.

Haverkamp, A. D., Orleans, M., Langendoerfer, S., et al.: A controlled trial of the different effects of intrapartum fetal monitoring. Am. J. Obstet. Gynecol. 134:395, 1979.

Hon, E. H., Khazin, A. F., and Paul, R. H.: Biochemical studies of the fetus. Obstet. Gynecol. 33:237, 1969.

Hon, E. H., and Quilligan, E. J.: The classification of fetal heart rate. II. A revised working classification. Conn. Med. 31:779, 1967.

Hon, E. H., Zannini, D., and Quilligan, E. J.: The neonatal value of fetal monitoring. Am. J. Obstet. Gynec. 122:508, 1975.

Krebs, H. B., Peters, R. E., and Dunn, L. J.: Intrapartum fetal heart rate monitoring. VIII, Atypical variable decelerations. Am. J. Obstet. Gynecol. 145:297, 1982.

Kubli, F. W., Hon, E. H., Khazin, A. F., et al.: Observations on fetal heart rate and pH in the human fetus during labor. Am. J. Obstet. Gynecol. 104:1190, 1969.

Low, J. A., Cox, M. J., Karchmar, E. J., et al.: The prediction of intrapartum fetal metabolic acidosis by fetal heart rate monitoring. Am. J. Obstet. Gynecol. 135:299, 1981.

Lumley, J., McKinnon, L., and Wood, C.: Lack of agreement and normal values for fetal scalp blood. J. Obstet. Gynaecol. Br. Commonw. 78:13, 1971.

Martin, C., and Gengerich, B.: Factors affecting the fetal heart rate: Genesis of FHR patterns. J.O.G.N. Nurs. 5(Suppl.):5, 1976.

Miller, F.: Prediction of acid-base values from intrapartum fetal heart rate data and their correlation with scalp and funic values. Clin. Perinatol. 9:2, 1982.

Modanlou, H. D., Yeh, S. Y., Hon, E. H., et al.: Fetal neonatal biochemistry and Apgar scores. Am. J. Obstet. Gynecol. 117:942, 1973.

Parer, J. T.: Handbook of Fetal Heart Rate Monitoring. Philadelphia, W. B. Saunders Co., 1983.

Paul, R. H., Suidan, A. K., Yeh, S. Y., et al.: Clinical fetal monitoring. III. The evaluation and significance of intrapartum baseline fetal heart variability. Am. J. Obstet. Gynecol. 123:206, 1975.

Renou, P., and Wood, C.: Interpretation of the continuous fetal heart rate record. Clin. Obstet. Gynecol. 1:191, 1974.

Saling, E.: A new method of safeguarding the life of the fetus before and during labor. J. Int. Fed. Gynecol. Obstet. 3:100, 1965.

Schifrin, B. S.: The case against the fetal monitor. South. Med. J. 71:9, 1978.

Schifrin, B. S.: Workbook in Fetal Heart Rate Monitoring. bpm, inc., Los Angeles, 1974.

Schifrin, B. S.: Fetal heart rate patterns following epidural anesthesia and oxytocin infusion during labor. J. Obstet. Gynaecol. Br. Commonw. 79:332, 1972.

Tejani, N., Mann, L. I., Bhakthavathsalan, A., et al.: Correlation of fetal heart rate–uterine contraction patterns with scalp blood pH. Obstet. Gynecol. 46:392, 1975.

The fetal heart rate W-sign. Letters to the Editors by Spencer, J. A., and Roux, J. F., with reply by Welt, S.: Obstet Gynecol. 65:298, 299, 1985; and by Krebs, H. B. (reply to Welt, S.): Obstet. Gynecol. 65:448, 1985.

Welt, S.: The fetal heart rate W-sign. Obstet. Gynecol. 63:405, 1984.

Wood, C., Ng, K. H., and Hounslow, D.: Time—an important variable in normal delivery. J. Obstet. Gynaecol. Br. Commonw. 80:295, 1973.

Young, D. C., Gray, J. H., Luther, E. R., et al.: Fetal scalp blood pH sampling: its value in an active unit. Am. J. Obstet. Gynecol. 136:276, 1980.

Zanini, B., Paul, R. H., and Huey, J. R.: Intrapartum fetal heart rate correlation with scalp pH in the preterm fetus. Am. J. Obstet. Gynecol. 136:43, 1980.

14

CESAREAN SECTION

MARY JO O'SULLIVAN
ABBE LOVEMAN
VICKI COLBURN

Twentieth century technology has produced many changes, with some of the most dramatic having occurred in medicine. In obstetrics, in particular, management of the pregnant mother and her fetus/neonate have undergone overwhelming changes.

Prior to the availability of anesthesia, suture material, antibiotics, and blood, the incidence of recorded cesarean section was low. Since the risks were excessive, with a maternal death rate of almost 100 percent, it is doubtful that the physician would have attempted such a risky procedure. Even at the beginning of this century, when suture material and chloroform were available, cesarean section was extremely rare.

Edith Potter's studies early in this century indicated that intracranial bleeding was the leading cause of perinatal mortality (Hoffman, 1982). Later, Friedman's work showed the relationship of prolonged labor and forceps delivery to poor perinatal outcome (Friedman, 1978). As a result of these and other studies, there has been a progressive decrease in the incidence of operative vaginal deliveries and a concomitant increase in the cesarean section rate. This is not a direct cause and effect relationship, since many other factors have also contributed to these changes. Changing attitudes toward infant survival, quality of life, and limited family size have resulted in continued changes in obstetric management. Neonatal intensive care units, and the development of the subspecialty areas of neonatology and maternal-fetal medicine, have also contributed considerably to these changing attitudes and improved survival rates.

What is not known is whether long-term infant morbidity will be affected by the increased cesarean section rate. By morbidity we refer to mental retardation, cerebral palsy, and birth trauma, which may or may not be directly labor related. Not to be ignored is the legal climate and the attitude of families toward complications during the course of pregnancy, labor, and delivery that may ultimately affect the outcome of the pregnancy. It should be noted that although abnormal outcomes are often attributed to events surrounding labor and delivery, the damage in fact may have occurred during the antenatal period.

Maternal Mortality and Morbidity

In the United States, maternal mortality associated with cesarean section was 2 percent for the period from 1933 to 1939, and decreased to 0.2 percent for the period from 1949 to 1956 (Cohen, 1982). This decline appears to be associated with (1) improved blood bank facilities, (2) antibiotics, (3) improved anesthesia, (4) change in surgical technique from the classical cesarean section to the low segment transverse procedure, and (5) improved maternal status prior to surgery. The 1967 PAS hospital survey in 1974 reported a maternal mortality of 0.08 percent from cesarean section as compared with an overall maternal mortality of 0.027 percent (Slee, 1976). Hemorrhage, hypertensive disorders with their associated cardiovascular complications, and infection account for the majority of the deaths. Interestingly, the classical cesarean section, which accounted for 4 percent of all cesarean sections, was performed in 13 percent of the patients who subsequently died. The Report of Confidential Enquiries into Maternal Deaths in England and Wales for 1973 in 1975 also quotes a mortality rate of 0.08 percent in cesarean sections compared with an overall maternal mortality rate of 0.01 percent during the same time period. Of these cesarean section mortalities, 25 percent were due to associated conditions and not to the operation per se.

Although mortality has been reduced, morbidity with cesarean section remains high (20 to 80 percent). In the majority of instances this morbidity is relatively benign (e.g., endomyometritis, urinary tract infection, anemia, wound infection, atelectasis); however, a small percentage of patients develop wound dehiscence, evisceration, pneumonia, thrombophlebitis, pulmonary embolus, and/or pelvic or abdominal abscesses. Most of the benign complications can be prevented by the routine use of prophylactic antibiotics. On the other hand, their use can be limited to specific instances that predispose to maternal morbidity, e.g., prolonged labor with ruptured membranes, in which the risk of infection is higher than it is in the routine elective repeat cesarean section. More recently, irrigation of operative wounds, including the uterine wound and uterine cavity, has been suggested as an alternative to prophylactic antibiotics. This can be done using saline or antibiotics (Jensen, 1985).

Definition and Incidence of Cesarean Section

Cesarean section in medical terms is the transabdominal delivery of an intrauterine fetus or fetuses weighing 500 grams or more through a uterine or cervical incision. More generally, to quote Webster, it is "the operation of taking a child from the uterus by cutting through the walls of the abdomen and the uterus."

The incidence of cesarean section has changed considerably over the last decades. In the 1930s and early 1940s, the cesarean section rate was 2.6 to 3.0 percent. Following World War II and throughout the 1950s the rate increased to 4 percent. However, from the early 1960s onward the increase was more precipitous, so that now in the 1980s the rate varies somewhere between 15 and 30 percent.

Types of Cesarean Section

Cesarean sections are categorized by the type of uterine incision, as follows (Fig. 14–1):

I. **Low Segment**—an incision in the isthmic or cervical portion of the uterus
   A. Transverse (Munro-Kerr)
   B. Vertical (Beck or Kronig)
II. **Classical**—an incision in the fundus of the uterus
   A. Longitudinal
   B. Transverse (rare)

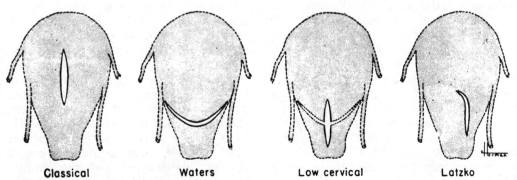

Classical   Waters   Low cervical   Latzko

Figure 14–1. Uterine incisions for cesarean sections. (From Quilligan, E., and Zuspan, F.: Douglas-Stromme Operative Obstetrics, 4th ed. New York, Appleton-Century-Crofts, 1982.)

III. **Extraperitoneal**—a low segment incision without entering the intraabdominal cavity
   A. Transverse (Waters)
   B. Vertical (Latzko)
IV. **Postmortem**—uterine incision, generally fundal, performed shortly after maternal death

Low segment. The lower uterine segment incision may be somewhat difficult technically, compared with the classical incision (discussed below). Nonetheless, in experienced hands, delivery occurs within 2½ to 3 minutes of operating time, in the absence of complications. There is less bleeding intraoperatively, because the blood supply and muscle thickness are less than in the fundus. The major advantage is that the uterine incision is retroperitoneal. This protects the peritoneal cavity from infection and decreases the incidence of adhesions forming postoperatively. Therefore, this is the procedure of choice for cesarean section. A technical disadvantage of the low segment incision is the risk of extension into the broad ligament, resulting in laceration of the uterine arteries. This risk can be minimized by using scissors to cut the lower segment, rather than separating it with the fingers. The advantage of finger separation is decreased blood loss generally. The low vertical incision is often indicated for the delivery of the premature breech, transverse lie, and anterior placenta previa. It has, however, the disadvantage of a risk of extension toward the vagina. Many times, because of poor development of the low segment, the incision must be extended into the upper segment of the uterus and becomes, therefore, a classical incision.

Classical. The classical cesarean operation was the standard procedure in the early part of the 20th century. By the late 1930s and mid 1940s the classical cesarean was being replaced by the low segment technique. Today, the classical procedure is seldom done. The low segment operation is preferred because of improved maternal results. The postoperative course is less morbid, and the chance of rupture of the lower segment is far less than that of rupture of the classical incision. Twenty-five percent of classical scar ruptures may occur prior to the onset of labor.

The advantage of the classical incision is rapid delivery of the infant. Disadvantages include a higher risk of infection, greater blood loss, a potentially more morbid postoperative course as a result of infection adhesions, and a greater risk (long-term) of rupture.

Nevertheless, although the classical procedure is seldom done today, it still has specific indications. Among these are (1) a transverse lie, especially in patients in whom development of the lower uterine segment is poor; (2) an anterior low lying placenta; (3) extensive lower uterine segment varicosities or myomas; (4) adhesions as a result of previous surgery, which makes exposure difficult; and (5) the rare situation in which the uterus is adherent to the anterior abdominal wall, making identification of the lower uterine segment impossible.

Extraperitoneal. The extraperitoneal section is rarely done in modern obstetrics, since, even in the presence of overt infection, the use of antibiotics appears to provide sufficient protection for the patient. The theoretical advantage of this procedure is protection of the intraabdominal cavity from exposure to contaminated or infected intrauterine contents. Its disadvantages include technical difficulty performing the operation, which involves staying outside the abdominal cavity and at the same time not entering the bladder. The procedure takes longer because of these difficulties. In spite of this, and even in the most careful hands, the peritoneum may be inadvertently entered. Few obstetricians today are trained to do the procedure.

Postmortem. The postmortem cesarean is also rarely performed. It is done within a short time of maternal death (10 to 20 minutes), to avoid the risk of fetal hypoxia. Anesthesia and sterile technique are unnecessary. Any scalpel or knife that will cut through the abdominal and uterine cavities can be used. The purpose is to deliver a live infant that has a reasonable chance of survival. Often, however, the decision is made too late to effect survival. Whenever there is a critically ill pregnant patient, preparations should be made for a postmortem section if there is any possibility the mother might die. Of course, when possible, the procedure should be discussed with the family. Attempts at resuscitation of the mother come before attempts at delivery of the infant.

However, unless an endotracheal tube is in place with adequate oxygenation of the mother, a period of greater than 10 minutes of resuscitation decreases the chances of delivering a liveborn normal infant.

Indications for Cesarean Section

The standard indications for abdominal delivery are listed in Table 14–1. Because of the potential risk of uterine scar rupture, previous cesarean section or any other operative procedure that involved entry into the uterine cavity through the myometrium (e.g., myomectomy, Strassman procedure, or hysterotomy) has been considered an indication for cesarean section.

Among the indications listed under Dystocia in Table 14–1, absolute cephalopelvic disproportion should be recognizable at initial clinical pelvimetry. Other conditions listed under this heading are often not discovered until after the onset of labor. Some may be obvious in early labor, e.g., malpresentations such as a transverse lie, or a tumor obstructing the birth canal. Others may not be diagnosed until the later stages of labor, such as relative cephalopelvic disproportion. In the latter case, even in the presence of borderline clinical pelvimetry, a trial of

Table 14–1. Standard Indications for Cesarean Section

1. *Previous Cesarean Section or Uterine Surgery*

2. *Dystocia*
   Cephalopelvic disproportion
   Pelvic contraction
   Malpresentation
   Uterine dysfunction
   Cervical dystocia
   Tumor obstructing birth canal

3. *Hemorrhage*
   Placenta previa
   Abruptio placentae
   Vasa previa

4. *Fetal Distress*
   Prolapsed cord

5. *Failed Induction*

6. *Miscellaneous*
   Premature rupture of membranes
   Hypertensive disorders of pregnancy
   Elderly primigravida
   Rh incompatibility
   Previous successful vaginal plastic surgery
   Invasive cervical cancer

labor is usually indicated to determine whether the fetus will negotiate the pelvis. Arrest of progress for 2 hours in active labor, in the presence of ruptured membranes, with no evidence of disproportion, and good uterine contractions with oxytocin stimulation, may be the result of uterine dysfunction, cervical dystocia, or even unrecognized positional cephalopelvic disproportion. Cervical dystocia is usually preceded by a history of cervical surgery, e.g., cone biopsy, encirclage, or surgical repair of previous cervical trauma, that has resulted in cervical fibrosis or scarring, which prevents progressive cervical dilatation despite good uterine activity in the absence of disproportion.

Malpresentations include transverse lie, brow, and persistent mentum posterior. A floating brow presentation in early labor, in the presence of intact membranes, may, with continued contractions, flex to a vertex, or further deflex to a face presentation. Once the membranes are ruptured, the aforementioned is unlikely. In a brow presentation, the diameter presenting to the pelvis is the occipitomental, which at term is approximately 13 cm. A fetus with this presentation is unlikely to get through the pelvis. For a persistent mentum posterior there is no mechanism of labor; therefore, the fetus must be delivered abdominally. However, this diagnosis cannot be made until late in labor, since the mentum does not rotate until it reaches the pelvic floor. Fortunately about two thirds of all fetuses presenting as a mentum posterior will rotate and deliver vaginally. In present-day obstetrics, there are some who believe that all primigravidas with a face presentation (mentum) in labor should be delivered abdominally, especially if the fetus is in the mentum posterior position, regardless of the station.

Placenta previa is usually diagnosed either as an incidental finding on routine sonography, or when the latter is indicated because of painless vaginal bleeding. These patients are generally managed as conservatively as possible, since most marginal or low-lying placentas seldom present a problem as gestation progresses. With progressive uterine growth, the placental location appears to rise as the lower uterine segment undergoes continued development. If bleeding is excessive and/or pregnancy is 37 weeks or greater, there is little room for procrastination, and one may proceed to double set-up (vaginal exam in the operating room with a team scrubbed for immediate cesarean section). Occasionally, going right to cesarean section without the double set-up in the presence of brisk vaginal bleeding is indicated, based on an ultrasound diagnosis alone. An obvious abruptio placentae, without labor, or in the presence of fetal distress, requires delivery by the most expeditious route, which is likely to be a cesarean section. A very rare cause of vaginal bleeding is vasa previa. This presents as fetal distress after amniotomy (spontaneous or artificial), associated with vaginal bleeding with no apparent evidence of abruption. The bleeding in such cases is fetal. Since the term infant's circulating fluid volume is only 350 to 375 cc, a significant loss would be 80 to 100 cc. The diagnosis should be suspected when bleeding occurs at amniotomy and can be confirmed by an Apt test.

Prior to the era of electronic monitoring, fetal distress was usually diagnosed on the basis of bradycardia and/or an irregular fetal heart rate, especially if associated with meconium. This was a rare indication for cesarean section. In fact, prolapsed cord was more commonly the cause of fetal distress, and therefore a more common indication for cesarean section. With the advent of electronic fetal monitoring, however, there has been a whole new approach to this area. The diagnosis of fetal distress is based now on fetal heart rate patterns, resulting in an increase in the number of abdominal deliveries performed for fetal distress.

Little has changed over the years with regard to the remaining indications listed in Table 14–1, and all are still acceptable reasons for performing a cesarean section.

Table 14–2, listing newer indications for cesarean section, reflects an increased awareness of the fetus and its chances of survival since the development of the fields of maternal fetal medicine and neonatology. Experience indicates that the better the condition of the neonate at delivery, the better its chances of survival without long-term handicaps. It is now generally accepted that the small premature breech is best delivered abdominally, although some controversy still exists because of the absence of well-controlled studies. One major reason is the hypoxia that might occur during vaginal delivery as a result of cord compression as the small body is delivered through the incompletely dilated cervix, which then results in further hypoxia and trauma as the

Table 14–2. Newer Indications for Cesarean Section

1. Breech presentation
   a. In primigravida
   b. With premature infant
   c. All breeches
2. Macrosomia (fetus greater than 4000 grams)
3. Herpes genitalis
4. Placental insufficiency
5. Severe preeclampsia or eclampsia with an unripe cervix
6. Multiple gestation
7. Failed progress in labor
8. Fetal distress, as indicated by:
   a. Fetal heart rate patterns
   b. Acid-base balance
9. Hydrocephaly

head is trapped behind the cervix. Premature neonates of less than 33 weeks' gestation have a higher incidence of intracerebral bleeding (ICB), probably because of immaturity of the subependymal vessels. Trauma, hypoxia, and changes in cerebral blood flow increase these risks. The most commonly associated factor with ICB is low gestational age; however, hyaline membrane disease is also known to be an associated factor, as are intubation and the administration of bolus fluids. There are some who believe that all small premature infants should be delivered by cesarean section to prevent ICB; however, this subject generates even more controversy than abdominal delivery of the breech. The best candidate for vaginal breech delivery is the term fetus with a frank breech presentation, a well-flexed head, no evidence of nuchal arms, weight of less than 4000 grams, and whose mother is a multipara, with normal gynecoid pelvic measurements, with the final key factor of being handling by an experienced obstetrician.

As the weight of the infant increases, the risks of trauma during vaginal delivery increase, and therefore it is recommended that macrosomic infants (birth weight over 4000 grams) might best be delivered by cesarean section. Macrosomia is associated with an increased incidence of shoulder dystocia, fractures of the clavicle or humerus, Erb-Duchenne paralysis (brachial plexus palsy), hypoxia, anoxia, and maternal trauma.

Herpes genitalis that is active at the time of delivery is associated with an increased risk of neonatal herpes, which has a high morbidity and mortality; thus active herpes is now an accepted indication for cesarean section regardless of the duration of ruptured membranes. Patients with previously active disease may deliver vaginally provided they have a negative culture or no lesion in the last few weeks prior to delivery.

Abdominal delivery of the fetus may be indicated when placental insufficiency, as assessed by biochemical or biophysical tests, implies deterioration of fetal well-being in the intrapartum period. However, in the presence of a nonreactive nonstress test and a positive contraction stress test, a trial of labor might be considered with a ripe cervix and a normal presentation, as these tests have a high false-positive rate. If evidence of fetal distress was found in labor, expeditious delivery would be desirable.

In the presence of an acute severe hypertensive disorder of pregnancy and/or eclampsia, in the interests of both mother and infant, rapid stabilization and control is essential, followed by delivery by the most expeditious route. If the cervix is inducible, then attempted vaginal delivery is preferable; otherwise, cesarean section may be the procedure of choice.

There are some who feel that all multiple gestations should be delivered abdominally. Certainly, when there is malpresentation of the first infant, or if there are more than two infants, there is general agreement that cesarean section is the procedure of choice. If twin A is a vertex, regardless of the presentation of twin B, and labor progresses normally, in the proper setting twin A should be allowed to deliver vaginally. The management of twin B will depend upon the presentation, fetal condition, and experience of the delivering physician.

Failed progress or secondary arrest, now one of the most common indications listed for cesarean section (in contrast to 15 to 20 years ago), appears to include the older standard indications of of uterine dysfunction, cervical dystocia, and possibly positional dystocia, which today are almost never listed as indications. Failed progress is diagnosed in a laboring patient with ruptured membranes and no evidence of cephalopelvic disproportion, who is having good uterine contractions but who has not progressed in 2 hours despite oxytocin augmentation. Because current obstetric practice favors the active management of labor, there is a reluctance to follow the older practice of resting such a patient with sedation for a few hours and then allowing her to resume labor to determine if she will go on and deliver vaginally.

Since the advent of electronic fetal monitoring, there has been an increase in the incidence of cesarean section for fetal distress. This is related to changes in the definition of fetal distress, and to our overall attitude toward the quality of the neonate. Unfortunately, abnormalities on electronic heart rate monitoring alone are not sufficient to make the diagnosis of fetal distress. They do alert the obstetrician to those infants who are likely to have acidosis, and therefore should be used wherever possible, in combination with fetal pH determinations. This results in a more accurate diagnosis and should decrease the incidence of overdiagnosis of fetal distress. Once the diagnosis of acute fetal distress is made, rapid delivery is essential. A delay of 10 to 15 minutes from decision to delivery doubles the perinatal mortality. If this interval is further increased to 15 to 30 minutes, the mortality doubles again (Choate and Lund, 1968). It is now accepted that the hydrocephalic infant with a large head is best delivered abdominally rather than by any procedure that would decompress the head of a live infant in labor. Despite the fact that at one time a cerebral plate of less than 1 cm was thought not to be salvageable, neurosurgeons today will shunt almost any infant. Therefore, destructive procedures are no longer acceptable.

Choice of Skin Incision

The choice of abdominal incision is dependent upon many factors, not the least of which is speed. The easier incision is a vertical, midline, or paramedian. The advantages of the vertical incision include decreased blood loss and operating time. The disadvantages are the cosmetic location of the scar and the minimal postoperative risk of decreased healing, resulting in either dehiscence and/or evisceration. In modern times, probably somewhat as a result of the popularity of bikini swimsuits, the transverse abdominal incision has gained increasing popularity. This incision is technically a little more difficult. There are two types of transverse incisions used obstetrically. One is the Pfannenstiel, which involves incising the skin and fascia transversely. The fascia is then dissected off the underlying rectus muscle. The muscle is separated in the midline and the peritoneum opened longitudinally. The other is the Joel-Cohen incision, in which, again, the abdomen is entered through a transverse incision in the skin and fascia. However, the fascia is not separated from the muscle, and the peritoneum is incised transversely. The latter is associated with a lower incidence of seromas, and less blood loss than the Pfannenstiel incisions.

Physical and Psychological Preparation of the Patient

Since some 15 to 30 percent of women are delivered by cesarean section, ideally, all should be prepared for this possibility. At times, the obstetrician can predict a cesarean delivery based upon the medical problems of the patient, her past obstetric performance, and the size of her pelvis and/or her infant. Once it becomes apparent during the course of pregnancy that cesarean section is likely, this should be expressed to the patient and her family. The patient and physician will then have time to discuss the procedure, the possible presence of a family member in the operating room, anesthesia choices, and operative risks. The patient may be given the opportunity to meet the anesthesiologist in order to discuss various anesthetic choices and their risks. Finally, she should have the opportunity to meet the nurses on the labor floor and, as a result, be familiar with those who will be providing direct care for her. Fortunately, many childbirth education courses include cesarean section in their format, which should be helpful for those patients who may come to abdominal delivery unexpectedly.

Some women look upon cesarean childbirth as a failure of their reproductive performance and as a result may be hostile and depressed. It is incumbent upon physicians and nurses to be aware of this, to provide adequate explanations, and to be understanding. There is even the rare patient who will refuse surgery under any circumstances, so that a court order may become necessary. While this may incite anger on the part of the staff dealing with her, one must accept the fact that understanding is far more important than anger, and gentle urging far more successful than force.

The type of anesthesia to be selected is greatly dependent upon the indication for surgery, the expertise of the anesthesiologist, and the preferences of the patient and her obstetrician. In cases of bleeding, e.g., placenta previa or abruptio, or when there is acute fetal distress, the choice of anesthesia would be general. Regional block is contraindicated because of the associated sympathetic blockade, which reduces the patient's ability to vasoconstrict her splanchnic vessels to compensate for blood loss.

Prior to any elective cesarean delivery, it is essential that fetal maturity be established. This can be based upon the last menstrual period, uterine size at the first prenatal visit, fetal heart tones at 20 weeks with a DeLee stethoscope, and an early ultrasound before 24 weeks. If these are compatible in an otherwise uncomplicated pregnancy, amniocentesis for fetal lung maturity is not essential. A grade III placenta at term is also compatible with a mature fetus. If, however, this is not the case, or the pregnancy is complicated by a maternal medical condition such as diabetes, then amniotic fluid studies for fetal lung maturity should be considered. Awaiting the spontaneous onset of labor, on the other hand, provides assurance that the fetus is as mature as possible. However, the unscheduled cesarean section may come at an inconvenient time and may increase the risk of aspiration during anesthesia if the mother has recently eaten.

The physician and nurse begin education and preparation of the patient during her prenatal course, especially when elective cesarean has been chosen. The amount, level of detail, and need for ongoing information increases the nurse's essential role after hospital admission in preparing the patient for her hospital stay and its associated events.

On admission, a thorough history is taken and a physical assessment done, including fetal heart rate and fetal position. This is a good time to assess the patient's understanding of her need for surgery, her expectations, and her overall attitude toward the procedure. The admission laboratory studies include a complete blood count, serology, blood type, Rh, antibodies where necessary, and a urinalysis. In some hospitals a crossmatch is routine, while in others type and screening is sufficient, but only in the absence of specific antibodies. If unusual antibodies are present, then cross-matched blood is necessary.

The patient should be oriented to her new environment in the hospital. She should be taught how to work the call light, the mechanics of her electric bed, where the bathrooms, showers, and lounges are located, and finally, she should be encouraged to visit the newborn nursery. Many hospitals provide a tour of the labor and delivery suite or operating room, so that the parturient can see where her surgery will be performed. A preoperative educational checklist (Table 14–3) can be helpful to make certain that patient education is completed.

Time should be set aside to prepare the patient psychologically for surgery, to ascertain her past surgical experience, and to start her preoperative teaching. Some hospitals have slide-tape presentations that give a step-by-step account of the cesarean section as experienced from the patient's viewpoint (Alley, 1981). If such a presentation is not available, a detailed description should be given regarding transport to the operating room, the intravenous infusion, the abdominal prep, and the Foley catheter. Some physicians like to have the Foley inserted before anesthesia, whereas others prefer to wait. The procedure for anesthesia should be described.

An abdominal "prep" includes washing and shaving the abdomen from below the breasts to above the symphysis pubis. An antibacterial soap is commonly used, and in some hospitals, a 20-minute scrub or a pHisoHex shower the night before surgery is routine. This "prep" is a source of controversy. Some shave the entire abdomen, while others shave only the area of the expected incision. Some shave the night before surgery, others just before surgery. The patient should be educated in the timing of these preparations, as she may be awake in the operating room during these preparatory procedures and have concern that she will not be asleep before the incision is made.

Preparing the patient for postoperative care and telling her of the necessity for deep breathing and coughing after surgery should also be done before the surgery is begun.

It is important to encourage the parturient to express her feelings about the upcoming surgical birth experience. Patients express a variety of feelings, such as fear of pain and disfigurement, and fear of being unable to mother their babies. Others express a sense of relief that the pregnancy is finally coming to an end so that motherhood can begin. It is safe to assume that patients will experience some preoperative anxiety; therefore, enough time should be provided for reassurance and to allow the patient to voice her concerns (Affonso and Stickler, 1978).

Often, a "significant other" may express concern for the safety of the mother and child. Some fathers have feelings of guilt or disappointment that childbirth cannot be achieved in the conventional manner (Clark and Affonso, 1979). Many couples express concern over the increased financial burden of a surgical delivery. Once again, parent education may help to allay these fears.

The birth experience should be as close to normal as possible. Many hospitals provide family-centered surgical births, allowing fathers to be present during the surgery to support the mothers and to hold their newborn baby. Mothers are also encouraged to hold their babies shortly after delivery, to facilitate bonding. When this has occurred, couples have described the experience very positively, and demonstrated a genuine enjoyment of the birth process (Gawse, 1982).

If this is the patient's first experience with surgery, it could be beneficial to introduce her to a woman who is 4 or 5 days postoperative, or to call a volunteer representative from the local chapter of the Cesarean Section Support Group or the Childbirth Education Association. Interaction with someone who has experienced surgical birth and perceives it in a positive fashion will help to set a favorable emotional climate (Conklin, 1977).

Table 14–3. Pre-op Teaching List

A. Preparation for O.R.
  1. Removal of cosmetics/glasses/contact lenses
  2. Catheter
  3. Pre-op medications
B. Location of delivery and transport
  1. Stretcher/wheelchair
  2. Waiting on call in operating/delivery area
C. Anesthesia—type and procedure
  1. General
  2. Regional
D. Involvement in birth process
  1. Patient
  2. Family/significant other
E. Recovery Room Procedures
  1. IV fluids
  2. Oxygen mask/inspirometer
  3. Return to postpartum area
F. Postpartum/operative care and expectations
  1. Respiratory assistance
  2. Ambulation
  3. Pain relief
  4. Engorgement/postpartum blues
G. Involvement in newborn care
  1. Bonding
  2. Feeding—breast/bottle

Ultimately, emphasis should be placed on a healthy, positive outcome for mother and baby. Since abdominal delivery has become so common for a large percentage of the population, it should be viewed simply as an alternative to vaginal birth. It is hoped that the emergence of this attitude will continue to open the surgical birth experience to those who wish a family-centered birth, with more hospitals, physicians, and nurses recognizing that couples should not be excluded from the shared fulfillment of childbirth, wherever and whenever possible (Donovan and Allen, 1977).

Intraoperative Care

Most hospitals use a preoperative checklist in order to ensure thorough preparation for surgery. All requirements must be fulfilled, including consent forms, history, and physical and lab work. Preparation of the patient for surgery often includes removal of dentures, contact lenses, jewelry, hairpins, and hairpieces or wigs. No nail polish or cosmetics should be worn, as these may give a false appearance of color to the lips, face, and nail beds and could confuse the anesthesiologist and the postanesthesia nurse. The patient should be wearing a hospital gown, and all underwear should have been removed. She should be "NPO" and the necessary "prep" completed. The patient should either void "on call" or have the Foley catheter inserted. Blood administration tubing should be used for the intravenous in case the need for blood arises.

Some of these preoperative procedures may be perceived as a threat to a young mother who is particular about her grooming and appearance. Simple explanations about what to expect are helpful before and during the procedures. Insertion of the Foley catheter and the intravenous line are sometimes described by patients as traumatic events (Affonso and Stickler, 1978). Many patients better express their worries and fears during these procedures, so it is advisable to encourage discussion during preparation (Anderson et al., 1975).

The patient's identification plate should be sent to the operating-delivery suite with the chart so that intraoperative financial charges and labels can be facilitated. In some hospitals, the intraoperative records will be generated and sent to the operating room along with baby bracelets and footprint sheets. These may be filled out in advance (except for the time of delivery and sex of the baby), thus reducing the amount of paperwork at the time of delivery. Upon arrival at the operating area, the preoperative checklist is again reviewed by the circulating nurse.

Many anesthesiologists order an antacid prior to surgery, to decrease the risk of Mendelson's syndrome (aspiration pneumonitis). A nonparticulate antacid such as sodium citrate is preferable to the colloidal antacids, since aspiration of the latter may contribute to the syndrome.

Before the patient enters the operating room, a preoperative inspection of the room is essential. The delivery table should be checked to make sure that the Trendelenberg

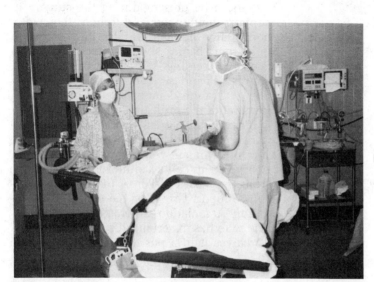

Figure 14–2. The patient is positioned in a lateral tilt to the left.

and lateral tilt positions work (Fig. 14–2). A safety strap and armrests should be available. The supply cupboard should have adequate quantities of intravenous and irrigating fluids, as well as a proper supply of sutures and the necessary surgical supplies. Irrigation solutions should be prewarmed. Ideally, a blood warmer should be available and functioning, and suction equipment should be functional.

The anesthesia cart and equipment should be inspected. Usually this is done by the anesthesia staff. Adequate supplies of drugs should be on hand. A separate compartment may be used to keep controlled drugs; these must be checked periodically for expiration dates and replacements made as necessary.

The infant laryngoscope, ambu bag, face mask, and airways and intubation equipment should be present and functioning. If the laryngoscope shows a yellow light, the batteries and/or the bulb should be replaced, until a white light shines. The necessary pediatric drugs and dosages should be available in case the need for them arises for

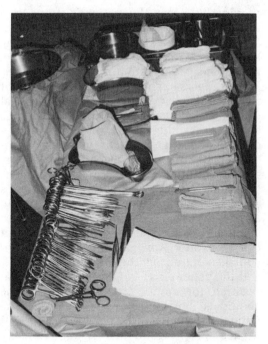

Figure 14–3. The back field.

emergency resuscitation (Bacon et al., 1981) (see Chapter 25). It is important to check the heating element in the infant warmer. The temperature should range from 96° to 99°F. A supply of prewarmed blankets should be ready to be used to dry the baby. The necessary equipment for infant identification procedures must be available.

Finally, surgical lamps should all be functioning, and the thermostat set at 72°F so that the patient and infant will not suffer from environmental hypothermia (Bacon et al., 1981). A pre-op room inspection checklist is shown in Table 14–4.

Once the room has passed scrutiny, the scrub technician can set up a sterile field and prepare the instruments and drapes for surgery (Fig. 14–3). The first count of sponges, instruments, and needles can be accomplished and recorded at this time (AORN, 1979).

When the patient is brought into the room, she should be assisted onto the table. The Foley catheter should be placed over the leg and the bag hung at the head of the table for monitoring of decreased output caused by anesthesia.

An epidural injection requires proper positioning and emotional support. Usually, the procedure is performed with the patient in the sitting position. A footrest should be

Table 14–4. Preoperative Room Inspection

	Yes	No
1. Suction equipment functional	☐	☐
2. Delivery table functional		
a. Trendelenberg	☐	☐
b. Lateral tilt	☐	☐
c. Foot of bed	☐	☐
d. Arm rests	☐	☐
3. Safety strap present	☐	☐
4. IV fluid stock level adequate	☐	☐
5. Irrigating fluid level adequate	☐	☐
a. Normal saline prewarmed	☐	☐
b. Sterile water	☐	☐
6. Suture stock level adequate	☐	☐
7. Blood warmer functional	☐	☐
8. Anesthesia cart properly stocked	☐	☐
9. Stock drugs not expired	☐	☐
10. Infant laryngoscope functional	☐	☐
11. Infant ambu bag—no holes or leaks	☐	☐
12. Preemie face mask	☐	☐
Term face mask	☐	☐
13. Pediatric emergency drugs in date		
a. Bicarbonate	☐	☐
b. Epinephrine	☐	☐
c. Calcium gluconate	☐	☐
d. Dextrose	☐	☐
e. Narcan	☐	☐
14. Infant endotracheal tubes in date		
a. 3.5	☐	☐
b. 3.0	☐	☐
c. 2.5	☐	☐
15. Infant heater at 96°–99°F	☐	☐
16. Infant blankets	☐	☐
17. Infant I.D. apparatus	☐	☐
18. Surgical lamps functional	☐	☐
19. Room temperature 70°–76°F	☐	☐

provided so that the patient's spine and upper legs form a 90° angle. Placing a pillow across the patient's abdomen and instructing her to sit without leaning to either side, putting her arms around the pillow, relaxes her shoulders and allows her to push out or round out her back. Many patients have great difficulty getting into this position because of tenseness due to anxiety, and subsequently they tighten their muscles. Additional support can be provided by having the patient put her chin against her chest as the nurse puts her hands on the patient's shoulders and instructs the patient to lean against her. This can be described as a therapeutic embrace (Fig. 14–4). The assistant can then offer words of instruction or encouragement during the procedure.

If the patient is to be placed in the lateral position for spinal anesthesia, the spine should be horizontal to the table and the patient instructed to put her chin and knees to her chest. Again, this is an extremely difficult position for a patient at term. Assistance can be given by placing one hand against the back of the patient's neck and the other behind her knees. Gentle pressure behind the knees and neck will help the patient to flex the spinal cord and open the intervertebral spaces (Reeder et al., 1980). Since this position places the assistant in very close proximity to the patient, verbal as well as physical reassurance is facilitated. Once the procedure is completed, the patient is returned to the supine position, a safety strap is applied, and the fetal heart is checked. A small towel can be placed under the mother's right hip to encourage blood flow to the uterus.

On the other hand, if general anesthesia is to be used, an assistant may be required to assist the anesthesiologist during induction and intubation. Prior to beginning the procedure, the safety strap should be securely placed over the patient's thighs. Ideally, someone should remain in physical contact with the patient until she is asleep, assisting the anesthesiologist by handing him or her the endotrachial tube and applying cricoid pressure according to the anesthesiologist's instructions. Once the tube is secure and assistance is no longer necessary, the fetal heart should be auscultated.

The timing of induction of general anesthesia varies. In the United States, most patients are draped prior to induction, whereas in Great Britain it is not unusual to induce anesthesia first and then drape the patient.

Either the doctor or the circulating nurse scrubs and paints the abdomen. The Association of Operating Room Nurses (AORN) standards advise a 5-minute scrub with an antibacterial agent, such as Betadine or a pHisoHex preparation. The scrub begins along the suture line and proceeds in gradually larger circles. The abdomen should then be dried with sterile towels and the antimicrobial paint applied in the same fashion.

DUTIES OF THE SCRUB NURSE

The duties of the scrub nurse or technician during a cesarean section are much the same as for any abdominal surgery. The nurse, however, must give special consideration to

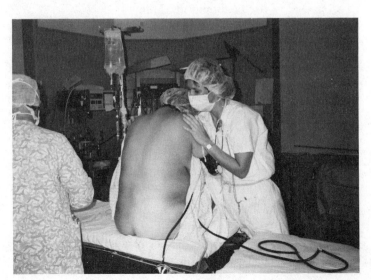

Figure 14–4. The therapeutic embrace—positioning for epidural anesthesia.

the fact that the fetus is totally dependent on its mother for ventilation, nutrition, excretion, and other vital functions, and therefore time is of the essence. Valuable time can be saved by anticipating the surgeon's needs during the procedure. For the most part, the surgery will follow certain predictable patterns.

In general, the scrub nurse is relied on to furnish the appropriate instruments, sutures, and sponges, and to monitor the sterile field and technique of all participants. She will assist in gowning and gloving the physicians and in draping the patient. As a rule, all laparotomy sponges should be moistened with warm normal saline. Commonly, two of these are kept on the surgical field at all times. The scrub nurse must keep track of any instruments, suture needles, and lap sponges placed on the field. Only items in use should be on the field. Instruments likely to be used should be kept on the Mayo stand. A list of instruments and what is necessary on the Mayo stand is given in Table 14–5. Those items least likely to be used should be accessible on the back table. Occasionally a hysterectomy is performed, and the additional instruments required for this procedure are listed in Table 14–6. Any laparotomy sponges that enter the abdominal cavity should be "tagged" or attached to a hemostat

Table 14–6. Extra Supplies for Hysterectomy

6 Ballantyne or heavy clamps
4 Straight Kocher long forceps
2 Curved Kocher long forceps
2 Péans
4 Carmalt
4 Curved Criles
6 Long right-angled clamps
4 Long tonsil clamps (Schnidt angled)
3 Long Babcock clamps
1 Single-toothed tenaculum
2 Long dissecting scissors (Mayo)
1 Long dissecting scissors (Metzenbaum)
2 10″ Mayo Hager needle holders
1 Bozeman vaginal packing forceps
1 Singley forceps
2 Long Russian forceps
2 Tissue forceps (smooth)
2 Tissue forceps (toothed)
1 Long #3 scalpel handle
1 Skin hook
1 Myoma screw
2 Sponge sticks
1 Balfour retractor

so that they can be identified and accounted for easily. A sterile towel can be made into a "pocket" for used suture materials, which can then be disposed of at the end of the case. A complete sponge and instrument count is performed before surgery begins, and the scrub nurse should be certain that the radiopaque tag is attached to each counted sponge (AORN, 1979). Once the patient is draped, the scrub nurse drops the proximal end of the suction tubing out of the sterile field, and the circulating nurse attaches it. The suction tube is then tested for proficiency. The Mayo stand and back table are moved into place, and surgery may begin.

For the skin incision, the surgeon needs a #21 blade. Once used, this is considered contaminated and is placed on a receptacle on the back table. Next, a #10 blade is used to incise the fat and nick a small hole in the fascia. The surgeon then needs a forceps with teeth and Mayo scissors (curved or straight) to open the remaining fascia. The instruments used to grasp the peritoneum prior to incising it may vary. Some surgeons use two Péans, while others use Kelly or toothed forceps. Once grasped, the peritoneum is usually incised with a knife, and the incision is extended with Metzenbaum scissors. Next, the bladder is dissected off the uterus. For this, the surgeon needs a smooth forceps and Metzenbaum scissors.

Table 14–5. Cesarean Section Instruments

Mayo Stand—Emergency Tray

2 Tissue forceps—smooth	1 #4 Scalpel handle
2 Tissue forceps—toothed	1 Bandage scissors
2 Short Russian forceps (5″)	1 Straight Mayo scissors
2 Adson forceps—toothed	1 Curved Mayo scissors
1 #3 Scalpel handle	2 Curved Kellys
	2 Péans
	4 Pennington clamps

Back Table

12 Towel clips	2 Straight Kocher forceps
4 Curved mosquitoes	2 Curved Kocher forceps
2 Straight mosquitoes	1 Singley forceps
6 Curved Kellys	1 Long smooth forceps
2 Straight Kellys	1 Long toothed forceps
6 Curved Péans	1 #4 Scalpel handle
6 Allis clamps	1 #3 Scalpel handle
2 Pennington clamps	1 Bladder blade retractor
2 Babcock clamps	1 Large Richardson
2 Curved Mayo scissors	1 Medium Richardson
1 Straight Mayo scissors	1 Pair Simpson forceps
8 Needle holders	
5 Sponge sticks	

The bladder blade is positioned so as to keep the bladder out of the way. In order to enter the uterus, the surgeon incises the myometrium with a #10 blade and either spreads the muscles manually or cuts them with a bandage scissors. It is very important that suction and lap sponges be available at this time. When the amniotic sac is ruptured, approximately 700 to 1000 cc of fluid will flow out of the uterus. For this reason, sterile towels may be draped around the wound for absorption. Sometimes the surgeon will require an Allis clamp to rupture membranes. The bladder blade is removed just before starting the delivery of the baby.

Once the baby's head is delivered, the physician will need a bulb syringe to suction the baby's mouth and nose. If meconium is noted in the amniotic fluid, a DeLee suction trap should be used to suction the baby. It is important that in disposing of the DeLee, the nurse take care not to contaminate the sterile field with the unsterile mouthpiece.

Following delivery, two straight Péan forceps are used to clamp the cord, and a pair of bandage scissors can be used to sever the cord between the clamps. The baby is then handed to the circulating nurse or pediatrician, with care taken to maintain sterility. Often before the placenta is delivered, the physician collects cord blood to be sent for analysis. (In multiple deliveries, each umbilical cord should be clamped with a different type of instrument so that one knows with delivery of the placentae which cord belongs to which baby. Obviously all tubes of cord blood should be properly identified.) Then the placenta is delivered into a basin and set on the back table. At this time the surgeon will need sponge sticks or Pennington clamps for removal of the membranes and to identify the uterine wound angles and the upper and lower portions of the uterine incision. The surgical field should be kept clear of excess blood, amniotic fluid, unused lap pads and towels. Dry sterile towels can be placed around the opening to help maintain a dry sterile field.

Next, the bladder blade is repositioned and uterine closure begun. Usually #0 or #1 atraumatic chromic sutures are used to suture the uterus in two layers. The surgeon also needs a toothed forceps for this step, and two hemostats are needed to "tag" these sutures until muscle closure is completed. After uterine closure, a count is needed to ensure that no lap pads or needles are left

behind. Next, the bladder flap is reapposed. The surgeon generally uses smooth forceps and a 2-0 chromic atraumatic suture. The bladder blade is now removed, and the tagged sutures are cut with a suture scissors.

A second sponge and instrument count is necessary before closing the parietal peritoneum. All lap sponges must be removed from the abdominal cavity. Some surgeons also remove blood clots and amniotic fluid from the abdomen. The abdomen may then be explored and the fallopian tubes and ovaries inspected. The peritoneum is usually identified with 3 Péan forceps, and sutured with a #0 chromic atraumatic suture. To appose the fascia, the surgeon needs a forceps with teeth and a #0 Vicryl or chromic but generally absorbable suture. If interrupted stitches are to be used, approximately 16 sutures will be needed. They are available with "pull-off" needles as a convenience. If a running stitch is to be used, two sutures on general closure needles will be required. Every time a surgeon uses sutures or ties, the suture scissors will be required to cut the excess material.

The fat is approximated using a toothed forceps and a 3-0 chromic or a plain catgut suture.

Skin closure may be accomplished by any of several different methods. If staples are chosen, the skin edges are usually held together during stapling with Adson forceps. A subcuticular suture of absorbable or nonabsorbable suture material may be used. The skin may also be closed using skin suture of nonabsorbable material, usually 3-0 or 4-0. Once the skin is closed, the nurse should provide a non-stick dressing, 4 × 4 gauze pads, and tape to dress the wound. A final sponge and instrument count is done following closure of the parietal peritoneum (AORN, 1979).

DUTIES OF THE CIRCULATING NURSE

The circulating nurse must record the following times when the patient entered the operating room; when anesthesia was started, when surgery was started; when delivery occurred; when surgery and anesthesia were completed; and when the patient left the room. This information becomes a permanent part of the patient's record, and should be accurate.

The circulating nurse may be asked by the anesthesiologist/anesthetist to apply pressure over the cricoid cartilage. Enough pressure should be applied to prevent vomitus from coming up from the stomach. This procedure is helpful in preventing aspiration, especially if the patient has eaten recently. However, it is usually recommended in all pregnant patients, because they have a slower rate of digestion.

Once surgery has begun, the circulating nurse should take a moment to scrutinize the environment, keeping the room neat. The lap bucket should be placed so that the technician can easily dispose of used laps for later counting and evaluation of blood loss. The AORN recommends that used laps be counted and placed in plastic bags as they accumulate (AORN, 1979). This helps to reduce splattering of blood and simplifies the counting process. Many hospitals require the bagging of laps by fives or tens. The circulating nurse should alert the anesthesiologist prior to bagging the blood-soaked laps so that blood loss can be accurately measured.

The nurse should make herself available for the care of the newborn before the uterine incision is made. In some hospitals, the infant warmer is covered with sterile drapes and the baby is placed directly into the warmer by the physician. In others, either the nurse or a pediatrician is covered with sterile drapes and the baby is handed directly to that person.

Resuscitation of the newborn proceeds as it would with a vaginal delivery. If the mother has received a general anesthetic, the baby might be lethargic and may have to be ventilated and stimulated until the ability to breathe spontaneously is demonstrated. The nurse should be able to respond quickly should the baby need to be intubated, in which case she must provide the doctor with the necessary equipment and assistance (Bacon et al., 1981).

Once the baby has been stabilized, it should be presented to the mother, if she is awake (Harmon et al., 1982) (Fig. 14–5). Eye drops and identification can be delayed until eye-to-eye contact has been accomplished. The mother should have her arms released so that she can hold and examine her infant. Bonding can proceed as it would with a vaginal delivery, provided the integrity of the sterile field is not violated. Some experts encourage breast-feeding at this time.

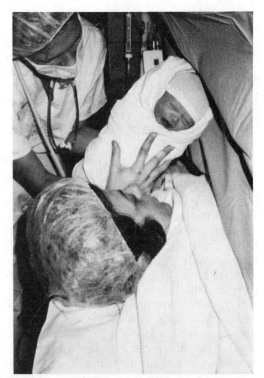

Figure 14–5. Bonding in the en face position can be accomplished even during surgery.

Once bonding is completed and eye drops are instilled, the baby can be sent to the nursery according to the usual hospital routine.

Lap pads, instruments, and needles should be counted by the scrub nurse as previously mentioned. The circulating nurse should observe sterile technique and report any breaches of technique. She should feel free to insist on a change of gloves, gowns, instruments, or drapes without fear of recrimination. She serves as a patient advocate and should recognize her role in reinforcing quality assurance in the operating room.

Upon completion of the surgery, the patient's abdomen should be cleansed before the dressings are applied. Since the patient may be lying in a pool of amniotic fluid and blood, the nurse will want to make sure that the patient is thoroughly bathed before moving her to a clean stretcher with a clean gown and peri pad. Many anesthesiologists agree that regardless of the type of anesthesia, the patient should be moved gently, preferably using a roller. Sudden changes in position or rough handling may result in hypotension.

In a family-centered birth experience, coordination with the anesthesiologist and surgeon is necessary with regard to when the support person may be allowed into the operating room. Some physicians prefer that significant others wait until the patient has been anesthetized and draped, whereas others prefer that the visitor be ushered in earlier to give support throughout the entire procedure.

Obviously, the support person should be in scrub attire with cap and mask. He or she is seated at the head of the table, close to the patient, so that physical contact and verbal intimacy can be enjoyed. If the father and mother wish to see the delivery, mirrors can be strategically placed. Frequently, the surgeon will instruct the father to stand up and watch as his baby is being delivered (Gawse, 1982).

If the couple requests a gentle birth experience following surgical delivery, adaptations can be made once the baby is stabilized. The father can be encouraged to act as mother surrogate in this case.

If the father has been excluded from the birth process, a message should be sent to him in the waiting room announcing the time of birth and the sex of the infant (Quinn and Sommers, 1974). The father will also appreciate reassurance that the surgery is proceeding as expected. He should be given a realistic idea as to when he, the baby, and the mother will be reunited.

Emergency Cesarean Section

Normal labor can suddenly and unpredictably become an obstetric emergency necessitating cesarean section. Some are true emergencies in which the surgery must be performed immediately, to avoid serious risk to the mother or the fetus, or both. Other situations may be characterized as semi-emergencies, e.g., secondary arrest, cephalopelvic disproportion, or determination of the need for a repeat section in early labor. The emergency cesarean section is defined as "surgical removal of the fetus from the womb specifically aimed at saving the baby or mother from life-threatening complications."

Indications for emergency cesarean delivery are: fetal distress, prolapsed cord, abruptio placentae with fetal distress, placenta previa accompanied by vaginal hemorrhage, and/or a transverse lie in active labor. Occasionally, a multiple gestation requires an emergency cesarean section.

Since time is of the essence, it is obvious that neither the physician, the nurse, nor the patient will have time to make elaborate plans. Thus, the emotional and educational preparation described previously will largely be eliminated. It is important to emphasize that *although physiologic needs must take priority during the emergency, psychologic needs must not be neglected, but unfortunately often are in the rush to get the infant delivered* (Schlosser, 1978). However, especially in a life-threatening crisis, any education and support to the patient and her family will be well appreciated.

The labor room nurse is expected to demonstrate considerable expertise in the interpretation and treatment of fetal distress. Since the advent of fetal monitoring, the nurse's role and responsibilities have increased. Once fetal distress or any other acute situation has been detected, and the necessity for cesarean birth established, the preparatory tasks will have to be performed expeditiously. Emergency cesarean section equipment should be conveniently located in every operating/delivery suite.

Although the patient may not have been specifically prepared for a cesarean, as mentioned earlier, information about cesarean delivery may have been included as part of her routine prenatal care and education. Again, during the "prep" and catheterization of the patient, an explanation of the problem should be given, along with supportive reassurance that under the circumstances, this is the best possible choice (Schlosser, 1978).

Everyone's anxiety level is increased during an emergency. Aimless rushing about serves only to increase confusion and results in unnecessary mistakes. Thus, it is necessary to minimize chaos and organize priorities of care to meet the life-threatening crisis.

Preparation for an emergency or semi-emergency cesarean should be a consideration for every patient admitted to Labor and Delivery. As a result, many obstetric services on admission routinely request permission for cesarean section, fetal scalp sampling, and blood administration. When consent for these procedures is requested, the patient should be advised that this is in order to save precious time later, in the event that surgical intervention becomes necessary. Permissions signed on admission, when stress is less than during an acute emergency and when the patient is not receiving any drugs, are more valid. Again, the prenatal course provides a good opportunity to inform the patient and her family about these forms; this is best included in the discussion on hospital admission procedures. The consent forms should be discussed clearly and in language the patient can comprehend (Quinn and Sommers, 1984). She should be reassured, however, that operative intervention will be undertaken *only* if absolutely necessary. If the patient is actively bleeding or is anemic, or if excessive blood loss is expected, then blood should be cross-matched. While preparing for the emergency or semi-emergency cesarean, all personnel will perform the same tasks practiced at a more leisurely pace during the planned cesarean. The difference is the time element and its impact on the emotions of all involved.

During a medical crisis, there is a tendency for people to congregate. All nonessential personnel should be told to leave the room. There is *no need* for more than two circulating nurses during an emergency cesarean. Ideally, all members of the operating room staff clearly understand the procedure and their responsibilities. It is advisable for only one person to give instructions; traditionally this is done by the surgeon, but if he or she is preoccupied, the assertive, experienced nurse should be the organizer. Talking should be kept at a minimum and limited to only necessary instructions.

The circulating nurse must prioritize her activities, starting by opening items that will be needed initially, such as gloves, gowns, drapes, and blades. Nonessential items clutter the operative table, confuse the technician, and waste time. Ideally, the operating room will have been scrutinized at shift change, and all equipment will be present and functional. Some hospitals have an emergency Mayo tray already prepared with everything needed to reach the baby (even the blades having been previously placed on the scalpel). Then, when time permits, another tray, with the remaining instruments needed, is opened for the back table.

It is imperative to realize that any emergency situation will have some traumatic effect on the patient. (Integration of the cesarean birth experience, 1980). Some patients express anger at the medical staff for neglecting labor pains during the preparations for emergency surgery. Others report they felt embarrassed by being stripped naked and "crucified." Fortunately, the majority express gratefulness and genuine admiration of the staff as they adeptly move through their paces. Finally, some express a sense of unreality described as a feeling of having their hands disengaged from their bodies!

It is important to remember that the patient will be watching the team spring into action. She is frightened and sensitive to facial expressions, tone of voice, and all movement going on in the room. By minimizing confusion and providing support, the staff can prevent her from becoming panicky. Patients frequently remember either that they were treated well during the crisis or that they were emotionally abandoned (Clark and Affonso, 1979). They respond very favorably to physical reassurance, such as holding of a hand or stroking of the face. Ideally a specific person should have responsibility for maintaining emotional contact with the patient; the importance of this support should not be underestimated (Schlosser, 1978).

Another emotion that a mother will recall is fear for the welfare of her baby and/or herself. As soon as the patient emerges from anesthesia she should be appraised of the status of the baby, and if the father or a "significant other" is nearby, he (or she) should be sent word as to the baby's and mother's well-being at the earliest possible time.

Some mothers will go through a grief reaction because of what they perceive as reproductive failure, and will need substantial emotional support later on. However, most accept that the cesarean was the best choice.

The Postanesthetic Period: The Fourth Stage of Labor

Once the patient has been moved to the Postanesthesia/Recovery Room, vital signs are taken; breath sounds are checked; the intravenous line, dressings, fundus, and lochia are inspected; and the Foley catheter is checked to make sure that it is draining. The patient's skin color and level of consciousness must also be noted. If the patient is recovering from regional anesthesia, she is asked to move her legs, and her level of activity is noted. While the patient is in the recovery room, her I & O should be recorded at a minimum of every hour.

Vital signs should be taken every 15 minutes for 1 or 2 hours or until the patient is stable. The patient should be fully alert and oriented (in the case of general anesthesia), or able to lift her knees against gravity (in the case of regional anesthesia) before discharge to floor care.

Postanesthesia care includes careful gentle assessment of uterine contractility and lochial flow. Should the uterus become boggy, resulting in excessive bleeding or accumulation of clots, gentle fundal massage and oxytocics should be instituted. Fundal massage is painful, so caution should be exercised and a very sympathetic explanation given as to its necessity. Postcesarean care combines postanesthetic and postpartum nursing skills.

Postoperative Care

Just as preoperative care and understanding of the procedure of cesarean section is important to the patient, so also is postoperative care. Most commonly, management is conservative. Patients are usually kept in bed until the Foley catheter is removed and/or the intravenous line is discontinued.

Upon transfer to the postpartum area, an overall physical, psychologic, and social assessment of the patient should be made and the information entered on a form such as the one shown in Figure 14–6 (Jenson et al., 1981; Olds, 1980). It is important to know the location and status of the neonate, since a sick neonate is a signal that the patient may need even more psychologic support than usual. Based on all of the aforementioned factors, a nursing care plan can be outlined. Since the mother may not be able to visit the intensive care nursery, a photograph of her baby will help her to initiate bonding. However, if there is a chance that the baby will die, the mother should be encouraged to visit the baby in the nursery, even if it is by wheelchair or stretcher.

Among the postpartum clinical problems is the potential for increased blood loss or hemorrhage. Vital signs should be taken at least every 4 hours for the first 48 to 72 hours. Any significant changes in the patient's pulse (rhythm and character) and/or blood pressure necessitates further investigation to determine what, if any, hemodynamic changes are occurring (Jenson et al., 1981; Olds, 1980). Other measures include observation of the lochia, of the number of pads used, of fundal height and firmness, and of the dressing, for evidence of increased bleeding. Oxytocin may be added to the intravenous line in an effort to control uterine bleeding, and manual pressure may be applied to the fundus in order to express blood clots from the uterus and vagina. If bleeding from the incision is noted, the wound should be inspected for defects and to determine the bleeding site. Postoperatively, there are usually orders for two blood counts, one within several hours of surgery, and one for the next day. These results should be reviewed to determine if there has been a drop in hematocrit, which would indicate blood loss (Olds, 1980).

The patient's respiratory status is an important key to her recovery. Breath sounds should be checked at least once every 8 hours, to make sure that they are clear and that there is no congestion. For the most part respiratory care is preventive. Breathing exercises such as blow bottles and volume inspirometers encourage deep breathing, helping to prevent postoperative atelectasis. Pillows may be used for splinting the incision site during coughing. Other respiratory treatments (e.g., chest physiotherapy, jet nebulizers, IPPB, and antibiotics) may be ordered, depending on whether respiratory complications, such as pneumonia, develop.

Alimentation is generally progressed gradually: The patient is kept NPO on the day of surgery; clear liquids are given the following day; and the patient gradually progresses to full liquids and then to a regular diet by about the 3rd postoperative day (Bleier, 1979). This gives the intestinal tract the chance to recover from major abdominal surgery. Intravenous therapy provides nutritional support and hydration during this time. When bowel sounds are present, a regular diet can be given.

A more aggressive approach may be taken, which includes feeding patients clear hot liquids in the recovery room postoperatively as early as 2 hours after general anesthesia or immediately following the operation if only a regional block was used. If the patient tolerates fluids without difficulty, and the

CESAREAN SECTION

PATIENT ASSESSMENT

Name _____Age_____Religion/Culture_____

G/P _____Allergies_____Language_____

C/S planned _____ _____Unplanned_____Emergency_____

Patient's perceptions of the procedure:
  (Before and/or after)

_____

_____

_____

_____

Significant medical OB history and complications:

Past _____

_____

Present _____

_____

Present Medications: _____

_____

Physical Assessment

Vital signs: Temperature _____ Pulse _____ Respirations_____

             B.P. _____

Breath Sounds: Clear _____ Congested _____

Bowel Sounds: Present _____ Absent _____

Elimination - Bladder: Foley _____   Voiding _____

                        Color _____   Consistency _____

Incision site: Dressing intact _____ Bloody _____ Drainage _____

Additional drains in place? _____

_____

Other pertinent observations: _____

_____

_____

Lochia: Profuse _____   Moderate _____Scanty_____

         Rubra_____   Serosa _____   Alba _____

Figure 14–6. Patient assessment form for cesarean section.

vast majority of patients do, she can be started on a regular diet for the next feeding if desired. Ambulating patients as early as 6 hours postoperatively, together with early feeding, stimulates gastrointestinal motility, is effective in the relief of gas pain, and decreases the need for narcotics. An antiflatulent or a Harris flush is also helpful in relieving discomfort from gas. Early ambulation may be even more important for those mothers whose babies are in the ICU, since visits to the ICU facilitate bonding and involvement in the infant's care. All patients should have had a bowel movement prior to discharge.

Urinary output should be monitored frequently and recorded at least every 4 hours, and should average 30 cc per hour. The catheter is often left in place for 6 to 12 hours postoperatively. After it has been discontinued, the patient's output should continue to be monitored for at least 8 hours, to verify that normal bladder/urinary tract function has returned.

Patients experience two different types of pain: incisional site and "afterbirth" pains. Pain perception is highly individualized because of vast differences in pain threshold. Patients may be medicated intramuscularly or orally. Pain relief is generally in the form of narcotics for the first 24 to 48 hours and in some cases even as long as 72 hours. Positioning, early ambulation, and general comfort measures can also help to relieve pain. Patients on pain medication can provide care to their newborns, provided they have proper supervision. In some areas of the country, a device called a transcutaneous nerve stimulator is being used to decrease the degree of postoperative pain felt by the patients.

Sutures or staples are removed on the 4th or 5th postoperative day, and a patient with an uncomplicated, uneventful course may be sent home on that day. Some patients who are fully ambulatory, able to care for themselves, and have help at home may be discharged as early as the second postoperative day. Of course, this also depends on the psychologic makeup of the patient—her initiative and drive—and on the absence of postoperative complications.

Infection is another concern in the postpartum period. An increasing temperature and/or pulse rate is a sign that an infectious process may be present.

The most common cause of postoperative infection is endomyometritis, usually as a result of prolonged labor, multiple pelvic examinations, and/or prolonged rupture of the membranes. Since postoperative infection most commonly results from a combination of aerobic and anaerobic bacteria, it is very difficult—even with good culturing techniques—to identify the offending organisms. Most of these infections respond to broad-spectrum intravenous antibiotics (e.g., penicillin and/or gentamycin) within 24 to 36 hours, but if they do not, then they will generally respond to the addition of clindamycin (Cleocin) or chloramphenicol (Chloromycetin), which covers *Bacteroides* organisms. The presence of infection, however, is not a reason to limit ambulation. Methylergonovine maleate (Methergine) intramuscularly or orally augments treatment of uterine infection by stimulating contractions and encouraging involution. Breast-feeding accomplishes the same purpose, but the nursery staff may be concerned about the possibility of neonatal sepsis if the mother is infected. So long as the patient does not have an open draining wound or a known bacteremia, and once she is sufficiently covered by antibiotics, there is certainly no contraindication to her breast-feeding unless certain antibiotics are used (see Chapter 6 for a complete list).

Other causes of postoperative fever include wound infections and urinary tract infections. Patients who are exposed to anesthesia, specifically general anesthesia, may develop atelectasis or pneumonia. Finally, although very rare, pelvic thrombophlebitis may also be a source of fever and may result in pulmonary emboli. Any patient who postoperatively has a persistent fever that does not respond to triple antibiotic therapy, and who has no other source of infection, should seriously be considered as having a suppurative venous thrombophlebitis, which will have to be treated with heparin. Of course, intraabdominal abscesses must also be ruled out. If she develops chest pain and/or shortness of breath in the postoperative period, pulmonary embolus is a distinct possibility. Patients diagnosed as having deep thrombophlebitis or pulmonary emboli should be treated with intravenous heparin. If the diagnosis is deep phlebitis without an embolus, heparin is continued for 10 days. If pulmonary embolus is diagnosed based on chest pain, dyspnea, and arterial blood gases, and is confirmed by ventilation perfusion lung scans, then treatment will also include warfarin (Coumadin) for 3 to 6 months. Patients receiving anticoagulants will require multiple lab tests to follow the coagulation studies. The Lee White or activated PTT is kept at 1½ to 2½ times normal to follow heparin, and the Pro-Time at 1½ to 2½ times normal to follow Coumadin for anticoagulation effect.

Continued family-centered maternity care can be fostered by allowing a significant other to participate (in the company of the patient) in those activities that the patient would normally do (Reeder et al., 1980), for example, feeding the baby or changing its diapers. Rooming-in during the first 48 hours, when the mother is the most uncomfortable, can be accomplished by means of surrogate care given in the patient's room. Bonding between mother and baby may be impeded as a result of the mother's immobility from pain, effects of narcotics, and so on. In such cases, bonding should be assisted by the nursing staff via frequent contacts with the baby and properly timed pain medication. When a patient who has undergone a cesarean section desires to breast-feed, assistance should be given in determining the easiest position for her. For those mothers whose infants are in the ICU, assistance in using the breast pump, manual or electric, will be necessary. This is also a good time to offer psychologic support to the mother with a sick neonate.

For those mothers not breast-feeding, suppressive therapy may or may not be used. If patients are allowed to lactate, they will need breast binders or tight bras and ice packs for the 24-hour period from day 3 to day 4, when engorgement occurs.

Tylenol around the clock every 3 hours is most helpful for pain relief and has decreased the incidence of postoperative thrombophlebitis as well.

Psychologic support for the mother is a continuing aspect of care. Encouraging the patient to express her feelings regarding the surgery is important to her psychologic well-being in the future. This is especially true if she has undergone an emergency cesarean section and therefore had little or no time to mentally prepare herself. Women who have had cesareans under emergency circumstances have reported feelings that range from fear to sensations of having been "attacked" (Quinn, 1974). Women whose infants are in the ICU are also in need of special psychologic support.

It has been found that holding postpartum support groups, either in the hospital or later in the postpartum period, has been beneficial in reducing fears for future pregnancies and in explaining the circumstances surrounding the actual delivery.

One of the most difficult days for the postpartum patient is the day of breast engorgement and postpartum blues, which occurs about the third day. During this period, she may be minimally depressed or in rare cases severely depressed. If she is made aware that this occurs and is normal, she will probably handle it much better. Making the family aware that the patient may be teary-eyed for approximately 24 hours certainly helps them to cope with the situation as well. One has to remember that these patients, in addition to their physical discomfort, are now learning to deal with a new infant and wondering how they will interrelate with the infant and husband or significant other.

Patient education should be an ongoing process during the hospital stay and should include both maternal and newborn care. Additionally, special guidelines for the cesarean section patient to follow after discharge should be given. These should include:

- A list of warning signs to alert them when to see their physician or go to the emergency room (e.g., if they develop a fever, chills, increased bleeding, problems with the incision site)
- A list of contraindications to performing certain activities; this should include no driving, lifting, housework, or exercises for 2 weeks, or for as long as the physician orders.
- Instructions to take showers instead of baths for a week when external incisional healing has taken place.
- Information about changes to expect in their lochia, which will change in color from red to brown to white.

Many cesarean section patients feel ready to return to work by 4 weeks post partum, and as long as all is well, they may do so. Certainly, from a medical point of view, there is no question that most mothers should be able to return to work by 6 weeks post partum.

Cesarean Hysterectomy

Rarely a patient may undergo a cesarean hysterectomy, either as a preplanned procedure or as an emergency procedure at the time of cesarean section for uncontrollable bleeding, infection, or the inability to close the uterus because of fibroids, for example. Such a patient loses her reproductive function. The patient who has an emergency procedure is totally unprepared for this loss. It is essential that physicians and nurses spend enough time with the patient and her family to ensure that they fully understand the need for the procedure and what its results will be. Although it is not necessarily the case for all patients, for some the loss of reproductive function results in a grieving process. Should this loss also be combined with the loss of a child, the situation becomes extremely difficult for the patient and her family to handle. The patient will need counseling over the next several days, whether it be by a nurse, a bereavement team, a psychologic social worker, or a psychiatrist. These patients may be especially difficult to treat because of their anger and sense of loss. It is incumbent upon the staff to try and understand the patient's anger and not to overreact to what they may perceive as a lack of cooperation on her part. (This applies to the physician as well.) Such patients are extremely challenging to deal with, but if one takes the time and effort, the vast majority will respond.

Vaginal Delivery in a Previous Cesarean Section Patient

One of the major contributing factors to the increased cesarean section rate has been the elective repeat procedure, which accounts for 25 to 30 percent of the increase in rates from 1970 to 1978, according to the National Institutes of Health Consensus Report (NICHD, 1980).

As mentioned earlier, in the first part of this century, the majority of abdominal deliveries were carried out through an incision in the fundal portion of the uterus. In a subsequent pregnancy, rupture was a real risk. Therefore, it became standard procedure to do elective repeat cesarean sections.

The risk of rupture of a classic scar is approximately 2.2 percent, which is 4 to 5 times greater than the risk of rupture with a lower uterine segment scar (0.5 percent). Rupture of either scar most commonly occurs following vaginal delivery. The classic

scar is 7 times more likely to rupture during labor and delivery than is the lower segment scar (8.9 vs. 1.2 percent). Maternal mortality from a fundal scar rupture is 5 percent, with a fetal mortality of 73 percent, as compared with the lower segment situation, in which maternal mortality is almost nonexistent and fetal mortality is approximately 12.5 percent (Dewhurst, 1957). Therefore, in terms of future obstetric performance, the lower segment transverse incision offers a better opportunity for a safe trial of labor, since the risk of rupture is considerably lower than that associated with a classic incision.

Numerous publications show that from 33 to 75 percent of all patients previously delivered abdominally can subsequently deliver vaginally, depending upon selection criteria. Since more primary cesareans are being done today because of a more liberal attitude toward total fetal and maternal outcome, it only stands to reason that if the risks are acceptable, more consideration should be given to allowing a subsequent trial of labor under carefully set criteria.

Repeat cesarean section increases the risk of maternal mortality to at least twice that of vaginal delivery. Health care costs also are considerably more. The NIH therefore has recommended that serious consideration be given to attempted vaginal delivery following a low segment transverse operation for a previous cesarean section.

Selection criteria will vary somewhat from hospital to hospital, as will exclusion criteria. However, one essential criterion is that facilities and staff be available for prompt emergency cesarean section. Other criteria for vaginal delivery in women with previous cesarean section may include the following:

1. Only one previous low segment procedure with no extension, as documented by hospital records and operative note.

2. Previous indication for the initial cesarean section no longer exists.

3. Patient acceptance after an explanation of the risks of delivery vaginally versus abdominally.

4. Clinically adequate pelvis for this baby.

5. No medical or obstetric problems.

6. No previous uterine rupture.

In view of the above listed inclusion criteria, *excluded* from a trial of labor would be patients for whom any of the following apply:

1. Any patient whose uterine incision was

other than a low segment transverse—e.g., "T", low segment vertical, classic, unknown incisions.

2. Inadequate facilities for a prompt emergency cesarean section.

3. Patient refusal.

4. Contracted pelvis or macrosomic infant.

5. Recurrent condition.

6. Medical or obstetric complications that may increase risks for either mother or infant, e.g., diabetes, multiple gestation, malpresentations, induction for preterm delivery.

When conducting a trial of labor, ideally, the onset of labor should be spontaneous. The patient should be instructed to report to the hospital as soon as she is suspicious that labor has begun. Once admitted to the hospital, blood should be drawn for routine studies and cross-match, IV fluids initiated, and permission obtained for cesarean section and possible hysterectomy. Continuous external monitoring should be instituted. Once membranes are ruptured and/or labor is active, a scalp electrode should be used. If an internal catheter for uterine contractility is not used, a hand should be kept on the abdomen so that uterine contractions can be carefully observed. The patient should not be left unattended under any circumstances; thus, a 1:1 nurse–patient ratio should be maintained. However, if an intrauterine catheter is in place, a minimum of a 1:2 ratio is acceptable. Labor should progress normally. This can be assessed through the use of a partogram. Vital signs must be carefully monitored every 15 to 30 minutes. Many physicians use oxytocin for induction and/or stimulation of labor in these cases. However, improper use of this drug has been associated with rupture of a previously non-scarred uterus; therefore, extreme caution should be exercised when using oxytocin in patients with a uterine scar.

The patient should be very carefully watched for the signs and symptoms of scar rupture listed in Table 14–7.

Analgesia should be selected, keeping the signs and symptoms of rupture in mind as well as the effects of analgesia on uterine contractility, pelvic floor relaxation, and the possibility of a subsequent need for instrument assistance in delivery, e.g., forceps or vacuum extractor.

It is essential that once the infant is delivered, the lower uterine segment be carefully

Table 14–7. Signs and Symptoms of Ruptured Cesarean Scar

	Classical	Low Segment
Pain	Continuous	+
	Tearing, then relief	±
Scar	Tenderness	+, suprapubic
Fetus	Extruded into abdomen	Rarely
		Irregularity or swelling suprapubically
	Fetal distress	Occasionally
	Fetal death	Rarely
Contractions	Frequently cease	Continue
Abdomen	Distention	Rarely
	Tenderness	±
Pulse	Tachycardia	+
Restlessness	+	±
Collapse	+	Rare
Cervical dilatation	Arrested	±
Vaginal bleeding	±	±/L late, first stage, postpartum
Hematuria	−	±

From O'Sullivan, M. J., Fumia, F., Holsinger, K. K., et al.: Vaginal delivery after cesarean section. Clin. Perinatol. 8:138, 1981.

examined to determine the presence or absence of a defect. Of course, the cervix and vagina should also be evaluated and checked for possible lacerations, regardless of whether delivery was assisted or spontaneous. Should a defect be palpable, indicating that the abdominal cavity and/or broad ligaments have been entered, then a laparotomy must be performed. A defect in which the abdominal cavity or broad ligaments have *not* been entered and which is not bleeding can be closely observed to determine if there is concealed bleeding. The development of tachycardia, restlessness, hypotension, thirst, tachypnea, air hunger, and/or abdominal pain is highly suggestive of concealed bleeding. If the fundus rises and is pushed to one side in the presence of an empty bladder, a broad ligament hematoma must be ruled out. On vaginal examination, fullness anteriorly (after bladder evacuation) or in either parametrial region also suggests bleeding and warrants further evaluation. Any abnormal bleeding, either associated with a defect or which is not easily explained or controlled, warrants laparotomy.

Before a trial of labor, all patients should be told that if a scar rupture occurs they may require a hysterectomy, although this is not always necessary. Neither the postpartum hospital stay nor febrile morbidity is affected by a previous section patient who is allowed a trial of labor that failed, compared with patients having primary cesareans for secondary arrest, cephalopelvic disproportion, etc. (O'Sullivan et al., 1981). The cost of care for patients who deliver vaginally following a trial of labor is considerably reduced, as are the number of postpartum hospital days. A patient who successfully delivers vaginally is not by any means immune from scar rupture in her next pregnancy. Each subsequent labor should be conducted as carefully as the first one following cesarean delivery. If a defect is palpable after delivery, but is asymptomatic, the woman's next delivery is better conducted abdominally.

Following a primary cesarean section, discussion should be held with the patient concerning her future method of delivery. If she is a candidate for vaginal delivery in the future she can be reassured this is the case, but if the physician feels she is not a candidate, he should tell her so. It is important that she know the type and location of her uterine incision, extensions if any, and the indication for her primary cesarean section. Careful documentation on the hospital chart is very important and helpful in future management. Also, a surgery summary may be given to the patient for her own records.

Conclusion

Obstetrics has changed radically over this century, and will continue to change. As providers of health care, we must be informed, sensitive to our patients, and adaptable to changes that are beneficial and important, but not too eager to jump on bandwagons.

The greatest gains in perinatal outcome have been made in cases of premature infants. Some of this is due to an increase in abdominal deliveries for these infants, but the greatest increase in cesarean sections has actually been in term pregnancies—without a concomitantly increased improvement in perinatal outcome. It is incumbent upon us all in the medical profession to provide good health care to the maternal-fetal unit, but at minimal risk, and to do no harm.

REFERENCES

Affonso, D., and Stickler, J.: Women's reactions to their cesarean births. Birth Family Journal 5:1, 1978.

Alley, A.: Pre-operative teaching for cesarean birth. AORN 34:846, 1981.

Anderson, B., Camacho M., and Stark, J.: Interruptions in family health during pregnancy. In The Childbearing Family, Vol. II. New York, McGraw-Hill, 1975.

AORN Standards of Practice Association of Operating Room Nurses, Inc., Denver, CO, 1979.

Bacon, K., Louch, G., Louch, K., et al.: Care of the neonate after cesarean section. AORN 34:860, 1981.

Bleier, I.: Bedside Maternity Nursing. Philadelphia, W. B. Saunders Co., 1979, pp. 210–211.

Choate, J. W., and Lund, C. J., Emergency cesarean section. Am. J. Obstet. Gynecol. 100:703, 1968.

Clark, A., and Affonso, D.: Childbearing: A Nursing Perspective, 2nd ed. Philadelphia, F. A. Davis, 1979, pp. 718–727.

Cohen, S. A.: The aspiration syndrome. Clin. Obstet. Gynaecol. 9:235, 1982.

Conklin, M., Discussion groups as preparation for cesarean section. JOGN Nurs. 6 (4):52, 1977.

Cox, B., and Smith, E.: The mother's self-esteem after a cesarean delivery. MCN 7:309, 1982.

Dewhurst, C. J.: The ruptured cesarean section scar. J. Obstet. Gynaecol. Br. Commonw. 74:113, 1957.

Donovan, B., and Allen, R.: The cesarean birth method. JOGN Nurs. 6:37, 1977.

Friedman, E.: Labor: clinical evaluation and management, 2nd ed. New York Appleton-Century-Crofts, 1978.

Gawse, R.: Fathers at the cesarean delivery. American Baby 44:32, 1982.

Harmon, R., Glicken, A., and Good, W.: A new look at maternal-infant bonding. Perinatol. Neonatol. 6:27, 1982.

Hoffman, N.: Edith Potter, M.D., Ph.D.: Pioneering infant pathology. JAMA 248:1551–1553, 1982.

Integration of the cesarean birth experience—the various adjustment cycles. Perinatal Press, 4:136, 1980.

Jenson, M., Benson, R., and Bobak, I.: Maternity Care—The Nurse and the Family. St. Louis, C. V. Mosby Co., 1981, pp. 518–529, 559–586.

Mann, L. I., and Galant, J. M.: Modern indications for cesarean section. Am. J. Obstet. Gynecol. 135:437, 1979.

NICHD: Consensus Report by the Task Force on Cesarean Childbirth. Bethesda, MD, NICHD, 1980.

Olds, S. B.: Obstetric Nursing. Reading, MA, Addison-Wesley, 1980, pp. 601–629.

O'Sullivan, M. J., Fumia, F., Holsinger K. K., et al.: Vaginal delivery after cesarean section. Clin. Perinatol. 8:131, 1981.

Quilligan, E., and Zuspan, F.: Douglas-Stromme Operative Obstetrics, 4th ed. New York, Appleton-Century-Crofts, 1982.

Quinn, N., and Sommers, A.: The patient's Bill of Rights. Nursing Outlook 22:240, 1974.

Reeder, S., Mastroianni, L., and Martin, L.: Maternity Nursing. Philadelphia, J. B. Lippincott Co., 1980, pp. 573–577, 723–724.

Schlosser, S.: The emergency C-section patient. Why she needs help . . . what you can do. RN 41:53, 1978.

Slee, V. N. (ed.): Cesarean sections in U.S. P.A.S. Reporter C.P.H.A., Ann Arbor, MI, 1976, p. 15.

ANESTHESIA IN PREGNANCY

CHARLES P. GIBBS

Introduction

DEFINITION OF TERMS

Before discussing obstetric anesthesia, commonly used terms in anesthesiology need definition. *Anesthesia* encompasses all the various techniques used by the anesthesiologist—for example, general anesthesia, analgesia, regional anesthesia, and local anesthesia.

General anesthesia implies not only loss of sensation but also loss of consciousness and varying degrees of motor and reflex activity. Traditionally, general anesthesia includes four stages, and only during the deeper stages will all of these losses occur. Stage I is *analgesia*, during which memory and sensitivity to pain fade, yet consciousness and protective reflexes, such as swallowing and laryngeal closure, are maintained. *Stage II*, the *excitement* stage, approaches the border between consciousness and unconsciousness. During this stage the patient may be markedly uncooperative as well as susceptible to laryngospasm, vomiting, and aspiration. Anesthesiologists avoid this stage by keeping the patient in Stage 1 or by passing rapidly to Stage 3 with the aid of fast-acting barbiturates and muscle relaxants. *Stage III*, the stage during which most surgical procedures are performed, has four planes. As the patient passes through them, anesthesia deepens, and the nervous, cardiovascular, and respiratory systems are progressively depressed. Also, laryngeal reflexes almost disappear. Thus, vomiting or regurgitation render the patient dangerously susceptible to aspiration unless her airway is protected by an endotracheal tube. *Stage IV* terminates in death.

Anesthesiologists can produce either analgesia or general anesthesia with nearly all inhalation agents and some intravenous agents, such as narcotics or ketamine. They select the proper dose, concentration, and combination of these agents according to the particular obstetric procedure. Nitrous oxide and enflurane are the inhalation agents most commonly used to produce analgesia. When used appropriately in low doses or concentrations, these agents do not produce enough anesthesia for surgery; they produce only analgesia. Without an accompanying pudendal block or local infiltration of the perineum, analgesia techniques have little effect except during spontaneous delivery without episiotomy.

Balanced anesthesia is general anesthesia that utilizes a thiobarbiturate (usually thiopental) or ketamine as an induction agent, succeeded by succinylcholine and nitrous oxide. An induction agent produces unconsciousness rapidly, so that paralysis and intubation can be performed without the patient's awareness; succinylcholine provides muscle relaxation for intubation and immobility during the procedure, and nitrous oxide produces analgesia (pain relief). Low-dose halothane or enflurance can add additional analgesia. Because laryngeal reflexes are obliterated, an endotracheal tube is necessary to protect the airway. Balanced anesthesia works effectively for any difficult or operative obstetric procedure, including cesarean section, but is not necessary for most vaginal deliveries. In those rare instances when uterine relaxation is necessary, higher concentrations of halothane may be added to the balanced general technique. Older agents, such as ether and cyclopropane, are flammable, dangerous, and no longer necessary.

Regional analgesia (although analgesia is the more correct term, anesthesia is commonly used in its place) uses local anesthetics to provide sensory as well as varying degrees of motor blockade over a specific region of the body. Pain during the first stage of labor results primarily from the dilating cervix and the contracting fundus. Painful sensations travel from the uterus along the sympathetic nerves and enter the spinal cord through the posterior segments of thoracic spinal nerves 11 and 12 (Fig. 15–1). Pain during the second stage of labor results from the distension of the pelvic floor and vaginal outlet by the presenting part. The sensory fibers of sacral nerves 2, 3, and 4, which make up the pudendal nerve, transmit the pain to the spinal cord (Fig. 15–1).

In obstetrics, regional analgesic techniques to block these pain impulses include major blocks, such as spinal (saddle), lumbar and caudal epidural, as well as paracervical, pudendal, and local infiltration (Fig. 15–1).

PERSONNEL

An *anesthesiologist* is a physician who has completed at least 3 years of postgraduate training in an approved residency program. A *nurse anesthetist* is a nurse who has completed at least 18 months in a training program sponsored by the American Association of Nurse Anesthetists. The word anesthetist is often used for either nurse anesthetist or anesthesiologist: In England, anesthesiologists are called anaesthetists. Because nurse anesthetists are not physicians, they must work under the supervision of a physician. Ideally, an anesthesiologist assumes this supervisory role, resulting in a very efficient anesthesiologist/anesthetist team. However, often the operating surgeon or obstetrician will, or must, assume the role of the physician supervisor to the nurse anesthetist. In these instances, the physician must be both surgeon and anesthesiologist.

Effects of Anesthetic Agents on the Newborn

It is safe to generalize about the placental transfer of anesthetic agents and say that all

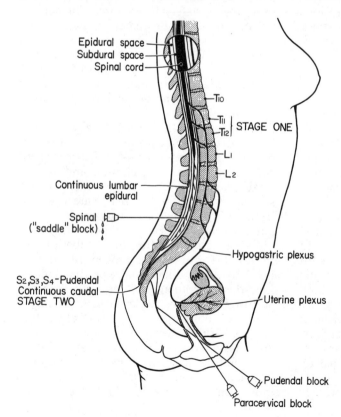

Epidural space —
Subdural space —
Spinal cord —

—T10

—T11 STAGE ONE
—T12

—L1

—L2

Continuous lumbar epidural —

Spinal ("saddle" block) —

Hypogastric plexus

S2,S3,S4–Pudendal
Continuous caudal
STAGE TWO

Uterine plexus

Pudendal block

Paracervical block

Figure 15–1. Obstetric pain pathways and anesthetic techniques used for blocking them. (Modified from Bonica, J. J.: An Atlas on Mechanisms and Pathways of Pain in Labor. Copyright 1960, Abbott Laboratories.)

cross the placenta to the fetus (Moya and Thorndike, 1962). Muscle relaxants, for clinical purposes, are the only important exception (Moya and Kvisselgaard, 1961). Despite this ready transfer, anesthesiologists, obstetricians, and physiologists over the years have combined their clinical and experimental efforts to provide anesthesia that does little, if any, harm to the newborn as evaluated by Apgar scores and acid-base and blood-gas status (Marx et al., 1970; Kosaka et al., 1969; Galbert and Gardner, 1972; James et al., 1977; Magno et al., 1976; Datta and Alper, 1980). These measurements, however, evaluate only brain stem function. They evaluate functions of a newborn necessary for physical well-being and survival but not functions of the higher cortical centers. For several years, psychologists have used tests such as the Brazelton, Prechtal, and Bientema to evaluate the newborn's and older infant's more subtle neurobehavioral activities and, occasionally, to evaluate drug effects. However, these tests, long and cumbersome, were not widely used in the early neonatal period. Therefore, Scanlon manufactured a neurobehavioral examination that included features from the neurologic examinations of Prechtal and Bientema as well as from behavioral testing of the Brazelton examination (Scanlon et al., 1974). The behaviors selected were considered easier to elicit during the first few hours and days of life:

1. Apgar score
2. State
   a. Awake
   b. Asleep
3. Response to pinprick
4. Tone evaluation
   a. Pull to sitting
   b. Arm recoil
   c. Truncal tone
   d. General body tone
5. Rooting
6. Sucking
7. Moro response
8. Response decrement to light in eyes
9. Response to sound
10. Placing
11. Alertness
12. General assessment

The Apgar score serves as an indicator of vital signs to begin the examination. Next, the general state of the fetus is recorded. This is scored by various states of wake or sleep of the infant. The fetal state is then recorded again before each of the specific tests. Each of these specific tests is scored from 0 to 3, with the higher number indicating a more alert, responsive newborn. To complete the scoring, general scores for alertness, overall assessment, predominant state, and lability of state are added to all of the above. Scores above 33 to 35 indicate a normal fetal condition, provided that points were not lost in one specific category, such as tone or adaptive capacity (Bonica, 1980).

Since the first appearance of Scanlon's test, many anesthetic agents and techniques have been found to have some effect according to this now widely accepted neurobehavioral scoring system (Hodgkinson, Bhatt, and Wang, 1978; Hodgkinson, Bhatt, Kim, et al., 1978; Corke, 1977; Hodgkinson et al., 1977; Scanlon et al., 1976). Although many, but not all, anesthetic agents alter these tests, the alterations are subtle and transient (Tronick et al., 1976). Infants of mothers who received regional analgesia had higher scores than did those whose mothers received general anesthesia. Ketamine as an induction agent produced better scores than did thiopental (Hodgkinson, Bhatt, Kim, et al., 1978; McGuinness, 1978).

Infants also seemed to do better when the local anesthetic used was chloroprocaine or bupivacaine as opposed to lidocaine or mepivacaine (Scanlon et al., 1974). However, more recent studies have exonerated lidocaine (Abboud et al., 1982).

I and many other obstetric anesthesiologists believe that the whole area of neurobehavioral testing can be summarized as follows:

1. Anesthetic agents alter neurobehavioral performance in newborns.
2. There is no evidence to suggest that these alterations have any effect on later development.
3. The results of such tests probably should not significantly influence the anesthesiologist's choice of anesthetic or technique.

Anesthesia for Labor

PSYCHOPROPHYLAXIS

Psychoprophylaxis for pain relief during labor is ostensibly simple but actually demands much preparation. The successfully implemented technique educates and prepares the patient for what will happen during labor and delivery. The patient eliminates fear and thus tolerates pain better. Throughout labor, the patient remains aware and can appreciate what happens around her. Depressant drugs do not obtund her or affect her fetus. When desired by the patient and when successful, the technique is satisfactory and rewarding, but there are disadvantages. First, not all patients are suited for such an effort. Others may not be able to find suitable instruction. Finally, the patient may need anesthesia because the labor is longer or more painful than expected, or the delivery requires forceps, or a cesarean section is necessary. In these instances, the patient should not be made to feel guilty; instead both she and her husband must realize that properly administered anesthesia during labor or delivery will not compromise the fetus. Occasionally, the enthusiasm of an instructor or husband for "natural" childbirth overshadows the genuine feelings of the mother—the person who actually experiences labor and delivery and whose feelings and concerns must be primary.

NARCOTICS

Narcotics may ease the pain of contractions and promote rest between contractions. They are easy to administer and, when given in appropriate doses, cause little, if any, fetal depression. They do not, however, provide total pain relief and may cloud the patient's awareness. Also, neonatal neurobehavioral scores are consistently altered (Hodgkinson, Bhatt, and Wang, 1978; Corke, 1977). Meperidine and alphaprodine are examples of frequently used narcotics. Preferably, one should give narcotics in small, intravenous doses (e.g., 25 to 50 mg meperidine), because larger doses may depress the fetus, the mother, or both. Although it is sometimes difficult to estimate the time of delivery, it is recommended that narcotics not be given during the last hour of labor before delivery. This will help to decrease newborn depression. It is important to remember, however, that depression caused by narcotics is not due to asphyxia; the infant is not acidotic or hypoxic but merely depressed. One need only stimulate or ventilate the infant to prevent the more substantial threat from as-

phyxia. Moreover, naloxone (Narcan) (0.01 mg/kg intravenously, intramuscularly, or subcutaneously) can easily reverse depression secondary to narcotics. Naloxone is not, however, a substitute for ventilation and thus should be used in conjunction with, not instead of, ventilation. Moreover, a person who administers naloxone for narcotic reversal should alert the nursery staff, because the antagonist effect of naloxone may wear off (by approximately 45 minutes) before the infant has metabolized the narcotic. If this happens, the infant may become drowsy again. Other agents often used with narcotics, such as barbiturates, promethazine, and hydroxyzine, also may cause fetal depression. There are no known antagonists for most of these other drugs; thus, their advantages and disadvantages should be carefully weighed.

DIAZEPAM

The major disadvantage of diazepam is that it disrupts temperature regulation in newborns, which renders them less able to maintain body temperature (Owen et al., 1972). The drug may persist in the fetal circulation for as long as 1 week (Cree et al., 1973). As with many drugs, beat-to-beat variability of fetal heart rate is reduced markedly, even with small intravenous doses (5 to 6 mg) (Hon, 1968). However, these doses have little effect on the acid-base or clinical status of the newborn (Yeh et al., 1974). Sodium benzoate, a buffer in the injectable form of diazepam, competes with bilirubin in binding to albumin. Thus, unbound bilirubin is increased and could be a threat to infants susceptible to kernicterus (Schiff et al., 1971).

SCOPOLAMINE

Scopolamine is not an analgesic but an anticholinergic that inhibits oral secretions and increases heart rate. Also, it is a cerebral depressant and an amnesic; however, it may cause excitement and hyperkinesis in some patients. These patients frequently become difficult to manage during labor and may even end up being ashamed of themselves. Therefore, it is doubtful that scopolamine has any place in modern obstetrics.

HAND-HELD INHALERS

Hand-held inhalers and "whistles" are devices in which 15 cc of the inhalation anesthetic methoxyflurane is placed (Dolan and Rosen, 1975; Clark et al., 1976). Either type of device is strapped to the patient's arm, and she inhales the agent through a mask (inhaler) or by sucking on the whistle during contractions. The degree of relief achieved by a particular patient is unpredictable and depends to some degree on such things as education and prior medication. The devices are calibrated to provide analgesic quantities of the agent. Although in most cases methoxyflurane so administered is not detrimental to the mother or the fetus, the devices should not be used in patients with renal disease, because of methoxyflurane's known capacity for producing high-output renal failure with extended use at high concentrations (Mazze et al., 1971). Also, an attendant should watch the patient at all times to ensure that she does not fall asleep with the mask on her face or the whistle in her mouth. Finally, some patients may find the sweet smell of methoxyflurane offensive.

PARACERVICAL BLOCK

Paracervical block analgesia is an effective, relatively simple method of relieving pain during labor. Basically, the technique uses a local anesthetic injected through the vaginal canal into the cervical tissue, at 3 and 9 o'clock or at 4 and 8 o'clock, which blocks the nerve fibers that make up the uterine plexus (Fig. 15–1). Although the technique is easy to perform and provides adequate pain relief in most instances, it does have three major disadvantages: (1) pain relief is brief, so the process must be repeated; (2) it provides no perineal or vaginal analgesia and therefore must be supplemented at the time of delivery; (3) fetal bradycardia occurs in 3 to 70 percent of cases (Weiss et al., 1977; Freeman and Arnold, 1975; Teramo and Widholm, 1967; Shnider et al., 1970). The incidence of bradycardia depends on the agent, the dosage, and the technique used. Mepivacaine is one of the major offenders, whereas 2-chloroprocaine, 2 percent, 5 to 6 cc per side, is effective and infrequently produces bradycardia (Weiss et al., 1977; Freeman and Ar-

nold, 1975; Teramo and Widholm, 1967). Using the minimal amount of drug necessary and using a needle guide to ensure only superficial penetration will minimize the occurrence of bradycardia. Careful fetal monitoring, preferably electronic, is mandatory. Usually, the bradycardia occurs within 15 minutes of the injection and lasts from 3 to 15 minutes. Although fetal asphyxia occurs more frequently in fetuses suffering bradycardia, asphyxia in an individual fetus is not predictable.

The cause of bradycardia is unknown, but a number of explanations are offered. Of these, one or all of the following seem plausible: (1) direct action of the local anesthetic on the fetal myocardium; (2) uterine hypertonus secondary to either the local anesthetic or trauma after the injection; (3) direct vasoconstriction of the uterine vessels by the local anesthetic (Ralston and Shnider, 1978; Gibbs and Noel, 1977). In an early study, Miller and colleagues found that paracervical block utilizing lidocaine produced not only an 11 percent incidence of fetal bradycardia but also a significant increase in fetal heart rate variability, which they interpreted as an early sign of hypoxia (Miller et al., 1978). More recently, by selecting patients carefully and keeping them in true lateral position for at least 30 minutes before and after injection, they found no paracervical block bradycardia. Therefore, they concluded that the block may be used safely in healthy patients (Van Dorsten et al., 1981). However, because of the potential for bradycardia and the increased fetal depression that may be associated with it, I feel that the use of paracervical block in normal patients is questionable and should be avoided in cases of acute fetal distress or chronic fetal compromise.

LUMBAR EPIDURAL VERSUS CAUDAL EPIDURAL ANALGESIA

In both of these blocks, local anesthetic is injected through a catheter into the epidural space, a space that is continuous along the entire course of the spine. For the lumbar epidural block, the anesthetic is injected into the lumbar area; for the caudal block it is injected into the sacral area (Fig. 15–1). Because the latter requires much more local anesthetic than the former and allows more perineal relaxation, many obstetric anesthesiologists now favor the lumbar approach. For both blocks, a 17-gauge needle is used to identify the epidural space; a small catheter is then threaded through the needle, the needle is removed, and the catheter is left in place. The physician tapes the catheter to the patient's back and injects the local anesthetic through the catheter. The catheter, in situ through labor and delivery, provides a means to reinject local anesthetic whenever the drug begins to wear off and thus allows continuous analgesia as long as desired. In most instances pain is totally relieved, yet the patient is awake and able to appreciate her labor and relate to those around her.

The ability to select the appropriate dose and concentration of local anesthetics makes these blocks even more desirable. Bupivacaine, 0.25 percent, 2-chloroprocaine, 2 percent, and lidocaine, 1 percent, block pain fibers but leave motor fibers relatively intact. Thus, the patient has no pain but does not feel paralyzed and can move about in bed. Both bupivacaine and chloroprocaine minimally transfer across the placenta, because bupivacaine is highly protein-bound, and 2-chloroprocaine, an ester, is broken down rapidly by cholinesterases (Ralston and Shnider, 1978; Tucker et al., 1970; Finster, 1976). Unfortunately, the reputations of chloroprocaine and bupivacaine have been tarnished somewhat in the recent past because both have been associated with rather serious complications in the mother. Chloroprocaine may produce severe and prolonged nerve damage (Covino et al., 1980; Moore et al., 1982), while high concentrations (0.75 percent) of bupivacaine injected intravascularly may cause arrhythmias and cardiovascular depression (Albright, 1979). While the scope of these problems is too great for adequate discussion in this chapter, suffice it to say that in the case of chloroprocaine, final conclusions regarding complications are not now available. Some experts have chosen to avoid one or both drugs, while others still use both. Most authorities now believe that chloroprocaine is no more dangerous than any other local anesthetic. However, some still believe the question has not been settled conclusively (deJong, 1981; Moore et al., 1982; Ravindran, 1980; Reisner, 1980; Rosen, 1983; Barsa, 1982; Gibbs and Munson, 1980). Some have chosen to use lidocaine, a drug tainted only by early reports indicating neonatal neurobehavioral depression (Scanlon et al., 1974). Recently, in a well-controlled study, Abboud and colleagues have reported that neurobehavioral depression of newborns whose mothers had received epidural analgesia with lidocaine was no greater than that of newborns whose mothers had received bupivacaine or no local anesthetic (Abboud et al., 1982).

The problems associated with epidural analgesia in general include its effects on labor and blood pressure, production of "total spinal" anesthesia in rare cases, and anesthetic toxicity or overdose. Normally, unless the block is administered before a good labor pattern is established or the pattern is irregular, the effects of epidural anesthesia on labor are minimal (Ralston and Shnider, 1978). During a normal labor, a transitory decrease in the frequency of contractions may occur immediately after the injection of the local anesthetic, but the original pattern resumes within minutes. An obstetrician who doubts the efficacy of a labor pattern during epidural analgesia can supplement a desultory labor with oxytocin or allow the anesthesia to wear off and then evaluate labor without having to take the effects of the epidural into account. The anesthesia can be reinstituted through the previously placed catheter when the labor pattern is satisfactory or the delivery begins. Although the incidence of forceps deliveries may increase with epidural analgesia (Hoult et al., 1977), this is not necessarily the case (Doughty, 1976). Optimum management of the epidural block and the delivery can result in a low incidence of forceps deliveries. Furthermore, with epidural analgesia, the application of indicated forceps and the delivery are facilitated, resulting in an easy, comfortable, and controlled delivery, thus minimizing risk to the fetus. With some infants, such as a small, premature one, such a delivery is desirable.

Although it is usually preventable, hypotension, the most common complication or side effect of epidural analgesia, occurs in approximately 4 to 5 percent of epidurals used for labor (McDonald et al., 1974). Hypotension results from sympathetic nerve blockade, which blocks not only pain sensation but also sympathetic control of blood vessels below the level of analgesia. Thus, with sympathetic blockade, there is widespread vasodilatation and subsequent pooling of blood in the lower extremities. These effects cause decreased cardiac return, which, in turn, causes decreased cardiac output and hypotension. Decreased cerebral and uterine blood flow may subsequently occur and jeopardize both mother and fetus. Although systolic blood pressures of 80 mm Hg are usually considered hypotensive, for the mother, a 20 to 30 percent reduction or systolic pressures below 100 mm Hg may threaten the fetus. Because of this complication, electronic fetal monitoring should be employed during this procedure. If external monitoring is used, it is imperative to maintain an adequate tracing. If the side-lying position makes this difficult or the belts interfere with the procedure, an internal monitor should be inserted.

Usually, effective prevention includes left uterine displacement to ensure that cardiac return is not mechanically impeded, together with administration of 1000 cc Ringer's lactate to help fill the enlarged vascular space created by the vasodilatation. Left uterine displacement can be accomplished either manually or by insisting that the patient remain on her left side, a good practice any time during labor. However, alternating sides will give the same effect and may produce a more even pain relief.

Treatment of hypotension consists of administering still more intravenous fluids and exaggerating the uterine displacement. In addition, one should lower the head of the bed to improve cerebral blood flow, and elevate the foot of the bed or legs to facilitate cardiac return of blood pooled in the lower extremities. If these maneuvers do not suffice, administration of ephedrine, 10 to 15 mg intravenously, is indicated. Rarely will this regimen not be effective. Ephedrine is an appropriate vasopressor to use, because much of its pressor activity is beta- rather than alpha-adrenergic; thus, the blood pressure increases without the widespread vasoconstriction (including that of uterine arteries) that characterizes many other vasopressor agents (Shnider et al., 1968). Hypotension treated rapidly in the above manner is not likely to harm the fetus (James et al., 1977). However, even brief periods of hypotension may be dangerous to the fetus that is already severely compromised, either acutely or chronically (Datta and Brown, 1977). Recently, Datta has suggested that any fall in blood pressure greater than 10 mm Hg is an indication for ephedrine. In following this guideline, he reported no hypoten-

sion in a series of patients receiving spinal analgesia for cesarean section (Datta et al., 1982).

"Total spinal" anesthesia after epidural anesthesia, meaning anesthesia to the C_5–C_6 level (affecting the shoulders and hands), occurs rarely; however, when it does occur, it must be treated effectively. A "total spinal" may compromise the patient's breathing by weakening the intercostal muscles and perhaps even the diaphragm. The anesthesiologist should reassure the patient and then maintain her airway with a mask and ambu-type bag or even endotracheal intubation until her muscle control returns. An extremely apprehensive patient may be sedated once her airway is secure. Hypotension in these cases, if present, should be treated as described earlier. Because there may be more to do than one person can handle, good judgment dictates calling for assistance. When treated appropriately, no serious or permanent damage should occur to the patient. The incidence of "total spinal" anesthesia after epidural analgesia varies from 0.03 to 0.06 percent (Ralston and Shnider, 1978).

Local anesthetic toxicity, a manifestation of excessively high blood levels of local anesthetic, usually results from intravascular injection or miscalculation of dosage. (Maximum recommended doses are found in all package inserts.) The symptoms range from excitement and mental confusion to convulsions to cardiovascular and respiratory depression. Although the blood levels at which central nervous system symptoms occur are high, they are usually considerably lower than those required to cause cardiovascular depression. Thus, the patient will usually manifest the central nervous system symptoms much before any cardiovascular symptoms. The recent controversy surrounding bupivacaine (as discussed earlier) is concerned with precisely this point. That is, there appears to be little separation between levels required to produce both central nervous system and cardiovascular effects (Albright, 1979; Morishima et al., 1983; deJong et al., 1983). Therefore, once a reaction begins, treatment may be more difficult because of accompanying arrhythmias and cardiovascular depression. Moreover, cardiac resuscitation may prove ineffective. Because of these concerns, several manufacturers have recommended that the 0.75 percent concentration of bupivacaine not be used for obstetrics and that the drug be contraindicated for paracervical block (Abbott Laboratories, Astra Pharmaceutical Products, Inc., Breon Laboratories, 1984).

In the usual case of local anesthetic toxicity, any sort of anxiety or abnormal behavior on the part of a patient should alert the physician to stop administering the drug if possible. If convulsions occur, they will usually subside spontaneously in a short period of time. Even so, it is imperative that oxygen be administered immediately, because these patients soon become severely hypoxic and acidotic. If the convulsions do not subside immediately, small doses of thiopental (25 mg) or diazepam (5 mg) can counteract them. However, the physician administering these drugs must be prepared to deal with a drug-depressed as well as postictally depressed patient. Thus, the ventilatory and circulatory systems may need support. Some authorities recommend avoiding these drugs completely. Instead, they recommend the use of succinylcholine, a muscle relaxant, to stop the convulsions (Moore et al., 1960; Moore and Bonica, 1985). Certainly this admonition seems prudent when bupivacaine has caused the reaction. If succinylcholine is used, endotracheal intubation and manual ventilation will be necessary. Also, it is extremely important to remember that during resuscitation of a pregnant patient for whatever reason, the uterus must be kept off the inferior vena cava and aorta. The incidence of local anesthetic overdose with epidural anesthesia varies from 0.03 to 0.5 percent (Ralston and Shnider, 1978).

During any major regional block, equipment in proper working order and drugs to treat complications must be available and should include a bag and mask for ventilation, oral and nasal airways, laryngoscope, endotracheal tubes, vasopressors, anticonvulsant drugs, oxygen, a suction apparatus, and equipment for intravenous therapy.

Another area of concern is the possibility of paralysis or permanent nerve damage after regional techniques. Ralston and Shnider (1978) discussed this problem in an excellent review of regional anesthesia in obstetrics. In over 31,000 epidural and caudal epidurals reviewed in the recent literature, the authors found no instance of permanent nerve damage. In 29,000 patients in whom spinal anesthetics were used, there were only two instances. Both of these patients experienced footdrop, which could have been of obstetric as well as anesthetic origin.

Thus, serious neurologic sequelae are indeed rare.

Firm contraindications to regional analgesia include:

1. Hemorrhage or hypovolemia, because the sympathetic blockade may attenuate the patient's compensatory mechanisms.

2. Anticoagulation or inadequate clotting mechanisms, because a punctured vein in the epidural space will not stop bleeding and may form a large hematoma, which could compress and compromise the spinal cord.

3. Infection at the site of puncture.

4. Allergy to the local anesthetic.

5. Patient refusal.

Other instances in which the risks and benefits of regional analgesia should be thoroughly evaluated are:

1. Fetal distress. If acute and severe, it is usually best to avoid regional analgesia.

2. Severe preeclampsia or eclampsia. Regional analgesia can be used safely and effectively in these patients if their condition is optimized before instituting the block. Volume status should be evaluated by means of a central line. Any deficit should then be corrected by appropriate fluid administration. In many patients an arterial line will be necessary for accurate continuous monitoring of blood pressure. Finally, clotting studies must be done to rule out a preeclampsia-induced coagulopathy.

3. Some forms of maternal heart disease that cannot tolerate hypotension, e.g., aortic stenosis.

4. Preexisting neurologic abnormality.

Anesthesia for Vaginal Delivery

PUDENDAL BLOCK

Pudendal block is probably the most popular form of obstetric anesthesia in the United States. Administered vaginally by the obstetrician, it is usually adequate for spontaneous vaginal and low forceps deliveries (Fig. 15–1). Although it is safe for mother and fetus, complications can arise from an overdose of the local anesthetic. As stated before, overdose most often results from an intravascular injection or miscalculation of dosage. The person administering the block must aspirate before injecting the local anesthetic and remember that a 1 percent solution contains 10 mg of the agent, not 1 mg. Before using any local anesthetic, one must also know the maximum safe dosage, which can always be found on the package insert. For example, the maximum safe dose of lidocaine without epinephrine is 4.5 mg/kg. The treatment of local anesthetic overdose has been discussed.

INHALATION ANALGESIA

Inhalation analgesia, also popular, uses subanesthetic concentrations of inhalation agents to produce Stage 1 anesthesia. As described in the introduction to this chapter, Stage 1 anesthesia provides various degrees of pain relief and amnesia but does not suppress consciousness or protective reflexes; thus, the patient is not exposed to the dangers of general surgical anesthesia. By itself, inhalation analgesia has minimal effect and is not surgical anesthesia; however, in conjunction with a good pudendal block, inhalation analgesia aids in the performance of spontaneous vaginal, low forceps, and some mid-forceps deliveries. Nitrous oxide is the agent most commonly used, but methoxyflurane and enflurane also work well (Abouleish, 1977). For those patients afraid of masks, 0.25 to 0.50 mg/kg of intravenous ketamine can be substituted for the inhalation agent (Akamatsu et al., 1974). To be effective, however, ketamine analgesia, like inhalation analgesia, must be given with a pudendal block or local infiltration. Again, for these techniques to be safe, the anesthesiologist must keep the patient conscious and in control of her reflexes. Therefore, constant patient supervision is mandatory.

SPINAL ANALGESIA

Spinal analgesia administered as a low spinal (analgesia to the umbilicus) or a saddle block (analgesia limited to the perineal or "saddle" area) can provide optimum conditions for nearly any vaginal delivery, spontaneous or operative. (It is almost always used during delivery, and not during labor.) The most commonly used local anesthetic for spinal anesthesia is 4 mg of 1 percent tetracaine. With adequate precautions taken, the incidence of hypotension is nearly nil (Phillips et al., 1959), but if hypotension should occur, the treatment is as described before. Although local anesthetic toxicity

does not occur, because of the small amount of drug used, "total spinals" do occur at a frequency of 0.1 percent (Ralston and Shnider, 1978). However, as with epidural anesthesia, when treated adequately, no serious sequelae will follow.

Spinal headache, most likely caused by spinal fluid leaking through the punctured dura, occurs in 2 to 4 percent of obstetric patients after spinal analgesia (Abouleish, 1977). The most consistent and diagnostic feature of the headache is that it is present only with the patient upright; lying down relieves the pain. Although rarely severe, the headache often troubles and depresses the patient at an otherwise happy time. Initial treatment consists of bedrest, fluids, abdominal binders, and analgesics. If these simple measures fail, and the headache is burdensome, a recently devised procedure, epidural blood patch, is indicated. For an epidural blood patch, the physician places 10 ml of the patient's own blood aseptically in the epidural space. The procedure, simple and with rare serious complications (such as infection), is 90 to 95 percent effective, and the patient may leave the hospital the same day (Abouleish, 1977; DiGiovanni et al., 1972).

LUMBAR AND CAUDAL EPIDURAL ANALGESIA

Lumbar and caudal epidural analgesia for vaginal delivery provide the same advantages and optimum working conditions as spinal analgesia. In addition, if instituted early, the patient has pain relief throughout both labor and delivery. Occasionally, a "single shot" caudal will be given at the time of delivery. In these instances, a catheter is not needed for continuous use, since the local anesthetic is injected directly through the needle. Pain relief and operating conditions are the same as with spinal analgesia, except that much more local anesthetic is necessary. On the other hand, the chance of developing a spinal headache is small because the dura is not punctured with epidural analgesia.

GENERAL ANESTHESIA

General anesthesia is rarely indicated for vaginal delivery. Spontaneous deliveries, low forceps deliveries, and low mid-forceps deliveries are easily accomplished with either regional analgesia or inhalation analgesia and pudendal block. Neither of these techniques carries the risks of general anesthesia. Except for cesarean deliveries (see below), instances in which general anesthesia might be necessary are increasingly rare in modern obstetrics. It may be required for a difficult breech delivery or a shoulder dystocia, or for a successful internal version of a second twin. (In rare instances, after delivery of the infant, general anesthesia may also be necessary to relax the uterus if it is inverted. Relaxation allows the uterus to be replaced.) In these few emergent cases, general anesthesia can help greatly by providing the obstetrician with the conditions necessary to accomplish the difficult task at hand. Otherwise, the risk is too great. Aspiration of gastric contents during general anesthesia still represents the number-one cause of anesthesia-related maternal mortality.

Anesthesia for Cesarean Section

Anesthesia for cesarean section with no complications can be done with either epidural or spinal analgesia or with a balanced general anesthesia technique. If properly administered, comparably favorable results for the fetus can be anticipated with each of these techniques (James et al., 1977; Datta and Brown, 1977). The risk to the mother, however, is probably greater with general anesthesia.

The main advantages of regional analgesia are that the patient is awake and thus experiences the birth of her infant and also has little, if any, risk of drug depression. Moreover, newborn neurobehavioral scores are better after regional than after general anesthesia (Hodgkinson, Bhatt, Kim et al., 1978). The disadvantages include inadequate block, hypotension, spinal headache, and possible local anesthetic toxicity. Of these, hypotension, the most frequent complication, occurs in 25 to 70 percent of patients administered a spinal or an epidural anesthetic—even when all prophylactic measures have been taken (James et al., 1977; Datta and Brown, 1977). However, as discussed in the section on epidural analgesia for labor, hypotension treated promptly and efficiently is not likely to harm either the mother or the fetus (James et al., 1977). Most

anesthesiologists are adept at treating hypotension secondary to regional analgesia.

General anesthesia also has certain advantages. Because many patients are afraid to be awake during an operation, one main advantage of general anesthesia is that it makes these patients unconscious for the entire procedure. General anesthesia also provides optimum operating conditions. Although the anesthetic agents do cross the placenta, there is little evidence to indicate that general anesthesia, when administered by competent personnel, will depress the infant (Marx et al., 1970; Kosaka et al., 1969; Galbert and Gardner, 1972; McDonald et al., 1972). Probably the most significant disadvantage of general anesthesia is the necessity for a rapid "crash" induction of anesthesia and rapid endotracheal intubation. This type of induction is necessary to minimize the threat of aspiration. Aspiration is a significant risk because many pregnant patients, even if they have not eaten recently, will have full stomachs, owing to the slow emptying of the stomach during pregnancy (Roberts and Shirley, 1976). Because general anesthesia obliterates the normally protective laryngeal reflexes, a cuffed endotracheal tube must be placed to prevent aspiration into the lungs in the event of regurgitation or vomiting. To accomplish the intubation quickly, the patient must be paralyzed, and while paralyzed, she is not breathing. Although intubation of the trachea is usually not difficult for the experienced anesthetist, there are times when it is quite difficult and may be impossible. In such instances, regurgitation and aspiration can occur. Furthermore, if the tube cannot be placed, or if it is improperly placed, ventilation may not be adequate, which results in hypoxia and even cardiac arrest. The two most common causes of anesthesia-related mortality are aspiration and failure to be able to intubate. Inexperienced personnel contribute to and compound both of these problems (Tomkinson et al., 1979). Thus, during induction, all personnel involved must realize that the endotracheal tube should be in place *before* the operation begins. If difficulty with intubation is encountered before the operation begins, the anesthesiologist most likely will allow the patient to awaken, and the situation will be reassessed. If, however, the operation was begun before the airway was secured and then the intubation is difficult, it is nearly impossible to awaken the patient and begin again. During this critical time, the obstetrician and anesthesiologist must cooperate to the utmost.

The dangers of aspiration and inadequate airway are also present at the time of extubation, requiring that the patient be in Stage 1 and conscious before the endotracheal tube is removed.

Because aspiration of partially digested food is particularly damaging to the lung (Schwartz et al., 1980), one should be forceful and convincing when advising patients not to eat before coming to the hospital. Also, because aspiration of acid gastric contents produces more lung damage than aspiration of nonacid contents, 30 ml of a clear, nonparticulate antacid should be administered prior to initiating general anesthesia. It is probably not necessary to administer antacids throughout labor. Clear, nonparticulate antacids are preferable to the particulate, chalky-type antacids, because laboratory studies have shown that the latter can produce significant pulmonary damage themselves when aspirated (Gibbs et al., 1979; Eyler et al., 1982). Sodium citrate, 0.3 M, prepared by the hospital pharmacy according to the formula shown below is appropriate (Gibbs et al., 1982). Also, Bicitra, a commercially available urinary alkalinizing agent, and Alka-Seltzer Gold have been found to be effective (Eyler et al., 1982; Gibbs and Banner, 1982).

Formula for 0.3 M Sodium Citrate:

Sodium citrate	88.2 g
Simple syrup	100.0 ml
Mint flavor	1.0 ml
H_2O q.s.	1000.0 ml

The cardiovascular changes that occur after intubation represent other problems with general anesthesia (Fox et al., 1977; Ueland et al., 1970). Stimulation of the oropharynx and trachea substantially increases cardiac output, heart rate, and blood pressure, and these increases are difficult, if not impossible, to obliterate. Although these changes are tolerated by the normal and healthy pregnant patient, they may drastically compromise the patient with severe preeclampsia or heart disease (Hodgkinson et al., 1980).

Thus, for cesarean sections, both regional and general anesthesia have good and bad features. Each must be weighed and considered for the individual patient and her needs, after which the proper choice can be made.

Some institutions are using lumbar epidural and subarachnoid narcotics for postoperative pain relief. Although these methods are effective, to prevent serious sequelae from respiratory depression, they require recovery room–like observation throughout the period of effectiveness of the agents.

Patient self-administered morphine

Table 15–1. Patient Care Summary for Anesthesia*

	Intrapartum	Postpartum
Regional Anesthesia		
BP, P, R	q 5 min × 20 min initially and after each reinjection. (q 5 min should be continued longer if patient is not stabilized in 20 min) After stabilization, q 15 min	q 15 min × 4 q 30 min × 2 then q 1 hr, then on discharge to PP
T	q 4 hr	On admission, then q 4 hr, then on discharge to PP
Position	Alternate side lying (right & left) initially. Once anesthetic effective, left lateral preferred, but can rotate	—
Fetal monitoring	Continuous FM during anesthesia, preferably with internal; without monitor, q 10–15 min	—
Contractions Frequency Duration Quality Resting tone	Continuous FM during anesthesia q 30 min	
I & O	q shift (if patient has no other complications). By anesthesia standards	
General Anesthesia (for cesarean section)		
BP, P, R		q 15 min × 4; if stable, then q 30 min ×2: if stable, then q 1 hr until stable; then q 4 hr
T		On admission to RR, then q 4 hr, then on discharge to PP
I & O		q shift in RR
Inhalants	Same as routine labor, 1:1 supervision	
Scopolamine	Not recommended for use in labor	

*Nurse–patient ratio = 1:1 until stabilization; 1:2 after stabilization.

through an IV pump has also been demonstrated to be useful in alleviating postoperative pain.

Conclusion

Pain relief during labor and delivery is an important part of modern obstetrics. More than providing personal comfort to the mother, it is a necessary part of good obstetric practice. Thoughtfully chosen analgesia improves labor, and proper anesthesia enhances the safety of difficult deliveries. On the other hand, poorly chosen or administered analgesia or anesthesia may compromise labor, depress the fetus, and contribute to maternal or fetal morbidity and even mortality.

The choice of analgesic and anesthetic techniques rests with the experience and knowledge of the anesthesiologist or anesthetist, on the personal preference of the obstetrician and patient, and on the circumstances of labor and delivery. Safe pain relief depends on a careful choice, proper selection, and skillful administration of the anesthetic. The anesthesiologist or anesthetist, in consultation with the obstetrician and after discussion with the patient, should plan the anesthesia as early as possible. Table 15–1 summarizes the general management scheme for care of the patient under anesthesia.

REFERENCES

Abbott Laboratories, Astra Pharmaceutical Products, Inc., Breon Laboratories, Inc.: Letter to doctors. Urgent new recommendations about bupivacaine. 1984.

Abboud, T.K., Khoo, S. S., Miller, F., et al.: Maternal, fetal, and neonatal responses after epidural anesthesia with bupivacaine, 2-chloroprocaine, or lidocaine. Anesth. Analg. 61:638, 1982.

Abouleish, E.: Pain Control In Obstetrics. Philadelphia, J.B. Lippincott Co., 1977.

Akamatsu, J., Bonica, J. J., Rehmet, R., et al.: Experiences with the use of ketamine for parturition. I. Primary anesthetic for vaginal delivery. Anesth. Analg. 53:284, 1974.

Albright, G. A.: Cardiac arrest following regional anesthesia with etidocaine or bupivacaine. Anesthesiology 51:285, 1979.

Barsa, J., Batra, M., Fink, B. R., et al.: A comparative in vivo study of local neurotoxicity of lidocaine, bupivacaine, 2-chloroprocaine, and a mixture of 2-chloroprocaine and bupivacaine. Anesth. Analg. 61:961, 1982.

Bonica, J. J.: Obstetric Analgesia and Anesthesia. Amsterdam, World Federation of Societies of Anaesthesiologists, 1980.

Clark, R. B., Beard, A. G., Thompson, D. S., et al.: Maternal and neonatal plasma inorganic fluoride levels after methoxyflurane analgesia for labor and delivery. Anesthesiology 45:88, 1976.

Corke, B. C.: Neurobehavioral responses of the newborn: the effect of different forms of maternal analgesia. Anaesthesia 32:539, 1977.

Covino, B. G., Marx, G. F., Finster, M., et al.: Prolonged sensory/motor deficits following inadvertent spinal anesthesia. Anesth. Analg. 59:399, 1980.

Cree, J. E., Meyer, J., and Hailey, D. M.: Diazepam in labour: its metabolism and effect on the clinical condition and thermogenesis of the newborn. Br. Med. J. 4:251, 1973.

Datta, S., and Alper, M. H.: Anesthesia for cesarean section. Anesthesiology 53:142, 1980.

Datta, S., and Brown, W. U.: Acid-base status in diabetic mothers and their infants following general or spinal anesthesia for cesarean section. Anesthesiology 47:272, 1977.

Datta, S., Kitzmiller, J. L., Naulty, J. S., et al.: Acid-base status of diabetic mothers and their infants following spinal anesthesia for cesarean section. Anesth. Analg. 61:662, 1982.

deJong, R. H.: The chloroprocaine controversy. Am. J. Obstet. Gynecol. 140:237, 1981.

deJong, R. H., Gamble, C. A., and Bonin, J. D.: Bupivacaine-induced cardiac arrhythmias and plasma cation concentrations in normokalemic cats. Regional Anesth. 8:104, 1983.

DiGiovanni, A. J., Galbert, M. W., and Wahle, W. M.: Epidural injection of autologous blood for postlumbar-puncture headache. II. Additional clinical experiences and laboratory investigation. Anesth. Analg. 51:226, 1972.

Dolan, P. F., and Rosen, M.: Inhalational analgesia in labour: facemask or mouthpiece. Lancet 2:1030, 1975.

Doughty, A.: Selective epidural analgesia and the forceps rate. Br. J. Anaesth. 41:1058, 1976.

Eyler, S. W., Cullen, B. F., Murphy, M. E., et al.: Antacid aspiration in rabbits. A comparison of Mylanta and Bicitra. Anesth. Analg. 61:288, 1982.

Finster, M.: Toxicity of local anesthetics in the fetus and newborn. Bull. NY Acad. Med. 52:222, 1976.

Fox, E. J., Sklar, G. S., Hill, C. H., et al.: Complications related to the pressor response to endotracheal intubation. Anesthesiology 47:524, 1977.

Freeman, D. W., and Arnold, N. I.: Paracervical block with low doses of chloroprocaine: fetal and maternal effects. JAMA 231:56, 1975.

Galbert, M. W., and Gardner, A. E.: Use of halothane in a balanced technic for cesarean section. Anesth. Analg. 51:701, 1972.

Gibbs, C. P., and Banner, T. C.: Effectiveness of Bicitra as a preoperative antacid. Anesthesiology 61:27, 1984.

Gibbs, C. P., and Noel, S. C.: Response of arterial segments from gravid human uterus to multiple concentrations of lignocaine. Br. J. Anaesth. 49:409, 1977.

Gibbs, C. P., Schwartz, D. J., Wynne, J. W., et al.: Antacid pulmonary aspiration in the dog. Anesthesiology 51:380, 1979.

Gibbs, C. P., Spohr, L., and Schmidt, D.: The effectiveness of sodium citrate as an antacid. Anesthesiology 57:44, 1982.

Hodgkinson, R., Bhatt, M., Kim, S. S., et al.: Neonatal neurobehavioral tests following cesarean section under general and spinal anesthesia. Am. J. Obstet. Gynecol. 132:670, 1978.

Hodgkinson, R., Bhatt, M., and Wang, C. N.: Double-blind comparison of the neurobehaviour of neonates following the administration of different doses of meperidine to the mother. Can. Anaesth. Soc. J. 25:405, 1978.

Hodgkinson, R., Farkhanda, J. H., and Hayashi, R. H.: Systemic and pulmonary blood pressure during caesarean section in parturients with gestational hypertension. Can. Anaesth. Soc. J. 27:389, 1980.

Hodgkinson, R., Marx, G. F., Kim, S. S., et al.: Neonatal neurobehavioral tests following vaginal delivery under ketamine, thiopental, and extradural anesthesia. Anesth. Analg. 56:548, 1977.

Hon, E.: An Atlas of Fetal Heart Rate Patterns. Hardy Press, New Haven, Connecticut, 1968, p. 231.

Hoult, I. J., MacLennan, A. H., and Carrie, L. E. S.: Lumbar epidural analgesia in labour: relation to fetal malposition and instrumental delivery. Br. Med. J. 1:14, 1977.

James, F. M., Crawford, J. S., Hopkinson, R., et al.: A comparison of general anesthesia and lumbar epidural analgesia for elective cesarean section. Anesth. Analg. 56:228, 1977.

Kosaka, Y., Takahashi, T., and Mark, L. C.: Intravenous thiobarbiturate anesthesia for cesarean section. Anesthesiology 31:489, 1969.

Magno, R., Kjellmer, I., and Karlsson, K.: Anaesthesia for cesarean section. III. Effects of epidural analgesia on the respiratory adaptation of the newborn in elective cesarean section. Acta Anaesth. Scand. 20:73, 1976.

Marx, G. F., Joshi, C. W., and Orkin, L. R.: Placental transmission of nitrous oxide. Anesthesiology 32:429, 1970.

Mazze, R. I., Trudell, J. R., and Cousins, M. J.: Methoxyflurane metabolism and renal dysfunction: clinical correlation in man. Anesthesiology 35:247, 1971.

McDonald, J. S., Bjorkman, L. L., and Reed, E. C.: Epidural analgesia for obstetrics. Am. J. Obstet. Gynecol. 120:1055, 1974.

McDonald, J. S., Mateo, C. V., and Reed, E. C.: Modified nitrous oxide or ketamine hydrochloride for cesarean section. Anesth. Analg. 51:975, 1972.

McGuinness, G. A., Merkow, A. J., Kennedy, R. L., et al.: Epidural anesthesia with bupivacaine for cesarean section: neonatal blood levels and neurobehavioral response. Anesthesiology 49:270, 1978.

Miller, F. C., Quesnel, G., Petrie, R. H., et al.: The effects of paracervical block on uterine activity and beat-to-beat variability of the fetal heart rate. Am. J. Obstet. Gynecol. 130:284, 1978.

Moir, D. D.: Obstetric Anaesthesia and Analgesia. London, Baillière Tindall, 1980.

Moore, D. C., and Bonica, J. J.: Convulsions and ventricular tachycardia from bupivacaine with epinephrine: successful resuscitation—congratulations! (Letter to the Editor) Anesth. Analg. 64:843, 1985.

Moore, D. C., and Bridenbaugh, L. D.: Oxygen: the antidote for systemic toxic reaction from local anesthetic drugs. JAMA 174:842, 1960.

Moore, D. C., Spierdijk, J., van Kleef, J. D., et al.: Chloroprocaine neurotoxicity: four additional cases. Anesth. Analg. 61:155, 1982.

Morishima, H. O., Pedersen, H., Finster, M., et al.: Is bupivacaine more cardiotoxic than lidocaine? Anesthesiology 59:A409, 1983.

Moya, F., and Kvisselgaard, N.: The placental transmission of succinylcholine. Anesthesiology 22:1, 1961.

Moya, F., and Thorndike, V.: Passage of drugs across the placenta. Am. J. Obstet. Gynecol. 84:1778, 1962.

Owen, J. R., Irani, S. F., and Blair, A. W.: Effect of diazepam administered to mothers during labour on temperature regulation of neonate. Arch. Dis. Child. 47:107, 1972.

Phillips, O. C., Nelson, A. T., Lyons, W. B., et al.: Spinal anesthesia for vaginal delivery: a review of 2016 cases using xylocaine. Obstet. Gynecol. 13:437, 1959.

Ralston, D. H., and Shnider, S. M.: The fetal and neonatal effects of regional anesthesia in obstetrics. Anesthesiology 48:34, 1978.

Ravindran, R. S., Bond, V. K., Tasch, M. D., et al.: Prolonged neural blockade following regional analgesia with 2-chloroprocaine. Anesth. Analg. 59:447, 1980.

Reisner, L. S., Hochman, B. N., and Plumer, M. H.: Persistent neurologic deficit and adhesive arachnoiditis following intrathecal 2-chloroprocaine injection. Anesth. Analg. 59:452, 1980.

Roberts, R. B., and Shirley, M. A.: The obstetrician's role in reducing the risk of aspiration pneumonitis: with particular reference to the use of oral antacids. Am. J. Obstet. Gynecol. 124:611, 1976.

Rosen, M. A., Baysinger, C. L., Shnider, S. M., et al.: Evaluation of neurotoxicity after subarachnoid injection of large volumes of local anesthetic solutions. Anesth. Analg. 62:802, 1983.

Scanlon, J. W., Brown, W. U., Weiss, J. B., et al.: Neurobehavioral responses of newborn infants after maternal epidural anesthesia. Anesthesiology 40:121, 1974.

Scanlon, J. W., Ostheimer, G. W., Lurie, A. O., et al.: Neurobehavioral responses and drug concentrations in newborns after maternal epidural anesthesia with bupivacaine. Anesthesiology 45:400, 1976.

Schiff, D., Chan, G., and Stern, L.: Fixed drug combinations and the displacement of bilirubin from albumin. Pediatrics 48:139, 1971.

Schwartz, D. J., Wynne, J. W., Gibbs, C. P., et al.: The pulmonary consequences of aspiration of gastric contents at pH values greater than 2.5. Am. Rev. Respir. Dis. 121:119, 1980.

Shnider, S. M., Asling, J. H., Holl, J. W., et al.: Paracervical block anesthesia in obstetrics. I. Fetal complications and neonatal morbidity. Am. J. Obstet. Gynecol. 107:619, 1970.

Shnider, S. M., deLorimier, A. A., Holl, J. W., et al.: Vasopressors in obstetrics. I. Correction of fetal acidosis with ephedrine during spinal hypotension. Am. J. Obstet. Gynecol. 102:911, 1968.

Teramo, K., and Widholm, O.: Studies of the effect of anaesthetics on foetus. I. The effect of paracervical block with mepivacaine upon foetal acid-base values. Acta Obstet. Gynecol. Scand. 46(Suppl. 2):1, 1967.

Tomkinson, J., Turnbull, A., Robson, G., et al.: Report on confidential enquiries into maternal deaths in England and Wales, 1973–1975. Dept. of Health and Social Security, Report on Health and Social Subjects #14. London, Her Majesty's Stationery Office, 1979, pp. 68–88.

Tronick, E., Wise, S., Als, H., et al.: Regional obstetric anesthesia and newborn behavior: effect over the first ten days of life. Pediatrics 58:94, 1976.

Tucker, G. T., Boyes, R. N., Bridenbaugh, P. O., et al.: Binding of anilide-type local anesthetics in human plasma. I. Relationships between binding, physicochemical properties, and anesthetic activity. Anesthesiology 33:287, 1970.

Ueland, K., Hansen, J., and Eng, M.: Maternal cardiovascular dynamics. Am. J. Obstet. Gynecol. 108:615, 1970.

Van Dorsten, J. P., Miller, F. C., and Yeh, S. Y.: Spacing the injection interval with paracervical block: a randomized study. Obstet. Gynecol. 58:696, 1981.

Weiss, R. R., Nathanson, H. G., Tehrani, M. R., et al.: Paracervical block with 2-chloroprocaine. Anesth. Analg. 56:709, 1977.

Yeh, S. Y., Paul, R. H., Cordero, L., et al.: A study of diazepam during labor. Obstet. Gynecol. 43:363, 1974.

16

PREMATURE RUPTURE OF THE MEMBRANES

KENNETH A. KAPPY

The optimal management of patients with premature rupture of the membranes (PROM) still remains unsettled. This is so because there are two main complicating factors that must constantly be kept in mind. The first is infection. Intact membranes act as a formidable barrier to infectious agents, preventing ascending infections. If the bag of waters is no longer intact, any of the normal vaginal flora may become serious pathogens and place both the mother and fetus in serious jeopardy. Therefore, an aggressive management scheme that may involve induction or augmentation of labor is called for to minimize the dangerous risk of infection.

The second complicating factor is prematurity. PROM frequently occurs in patients who are carrying premature infants. A lack of functional maturity in a fetus may cause devastating complications that can easily result in great expenditures of time, money, and energy. To minimize this risk, a conservative management scheme may be appropriate, to allow intrauterine development to progress for as long as possible.

Therefore, each patient with PROM presents a dilemma, namely: Which is a more serious complicating factor, the risk of infection or that of prematurity? The optimal management protocol must take both of these factors, plus others, into consideration and weigh each separately to make a logical decision for each patient.

Definition and Incidence

A definition of PROM is not universally agreed upon. Some authors will make the diagnosis whenever the bag of waters ruptures before the onset of true labor. The time interval between rupture and labor is defined as the "latent period." Other authors require that a specific minimal latent period elapse before a diagnosis of PROM can be made. This may vary from 1 to 12 hours depending upon the study (Burchell, 1964; Taylor et al., 1961).

Latent periods tend to vary with the length of the gestation. The general rule is that the more premature the pregnancy, the longer the latent period. In a study by Kappy et al., 85 percent of the patients at term had latent periods of less than 24 hours, whereas 57 percent of patients at less than 37 weeks' gestation went more than 24 hours before labor commenced (Kappy et al., 1979). These values are consistent with those reported in other studies (Gunn et al., 1970).

The exact incidence rate of PROM varies with each study. Most studies report a rate of 7 to 12 percent, but the range can be anywhere from 2.7 to 17 percent (Gunn et al., 1970). This wide range may be due to a number of variables, such as the exact diagnosis and the investigator's definition of the latent period. In our referral center,* PROM in a premature pregnancy accounts for more than 50 percent of our referred cases. This obviously affects the incidence rates in many individual hospitals.

Etiology

The exact etiology of PROM remains unknown. There have been many postulated

---

*Newark Beth Israel Medical Center, Newark, NJ.

causes, but a single common denominator has not yet been found. Possible predisposing factors that have been suggested are incompetency of the cervical os, cervicitis, amnionitis, placenta previa, genetic abnormalities, fetal malpresentation, increased uterine tension as in multiple pregnancies or hydramnios, trauma, previous induced abortions, abruptio placentae, and vaginal infections (Sweet, 1981).

Others have suggested that the membranes themselves may have an inherent weakness that predisposes to PROM. Sbarra (1978) has been working on a theory that local bacterial action may produce a peroxidase that may weaken the membranes and cause PROM. However, other studies have failed to verify such a weakness (Danforth et al., 1953; Polishuk et al., 1962; Al-Zaid, 1980). Nutritional deficiencies have also been implicated. Wideman has postulated that an ascorbic acid deficiency predisposes the membranes to premature rupture (Wideman et al., 1964).

Infection has always been a leading contender as a cause of PROM. It has been postulated that the infection may act on the membranes directly, via an ascending route from the vagina or an intraamniotic fluid infection (Naeye and Peters, 1978; Naeye, 1977; Naeye and Peters, 1980).

Diagnosis

The correct diagnosis of PROM is obviously of great importance. The false-positive diagnosis threatens the patient with a nonindicated intervention involving a potential early delivery or a surgical delivery. The false-negative diagnosis places the infant and mother at an increased risk of infection that may be life-threatening to one or both. Therefore, every attempt should be made to diagnosis this condition as quickly and as accurately as possible. To do this, one or all of the following factors may be considered.

History. The patient's history is of importance but may be quite erroneous. Every patient who presents with a story of "feeling wet," or having a "sudden gush of fluid from the vagina" is a potential case of ruptured membranes, but frequently is found not to be so. In many cases, a thorough history of recent sexual intercourse, vaginitis, urinary incontinence or excessive fetal activity may

point to other sources of excessive vaginal moisture. Therefore, all cases require objective documentation of ruptured membranes before a definitive diagnosis can be made.

Physical Exam. After a complete history is obtained, the vulva should be examined. Any sample of moisture should be inspected for color, consistency, odor, and pH. The fluid may be urine or vaginal secretions. The pH of the fluid can be evaluated by the use of a nitrazine paper analysis (Abe, 1940). The vaginal secretions of the pregnant female are normally acidic with a pH of 4 to 5. This pH will not turn nitrazine paper from its normal yellow color. However, amniotic fluid with a pH of 7 to 7.5 will change nitrazine paper to a blue color. If blood is present in the fluid sample, it may also change the nitrazine paper to a blue color because of its higher pH.

No matter what the results of the vulvar inspection are, a sterile speculum examination should also be carried out. This permits inspection of the vaginal canal, the posterior vaginal pool, and the cervix itself. Direct visualization of fluid leaking from the cervical os is the most reliable diagnosis of PROM. If gross leakage is not seen spontaneously, then fundal pressure can be applied or the patient can be asked to cough or strain down (Valsalva maneuver) to help demonstrate leakage of fluid. If these maneuvers still do not produce leakage of fluid, then further evaluation should be made of the cervix and vagina. A sterile cotton swab can be placed at the external cervical os or the posterior vaginal vault to gather moisture which is then transferred to nitrazine paper. If the paper turns blue, it is presumptive evidence of PROM; however, on occasion the secretions within the canal itself may be more basic than those of the vagina, and this can lead to an incorrect diagnosis of PROM. Therefore, the posterior vaginal vault is a better area to sample. If gross fluid is not seen and the nitrazine test is positive, then a "fern" test should also be done (Tricomi et al., 1966). This is accomplished by placing a sample of the vaginal secretions onto a glass slide and allowing it to air dry. The slide is then inspected under a low-power microscope to look for crystallization or a ferning pattern. Vaginal secretions will not show the ferning pattern during pregnancy, but if amniotic fluid is present, the fern pattern will be seen. This is due to an increased concentration of protein and electrolytes within the fluid. The combination of these two tests should provide a correct diagnosis in over 90 percent of cases.

If there is still some question as to the diagnosis of PROM because of a very suggestive history but inability to confirm it by physical examination, the patient should be asked to ambulate. This change in position may allow fluid to drain from the cervix, and a repeat examination may confirm the diagnosis. If there is still some question of the diagnosis, amniocentesis with injection of 1 cc of indigo carmine may prove helpful. However, this procedure is invasive and should be used in relatively few cases. To document leakage in these patients, a sterile tampon should be placed in the vagina and the patient asked to ambulate. After a few hours, the tampon should be removed and the internal end inspected. If it is blue, the diagnosis is confirmed. However, since the dye is excreted mainly through the maternal urine, one must be careful not to make an erroneous diagnosis of PROM when the patient urinates and stains the external end of the tampon. Ultrasound may also assist in making the diagnosis by demonstrating oligohydramnios. However, it must be kept in mind that oligohydramnios may be caused by conditions other than PROM. Ultrasound is also useful for obtaining information on gestational age and presentation of the infant. These parameters will help in making a decision on the timing and route of the delivery.

Other Diagnostic Measures. During the sterile speculum examination, it is imperative to take a culture of the cervix if a diagnosis of PROM is made or even if it is suspected. This allows for early identification of potentially serious pathogens such as *E. coli* and group B beta-hemolytic streptococci. These pathogens will be discussed further when the infectious risks of PROM are dealt with later in this chapter.

One final point must be made. Careful consideration must be given to deciding whether or not a bimanual examination should be carried out in patients with PROM. In the premature patient not in labor, vaginal examination is usually unnecessary and rarely alters the early management of patients with PROM (Kappy et al., 1979; Gunn, 1970). It may even be deleterious in that the examining finger may inoculate the

lower uterine segment with the normal vaginal flora. These organisms can quickly and easily become serious pathogens. The digital examination should be performed only in those patients with PROM in whom labor has begun spontaneously or for whom labor induction is to begin. The total number of examinations should be kept to a minimum even in these cases.

Many other tests have been used for the diagnosis of PROM. Smith (1976) has reviewed the use of such tests as the Papanicolaou smear, Nile blue sulfate stain, fluorescein staining test, Sudan stains and even lanugo hair identification, and has reported varied results.

Initial Evaluation

When the diagnosis of PROM is made, an initial evaluation must be done to ascertain the status of the patient. Gestational age is very important. To determine this accurately, a thorough history and chart review is mandatory. Information must be obtained concerning last menstrual period, regularity of menstrual cycles, initial pelvic examination, availability of an early pregnancy test, date of quickening, date the fetal heart tones were first heard with a fetoscope, growth of the fundus, abdominal examination, and results of any ultrasound examinations that may have been done. All of these parameters will help identify the due date.

Gestational age alone may not be a reliable indicator of fetal maturity. For this reason, amniotic fluid can be used for an evaluation of fetal lung maturity. There has been some skepticism of the results of fetal lung maturity studies based on amniotic fluid collected from the vagina. The argument has been that the vaginal and cervical secretions in some way alter the L/S ratio, giving erroneous results. However, recent data shows that amniotic fluid collected vaginally is a reliable indicator of fetal lung maturity (Sbarra et al., 1981). We have compared vaginally collected amniotic fluid with that collected from transabdominal amniocentesis and found them to have good correlation (Kappy, unpublished data). Investigators have recently evaluated phospholipids such as phosphatidylglycerol (PG) to determine fetal lung maturity. There are currently reports in the literature of PG being used in cases of PROM to accurately predict fetal lung maturity, based on analysis of vaginally collected fluid (Stedman et al., 1981).

Part of the initial examination must be directed toward ruling out chorioamnionitis. Possible indicators of this serious infectious problem are maternal fever, maternal or fetal tachycardia, uterine tenderness to palpation, uterine contractions, odoriferous vaginal discharge, and elevated white blood cell counts with a shift in the differential.

All patients should also have external electronic fetal heart rate monitoring as part of an initial evaluation. This may show a fetal tachycardia or variable decelerations that may indicate occult cord prolapse or fetal compromise. Early labor can also be diagnosed by using the fetal monitor. A nonstress test can also be performed during the initial exam, to evaluate fetal well-being.

At the time of the sterile speculum examination, attention should be given to the condition of the cervix itself. On visual inspection, the examiner should be able to give a rough estimate of whether the cervix is (a) dilated or tightly closed, (b) anterior or posterior in the vagina, and (c) markedly effaced or very long. In other words, an estimate of inducibility may be obtained by visual inspection. This will not be as accurate as a bimanual examination, but it will provide a good estimate without exposing the patient to an added risk of infection. A prolapsed cord might also be seen at this time.

Subsequent Management Variables

Once the diagnosis of PROM has been made and an initial evaluation has been carried out, other variables must be considered. These would include such complicating factors as risk of respiratory distress syndrome (RDS), risk of infection, and cervical inducibility. Each of these variables should be considered for each patient before an individualized plan of management can be made.

RISK OF RDS

Aggressive management would be the ideal if there were some assurance that the infant was mature and that the attempted delivery would not put the infant and mother at an increased risk of morbidity or mortality. A good estimate of maturity can be made with increasing gestational age, but even term newborns may show RDS if complicating factors—such as maternal illnesses (e.g., diabetes), birth trauma, or hypoxia—are present.

With PROM in a pre-term gestation, there is always a risk of RDS. In fact, RDS is the major cause of neonatal morbidity and mortality. It is a far greater threat to the newborn than is neonatal sepsis. This risk has been shown to decrease, however, with antepartum exogenous steroid administration to the mother (Liggins and Howie, 1972). It is also possible for naturally occurring steroids to be an aid in fetal lung maturation. A stimulus for steroid release is stress. Whether this stress is from the loss of amniotic fluid, subclinical infection, or compression of the fetus in utero, the result is the same. A number of studies have shown an increased level of cortisol in patients with PROM as compared with normal patients. These studies have shown increased cortisol in the maternal serum in as short a time as 16 hours (Bauer et al., 1974) and in amniotic fluid after 24 hours of ruptured membranes (Cohen et al., 1976). Many investigators have demonstrated that this stress accelerates fetal lung maturity (Worthington et al., 1977; Sell and Harris, 1977; Berkowitz et al., 1978; Richardson et al., 1974). The length of the latent period required for this pulmonary maturation ranges from as little as 16 hours to 72 hours. Others have suggested that the pulmonary maturation actually precedes rather than results from the PROM (Worthington et al., 1977). An increased L/S ratio has also been shown in patients with PROM for more than 24 hours (Richardson et al., 1974; Morrison et al., 1977; Verder et al., 1978).

There are however, other studies that have not been able to show an accelerated fetal lung maturation in patients with PROM when compared with matched controls (Christensen et al., 1976; Barrada et al., 1977; Jones et al., 1975). The largest review of cases has been done by Jones and coworkers (1975). In their report, a review of 16,458 neonates weighing greater than 500 grams delivered from patients with and without PROM, was carried out to evaluate the effect that PROM for greater than 24 hours before delivery had on the eventual development of RDS. There was no significant difference between the two groups when infants of the same gestational age were compared. The different conclusions in these studies may be due to a number of factors. One may be that a study with a large number of cases may provide for more equal distribution of patients into smaller subgroups, thereby eliminating confounding variables. Another is that none of the studies routinely used the same variables, such as definition of ruptured membranes, length of latent period, and definition of RDS. These variations make it difficult to compare individual results and conclusions. Therefore, at this time it must be considered that PROM does *not* give definite protection against RDS.

One must also remember that lung maturity does not mean fetal maturity. A mature L/S ratio with the presence of PG indicates lung maturity alone. It does not tell about the central nervous system, liver function, or other organ systems. Premature infants who do not have problems with RDS may still have serious problems, such as necrotizing enterocolitis, hyperbilirubinemia, or intracerebral bleeding. A mature L/S ratio does *not* mean that a 33-week fetus should be delivered without concern. Continued intrauterine development in these premature patients may be of considerable importance and benefit.

INDUCIBILITY

Labor inductions are frequently carried out in patients with PROM who are thought to be at term. Frequently, this occurs in a patient whose cervix is not inducible, and thus attempted inductions may fail, since the cervix may not be ready to respond to oxytocin. This has been reported in the past with term patients with PROM (Kappy et al., 1979), and a more recent analysis reconfirms it (Kappy et al., 1982). In those patients in whom labor inductions were carried out because of PROM, as compared with those who began labor spontaneously, there was a higher risk of cesarean birth (39 vs. 19 percent) owing to lack of progress of labor. In many cases this occurred in patients who had delivered larger infants in prior pregnancies; therefore, bony cephalopelvic disproportion could not be the cause. It is also well known that patients who undergo cesarean sections have a higher morbidity and mortality than those who deliver vaginally.

This may be due to anesthesia, operative complications, or infection. If you add to this the increased risk of infection from multiple bimanual examinations to evaluate progress during the induction (Burchell, 1964), the total risk may outweigh the benefits of the induction.

RISK OF INFECTION

The major maternal complication with PROM is the development of chorioamnionitis, which may progress to general sepsis. The incidence of chorioamnionitis seems to be related to the length of the latent period and the route of delivery. Bryans (1965) reported that 6.4 percent of patients with PROM showed clinical infection within 24 hours but that this increased to 30 percent of patients beyond 24 hours. Others have shown similar data, with chorioamnionitis reported in 26 to 28 percent of patients with a latent period of greater than 24 hours (Lanier et al., 1965; Schreiber and Benedetti, 1980). As already discussed, cesarean sections place the mother at increased risk, especially for postpartum endometritis and bacteremia (Kappy, 1979; Bada et al., 1977; Mead and Clapp, 1977). These infections are frequently mixed bacterial infections with anaerobic organisms. Maternal outcome, however, tends to be good according to most studies.

Besides RDS, the major *fetal* complication associated with PROM is infection leading to sepsis. The risk of infection has long been considered to be in direct relationship to the length of the latent period. Gunn demonstrated an increased perinatal mortality rate after 48 hours of PROM and advocated early delivery (Gunn et al., 1970). However, the length of the latent period alone may not entirely account for the degree of risk of infection. It is probable that gestational age and maturation also play a role.

What factors influence the risk of infection? Clearly there are at least two: (1) the infectivity of the offending organism and (2) the available host defenses.

The normal bacteria flora of the vagina and cervix consists of many different organisms, both aerobic and anaerobic. Lactobacilli are the most common, but staphylococci, streptococci, E. coli, *Klebsiella* spp., clostridia, peptococci, and *Bacteroides* spp. have been identified. As a normal pregnancy progresses through the 2nd and 3rd trimesters, there is a decreasing number of anaerobic bacteria in the cervical flora, followed by an increase during the 1st week postpartum. The total number of bacteria returns to the level of the 1st trimester by the 6th postpartum week (Goplerua et al., 1976). The bacteria found in the uterus during labor or post partum can be any of these normally occurring bacteria.

An organism that is of grave concern is the group B beta-hemolytic streptococcus. It has been shown that 80 percent of newborn infants with early-onset group B streptococcus sepsis are of low birth weight and that 62 percent were born after a prolonged latent period following rupture of the membranes (Baker and Barrett, 1973). Part of the problem with group B streptococci is that they have been found to colonize in 5 to 27 percent of asymptomatic women (Sweet and Ledger, 1973), and these women may be at increased risk of PROM and premature labor (Regan et al., 1981). Rapid treatment with broad-spectrum antibiotics is indicated if group B beta-hemolytic streptococci chorioamnionitis is suspected. Many experts recommend initiating intravenous penicillin and inducing labor if gestational age is more than 32 weeks.

Amniotic fluid itself may have an antimicrobial property. According to the data of several investigators, there is a phosphate-sensitive bacterial growth inhibitor in amniotic fluid (Larsen, 1980; Schlievert et al., 1977). This substance is inactivated by phosphate and is dependent upon zinc for its activity. It is also inactivated by large numbers of bacteria and seems to reach its peak activity in term pregnancies. Amniotic fluid seems to be bacteriostatic near term. This explains why occult bacterial contamination can exist without evidence of sepsis at term. However, if PROM permits further contamination of the amniotic fluid and bacterial numbers reach a critical level, then bacterial growth will not be inhibited and sepsis will develop. Unfortunately, the action of the amniotic fluid's inhibitory substances against anaerobic organisms may be only temporary (Thadepalli et al., 1977). This inhibition may also be related to diet and could explain why patients of low socioeconomic class have an increased risk of infection.

Other antimicrobial substances have also been identified in the amniotic fluid. One is a bactericidal protein, a beta lysin that is believed to be present in pregnancies greater than 14 weeks and which acts against the cytoplasmic membranes of gram-positive bacteria (Ford et al., 1977). Lysozyme, another inhibitory substance that is normally contained in phagocytic leukocytes, may also provide bacteriolytic activity. The function of lysozyme remains unclear, but it may provide nonspecific resistance to bacterial infection. This substance also seems to increase from 25 weeks until term (Bratlid and Linoback, 1978).

DIAGNOSIS OF CHORIOAMNIONITIS

The diagnosis of chorioamnionitis once it is fulminant is not very difficult. Clinically one may see fetal or maternal tachycardia, maternal fever, uterine tenderness, foul vaginal or cervical discharge, and uterine contractions. A leukocytosis with a shift in the differential is also frequently seen. However, the early signs of chorioamnionitis are not as easily identified. In fact, none of the signs of chorioamnionitis are very reliable indicators of early infection. When these signs are compared with bacteriologic identification of the offending organisms or pathologic evidence of infection on microscopic examination of the placenta, more than 50 percent of the cases are false-positive (Townsend et al., 1966).

In an effort to make a more correct diagnosis in these cases, alternative parameters have been examined. One such parameter is microscopic examination of the amniotic fluid for the presence of leukocytes or bacteria. However, this determination is controversial. Some have reported that the presence of bacteria in an amniotic fluid sample shows an increased risk of infection (Bobitt and Ledger, 1978; Garite et al., 1979). Some of these amniotic fluid samples, however, were obtained by using an intrauterine pressure catheter or by transcervical amniocentesis, and both of these methods are unreliable for obtaining samples free of cervical contaminants. Similarly, other studies in which fluid was obtained by the same routes have shown that leukocytes are more indicative of risk than are bacteria (Larsen et al., 1974). Another study shows that neither bacteria nor leukocytes correlate to the potential for infection (Listwa et al., 1976). Any study, however, that uses leukocytes in amniotic fluid for predicting infection has a drawback. These white blood cells could be a contaminant from the cervix or blood or may be present as a result of the mechanical effects of labor.

Another potential sign of impending infection is an elevated level of C-reactive protein (CRP). In one study based on this indicator, there were no false-positives and only 10 percent false-negative results (Evans et al., 1980). This test has the obvious advantage of dealing with factors from maternal serum, making it preferable to a more invasive test such as amniocentesis.

The correct early diagnosis of fetal maturity and chorioamnionitis is of obvious importance. If a test can be used to accurately predict which fetuses are mature and which are at increased risk of infection, rapid delivery can be accomplished before the morbidity and mortality rates increase. These tests will probably involve amniotic fluid, thereby necessitating amniocentesis. Amniocentesis is a relatively simple procedure, but it does carry some risks, even in patients with intact membranes. The procedure carries the risk of trauma, bleeding, initiation of labor, and infection. Once the patient has PROM with leakage of varying amounts of fluid, the risk increases. In our experience and in that of others (Garite et al., 1979), the success rate for obtaining fluid in PROM patients was only 50 percent even with ultrasonic guidance.

ANTIBIOTIC USE

Antibiotic prophylaxis has been shown to be of value in certain obstetric and gynecologic procedures. However, in patients with PROM the benefits have ranged from small to none at all (Bobbitt and Ledger, 1978). The consensus is that although there may be a decrease in postpartum fever due to genitourinary infection, perinatal mortality is not decreased (Lebherz et al., 1963; Gordon and Winegold, 1974). Prophylaxis may also increase the risk of more serious nosocomial infections and may interfere with culture reliability in the neonate. If chorioamnionitis is present, therapeutic doses of antibiotics are given with delivery, which should be accomplished as soon as possible by the least traumatic route.

USE OF ANTEPARTUM STEROIDS

The use of antepartum steroids to accelerate fetal lung maturity has become widespread since it was originally described by Liggins and Howie (Liggins and Howie, 1972). Although there have been no significant adverse effects reported by these examiners, others have reported neurologic and electroencephalographic (EEG) abnormalities in the offspring (Fitzharding et al., 1974). The use of steroids in patients with PROM is also somewhat controversial because of the potential suppression of the immune system, with possible increased infectious risk for mother and fetus (Garite et al., 1981; Collaborative Group on Antenatal Steroid Therapy, 1981). However, in patients with PROM it appears that the major risk to the fetus is from RDS and prematurity rather than from infection. Therefore, steroids may be of benefit for these patients. Using this logic, Mead administered steroids and then delivered patients after 24 hours. He showed a significant reduction in neonatal morbidity and mortality, mainly as a result of a decreased incidence of RDS without an increase in maternal infectious morbidity (Mead and Clapp, 1977). Our studies and others would support this (Kappy et al., Quirk et al., 1979).

USE OF TOCOLYTICS

The use of tocolytics in patients with PROM is also controversial. Labor can be one of the signs of chorioamnionitis. Because of this, many feel that if labor occurs, no effort should be made to stop it, since if tocolytics are used, an infection problem may go unrecognized and worsen. Others say that since prematurity is such a serious problem in these patients, steroids should be used for lung maturation with concomitant tocolytics if needed, to prolong the pregnancy for 24 to 48 hours. This allows enough time for the steroids to work (Mead and Clapp, 1977). At the end of that time, either labor can be induced, or tocolytics can be stopped and labor allowed to ensue. Tocolytics themselves are less effective in patients with PROM. Frequently a delay of only 24 hours can be obtained by using tocolytics in these patients (Wesselius deCasparis et al.; Christensen et al., 1980).

ROUTE OF DELIVERY

Various opinions are held regarding the route of delivery in patients with PROM. As mentioned previously, patients with PROM who undergo cesarean section have an increased risk of infection. These infections not only occur more frequently but are also more serious, with more aggressive bacteria as causative agents. A vaginal delivery would diminish this risk (Ledger, 1979). In contrast, there are those, like Quirk, who believe that the route of delivery should be dictated by the risks to the fetus, especially in the premature infant (Quirk et al., 1979). In his study of predominantly lower socio-economic patients, every effort was made to achieve a nonhypoxic, nonstressful, atraumatic labor and delivery, along with the use of steroids for induction of pulmonary maturity. If an induction was not considered to be easy, or if there were signs of fetal distress, a cesarean section was carried out. This very strict surveillance resulted in a cesarean section rate of 40 percent. In this study, in which the mean gestational age was 31 weeks, there was a 15 percent incidence of RDS and an 88 percent survival rate.

In a similar study, Nochimson and co-workers (1980), using a middle-class population, showed comparable results. The study group consisted of patients pregnant for less than 34 weeks with PROM who were treated with steroids. If labor began within 24 hours, magnesium sulfate was started as a tocolytic agent until at least a 24-hour delay of labor was obtained after steroid administration. Elective delivery was then carried out by the least traumatic route. The control group was treated conservatively, without steroids, and delivered whenever spontaneous labor began, or when infection was found. In the study group, 11.9 percent of the fetuses developed RDS, and 16.6 percent were delivered by cesarean section. In the control group, 31.1 percent developed RDS and 9.8 percent were delivered by cesarean section. There was a mortality of 4.8 percent in the study group, compared with a 9.8 percent rate in the control group. The authors concluded that a nonconservative, dynamic management plan, with avoidance of delivery trauma, improved neonatal survival. The emphasis was on the avoidance of intrapartum stress, hypoxia, and trauma.

NEONATAL DEFORMITIES

One of the areas that must be considered in treating patients with PROM is the effect of decreased amniotic fluid on the further structural development of the fetus. Graham believes that limb reduction anomalies can occur from early in utero limb compression as seen in cases of PROM (Graham et al., 1980). This may be from the formation of amniotic bands from the amnion to fetal parts, particularly the limbs and digits (Torpin, 1965). These bands may produce amputation defects of limbs and digits. Similarly, band-induced craniofacial defects have also been described (Jones et al., 1974). These defects may be caused not only by bands of adhesions but also by compression of the fetal parts (Fig. 16–1). Kennedy and Persaud (1977) believe that compression may cause a vascular insult within the developing limb, resulting in necrotic absorption and loss of previously normal tissue. These defects would be considered non-band limb reductions defects. Limb-body wall defects have also been described by Miller and colleagues (1981). They postulate that all of these defects fit a spectrum of abnormalities that may occur with PROM, which they have named the "amnion rupture sequence." There is a recent review of this subject by Seeds that goes into greater detail (Seeds et al., 1982).

In premature infants of less than 28 weeks' gestation, when PROM was prolonged for greater than 24 hours, a higher incidence of positional foot deformities, congenital dislocations of the hips, and hypoplastic lungs was demonstrated in comparison with other newborns (Kanjanapone et al., 1979). This is believed to be related to the lack of adequate amniotic fluid to allow free motion of the fetus in utero.

A Management Plan

There is no ideal management for *all* patients with PROM. The management will vary depending upon gestational age, risk of infection, presence of labor contractions, and the specific patient population. In other words, a management scheme that works in a private institution dealing with well-educated, well-nourished patients may not be the same one used to manage indigent pa-

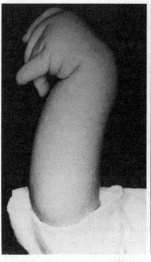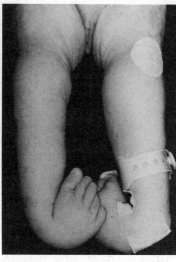

Figure 16–1. This neonate presented with arthrogryposis after prolonged rupture of the membranes. (Courtesy of University of South Florida, College of Medicine, Tampa, FL.)

tients in an inner-city hospital. The former patients may have a minimal risk of infection, while the latter may be at such a high risk for morbidity and mortality due to infection that any attempt at conservative management may be completely out of the question. With these factors in mind, a scheme for the *average* patient may be outlined.

Initially, it is of utmost importance that a correct diagnosis of PROM be made. A combination of history, sterile speculum examination, nitrazine paper test, fern test, and instillation of a dye into the amniotic fluid may be necessary for a truly accurate diagnosis. Reliance on only one of these parameters may easily result in an erroneous diagnosis. Of special note is that only a sterile speculum examination should be done. The amount of information gained by the digital examination over the visual inspection of the cervix is not sufficient to add the extra risk of infection that is inherent with this procedure. A bimanual examination should never be done unless the patient is in labor or thought to be already infected, with an induction of labor forthcoming. Patients with documentation of PROM should then be admitted to the hospital for evaluation.

The initial examination must evaluate the fetal status. Fetal monitoring for signs of occult cord prolapse (variable decelerations) or infection (fetal tachycardia) is mandatory. An estimation must be made of gestational age, based on information on the last menstrual period, early examination, early pregnancy test, date of quickening, date of first fetal heart tones oscultated with a DeLee

fetoscope, ultrasound examinations, and uterine growth rates, all of which should be verified if possible. Despite all of the sophistication of some of these parameters, a reliable date of the last menstrual period is still the best indicator of gestational age. The presence of infection must also be evaluated on the initial examination. A high white blood cell count with a shift in the differential, maternal fever, maternal or fetal tachycardia, uterine tenderness, a foul vaginal discharge, or labor may indicate infection. A transabdominal amniocentesis with fluid analysis for bacteria or white blood cells may give helpful information as to the risk of infection. An initial cervical bacterial culture and sensitivity should be obtained at the time of the sterile speculum examination, to obtain information on the cervical flora. Fetal lung maturity should be determined if feasible; amniotic fluid from an amniocentesis or from the vaginal pool may be reliably used for this purpose.

If there are signs of chorioamnionitis, an aggressive approach with delivery as soon as possible is indicated. In all such cases, broad-spectrum antibiotics in high doses should be started as soon as the initial cultures are obtained. If a cesarean section is deemed necessary, it should be carried out after the antibiotics are begun.

For the patient with PROM who shows no signs of infection, labor, or fetal distress, a conservative approach may be followed. This should consist of bedrest in the hospital with daily CBCs and differentials; vital signs and temperature every 4 hours while awake;

daily evaluation of uterine tenderness; and weekly antepartum fetal heart rate evaluations (NST/CST). This approach is followed in the hospital for as long as the patient is leaking fluid. If the leaking stops, even with increased ambulation, the patient may be given vaginal precautions (no sexual intercourse, douching, or tampons) and sent home. She is told to take her temperature 3 to 4 times a day and to report if there is any elevation of the temperature or if there is uterine tenderness, decreased fetal motion, or a foul vaginal discharge. Weekly antepartum fetal heart rate assessment should be continued. If at any time an infection is suspected, no matter what the gestational age, an aggressive approach is taken. Antibiotics are given and the patient should be delivered. Prophylactic antibiotics and tocolytics have no place in the routine care of patients with PROM, however. It is our feeling that labor may be an initial sign of chorioamnionitis and should not be ignored or suppressed.

This general management scheme, however, is modified depending on the gestational age of the patient. Patients of less than 20 weeks' gestation may be managed in either of two ways. First, because of the risk of infection and the need for intrauterine development to reach a minimal age of viability, the patient may choose to have a termination of pregnancy. This route should be favored if the risk of infection is high. On the other hand, some patients may be treated conservatively even at this early stage of gestation, for the amniotic sac may seal over and the pregnancy continue. If the patient continues to leak fluid, however, the fetus may be at increased risk of having compression deformities. In general, most of these early pregnancies are interrupted because of these risks.

In PROM patients with a gestational age of 20 to 27 weeks, conservative management is advised. All of these patients should be kept at bedrest and followed closely for as long as they continue to leak fluid.

Patients with a gestational age of 28 to 32 weeks who have PROM should be offered the benefits of antepartum steroid therapy to promote fetal lung maturation. This may consist of betamethasone given in a dose of 12 mg intramuscularly initially with a repeat dose in 24 hours. Further repeat injections are not indicated.

Between 32 and 36 weeks' gestation, the fetus still benefits from continued intrauterine development. Patients at this stage should be followed conservatively in the hospital, and signs of chorioamnionitis should be sought. The use of labor inductions in this group may lead to unnecessary problems with RDS or other prematurity complications. If an analysis of the amniotic fluid has shown fetal lung maturity, then labor induction may be carried out in patients who are at high risk for infection. All other may be allowed to wait for spontaneous labor, so that the fetus may benefit from continued intrauterine development.

Infants delivered at greater than 36 weeks' gestation, infrequently have RDS, or if they do, it is usually very mild. Thus, for patients with PROM at this gestational stage, delivery is indicated. The timing of the delivery should be based upon an estimate of inducibility of the cervix. If visualization of the cervix at the time of the sterile speculum examination shows an inducible cervix (effaced, anterior, and partially dilated), then an induction can be carried out immediately. If the cervix is not favorable, then observation for 24 to 48 hours should follow. Of the patients at term with PROM, approximately 90 percent will begin spontaneous labor during this period. If, at the end of this time, labor has not started, then an induction may be attempted if deemed appropriate.

The use of neonatal support systems is mandatory with all deliveries of premature infants. The possibility of concomitant infection in these infants further increases their risks of morbidity and mortality. Therefore, they should be delivered in a tertiary perinatal center where neonatal support is available in the form of skilled personnel and high-tech equipment.

It must be emphasized that the management schemes described here are those that work for us in our institution, at the current time, and with our current population. Each physician must be flexible enough to modify this approach to fit his or her patients. (Table 16–1 summarizes the general management scheme for the patient with premature rupture of the membranes.) As more and more information is obtained regarding patients with PROM, our management will become more ideal. Analysis of infection risks, host resistance factors, and neonatal complications will further refine our management to allow a delivery at the most appropriate time and by the most appropriate route.

Table 16–1. Patient Care Summary for Premature Rupture of the Membranes*

| | Antepartum | | Intrapartum | Postpartum |
	Outpatient	Inpatient		
Blood pressure	Weekly	q shift (except during the night)	q 1 hr	q 15 min × 4; then q 30 min × 2; then q 1 hr until stable; then on discharge to PP; then q shift
Pulse, Respiration	Weekly	q shift	q 1 hr	q 15 min × 4; then 30 min × 2; then q 1 hr until stable; then on discharge to PP; then q shift
Temperature	Weekly	q shift	q 2 hr	q 15 min × 4; then 30 min × 2; then q 1 hr until stable; then on discharge to PP; then q shift
Bedrest	Yes	Yes	Yes	
Fetal monitoring	NST/CST weekly starting at 32 weeks	NST/CST weekly starting at 32 weeks; FHR q shift	Continuous during labor, preferably internal Without monitor, q 15–30 min listening through 2–3 contractions	—
Monitoring of contractions Frequency Duration Quality Resting tone	Daily by patient at home	q shift, prn	Continuous during labor, preferably internal Without monitor, q 1 hr	—
I & O			q shift	—
Sonogram	q 2 weeks	q 2 weeks		—
Amniocentesis	May be done for gestational age	Depends on availability of fluid	—	—
Chemistry blood count	Weekly	CBC with differential daily	On admission	On admission to pp; then prn per infection
Sexual counseling	No intercourse	No intercourse	—	—
Check for uterine tenderness, foul vaginal discharge, cervical discharge	Weekly	q shift	Continuous assessment for changes	—
Amniotic fluid cultures	Depends on protocol	Depends on protocol	—	—

*Nurse–patient ratio is 1:6–8 antepartum; 1:2 intrapartum.

REFERENCES

Abe, T.: The detection of the rupture of fetal membranes with the nitrazine indicator. Am. J. Obstet. Gynecol. 39:400, 1940.

Al-zaid, N. S., Bou-Resli, M. N., Goldspink, G.: Bursting pressure and collagen content of fetal membranes and their relation to premature rupture of the membranes. Br. J. Obstet. Gynecol. 8:227, 1980.

Bada, H. S., Alojipan, L. C., and Andrews, B. F.: Premature rupture of membranes and its effect on the newborn. Pediatr. Clin. North Am. 24:491, 1977.

Baker, C. J., and Barrett, F. F.: Transmission of group B streptococci among parturient woman and their neonates. Pediatrics 83:919, 1973.

Barrada, M. I., Virnig, N. L., Edwards, L. E., et al.: Maternal intravenous ethanol in the prevention of respiratory distress syndrome. Am. J. Obstet. Gynecol. 128:25, 1977.

Bauer, C. R., Stern, L., and Collie, E.: Prolonged rupture of membranes associated with a decreased incidence of respiratory distress syndrome. Pediatrics 53:7, 1974.

Berkowitz, R. L., Kantor, R. D., Beck, G. J., et al.: The relationship between premature rupture of the membranes and the respiratory distress syndrome: an update and plan of management. Am. J. Obstet. Gynecol. 131:503, 1978.

Bobitt, J. R., and Ledger, W. J.: Amniotic fluid analysis: its role in maternal and neonatal infection. Obstet. Gynecol. 51:56, 1978.

Bratlid, D., and Linoback, T.: Bacteriolytic activity of amniotic fluid. Obstet. Gynecol. 51:63, 1978.

Bryans, C. I., in discussion, Lanier, L. R., et al.: Incidence of maternal and fetal complication associated with rupture of the membranes before onset of labor. Am. J. Obstet. Gynecol. 93:403, 1965.

Burchell, R. C.: Premature spontaneous rupture of the membranes. Am. J. Obstet. Gynecol. 88:251, 1964.

Christensen, K. K., Christensen, P., Ingemarsson, I., et al.: A study of complications in preterm deliveries after prolonged premature rupture of the membranes. Obstet. Gynecol. 48:670, 1976.

Christensen, K. K., Ingemarsson, I., Leidenman, T., et al.: Effect of ritodrine on labor after premature rupture of the membranes. Obstet. Gynecol. 55:187, 1980.

Cohen, W., Fencl, M. M., and Tulchinsky, D.: Amniotic fluid cortisol after premature rupture of membranes. J. Pediatr. 88:1007, 1976.

Collaborative Group on Antenatal Steroid Therapy: Effect of antenatal dexamethasone administration on the prevention of respiratory distress syndrome. Am. J. Obstet. Gynecol. 141:276, 1981.

Danforth, O. N., McElin, T. W., and States, M. N.: Studies on fetal membranes. Am. J. Obstet. Gynecol. 65:480, 1953.

Evans, M. I., Hajj, S. N., Devoe, L. D., et al.: C-reactive protein as a predictor of infectious morbidity with premature rupture of membranes. Am. J. Obstet. Gynecol. 138:648, 1980.

Fitzharding, P. M., Eisen, A., Lehtenyi, C., et al.: Sequela of early steroid administration of the newborn infant. Pediatrics 53:877, 1974.

Ford, L. C., Delance, R. J., and Lebherz, T. B.: Identification of a bactericidal factor (B-Lysin) in amniotic fluid at 14 and 40 weeks gestation. Am. J. Obstet. Gynecol. 127:788, 1977.

Garite, T. J., Freeman, R. K., Linzey, E. M., et al.: Prospective randomized study of corticosteroids in the management of premature rupture of the membranes and the premature gestation. Am. J. Obstet. Gynecol. 141:508, 1981.

Garite, T. J., Freeman, R. K., Linzey, E. M., et al.: The use of amniocentesis in patients with premature rupture of membranes. Obstet. Gynecol. 54:226, 1979.

Goplerud, C. P., Ohn, M. J., and Galask, R. P.: Aerobic and anaerobic flora of the cervix during pregnancy and puerperium. Am. J. Obstet. Gynecol. 126:858, 1976.

Gordon, M., and Winegold, A. B.: Treatment of patients with premature rupture of the fetal membranes: a) Prior to 32 weeks; b) After 32 weeks. *In* Reid, D. E., and Christian, C. D. (eds.): Controversy in Obstetrics and Gynecology. Philadelphia, W. B. Saunders Co., 1974.

Graham, J. M., Miller, M. E., Stephan, M. J., et al.: Limb reduction anomalies and early in utero limb compression. J. Pediatr. 96:1952, 1980.

Gunn, G. L., Mishell, D. R., and Morton, D. G.: Premature rupture of the membranes: a review. Am. J. Obstet. Gynecol. 106:469, 1970.

Jones, M. D., Burd, L. I., Bowes, W. A., et al.: Failure of association of premature rupture of membranes with respiratory distress syndrome. N. Engl. J. Med. 292:1253, 1975.

Jones, K. L., Smith, D. W., Hall, B. D., et al.: A pattern of craniofacial and limb defects secondary to aberrant tissue bands. J. Pediatr. 84:90, 1974.

Kanjanapone, V., Kappy, K. A., Herschel, M. J., et al.: The influence of prolonged premature rupture of membranes on the fetus. Pediatr. Res. 12:528, 1979.

Kappy, K. A.: Unpublished data.

Kappy, K. A., Cetrulo, C. L., Knuppel, R. A., et al.: Premature rupture of the membranes: a conservative approach. Am. J. Obstet. Gynecol. 134:655, 1979.

Kappy, K. A., Cetrulo, C. L., and Knuppel, R. A.: Premature rupture of the membranes at term: a comparison of induced and spontaneous labors. J. Reprod. Med. 27:29, 1982.

Kennedy, L. A., and Persaud, T. V. N.: Pathogenesis of developmental defects induced in the rat by amniotic sac puncture. Acta Anat. 97:23, 1977.

Lanier, R. L., Scarbrough, R. W., Fillingim, D. W., et al.: Incidence of maternal and fetal complication associated with rupture of the membranes before onset of labor. Am. J. Obstet. Gynecol. 93:398, 1965.

Larsen, B.: How does amniotic fluid protect mother and fetus against infection? Contemp. Obstet. Gynecol. 15:127, 1980.

Larsen, J. W., Goldhrand, J. W., Hanson, T. M., et al.: Intrauterine infection on an obstetric service. Obstet. Gynecol. 43:838, 1974.

Lebherz, T. B., Hallman, L. P., Madding, R., et al.: Double-blind study of premature rupture of the membranes. Am. J. Obstet. Gynecol. 87:218, 1963.

Ledger, W. J.: Premature rupture of membranes and maternal-fetal infection. Clin. Obstet. Gynecol. 22:329, 1979.

Liggins, G. C., and Howie, R. N.: A controlled trial of antepartum glucocorticoid treatment for prevention of the respiratory distress syndrome in premature infants. Pediatrics 50:515, 1972.

Listwa, H. M., Dobek, A. S., Carpenter, J., et al.: The predictability of intrauterine infection by analysis of amniotic fluid. Obstet. Gynecol. 48:31, 1976.

Mead, P. B., and Clapp, J. E.: The use of betamethasone and timed delivery in management of premature rupture of the membranes in the preterm pregnancy. J. Reprod. Med. 19:3, 1977.

Miller, M. E., Graham, J. M., Higginbottom, M. C., et al.: Compression-related defects from early amnion rupture: evidence for mechanical teratogenesis. J. Pediatr. 98:292, 1981.

Morrison, J. C., Whybrew, W. D., Bucovaz, E. T., et al.: The lecithin/sphingomyelin ratio in cases associated with fetomaternal disease. Am. J. Obstet. Gynecol. 127:363, 1977.

Naeye, R. L.: Causes of perinatal mortality in the United States: collaborative perinatal project. JAMA 238:229, 1977.

Naeye, R. L., and Peters, E. C.: Amniotic fluid infection with intact membranes leading to prenatal death: a prospective study. Pediatrics 61:171, 1978.

Naeye, R. L., and Peters, E. C.: Causes and consequences of premature rupture of fetal membranes. Lancet 1:192, 1980.

Nochimson, D. J., Petrie, R. H., Shah, B. L., et al.: Comparison of conservative and dynamic management of premature rupture of membranes/premature labor syndrome. Clin. Perinatol. 7:17, 1980.

Polishuk, W. Z., Hohane, S., and Peranio, A.: The physical properties of the fetal membranes. Obstet. Gynecol. 20:204, 1962.

Quirk, J. G., Raker, R. K., Petrie, R. H., et al.: The role of glucocorticoids, unstressful labor and atraumatic delivery in the prevention of respiratory distress syndrome. Am. J. Obstet. Gynecol. 134:768, 1979.

Regan, J. A., Chao, S., and James, L. S.: Premature rupture of membranes, preterm delivery and group B streptococcal colonization of mothers. Am. J. Obstet. Gynecol. 141:184, 1981.

Richardson, C. J., Pomerance, J. J., Cunningham, M. D., et al.: Acceleration of fetal lung maturation following prolonged ruptures of the membranes. Am. J. Obstet. Gynecol. 118:1115, 1974.

Sbarra, A. J., Blake, G., Cetrulo, C. L., et al.: The effect of cervical/vaginal secretions on measurement of lecithin/sphingomyelin ratio and optical density at 650 mm. Am. J. Obstet. Gynecol. 140:214, 1981.

Sberra, A. J.: Personal communication, 1978.

Schlievert, P., Johnson, W., Jalask, R. P.: bacterial growth inhibition by amniotic fluid. VII. The effect of zinc supplementation on bacterial inhibitory activity of amniotic fluids from gestations of 20 weeks. Am. J. Obstet. Gynecol. 127:603, 1977.

Schreiber, J., and Benedetti, T.: Conservative management of preterm premature rupture of the fetal membranes in a low socioeconomic population. Am. J. Obstet. Gynecol. 136:92, 1980.

Seeds, J. W., Cefalo, R. C., and Herbert, W. N.: Amniotic band syndrome. Am. J. Obstet. Gynecol. 144:243, 1982.

Sell, E. J., and Harris, Z. R.: Association of premature rupture of membranes with idiopathic respiratory distress syndrome. Obstet. Gynecol. 49:167, 1977.

Smith, R. P.: A technic for the detection of rupture of the membranes: a review and preliminary report. Obstet. Gynecol. 48:172, 1976.

Stedman, C. M., Crawford, S., Staten, E., et al.: Management of preterm premature rupture of membranes: assessing amniotic fluid in the vagina for phosphatidylglycerol. Am. J. Obstet. Gynecol. 140:34, 1981.

Sweet, R. L.: Perinatal infections: bacteriology, diagnosis and management. In Iffy, L., and Kaminetzky, H. (eds.): Principles and Practice of Obstetrics and Perinatology. New York, Wiley Medical Publications, 1981, pp. 1035–1071.

Sweet, R. L., and Ledger, W. J.: Puerperal infectious morbidity: a two year review. Am. J. Obstet. Gynecol. 117:1093, 1973.

Taylor, E. S., Morgan, R. L., Bruns, P. D., et al.: Spontaneous premature rupture of the fetal membranes. Am. J. Obstet. Gynecol. 82:1341, 1961.

Thadepalli, H., Appleman, M. D., and Maidman, J. E., et al.: Antimicrobial effect of amniotic fluid against anaerobic bacteria. Am. J. Obstet. Gynecol. 127:250, 1977.

Torpin, R.: Amniochorionic mesoblastic fibrous strings and amniotic bands: associated constricting fetal malformations or fetal death. Am. J. Obstet. Gynecol. 91:65, 1965.

Townsend, L., Aickin, D. R., and Fraillon, J.: Spontaneous premature rupture of the membranes. Aust. NZ Obstet. Gynecol. 6:226, 1966.

Tricomi, V., Hall, J. E., Bittar, A., et al.: Arborization test for the detection of ruptured fetal membranes. Obstet. Gynecol. 27:275, 1966.

Verder, H., Fonseca, J., Falck, L., et al.: Lecithin/sphingomyelin ratio in eight cases of premature rupture of the membranes. Dan. Med. Bull. 25:218, 1978.

Wesselius deCasparis, A., Thiery, M., Yo Le Sian, A., et al.: Results of a double-blind, multicenter study with ritodrine in premature labor. Br. Med. J. 3:144, 1971.

Wideman, G. L., Baird, G. H., and Baldin, O. T.: Ascorbic acid deficiency and premature rupture of fetal membranes. Am. J. Obstet. Gynecol. 88:592, 1964.

Worthington, D., Maloney, A. H. A., and Smith, B. I.: Fetal lung maturity. I. Mode of onset of premature labor: influence of premature rupture of the membranes. Obstet. Gynecol. 49:275, 1977.

17

PRETERM LABOR

JEFFREY LIPSHITZ
REBECCA L. BROWN

Preterm delivery, which accounts for over 75 percent of all cases of perinatal morbidity and mortality, remains the most important obstetric problem in the world today. Although ritodrine hydrochloride was introduced as the first FDA-approved drug for the treatment of preterm labor in the United States, it is far from a panacea and has resulted in serious iatrogenic problems such as maternal pulmonary edema and death. Part of the problem has been due to a poor understanding of the diverse nature of preterm labor, poor selection of patients for tocolytic therapy, the widespread metabolic and cardiovascular effects of the β-agonists (β-stimulators), and a failure to recognize the dangers and pitfalls associated with the use of these drugs in the treatment of preterm labor. This chapter is written with these issues in mind.

Definition and Incidence

In the past, the term *premature* was used to describe babies born before 37 or 38 weeks as well as those with a weight of less than 2500 grams. This is confusing, as approximately 40 percent of these babies, although they weigh less than 2500 grams, have a gestational age of greater than 37 weeks. The term premature should no longer be used, and infants should be described in terms of either birth weight or gestational age. The World Health Organization (WHO) recommendation is that infants delivered at less than 37 completed weeks (less than 259 days) gestation from the first day of the last menstrual period be defined as preterm, and infants weighing less than 2500 grams be classified as low-birth-weight (Anderson,

1977). Most statistics, however, refer to birth weight, as gestational age is often difficult to determine.

The incidence of low-birth-weight babies in the United States decreased from a peak of 8.3 percent in 1965 and 1966 to a low of 7.4 percent in 1974 (Chase, 1977). The incidence was higher in black women (13.1 percent) than in white women (6.3 percent).

Consequences of Preterm Birth

Preterm birth is the leading cause of early neonatal death. This is well shown in a study from England (Rush et al., 1976). Although the preterm birth rate was only 5.1 percent, 85 percent of early neonatal deaths not due to lethal deformity occurred in these newborns. Preterm newborns born alive had a chance of survival 120 times lower than that of newborns born later in gestation. The introduction of specialized neonatal intensive care units has greatly improved the prognosis for the small newborn from the depressing outcomes of the 1940s and 1950s, when the survival expectation for the neonate under 1500 grams was less than 20 percent, and up to 70 percent of the survivors had significant developmental handicaps. The incidence of major handicap is still approximately 10 percent (Stewart, 1977; Fitzhardinge, 1975; Sabel et al., 1976). Because of a decrease in the size of the family unit, there has been a shift of emphasis from mere survival to greater expectations for *quality* of life. Therefore, the goal is not just to ensure survival but also to decrease handicaps.

Data from the National Collaborative Perinatal Study of the National Institute of Neurological and Communicative Disorders and Stroke, in which children were followed to age 7 or 8 years, indicates a relationship between birth weight and gestational age statistics and later IQ scores and incidence of neurologic abnormalities (Hardy and Mellits, 1977). Preterm babies and low-birthweight babies had subsequent lower IQ scores and a higher incidence of neurologic abnormalities.

Parents are usually emotionally unprepared for the birth of a preterm infant. Anxiety about survival of the infant is accompanied by feelings of guilt, anger, and depression. These usual feelings of parents after the birth of a preterm infant are symptomatic of grief for the expected healthy, full-term infant that they didn't have, and of the realistic fear of the loss of the newborn (Taylor and Hall, 1979). The psychologic counseling of the parents will be dealt with in greater detail later in this chapter. The recognition of the importance of parent-infant bonding has led to parents no longer being excluded from the neonatal intensive care unit.

The financial drain caused by the delivery of a preterm infant is enormous. Pomerance and coworkers (1978) reported that the average daily cost for surviving infants was $450.00, and for those who died, $825.00. The cost per "normal" survivor, which is probably higher now, was $88,058.00.

Initiation of Labor

The sequence of events leading to the initiation of labor has been well documented in the sheep, in which it is the *fetus* that initiates the onset of parturition through activation of its hypothalamic-pituitary-adrenal axis (Lipshitz, 1980). A prelabor rise in fetal cortisol is the key to the fetal control of the onset of parturition in the sheep. Fetal cortisol, which increases during the last 8 to 10 days of gestation, stimulates a placental enzyme (17-α-hydroxylase) that decreases the level of progesterone and at the same time increases the level of estrogen. Estrogens are potent stimulators of prostaglandin (PG) production, whereas the fall in progesterone enables the release of PG to occur. Figure 17–1 details this sequence of events. The cortisol has a dual role in the sheep, in

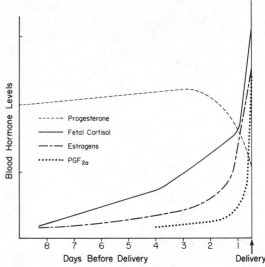

Figure 17–1. Sequence of events leading to the initiation of labor in the sheep.

which it not only stimulates the onset of parturition but also prepares the fetus for extrauterine life, e.g., by the induction of fetal lung maturity.

If, as in the sheep, the human fetus initiated labor and at the same time prepared itself for extrauterine survival, babies born prematurely would rarely get respiratory distress syndrome (RDS), and it would almost never be necessary to use drugs to inhibit preterm labor. However, it is obvious from clinical practice that this is not the case.

Although many studies have been reported on maternal and fetal cortisol levels, it has thus far not been shown that a sharp rise in maternal or fetal cortisol precedes the onset of labor in the human. Although an increase in the estrogen/progesterone ratio associated with the onset of labor has been described, the data in humans remain contradictory and confusing (Lipshitz, 1980).

The local production of prostaglandins, from precursors located in the fetal membranes and decidua, appears to be the primary mechanism by which labor is initiated in the human. The fetal membranes contain glycerophospholipids highly enriched with arachidonic acid. An enzyme, phospholipase A_2, is required to split off the arachidonic acid from the phospholipids. However, this enzyme is contained in the lysosomes, and its activity depends on release from them.

Schwarz and colleagues (1976) described a progesterone-binding substance in fetal membranes near term that competes with lysosomes for progesterone. As a conse-

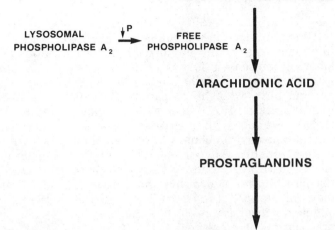

Figure 17–2. Initiation of labor in the human.

GLYCEROPHOSPHOLIPIDS

LYSOSOMAL PHOSPHOLIPASE A_2 → P → FREE PHOSPHOLIPASE A_2

ARACHIDONIC ACID

PROSTAGLANDINS

UTERINE CONTRACTIONS

quence, the lysosomes become more unstable and their contents leak out. Milewich and coworkers (1977) showed that progesterone metabolism was decreased in fetal membranes several weeks before normal labor when compared with the progesterone in midtrimester fetal membranes. Thus, there is a local withdrawal of progesterones in the membranes independent of maternal plasma levels.

The phospholipase A_2, which is released from the lysosomes, strips off arachidonic acid from the phospholipids. This results in an increased local production of prostaglandins, which diffuse to the myometrium and initiate uterine contractions (Fig. 17–2).

Etiology of Preterm Labor

The etiology of preterm labor is multifactorial and poorly understood. It can be broadly classified under four headings: Complications of Pregnancy, Epidemiologic Factors, Iatrogenic Factors, and Unknown Causes (Table 17–1).

A retrospective analysis of 486 preterm infants revealed that spontaneous labor of unknown cause accounted for 38 percent of all preterm deliveries and 35 percent of all preterm early neonatal deaths (Rush et al., 1976). Spontaneous labor associated with complications occurred in 24 percent of the preterm deliveries and accounted for 29 percent of the deaths. The most common complication was antepartum hemorrhage, followed by fetal growth retardation, cervical

incompetence, and hypertension. Multiple pregnancy accounted for 10 percent of the preterm deliveries and 27 percent of the preterm early neonatal deaths. The final 28 percent of preterm deliveries were accounted for by elective obstetric intervention due to complicating maternal or fetal factors. This group accounted for only 9 percent of the preterm early neonatal deaths. Thus, spontaneous preterm delivery was associated with either no apparent cause or with multiple pregnancy in almost 50 percent of the infants.

Table 17–1. Etiology of Preterm Labor

Factors in Pregnancy
   Infection
   Uterine bleeding
   Multiple pregnancy and hydramnios
   Uterine abnormalities
   Incompetent cervix
   Maternal illness
   Premature rupture of the membranes
   Fetal growth retardation
   Fetal anomalies

Epidemiologic Factors
   Maternal age
   Height and weight
   Socioeconomic status
   Race
   Antenatal care
   Smoking
   Psychologic factors
   Coitus
   Previous obstetric history
   Unwanted pregnancies

Iatrogenic Factors

Unknown Causes

COMPLICATIONS OF PREGNANCY

Although infection undoubtedly plays an important role in the etiology of preterm labor, at present it is unknown to what extent unrecognized infection contributes to preterm birth when no apparent cause is found (Lipshitz, 1977). Roos and coworkers (1980) were able to culture bacteria from the intrauterine environment in 72 percent of 56 preterm infants. An understanding of the factors that initiate parturition has clarified the possible mechanism by which bacteria may initiate preterm labor. The bacterial endotoxin itself is unable to stimulate the pregnant rat uterus (Wren, 1970). Bejar and colleagues (1979) have shown that the organisms associated with preterm labor have specific activity of phospholipase A_2 higher than that of the intracellular phospholipase A_2 of the amnion and chorion. Also, intact gram-positive and gram-negative bacteria were able to release stable prostaglandin E_2 and $F_{2\alpha}$ in the presence of arachidonic acid (Gulbis et al., 1979).

Placenta previa and abruptio placentae both commonly result in the delivery of preterm infants (Niswander, 1977). Threatened abortion in early pregnancy, and antepartum uterine bleeding that is *not* due to placenta previa or abruptio placentae, are both associated with an increased risk of preterm labor (Turnbull, 1977).

Maternal uterine abnormalities increase the risk of both spontaneous abortion and preterm delivery (Craig, 1977; Gibbs, 1973). The chance of a woman with Asherman's syndrome carrying a pregnancy to term is less than 50 percent (Forssman, 1965). Cervical incompetence results in repeated abortions as well as preterm deliveries. Cervical suture is usually successful if used for the correct indication. However, it is a procedure not without risk and will commonly be unsuccessful when used for conditions other than cervical incompetence (Lipshitz, 1975).

Chronic systemic diseases such as diabetes mellitus, hypertension, and chronic renal disease may result in preterm delivery, as a result of either spontaneous labor or obstetric intervention (Rush et al., 1976). Almost any severe maternal illness, as well as endocrine disorders such as untreated hypothyroidism (Mestman et al., 1974) and hyperparathyroidism (Johnstone et al., 1972), is associated with preterm labor.

EPIDEMIOLOGIC FACTORS

Epidemiologic factors are merely associations of preterm labor, and there is no evidence that they actually *cause* preterm labor. Great care needs to be taken when interpreting specific epidemiologic factors, as the apparent effect may be due to other associated variables. For example, it has been shown that, when analyzed separately, both maternal height and weight influence the weight of the infant (Hardy and Mellits, 1977) as well as the rate of preterm delivery (Fedrick and Anderson, 1976). However, when these two factors were examined simultaneously, it became obvious that maternal weight, but not height, was of importance to the rate of preterm delivery (Fedrick and Anderson, 1976). The preterm birth rate was almost 3 times as high in mothers who weighed less than 112 pounds at the start of their pregnancies than in mothers who weighed more than 126 pounds.

It has been shown that the younger the mother, the lighter the baby (Hardy and Mellits, 1977) and the higher the rate of preterm delivery (Fedrick and Anderson, 1976).

Women in lower socioeconomic groups have a 50 percent higher rate of spontaneous preterm births than do those in the higher socioeconomic groups. The rate for unmarried mothers is even greater (Fedrick and Anderson, 1976).

In the United States, the preterm birth rate among blacks is twice is high as among whites (Chase, 1977; Garn et al., 1977). This may in part be due to socioeconomic factors. As socioeconomic status increases, the prevalence of low-birth-weight and preterm deliveries markedly decreases. However, at equivalent socioeconomic levels, the incidence of low-birth-weight black neonates is still twice that of white neonates (Garn et al., 1977).

It has been shown that patients who have poor antenatal care have a higher incidence of preterm deliveries (Fedrick and Anderson, 1976; Schwartz, 1962).

The increased rate of preterm deliveries associated with smoking is directly proportional to the number of cigarettes smoked per day, being much worse in mothers who smoke more than 20 cigarettes per day (Meyer, 1977).

Several retrospective studies have reported that sexual orgasm is more frequent in mothers of preterm infants (Goodlin, 1969; Wagner et al., 1976). The prostaglandins implicated in the mechanism of orgasm, as well as their presence in the seminal fluid, may lead to preterm labor in certain susceptible individuals. A more detailed discussion of this subject is presented in Chapter 10.

Of all the epidemiologic factors, a history of previous preterm delivery correlates the most strongly with spontaneous preterm birth. Patients with one previous spontaneous preterm delivery have a 37 percent risk of having a second, and those with two or more preterm deliveries have a 70 percent risk of again delivering preterm (Keirse et al., 1978).

IATROGENIC FACTORS

It has been reported that 10 to 15 percent of neonatal intensive care unit admissions have resulted from elective or otherwise inappropriate obstetric intervention (Hack et al., 1976; Maisels et al., 1977). It is hoped that the wider use of fetal lung maturity testing will reduce this unnecessary and sometimes tragic cause of preterm delivery.

Specific Treatment of Preterm Labor

A significant number of patients in so-called "preterm labor" will respond to placebo treatment. This has resulted in claims of success for numerous regimens and therapeutic agents ranging from bedrest, sedatives and analgesics, alcohol, magnesium sulfate, progesterone, calcium inhibitors, aminophylline, diazoxide, antiprostaglandin drugs, and the β-sympathomimetic agents. Unfortunately, there are very few randomized, placebo-controlled trials with large enough numbers to draw valid conclusions for most of these therapies.

BEDREST AND INTRAVENOUS FLUIDS

It is not known whether patients who respond to bedrest and intravenous fluids were originally in true preterm labor or in "false labor." Bedrest increases uterine blood flow and reduces myometrial activity, while the infusion of water inhibits the secretion of antidiuretic hormone and may also inhibit the secretion of oxytocin. Bedrest and intravenous fluids may be used in the patient who has no evidence of cervical changes, in order to avoid the unnecessary use of potent drugs. However, once the preterm labor appears to be progressing, as evidenced by cervical change, this regimen cannot be relied upon to prevent preterm delivery, as evidenced by the large number of patients who deliver preterm infants while "at bedrest."

ANALGESICS, NARCOTICS, AND SEDATIVES

Because of their effect on the central nervous system, drugs such as meperidine, morphine, promethazine, and phenobarbital have been used in attempts to relax the uterus. However, these agents do not seem to significantly reduce uterine activity (Petrie et al., 1976; Riffel et al., 1973), and they may cause depression and respiratory difficulties in the preterm baby.

MAGNESIUM SULFATE

The administration of a 2-g intravenous dose of magnesium sulfate to women in labor has been found to decrease uterine activity by approximately 10 percent (Petrie et al., 1976). Steer and Petrie (1977) compared magnesium sulfate and alcohol in the treatment of preterm labor. In patients with a cervical dilatation of 1 cm or less, magnesium sulfate was found to inhibit contractions for 24 hours in 96 percent of the patients, compared with 72 percent for alcohol. However, when the cervix was more than 1 cm dilated, only 25 percent of the patients responded to magnesium sulfate and only 8 percent to alcohol. The dosage of magnesium sulfate used was a 4-g loading dose administered as a slow intravenous infusion, followed by a maintenance dose of 2 g per hour.

Following magnesium sulfate administration, the mother may experience a sensation of warmth and flushing owing to peripheral vasodilatation. Transient nausea and headache and palpitations may occur after rapid intravenous injection. Overdosage is followed by disappearance of the knee-jerk reflex, and as the plasma concentration increases, depression of respiration and eventually cardiac arrest may occur. McCubbin and coworkers (1981) reported on a patient who inadvertently received a 20-g loading dose of magnesium sulfate with resultant cardiopulmonary arrest. Of interest was the fact that although spontaneous uterine contractions ceased immediately, they resumed spontaneously at a serum magnesium level of 11.6 mg/dl, a level far in excess of that achieved on a normal therapeutic regime.

As the kidney is the primary route of elimination, caution is required in patients with renal disease. The patellar reflex and urinary output should be regularly checked, at least once every hour.

It is rare for magnesium therapy to depress the fetus, although neonatal depression due to magnesium has been reported, particularly after prolonged intravenous therapy and in cases in which high doses have been given close to delivery (Stone and Pritchard, 1970; Lipsitz, 1971).

ETHANOL

In the United States during the 1970s, ethanol was widely used to treat preterm labor. This treatment modality was pioneered by Fuchs, who used rabbits to demonstrate that oxytocin, which could be centrally inhibited by ethanol, was important in the initiation of labor and that ethanol could thus delay parturition (Fuchs, 1963, 1964; Fuchs et al., 1967). Fuchs and his coworkers showed that ethanol was also effective in inhibiting preterm labor in humans, provided the fetal membranes were intact (Fuchs et al., 1967; Zlatnick and Fuchs, 1972).

Several subsequent studies have failed to demonstrate that alcohol is effective in the treatment of preterm labor (Watring et al., 1976; Castren et al., 1975; Graff, 1971). Other studies have reported that both magnesium sulfate (Steer and Petrie, 1977) and ritodrine (Lauersen et al., 1977) are more effective agents in preterm labor management. These results may be due to the fact that oxytocin does not appear to play a major role in the initiation of labor in humans (Lipshitz, 1980).

Common maternal side effects of ethanol are nausea, vomiting, headache, diuresis, incontinence, restlessness, dizziness, and disorientation. More serious side effects, such as severe lactic acidosis (Ott et al., 1976) and aspiration pneumonia (Greenhouse et al., 1969), have also been reported. The inebriated patient requires constant nursing supervision.

Alcohol freely crosses the placenta, and blood concentrations in the fetus are similar to those in the mother (Idänpään-Heikkilä et al., 1972). Neonates, and especially preterm infants, have a reduced rate of ethanol clearance compared with adults (Cook et al., 1975; Wagner et al., 1970). Animal studies, which do not necessarily reflect human experience, have shown fetal asphyxia, acidosis, and depression of the electroencephalogram with ethanol administration (Mann et al., 1975a and b). Although the infant may be intoxicated at birth, ethanol does not usually cause significant problems in the human neonate. It has been reported that infants born within 12 hours of the administration of ethanol had a significantly lower 1-minute Apgar score and a higher incidence of respiratory distress syndrome than matched-control infants (Zervoudakis et al., 1980). Acute alcohol withdrawal syndrome has been reported in the newborn of an alcoholic mother (Nichols, 1967). Maternal alcohol consumption in early pregnancy may adversely affect subsequent fetal growth and morphogenesis (Hanson et al., 1978) as well as intelligence and behavior (Streissguth et al., 1978). It is not known whether the administration of alcohol in the late second trimester or early third trimester is completely safe, especially with regard to the more subtle effects of alcohol—e.g., its associations with developmental and psychological problems such as hyperactivity, delayed psychomotive development, and school behavioral problems, seen in what is referred to as the "expanded fetal alcohol syndrome" (Shaywitz, 1978).

PROSTAGLANDIN SYNTHETASE INHIBITORS

As already discussed, the prostaglandins play a central role in the initiation of labor, and thus it is not unexpected that drugs such as aspirin and indomethacin, which inhibit prostaglandin synthetase, would affect the labor process. These drugs have minimal maternal effects and would be attractive agents in the treatment of preterm labor if not for the possible adverse fetal effects.

Retrospective surveys of patients who had chronically ingested high doses of acetylsalicylic acid during pregnancy revealed that they had a highly significant increase in the average length of gestation, the frequency of postdates pregnancy, and the mean duration of spontaneous labor (Lewis and Schulman, 1973; Collins and Turner, 1973). Maternal ingestion of this drug during pregnancy may interfere with both neonatal and maternal hemostatic mechanisms. Computed tomographic scanning performed on 108 infants born at 34 weeks' gestation or earlier, and weighing 1500 grams or and less, revealed a higher incidence of intracranial hemorrhage in the infants whose mothers had ingested aspirin, compared with controls and with infants whose mothers had ingested acetaminophen (Rumack et al., 1981). A recent study revealed that of 10 mothers who ingested acetylsalicylic acid within 5 days of delivery, 6 mothers and 9 infants had bleeding tendencies; the same study found that of 7 maternal-neonatal pairs in which the mothers ingested aspirin 6 to 10 days before delivery, all were free of clinical bleeding (Stuart et al., 1978). The neonatal hemostatic abnormalities seen in the first group included numerous petechiae over the presenting part, hematuria, cephalhematoma, subconjunctival hemorrhage, and bleeding from a circumcision. The authors concluded that aspirin should be avoided during pregnancy, and that if ingestion has occurred within 5 days of delivery, the neonate should be evaluated for the presence of bleeding (Stuart et al., 1982).

Several clinical studies have described the use of indomethacin to treat preterm labor. Zuckerman and associates (1974) were the first to report on this treatment modality, and in an uncontrolled study they reported an 80 percent success rate in 50 patients. Wiqvist and coworkers (1975) confirmed that indomethacin was useful in the treatment of 6 patients in preterm labor and showed that the drug produced a reduction in the metabolites of prostaglandin $F_{2\alpha}$. Niebyl and colleagues (1980) showed that indomethacin was significantly more effective than placebo in the inhibition of preterm labor during a 24-hour course of therapy. They also showed that indomethacin mark-edly reduced the prostaglandin $F_{2\alpha}$ metabolite. No indomethacin-related adverse neonatal effects were described in any of the above studies.

Since prostaglandins are important in fetal cardiovascular homeostasis, and since indomethacin crosses the placenta without difficulty, it is not surprising that there have been several case reports of untoward neonatal cardiovascular effects. These consist mainly of narrowing of the fetal ductus arteriosus and persistent fetal circulation (primary pulmonary hypertension). These effects have been reported mainly in mothers who have received indomethacin for prolonged periods of time or in large doses, and in cases in which they have been treated close to term. That the response of the ductus arteriosus depends on gestational age was demonstrated by studies on rats. It was shown that a large dose of indomethacin given to the mother within 18 hours of term delivery resulted in intrauterine narrowing of the fetal ductus arteriosus (Sharpe et al., 1974), whereas this did not occur when the drug was administered several days prior to term (Sharpe et al., 1975).

Although these drugs cannot be recommended for general use in preventing preterm labor, in the early third trimester, in selected patients in whom conventional agents are contraindicated, a short course of antiprostaglandin drugs may have a favorable benefit-to-risk ratio.

BETA-ADRENERGIC AGONISTS

During the first half of this century, studies with epinephrine, the parent compound of the β-adrenergic agonists, produced perplexing and contradictory results. In certain animal species, epinephrine produced relaxation of the uterus, whereas in other species it produced contraction. In some animals it produced relaxation in the pregnant as well as nonpregnant uterus, while in others it produced contractions in both the gravid and nongravid uterus. It was left to Ahlquist, in 1948, to clarify these seemingly contradictory effects of epinephrine on the uterus. He showed that the adrenergic agonists produced their effects through two receptors, which he called α-adrenergic and β-adrenergic. Depending on dose, species, and hormonal status, epinephrine could stimulate

ADRENERGIC RECEPTORS

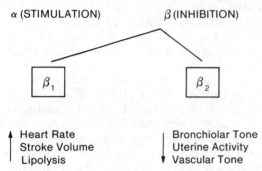

Figure 17–3. Physiologic effects of the adrenergic receptors.

either the α-receptors, which produced stimulation of the uterus, or the β-receptors, which produced uterine relaxation. In 1967, Lands further subdivided the β-receptors into β_1 and β_2 (Lands et al., 1967). The β_1-receptors mediate the increase in rate and force of the heart and produce lipolysis. The β_2-receptors cause relaxation of the smooth muscles of the bronchi, uterus, and arterioles (Fig. 17–3). There are, however, no "pure" β_1 or β_2 stimulants. Although a particular drug may effect mainly one type of receptor, there is usually some degree of overlap. Thus, when comparing the different drugs, the most β_2-selective agonists tend to have the least β_1 effects.

Isoxsuprine was the first β-sympathomimetic drug to be widely used as a tocolytic agent in the treatment of preterm labor (Hendricks, 1964). In 1970, Baillie and coworkers showed that metaproterenol (Orciprenaline) was also an effective tocolytic agent. The therapeutic usefulness of these drugs was somewhat compromised by their significant degree of cardiovascular β_1 effects. They have been replaced by a second generation of selective β_2-sympathomimetic drugs that have lesser β_1 effects, a listing of which follows:

1. Fenoterol (Th 1165, Berotec, Partusisten)
2. Hexoprenaline (Ipradol, Delaprem)
3. Ritodrine (Du 21220, Yutopar)
4. Salbutamol (albuterol, Ventolin)
5. Terbutaline (Brethine, Bricanyl)

Comparison of Beta$_2$-Sympathomimetic Drugs

To determine if any of the β_2-sympathomimetic drugs exhibit increased uterine selectivity (increased β_2-selectivity), fenoterol, hexoprenaline, ritodrine, and salbutamol were compared in dosages having equivalent uterine effects in pregnant patients at term who were undergoing oxytocin-induced labor (Lipshitz et al., 1976; Lipshitz and Baillie, 1976). For an equivalent uterine response, hexoprenaline had significantly less effect ($p < 0.001$) on the maternal rate heart than the other three drugs.

Hexoprenaline and fenoterol were compared in prostaglandin $F_{2\alpha}$–induced labor, and once again hexoprenaline was shown to produce significantly less effect on the maternal heart rate than fenoterol ($p = 0.005$). The tocolytic effects of the drugs were just as good in the prostaglandin $F_{2\alpha}$–induced as in the oxytocin-induced uterine contractions (Lipshitz and Lipshitz, 1983).

Preliminary data from the United States Multicenter Study comparing hexoprenaline and ritodrine in the treatment of preterm labor reveal the following: (1) hexoprenaline had significantly less effect on the maternal heart rate and blood pressure than did ritodrine; (2) serious untoward effects of the drugs, such as chest pain and dyspnea, occurred significantly less with hexoprenaline than with ritodrine; and (3) the drugs had to be discontinued owing to cardiovascular manifestations in 4.5 percent of the hexoprenaline patients, as compared with 15.4 percent of the ritodrine patients ($p < 0.01$) (Lipshitz et al., 1983). Since it is mainly the maternal cardiovascular effects of these drugs that limit their therapeutic application, hexoprenaline appears to be the safest and best tolerated of the β_2-sympathomimetic drugs.

Mechanism of Action

A detailed review of this subject has recently been published by Huszar and Roberts (1982). Uterine contractions occur when actin-myosin interaction takes place. This interaction is regulated through enzymatic phosphorylation or dephosphorylation of the myosin light chain. Myosin light chain phosphorylation depends on the activity of an enzyme, myosin light chain kinase. Relaxation of the uterine smooth muscle occurs when another enzyme, myosin light chain phosphatase, removes the phosphate group from the myosin light chains. Thus, uterine activity depends on the ratio of myosin light chain kinase and myosin light chain phosphatase (Fig. 17–4). Myosin light chain ki-

THE SMOOTH MUSCLE CELL

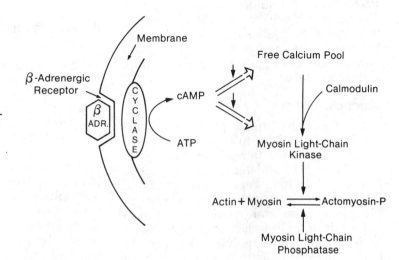

Figure 17-4. Mechanism of action of the β-adrenergic drugs.

nase, the key regulator of uterine contractility, is dependent upon an adequate supply of free intracellular calcium, which binds with a protein, calmodulin.

The β-adrenergic agonists interact with β-adrenergic receptors located on the outer surface of the cell membrane. This interaction then activates adenyl cyclase, an enzyme located on the internal surface of the plasma membrane of the cell. This stimulates the conversion of adenosine triphosphate to cyclic AMP (cAMP), which increases in concentration. The increase in cAMP stimulates a protein kinase, which results in phosphorylation of specific membrane proteins. This process produces uterine relaxation via two mechanisms:

1. A decrease in free intracellular calcium ions. The activation of cAMP-dependent protein kinases results in the phosphorylation of a protein associated with the sodium pump. Thus, Na^+ is pumped out of the cell in exchange for K^+, which enters the cell. This may partially explain the mechanism for the decrease in serum potassium that occurs with the use of the β_2-agonists. The increased Na^+ gradient also accelerates the rate of Na^+/Ca^{++} exchange, resulting in increased calcium efflux from the cytoplasm and sequestration of calcium by the sarcoplasmic reticulum.

2. Direct inhibition of the activity of myosin light chain kinase as a result of the cAMP-mediated phosphorylation (Fig. 17-4).

Cardiovascular Effects

Administration of the β-adrenergic agonists produces a consistent, dose-related increase in maternal heart rate. These drugs relax the smooth muscle in the vascular wall of resistant vessels, resulting in lowered peripheral vascular resistance. A decrease in diastolic pressure occurs that facilitates venous return and results in an increased stroke volume and a rise in systolic and pulse pressures (Bieniarz, 1977) (Table 17-2). Bieniarz (1977) described a consistent increase in maternal cardiac output in five patients receiving ritodrine for the treatment of preterm labor. As diastolic blood pressure tends to decrease more than the systolic pressure increases, the mean blood pressure tends to decrease slightly (Lipshitz and Baillie, 1976; Miller et al., 1976).

Direct measurement of uteroplacental blood flow in the human is not possible, but indirect evidence suggests that it is favorably influenced by these drugs, especially when

Table 17-2. Cardiovascular Effects of
β-Sympathomimetic Drugs

Decreased
Vascular resistance
Increased
Heart rate
Stroke volume
Pulse pressure
Venous return
Cardiac output
? Uteroplacental blood flow

vasospasm has resulted in a decrease in perfusion (Lippert et al., 1976; Brettes et al., 1976). Data from studies in sheep are conflicting, which may be because in the sheep the vessels may already be fully dilated. Hexoprenaline increases placental blood flow on day 14 of gestation in the rat (Lipshitz et al., 1982).

Metabolic Effects

The metabolic effects produced by the administration of β-adrenergic agonists are due, in part, to the increase in cyclic AMP (see Table 17–3). Maternal hyperglycemia results mainly from hepatic glycogenolysis. Since muscle does not contain glucose-6-phosphatase, an end product of glycogenolysis in muscle is lactate, which causes hyperlactacidemia. Lipolysis results in the outpouring of free fatty acids and glycerol into the bloodstream. In a study of the metabolic changes that occur in response to an intravenous bolus of hexoprenaline, it was found that the maximum increase in insulin and glucagon concentrations occurred before the peak in glucose and free fatty acid levels, which suggests a direct action on the α- and β-cells of the maternal pancreas (Lipshitz and Vinik, 1978).

Although plasma potassium concentration is reduced, urinary potassium and excretion is unchanged (Smith and Thompson, 1977), which is compatible with redistribution from the extracellular to the intracellular compartment. Electrocardiograms performed in a few patients showed no evidence of hypokalemia or disturbances in rhythm (Thomas et al., 1977). Potassium supplementation is not recommended, as no adverse effects have been reported and the change is of a temporary nature, with a return to normal within 24 hours.

Adverse Reactions

In the United States trials, intravenous ritodrine was associated with palpitations in one third of the patients (New Drug Application No. 18280). Tremor, nausea, vomiting, headache, and erythema was observed in 10 to 15 percent of patients. Nervousness, jitteriness, restlessness, emotional upset, or anxiety was reported in 5 to 6 percent of patients. Cardiac symptoms, including chest pain or tightness (rarely associated with abnormalities in the ECG) and arrhythmia, were reported in 1 to 2 percent of patients. Other infrequently reported maternal effects included anaphylactic shock, rash, epigastric distress, ileus, bloating, constipation, diarrhea, dyspnea, hypoventilation, sweating, and weakness.

A rare but serious complication of β-agonist therapy is *pulmonary edema*. The widespread use of ritodrine in the United States has resulted in several maternal deaths due to pulmonary edema associated with this therapy in the treatment of preterm labor. Although the exact mechanism for the occurrence of pulmonary edema is unknown, several high-risk factors have become apparent:

1. Fluid overload, which may be due to iatrogenic overvigorous hydration during therapy, as well as to the antidiuretic effect of the β-agonists, which results in gradual water retention with prolonged intravenous therapy.

2. Patients with a multiple gestation, in which there is a natural volume overload, are at increased risk of developing pulmonary edema.

3. Corticosteroids used in combination with the β-agonists have been implicated in the development of pulmonary edema, but convincing evidence is lacking.

4. The maintenance of maternal tachycardia for prolonged periods of time. Pulmonary edema does not usually develop within the first 24 hours of intravenous therapy. Maternal tachycardia results in a shortening of the diastolic filling time of the heart, which over a prolonged period of time may result in the slow accumulation of fluid in the lungs.

5. The patient with unrecognized subclinical amniotic fluid infection may be at par-

Table 17–3. Metabolic Effects of the β-Adrenergic Agonists

Increased	Unchanged	Decreased
cAMP	Pituitary hormones	Serum iron
Glucose	Calcium	Transferrin
Insulin	Phosphorus	TIBC
C-peptide	Cortisol	Potassium
Glucagon	Bilirubin	Cholesterol
Free fatty acids	Haptoglobin	Alanine
Triglycerides	Creatinine	Estriol
Lactate	Uric acid	Bicarbonate
Pyruvate	Sodium	
Glycerol	Chloride	
β-	HPL	
Hydroxybutylate	pH	
Acetoacetic acid		
Renin		

ticular risk for the development of pulmonary edema (Benedetti, et al., 1982).

Acute cerebral ischemic episodes during terbutaline therapy have recently been reported in two patients with a history of migraine headaches (Rosen et al., 1982). Thus, these drugs should probably not be used in patients with a history of migraine headache.

Because of the metabolic effects of these drugs, the patient with diabetes requires careful blood glucose monitoring and usually needs increased insulin administration during treatment of preterm labor. We have found that a continuous intravenous infusion of insulin, adjusted to the patient's blood glucose level, gives the most satisfactory results. Use of the β-agonists may result in ketoacidosis in the unrecognized diabetic patient.

Fetal and Neonatal Effects

Possible fetal effects of β-agonists can occur via two mechanisms: (1) direct action of the active drug on the fetus, and (2) indirect effects secondary to maternal changes, such as a raised plasma glucose or alterations in uteroplacental blood perfusion. Differences in the physical properties of the various β-adrenergic agonists may account for the differences in placental transfer of these drugs. Ritodrine has been shown to cross to the fetus in both sheep (Kleinhout et al., 1974) and humans (Gandar et al., 1980), although fetal levels are usually less than maternal levels. The fetus seems to be protected from the direct effect of fenoterol because of two mechanisms: first, placental transfer of the active substance is minimal (Meissner and Klostermann, 1976), and second, the small amount that is transferred to the fetus is further inactivated by conjugation at the time of passage (Kords, 1977). In animal experiments on ^{14}C-hexoprenaline it was found that none of this drug crossed the placenta to the fetus, perhaps because hexoprenaline is not fat-soluble (Lipshitz et al., 1982). No adverse effects of ritodrine have been described either in the newborn (Freysz et al., 1973; Blouin et al., 1976) or in follow-up studies on infants between 1 and 3 years of age (Freysz et al., 1977).

In a retrospective study, isoxsuprine was associated with neonatal hypoglycemia, hypocalcemia, ileus, hypotension, and death (Brazy and Pupkin, 1979). However, the isoxsuprine was administered as an intravenous bolus and produced hypotension or marked tachycardia in 58 percent of the mothers. Hypotension and death occurred mainly in those infants who were in the 26- to 31-week gestational age group and whose mothers had only a short interval from loading dose to delivery and/or developed hypotension and tachycardia. Maternal hypotension and resultant decreased uteroplacental blood flow is a serious risk with bolus injection of isoxsuprine because of its poor β$_2$-selectivity.

Patient Management
(Tables 17–4 and 17–5)

ANTEPARTUM OUTPATIENT MANAGEMENT

Many preterm births occur not because of the lack of effective tocolytic agents, or maternal contraindications to the use of these drugs, but because by the time the mother arrives at the hospital her labor has progressed to a stage (cervix dilated > 4 cm) at which it is too late to treat the preterm labor. This happens when the patient either ignores or does not recognize the early warning signs of preterm labor. At the E.H. Crump Women's Hospital and Perinatal Center in Memphis, approximately 25 percent of preterm deliveries occur solely because the patient has arrived too late for treatment. Thus, an extremely important part of the treatment of preterm labor should begin before the patient is actually in labor. This involves education of the patients, the nurses, and medical staff dealing with these patients. The early signs of preterm labor are as follows:

- Change of Braxton Hicks contractions from an irregular pattern to a regular pattern. Medical attention should be sought whenever contractions are gradually increasing in intensity, duration, and frequency and are occurring 10 minutes apart or closer.
- Abdominal cramping, sometimes associated with diarrhea.
- Menstrual-like cramps.
- Low backache, often of a different character than that previously felt. This may come and go or be constant.
- Intermittent pressure in the pelvis.
- Change in the character or amount of vaginal discharge. This is especially ominous when the discharge becomes bloody.

Table 17–4. Patient Care Summary for Preterm Labor

		Antepartum		Intrapartum	Postpartum
	Outpatient	Inpatient			
		IV Meds	Oral Meds		
BP, P, R	Weekly	q 15 min while increasing dose; then q 30 min maintenance MP should be <140; FP should be <180	On admission; then q 4 hr (except during the night) Adjust PO; check pulse before PO administration (P should be <140)	q 1 hr	On admission to RR; then q 15 min × 4; then q 30 min × 2; then q 1 hr until stable; then on discharge to PP floor; then q shift
T	Weekly	q 4 hr	On admission, then q 4 hrs	q 4 hr	On admission; then q 4 hr; then on discharge to PP floor; then q shift
Bedrest	Yes	Yes	Yes	Yes	
Fetal heart rate monitoring	NST weekly starting at 30–32 weeks (may discontinue when fetus mature or medications discontinued)	Continuously during tocolysis, chart q 15 min Without monitor, q 15 min listening through 2–3 contractions		Continuous during labor, preferably internal Without monitor, q 30 min listening through 2–3 contractions	
Contractions	Observe weekly (if indicated)	Continuously during tocolysis, chart q 1 hr Without monitor, q 15 min	q shift	Continuously during labor, preferably internal Without monitor, q 30 min	
I & O		q 1 hr	q shift	q shift	While in RR
Amniocentesis					
Chemistry Blood sugars Electrolytes	Weekly Weekly		With IV ritodrine, on admission and prn		
EKG	—		Baseline before administration of ritodrine	—	—
Sexual counseling	No intercourse No orgasm No breast stimulation				

Table 17–5. Medication Summary for Preterm Labor

Medication	Action	Route	Dose	Pregnancy Precautions	Side Effects	Nursing Considerations	Fetal/ Neonatal	Breast-Feeding
β-Adrenergic agonists	Prevents smooth muscle contractions by inhibiting actin and myosin interaction through two mechanisms: (a) decrease of free calcium pool, (b) inhibition of myosin light-chain kinase (Fig. 17–4)	IV & PO	Start infusion at recommended initial dose and increase every 10–20 min Titrate against contractions, pulse, and side effects keep maternal pulse less than 140 beats/min Generally continued for 6–12 hr after cessation of contractions Give first PO tablet, then discontinue IV medication 30 min later Usual PO dose is 1 tab every 2 hr for 24 hr, followed by 1–2 tabs every 3–6 hr depending on contractions, pulse, and side effects Continue until fetal maturity	Not indicated in the first half of pregnancy	Tachycardia, nervousness, anxiety, tremor, palpitations, nausea, vomiting, sweating, headache, chest pain, dyspnea, pulmonary edema, widened pulse pressure, metabolic effects, water retention	*DO NOT* fluid overload these patients, because of cardiovascular changes and water retention Strict I & O Contraindicated: before 20 weeks, antepartum hemorrhage, eclampsia, fetal death, IUGR, chorioamnionitis, maternal cardiac disease, pulmonary hypertension, maternal hyperthyroidism, uncontrolled diabetes Maternal and fetal vital signs every 15 min on IV dose Do not use if solution is discolored or has a precipitate Keep patient in left lateral position If stable, other positions can be tried	Observe for hypoglycemia; fetal tachycardia	No information is available about excretion in breast milk These agents not indicated after delivery The half-life is short and therefore should not cause problems for nursing mothers.
Magnesium Sulfate	Central nervous system depressant Diminishes excitability of muscle fibers and relaxes the uterus	IV	Loading dose 4–6 g Titration dose 2 g/hr Maintenace dose 1 g/hr Continue 24 to 72 hr after cessation of contractions	None	Sweating, drowsiness, depressed reflexes, flaccid paralysis, hypothermia, hypotension, depressed cardiac function, heart block, respiratory paralysis, hypocalcemia	Use cautiously in patients with impaired renal function, myocardial damage, heart block; have IV calcium gluconate (1 g) available to reverse MgSO$_4$ Monitor maternal vital signs q 1 hr; FHR q 15 min; I&O q 1 hr; urinary output should be over 30 cc/hr Reflexes q 1 hr Signs of hypermagnesemia begin to appear at blood levels of 4 mEq/liter	Crosses placenta, producing hypotonia lethargy, weakness, and low Apgar scores	Not indicated after delivery

As many of these symptoms frequently occur throughout gestation, the importance of any change or increase is stressed.

It is important to teach patients at risk how to palpate for uterine contractions. The patient should be taught how to feel the contractions with her fingertips placed on the fundus of her uterus. She should be taught to recognize a contraction as a tightening or hardening of the uterus, which then relaxes. If these contractions are recognized at home, the patient should be encouraged to lie in the partial left lateral position, and to time the contractions from the beginning of one contraction to the beginning of the next. She should time the contractions for 1 hour. If the contractions occur at a frequency of 10 minutes or less for a period of 1 hour, she should seek medical attention and *not* wait for them to disappear, as cervical dilatation may become advanced, which jeopardizes her chances of successful treatment. New in-home monitors that allow the mother to assess contractions at home and send the tracings to the physician's office for early detection of uterine contractions look promising (Katz et al., 1985).

During the antepartum period it is extremely important to obtain an accurate assessment of gestational age. If there is any discrepancy between dates and size, an ultrasonic examination should be obtained. It is important that the patient's weight gain be checked at each visit and that she be adequately informed about correct nutrition. If she smokes, the risks of preterm birth should be explained to her and she should be strongly encouraged to stop smoking.

ANTEPARTUM INPATIENT MANAGEMENT

The patient who presents with a diagnosis of possible preterm labor should receive prompt evaluation and treatment, since any delay may result in the progression of labor to a stage at which any attempted treatment is doomed to failure. It is tragic enough when the patient at risk delays seeking treatment for preterm labor because she ignores the signs of early labor that appear weeks before she expects them, but it is even worse when the delay is due to negligence by the medical staff.

Requirements to Treat Preterm Labor

For a physician to undertake the treatment of a patient in preterm labor, the following should be present:

1. The personnel and equipment necessary to assess the mother.

2. The personnel and equipment necessary to assess the fetus.

3. The facilities to perform an amniocentesis and to do fetal lung maturity studies on the amniotic fluid. The introduction of the Lumadex-FSI test makes this possible even in the smallest hospital (Lipshitz et al., 1984).

4. Close access to a neonatal intensive care unit.

As the treatment of preterm labor is not always successful, and as the resultant degree of infant morbidity and mortality is directly related to the quality of subsequent neonatal care and expertise, if a neonatal intensive care unit is not available, it is better to transfer the infant in utero than after delivery.

Selection of Patients for Tocolytic Therapy

It is often extremely difficult to distinguish between true preterm labor and so-called false labor. Often, the diagnosis of preterm labor can be made only in retrospect. No more than 50 percent of patients with regular painful contractions proceed to preterm delivery (Anderson, 1977). Thus, if all patients presenting with regular uterine contractions are treated, many will receive unnecessary pharmacologic treatment, the side effects of which may be life threatening. With false labor there is often no progressive cervical change, and the contractions cease spontaneously. However, the frequency, regularity, or pain of the contractions may not necessarily distinguish true labor from false labor.

Patients admitted without any evidence of cervical changes, i.e., whose cervix is found to be posterior, long, and closed, can safely be observed with regular pelvic assessments by the same examiner. During this interval the patient should be placed at bedrest in the partial left lateral position and an intravenous crystalloid infusion begun. In many such cases the contractions will stop before any changes in the cervix occur. This is especially important in research trials on new modalities of therapy. If patients are selected for therapy on the basis of contractions alone, a high success rate will be achieved no matter which therapy is employed.

Many of the epidemiologic factors associated with preterm labor are also found in patients who have growth-retarded fetuses. Thus, it is often in the case of the low-socioeconomic, high-risk, indigent patient, who may have unreliable dates, that a decision has to be made as to whether she is in preterm labor or whether the small fetus is in fact mature but growth-retarded. A single ultrasound examination at this stage is of very little value. The intrauterine growth-retarded fetus has an increased risk of asphyxia and stillbirth. It is thus unwise to use tocolytic drugs to maintain these fetuses in an unfavorable intrauterine environment. An excellent way to distinguish the mature growth-retarded fetus from the small pre-

term fetus is by performing an amniocentesis and analysing the fluid for fetal lung maturity. The potential complications of amniocentesis are minimal compared with the benefits gained (Dancis, 1979). In the presence of frequent contractions, tocolytic agents are used to inhibit the contractions until the results of pulmonary maturity studies are known. Another important reason to perform an amniocentesis is the fact that unrecognized chorioamnionitis may lead to preterm labor, and if β-adrenergic agonists are used in these patients, pulmonary edema is more likely to occur (Benedetti et al., 1982). Caution must also be used if the patient is to receive corticosteroids for lung maturity.

Figure 17–5 summarizes the selection of patients for tocolytic therapy developed for our hospital and used in the United States Multicenter Trial comparing hexoprenaline to ritodrine in the treatment of preterm labor. We have since found that the Lumadex-foam

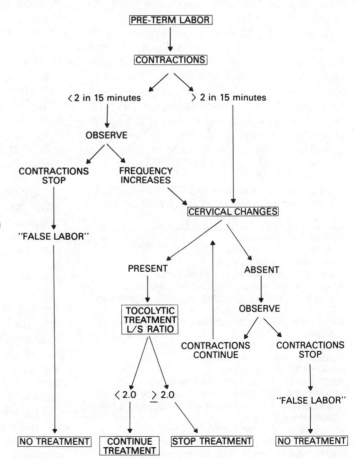

Figure 17–5. Protocol for the selection of patients for tocolytic therapy.

stability index test is more accurate than the L/S ratio in diagnosing the very small growth-retarded fetus (Lipshitz et al., 1983).

Patient Assessment

A full history and physical examination should be performed to evaluate the patient's suitability for receiving β-adrenergic drugs. The history should include details of the patient's past reproductive performance. Details should be sought regarding previous episodes of preterm labor, premature rupture of the membranes, number of preterm, low-birth-weight, and stillborn infants delivered, and previous infants with RDS or other problems. A history of allergies, longstanding medical diseases, and any relative or absolute contraindications to tocolytic therapy should be listed. Special attention should be paid to symptoms of cardiac disease, which should be outlined for the patient. A social history should include the consumption of alcohol, drugs, and tobacco, and other factors epidemiologically associated with the onset of preterm labor.

A detailed physical examination should be performed to recognize any possible contraindication to the use of β-sympathomimetic drugs (Table 17–6). It is especially important to examine the cardiovascular system very carefully to exclude any heart disease. If membranes are intact, a pelvic examination should be performed. The cervix should be examined for any evidence of

Table 17–6. Recommended Contraindications for the Administration of the β-Adrenergic Agonists

Gestation < 20 weeks
Maternal cardiac disease
Eclampsia or preeclampsia
Significant hypertension of any etiology
Abruptio placentae, severe bleeding with placenta previa, or significant vaginal bleeding of unknown cause
Intrauterine infection and probably fever of unknown origin
Fetal mortality or significant abnormality
Significant fetal growth retardation
Maternal hyperthyroidism
Uncontrolled maternal diabetes mellitus
Maternal medical conditions that would be seriously affected by the pharmacologic properties of the β-adrenergic agonists
Any obstetric or medical condition that contraindicates prolongation of pregnancy
Known hypersensitivity to any component of the product
Possibly migraine headache

effective uterine action. These changes are: (a) *position*—the cervix moves from a posterior to an anterior position during early labor; (b) *effacement*—the cervix becomes shorter before significant dilatation occurs; (c) *dilatation* of the cervix, which usually follows effacement. Effacement of the cervix associated with uterine contractions usually indicates the onset of preterm labor, and treatment should be instituted before any significant dilatation of the cervix.

If the patient gives a history of having ruptured her membranes, no pelvic examination should be performed. Instead a sterile speculum examination should be carried out to confirm whether the membranes are indeed ruptured and to assess the state of the cervix. Although it is a controversial practice, we use tocolytic drugs in the patient with ruptured membranes if the following criteria are met: (1) regular uterine contractions are present; (2) there is no evidence of infection; and (3) fetal lung immaturity is documented.

Criteria for the Use of Tocolytic Drugs

1. Gestational age is between 20 and 36 weeks.

2. At least two uterine contractions have occurred in a 15-minute period of time.

3. Cervical effects of contractions are present.

4. The cervix is dilated less than 5 cm.

5. If there is any doubt about gestational age, or if there is a possibility of fetal growth retardation or unrecognized chorioamnionitis, an amniocentesis should be performed.

6. There should be no contraindications to the use of β-adrenergic agonists (see Table 17–6).

7. The patient should be fully informed about the plan of action as well as the possible side effects of the drugs.

Special Investigations

1. A clean-catch specimen of urine should be examined for bacteriuria. This is mandatory in all patients, as there is an association between asymptomatic bacteriuria and preterm labor. When appropriate antimicrobial therapy is instituted at the time of treating the preterm labor, excellent results usually follow. However, if a urinary tract infection is missed, the patient may continue having episodes of preterm labor that will require prolonged tocolytic therapy, with the concomitant increased risk of untoward effects.

2. Blood sugars should be checked to exclude unrecognized diabetes.

3. It is recommended that baseline electrolytes be obtained.

4. If possible, an ECG should be obtained before starting therapy.

5. Hematocrit.

6. A full blood count to exclude unrecognized infection.

Administration of Drugs

Intravenous Administration

Our protocol for the administration of hexoprenaline sulfate and ritodrine hydrochloride is as follows:

1. Dilute 150 mg ritodrine hydrochloride (3 ampules) in a 500-ml solution of 5 percent w/v dextrose, which yields a final concentration of 0.3 mg/ml. To administer hexoprenaline, 150 mcg (6 ampules) is added to 500 ml of fluid, which yields a final concentration of 0.3 mcg/hml. An intravenous microdrip chamber (1 ml = 60 drops) provides a convenient range of infusion rates within the recommended dosages of these drugs.

2. The patient is kept in the partial left lateral recumbent position, and a large-bore indwelling catheter is kept open by a slow intravenous infusion.

3. Baseline values for maternal heart rate, respirations, blood pressure, uterine contractions, and fetal heart rate are determined.

4. The drug infusion is "piggy-backed" onto the main intravenous line, using a controlled infusion device to adjust the rate of flow in drops per minute (60 microdrops = 1 ml).

5. The drug infusion is started at 20 microdrops per minute (ritodrine, 0.1 mg/min; hexoprenaline, 0.1 mcg/min) and increased usually by increments of 10 microdrops (ritodrine, 0.05 mg/min; hexoprenaline, 0.05 mcg/min) every 10 to 15 minutes.

6. Maternal heart rate, blood pressure, respirations, and uterine contractions, as well as fetal heart rate, should be recorded immediately before the rate of the infusion is increased. These vital signs should be recorded every 15 minutes until the correct dose of the intravenous infusion is achieved, and then every 30 minutes throughout the intravenous infusion.

7. A strict intake/output chart should be maintained throughout the intravenous infusion. The total amount of intravenous fluid should not exceed 100 ml per hour.

8. The rate of the infusion is increased until one of the following occurs:
   a. Uterine contractions have stopped completely, or are reduced to less than one contraction per 15-minute period. If contractions occur less frequently than one per 15-minute period, it is advisable not to increase the dose of the drug further in an attempt to totally inhibit all uterine contractions.
   b. Maternal heart rate reaches 140 beats per minute. If the heart rate increases beyond this, the dosage of the drug should be reduced.
   c. Unacceptable side effects develop. The drug infusion may have to be reduced or discontinued.

9. We do not use an arbitrary maximum dosage of a particular drug, as the patient's sensitivity to the drugs may vary widely. Instead, once the maternal heart rate reaches 140 beats per minute, this is regarded as the maximum dosage for that particular patient, and the rate of the infusion is not increased any further. It is rare for a patient to require more than 350 mcg/min (0.35 mg/min) of ritodrine or more than 0.5 mcg/min of hexoprenaline.

10. We have found that the mean maximum dosage required to treat preterm labor is approximately 0.32 mcg/min for hexoprenaline and 270 mcg/min (0.27 mg/min) for ritodrine. However, dosages may vary widely among individual patients.

11. If a patient is sensitive to the drug and exhibits a rapid increase in heart rate, or experiences undesirable side effects, the dosage should be increased more slowly.

12. Upon effective inhibition of uterine contractions (or the reduction to less than one contraction per 15-minute period), the infusion should be continued at the same flow rate for 6 hours.

13. At the end of the 6-hour period, weaning should be commenced by reducing the infusion rate in decrements of 10 drops per minute at half-hour intervals. When the maternal heart rate decreases to 100 beats per minute, 1 tablet of hexopren-

aline or ritodrine should be administered by mouth and the infusion stopped 30 minutes later.

14. The intravenous infusion may be repeated if necessary, as long as the patient still meets the selection criteria.

Oral Administration

Following the initial administration of 1 tablet of ritodrine or hexoprenaline, further oral therapy consists of the administration of 1 to 2 tablets every 2 to 6 hours until it is decided to let the patient deliver. Tablet dosage must be tailored to individual patient needs, based on maternal heart rate, uterine activity, and undesirable subjective effects. Ideally, resting maternal heart rate should be maintained between 100 and 110 beats per minute. If the uterus remains relaxed, it may become unnecessary to disturb the patient during the night, and drug administration may be limited to her waking hours. Undesirable effects may be reduced, both in occurrence and intensity, by administering the tablets with meals.

Administration of the β-agonists, whether by intravenous infusion or by mouth, should be discontinued in any patient presenting with chest pain or dyspnea. An ECG should be recorded immediately and a chest x-ray taken. The patient should be evaluated for the presence of pulmonary rales or other pertinent clinical manifestations of incipient pulmonary edema.

Clinical Significance of the Maternal Pulse Rate

Whether the β-adrenergic agonists are administered as an intravenous bolus (Lipshitz et al., 1976), intravenous infusion (Lipshitz and Baillie, 1976a), oral tablet (Lipshitz, 1977), or aerosol (Lipshitz and Baillie, 1976b). There is a close correlation between the time of onset of the uterine inhibitory effect and the time of increase in the maternal pulse rate. The same correlation holds true for the time taken for uterine activity to return to normal after stopping the drugs, and the time taken for the heart rate to return to normal. Thus, the maternal pulse rate is an important clinical parameter during the administration of the β-agonists. The drug infusion is titrated against the patient's contractions as well as against the rise in maternal pulse rate. Conversely, if contractions recur during intravenous administration at close to "maximum" dosages, then, provided the maternal pulse rate is slow, the

dose can usually be increased further. The maternal pulse rate should also be used to adjust the oral dosage of the β-agonists.

Psychologic Aspects of Treatment

The psychologic effects of prolonged hospitalization and the emotional needs of the patient are often overlooked by the busy physician. Thus, this important aspect of the patient's treatment usually becomes a nursing responsibility. In addition to suffering the untoward effects of the drugs, the patient very seldom has an undisturbed night's sleep, which can result in chronic fatigue. The patient very often has guilt feelings from thinking that the preterm labor is due to something that she has done or not done. It is important that she be reassured that the preterm labor is not her fault. Although many pregnant women fear that their baby will not be normal, this is of even greater concern to many patients in preterm labor. Health care providers are occasionally faced with the patient who refuses further treatment and expresses the desire to end the pregnancy, although it has been explained to her that this may result in the loss of her baby. This is a normal part of the ambivalence that patients who have to be hospitalized for a long period of time feel toward their pregnancy. The patient blames the baby for the fact that she is confined to bed, separated from the rest of her family, and unable to conduct her life as she normally would. It should be explained to the patient that these are normal feelings faced by many women in preterm labor, and that these feelings do not make them an uncaring and unloving mother. Some patients have great difficulty confining themselves to bed when they do not feel ill, and these patients should be encouraged to develop activities that can be done in bed, such as knitting, embroidering, and reading.

It is not unexpected that the patient who is confined to bed in a hospital setting for a lengthy period of time would have periods of depression. Correct counseling and emotional support thus play a very important part in the patient's treatment for preterm labor.

Postpartum Management

The patient who has delivered a preterm baby will require intensive emotional support during the postpartum period. The preterm birth cuts short a normal developmental process of adjustment and attachment to the fetus. By the time the pregnancy has progressed to the stage of viability, the parents have made a significant psychologic and emotional investment in the fetus.

Preterm delivery represents a family crisis. Grief, guilt, and anxiety are the primary emotional responses to the preterm birth. The parents experience all the elements of grief, first because they did not have the baby that they expected, and then possibly anticipatory grief for the potential threats to their vulnerable newborn. At the same time, they are attempting to relate to their baby. It is important to allow and encourage them to see their newborn as soon as possible. The sooner they see their baby, the sooner they can work through their feelings and begin the process of relating to the baby. If visiting is impossible because of transport of the baby or the mother's condition, it is a good idea to provide the parents with a picture of their baby, which can help them deal with the real baby. The father and grandparents should be encouraged to visit the baby if the mother is unable to do so. They can give support to the mother as well. To help reduce anxiety, it is essential that the medical staff communicate with the family about the baby's condition. The elements of grief are essentially the same, regardless of the cause. They have been described as shock, denial, anger, bargaining, and acceptance. Parents of preterm babies exhibit varying degrees of these emotions at one time or another.

The initial emotion exhibited by the mother and family of the preterm baby is usually *shock*. The patient can expect to have periods of crying and silence, and to experience emotional numbness at times. The patient should be allowed to express her feelings and not to have sedation prescribed in order to help her deal with the seemingly negative emotions which will need to be dealt with eventually.

The *denial* phase is generally the longest and is probably the most troublesome response for the nursing and medical staff to deal with. During this phase the family apparently refuses to grasp and understand what is told to them about the baby's condition. Denial is a normal self-defense mechanism that the family uses to cope during such a crisis. This enables the family to feel that they are maintaining control and also

enables them to cushion themselves against the pain of the reality of the circumstances. Denial dosen't necessarily mean that the family does not hear what they are told by the staff. During this time, the staff will be called upon to give repeated explanations regarding the condition of the baby. During each meeting with the family, the staff should provide accurate information and prevent confrontation.

Anger is another common response to the birth of a preterm baby. The anger and hostility of the family is often directed at the physicians and hospital staff, especially the nurses who care for the baby. The mother may express jealousy of the nurses who are caring for her baby while she cannot. To alleviate this situation, the nurses should allow the mother to participate in as much of the infant's care as possible.

The mother may experience a period of *bargaining*, which is usually done in a religious context. The staff should withhold their personal feelings during this time and continue to provide emotional support without setting unrealistic expectations for the patient regarding the baby's condition. The easiest phase of grief for the nursing and medical staff to deal with is when the family members begin to *accept* the circumstances and ask pertinent questions on how to handle their situation.

Each of these responses is a phase. The phases may not occur in any particular order, and families may have different responses at different times. It is important that the staff be supportive and allow family members to express their feelings and ask questions, while at the same time correcting the parents in areas in which they are misguided with regard to their child's condition.

The mother of the preterm infant may feel guilty that she has failed to produce a healthy, full-term infant. She may ask the staff repeated questions in her search for something that she possibly did wrong and which may have resulted in her preterm delivery. The father may also have guilt feelings with regard to whether something he did, or failed to do, contributed toward the preterm delivery. Siblings may worry that their jealousy or fantasies were what caused the problem. The entire family needs to be listened to and reassured that they were not responsible for the preterm delivery.

The postpartum nursing staff and the neonatal intensive care unit staff should expect the family to experience episodes of severe anxiety in response to the daily fluctuations in the infant's condition. The family may experience fear and anxiety about their infant's prognosis; in addition to this there may be a great concern about the financial consequences of the neonate's prolonged hospitalization. The mother may feel inadequate and lack confidence in her ability to care for the baby in the neonatal intensive care unit. These feelings of inadequacy may be intensified by her lack of understanding of the medical terminology being used in reference to her baby's condition, as well as of the various life support systems and monitors in the ICU. Antepartum visits to the ICU may help to decrease the mother's anxiety.

The medical and nursing staff can be invaluable when they provide for both the emotional and physical well-being of the mother during the postpartum period. Explanations regarding the infant's condition should be given in simple terms to the patient and her family. Responses to the grief, guilt, and anxiety of the family should be expected, viewed as normal by the nurses, and dealt with in a professional manner. Without disregarding the physical condition of the patient, it is imperative that staff members exhibit an empathetic and nonjudgmental attitude as well as paying close personal attention to the emotional well-being of the patient. In this situation, as in all nursing situations in which interrelationships are so important, the key word is "caring."

Finally, when a mother has had preterm labor, she should be counseled that she is at risk for another preterm labor. She should be advised that with subsequent pregnancies she should seek medical care as soon as she knows that she is pregnant and advise the practitioners that she has had a previous preterm labor. She should also be told that she should seek prenatal care at a center in which comprehensive services are available.

REFERENCES

Ahlquist, R. P.: A study of the adrenotropic receptors. Am. J. Physiol. 153:586, 1948.

Anderson, A. B. M.: Pre-term labour: definition. In Anderson, A. B. M., et al. (eds.): Proceedings of the Fifth Study Group of the Royal College of Obstetricians and Gynaecologists. London, Royal College of Obstetricians and Gynaecologists, 1977.

Baillie, P., Meehan, P. P., and Tyack, A. J.: Treatment of premature labour with orciprenaline. Br. Med. J. 4:154, 1970.

Bejar, R., Cuberlo, V., Davis, C., et al.: Premature labor: infections as possible triggers. Twenty-sixth Annual Meeting of the Society for Gynecologic Investigation. San Diego, March 1979, Abstract No. 285.

Benedetti, T. J., Hargrove, J., and Rosene, K. A.: Maternal pulmonary edema during premature labor inhibition. Obstet. Gynecol. 59(Suppl.):33, 1982.

Bieniarz, J.: Cardiovascular effects of beta-adrenergic agonists. In Anderson, A. B. M., et al. (eds.): Proceedings of the Fifth Study Group of the Royal College of Obstetricians and Gynaecologists. London, Royal College of Obstetricians and Gynaecologists, 1977.

Bishop, E. H., and Woutersz, T. B.: Arrest of premature labor. JAMA 178:116, 1961.

Blouin, D., Murray, M. A. F., and Beard, R. W.: The effect of oral ritodrine on maternal and fetal carbohydrate metabolism. Br. J. Obstet. Gynaecol. 83:711, 1976.

Brazy, J. F., and Pupkin, M. G.: Effects of maternal isoxsuprine administration on preterm infants. J. Pediatr. 94:444, 1979.

Brettes, J. P., Renaud, R., and Gandar, R.: A double-blind investigation into the effects of ritodrine on uterine blood flow during the third trimester of pregnancy. Am. J. Obstet. Gynecol. 124:164, 1976.

Castren, O., Gummerus, M., Saarikoski, S.: Treatment of imminent premature labour: a comparison between the effects of nylidrin chloride and isoxsuprine chloride as well as ethanol. Acta Obstet. Gynecol. Scand. 54:95, 1975.

Chase, H. C.: Time trends in low birth weight in the United States, 1950–1974. In Reed, D. M., et al. (eds.): The Epidemiology of Prematurity. Baltimore, Urban and Schwarzenberg, 1977, pp. 17–34.

Collins, E., and Turner, G.: Salicylates and pregnancy. Lancet 2:1494, 1973.

Cook, L. N., Shott, R. J., and Andrews, B. F.: Acute transplacental ethanol intoxication. Am. J. Dis. Child. 129:1075, 1975.

Craig, C. J. T.: Congenital abnormalities of the uterus and foetal wastage. S. Afr. Med. J. 49:2013, 1975.

Dancis, J.: Task force of predictors of fetal maturity. Washington, D.C., United States Department of Health, Education, and Welfare, Public Health Service, National Institutes of Health, 1979.

Fedrick, J., and Anderson, A. B. M.: Factors associated with spontaneous preterm birth. Br. J. Obstet. Gynaecol. 83:342, 1976.

Fitzhardinge, P. M.: Early growth and development in low birth weight infants following treatment in an intensive care nursery. Pediatrics 56:162, 1975.

Forssman, L.: Posttraumatic intrauterine synechiae and pregnancy. Obstet. Gynecol. 26:710, 1965.

Freysz, H., Willard, D., Berland, H., et al.: Effets lointains de la thérapeutique sur le foetus: répercussions sur le métabolisme hydrocarbone et les fonctions hépatiques du nouveau-né d'un traitement beta-mimique (ritodrine ou PrePar) administré au cours de la gestation. J. Gynecol. Biol. Repr. 2:987, 1973.

Freysz, H., Willard, D., Lehr, A., et al.: A long term evaluation of infants who received a beta-mimetic drug while in utero. J. Perinat. Med. 5:94, 1977.

Fuchs, A. R.: Oxytocin and the onset of labour in rabbits. J. Endocrinol. 30:217, 1964.

Fuchs, A. R.: The inhibitory effect of ethanol on the release of oxytocin during parturition in the rabbit. J. Endocrinol. 35:125, 1966.

Fuchs, A. R., and Wagner, G.: Effect of alcohol on release of oxytocin. Nature 198:92, 1963.

Fuchs, F., Fuchs, A. R., Poblete, V. F., et al.: Effect of alcohol on threatened premature labor. Am. J. Obstet. Gynecol. 99:627, 1967.

Gandar, R., de Zoeten, L. W., and van der Schoot, J. B.: Serum level of ritodrine in man. Eur. J. Clin. Pharmacol. 17:117, 1980.

Garn, S. M., Shaw, H. A., and McCabe, K. D.: Effects of socioeconomic status and race on weight-defined and gestational prematurity in the United States. In Reed, D. M., et al. (eds.): The Epidemiology of Prematurity. Baltimore, Urban and Schwarzenberg, 1977, pp. 127–140.

Gibbs, C. E.: Diagnosis and treatment of uterine conditions that may cause prematurity. Clin. Obstet. Gynecol. 16:159, 1973.

Goodlin, R. C.: Orgasm and premature labor. Lancet 2:646, 1969.

Graff, G.: Failure to prevent premature labor with ethanol. Am. J. Obstet. Gynecol. 110:878, 1971.

Greenhouse, B. S., Hook, R., and Hehre, F. W.: Aspiration pneumonia following intravenous administration of alcohol during labor. JAMA 210:2393, 1969.

Gulbis, E., Marion, A. M., Dumont, J. E., et al.: Prostaglandin formation in bacteria. Prostaglandins 18:397, 1979.

Hack, M., Fanaroff, A. A., Klaus, M. H., et al.: Neonatal respiratory distress following elective delivery: a preventable disease? Am. J. Obstet. Gynecol. 126:43, 1976.

Hanson, J. W., Streissguth, A. P., and Smith, D. W.: The effects of moderate alcohol consumption during pregnancy on fetal growth and morphogenesis. J. Pediatr. 92:457, 1978.

Hardy, J. B., and Mellits, E. D.: Relationship of low birth weight to maternal characteristics of age, parity, education and body size. In Reed, D. M., et al. (eds.): The Epidemiology of Prematurity. Baltimore, Urban and Schwarzenberg, 1977, pp. 105–117.

Hendricks, C. H.: The use of isoxsuprine for the arrest of premature labor. Clin. Obstet. Gynecol. 7:687, 1964.

Huszar, G., and Roberts, J. M.: Biochemistry and pharmacology of the myometrium and labor: regulation at the cellular and molecular levels. Am. J. Obstet. Gynecol. 142:225, 1982.

Idänpään-Heikkilä, J., Jouppila, P., Akerblom, H. K., et al.: Elimination and metabolic effects of ethanol in mother, fetus and newborn infant. Am. J. Obstet. Gynecol. 112:387, 1972.

Johnstone, R. E., II, Kreindler, T., and Johnstone, R. E.: Hyperparathyroidism during pregnancy. Obstet. Gynecol. 40:580, 1972.

Katz, M., Newman, R. B., and Gill, P. J.: Assessment of uterine activity in ambulatory patients at high risk of preterm labor and delivery. Paper presented at Annual Meeting of Society of Perinatal Obstetricians, Las Vegas, Nevada, February, 1985.

Keirse, M. J. N. C., Rush, R. W., Anderson, A. B. M., et al.: Risk of preterm delivery in patients with previous preterm delivery and/or abortion. Br. J. Obstet. Gynaecol. 85:81, 1978.

Kleinhout, J., Stolte, L. A. M., and Veth, A. F. L.: Passeert ritodrine de placenta? Med. T. Geneesk. 118:1248, 1974.

Kords, H.: Pharmacology and pharmacokinetics of Partusisten (fenoterol). In Weidinger, H. (ed.): Labour Inhibition Betamimetic Drugs in Obstetrics. New York, Gustav Fischer Verlag, 1977, pp. 41–46.

Lands, A. M., Arnold, A., McAuliff, J. P., et al.: Differentiation of receptor systems activated by sympathomimetic amines. Nature 214:597, 1967.

Lauersen, N. H., Merkatz, I. R., Tejani, N., et al.: Inhibition of premature labor: a multicenter comparison of ritodrine and ethanol. Am. J. Obstet. Gynecol. 127:837, 1977.

Lewis, R. B., and Schulman, J. D.: Influence of acetylsalicylic acid, an inhibitor of prostaglandin synthesis, on the duration of human gestation and labour. Lancet 2:1159, 1973.

Lippert, T. H., De Grandi, P. B., and Fridrich, R.: Actions of the uterine relaxant fenoterol on uteroplacental hemodynamics in human subjects. Am. J. Obstet. Gynecol. 125:1093, 1976.

Lipshitz, J.: Cerclage in the treatment of incompetent cervix. S. Afr. Med. J. 49:2013, 1975.

Lipshitz, J.: Initiation of labor. In Givens, J. R. (ed.): Endocrinology of Pregnancy. Chicago & London, Year Book Medical Publishers, Inc., 1980, pp. 133–151.

Lipshitz, J.: Preventing premature delivery. S. Afr. Med. J. 52:1110, 1977.

Lipshitz, J.: The uterine and cardiovascular effects of oral fenoterol hydrobromide. Br. J. Obstet. Gynaecol. 84:737, 1977.

Lipshitz, J., Ahokas, R. A., and Broyles, K.: Effect of hexoprenaline on utero-placental blood flow. Proceedings of the Second Annual Scientific Meeting of the Society of Perinatal Obstetricians. San Antonio, TX, 1982.

Lipshitz, J., Anderson, G. D., and Whybrew, W. D.: Accelerated pulmonary maturity as measured by the Lumadex-foam stability index test. Obstet. Gynecol. 62:31, 1983.

Lipshitz, J., and Baillie, P.: The uterine and cardiovascular effects of beta$_2$-selective sympathomimetic drugs administered as an intravenous infusion. S. Afr. Med. J. 50:1973, 1976a.

Lipshitz, J., and Baillie, P.: The effects of fenoterol hydrobromide (Partusisten) aerosol on uterine activity and the cardiovascular system. Br. J. Obstet. Gynaecol. 83:864, 1976b.

Lipshitz, J., Baillie, P., and Davey, D. A.: A comparison of the uterine beta$_2$-adrenoreceptor selectivity of fenoterol, hexoprenaline, ritodrine and salbutamol. S. Afr. Med. J. 50:1969, 1976.

Lipshitz, J., Broyles, K., and Whybrew, W. D.: Placental transfer of 14C-hexoprenaline. Am. J. Obstet. Gynecol. 142:313, 1982.

Lipshitz, J., Depp, R., Hauth, J., et al.: Comparison of the cardiovascular effects of hexoprenaline and ritodrine in the treatment of preterm labor. Proceedings of the Third Annual Scientific Meeting of the Society of Perinatal Obstetricians. San Antonio, TX, 1983.

Lipshitz, J., and Lipshitz, E. M.: Uterine and cardiovascular effects of fenoterol and hexoprenaline in prostaglandin F$_{2\alpha}$ induced-labor in the human. Obstet. Gynecol. 63:396, 1984.

Lipshitz, J., and Vinik, A. I.: The effects of hexoprenaline, a β$_2$-sympathomimetic drug, on maternal glucose, insulin, glucagon and free fatty acid levels. Am. J. Obstet. Gynecol. 130:761, 1978.

Lipshitz, J., Whybrew, W. M. S., and Anderson, G. D.: Comparison of the Lumadex-foam stability index test, lecithin:sphingomyelin ratio, and simple shake test for fetal lung maturity. Obstet. Gynecol. 63:349, 1984.

Lipsitz, P. J.: The clinical and biochemical effects of excess magnesium in the newborn. Pediatrics 47:501, 1971.

Maisels, M. J., Rees, R., Marks, K., et al.: Elective delivery of the term fetus: an obstetrical hazard. JAMA 238:2036, 1977.

Mann, L. I., Bhakthavathsalan, A., Liu, M., et al.: Effect of alcohol on fetal cerebral function and metabolism. Am. J. Obstet. Gynecol. 122:845, 1975.

Mann, L. I., Bhakthavathsalan, A., Liu, M., et al.: Placental transport of alcohol and its effect on maternal and fetal acid-base balance. Am. J. Obstet. Gynecol. 122:837, 1975b.

McCubbin, J. H., Sibai, G. M., Abdella, T. M., et al.: Cardiopulmonary arrest due to acute maternal hypermagnesaemia [letter]. Lancet 1:1058, 1981.

Meissner, J., and Klostermann, H.: Distribution and diaplacental passage of infused ³H-fenoterol hydrobromide (Partusisten) in the gravid rabbit. Int. J. Clin. Pharmacol. Biopharm. 13:27, 1976.

Mestman, J. H., Manning, P. R., and Hodgman, J.: Hyperthyroidism and pregnancy. Arch. Intern. Med. 134:434, 1974.

Meyer, M. B.: Effects of maternal smoking and altitude on birth weight and gestation. In Reed, D. M., and Stanley, F. J. (eds.): The Epidemiology of Prematurity. Baltimore, Urban and Schwarzenberg, 1977, pp. 81–101.

Milewich, L., Gant, N. F., Schwarz, B. E., et al.: Initiation of human parturition. VIII. Metabolism of progesterone by fetal membranes of early and late human gestation. Obstet. Gynecol. 50:45, 1977.

Miller, F. C., Nochimson, D. J., Paul, R. H., et al.: Effects of ritodrine hydrochloride on uterine activity and the cardiovascular system in toxemic patients. Obstet. Gynecol. 47:50, 1976.

New Drug Application No. 18280, for ritodrine hydrochloride, submitted to the FDA on March 8, 1979, by Mid-West Medical Research, Inc., Columbus, Ohio, on behalf of Philips-Duphar, BV, Weesp, The Netherlands.

Nichols, M. M.: Acute alcohol withdrawal syndrome in a newborn. Am. J. Dis. Child. 113:714, 1967.

Niebyl, J. R., Blake, D. A., White, R. D., et al.: The inhibition of premature labor with indomethacin. Am. J. Obstet. Gynecol. 136:1014, 1980.

Niswander, K. R.: Obstetric factors related to prematurity. In Reed, D. M., and Stanley, F. J. (eds.): The Epidemiology of Prematurity. Baltimore, Urban and Schwarzenberg, 1977, pp. 249–264.

Ott, A., Hayes, J., and Polin, J.: Severe lactic acidosis associated with intravenous alcohol for premature labor. Obstet. Gynecol. 48:362, 1976.

Petrie, R. H., Wu, R., Miller, F. C., et al.: The effects of drugs on uterine activity. Obstet. Gynecol. 48:431, 1976.

Pomerance, J. J., Ukrainski, C. T., Ukra, T., et al.: The cost of living for infants weighing 1,000 grams or less at birth. Pediatrics 61:908, 1978.

Riffel, H. D., Nochimson, D. J., Paul, R. H., et al.: Effects of meperidine and promethazine during labor. Obstet. Gynecol. 42:738, 1973.

Roos, R. J., Malan, A. F., Woods, D. L., et al.: The bacteriological environment of preterm infants. S. Afr. Med. J. 57:347, 1980.

Rosen, K. A., Featherstone, H. J., and Benedetti, T. J.: Cerebral ischemia associated with parenteral terbutaline use in pregnant migraine patients. Am. J. Obstet. Gynecol. 143:405, 1982.

Rumack, C. M., Guggenheim, M. A., Rumack, V. H., et al.: Neonatal intracranial hemorrhage and maternal use of aspirin. Obstet. Gynecol. 58:52S, 1981.

Rush, R. W., Keirse, M. J. N., Howat, P., et al.: Contribution of preterm delivery to perinatal mortality. Br. Med. J. 2:965, 1976.

Sabel, K. G., Olegard, R., and Victorin, L.: Remaining sequelae with modern perinatal care. Pediatrics 57:652, 1976.

Schwartz, S.: Prenatal care, prematurity and neonatal mortality. Am. J. Obstet. Gynecol. 83:591, 1962.

Schwarz, B. E., Milewich, L., Johnston, J. M., et al.: Initiation of human parturition. V. Progesterone binding substance in fetal membranes. Obstet. Gynecol. 48:685, 1976.

Sharpe, G. L., Larsson, K. S., and Thalme, B.: Studies on closure of the ductus arteriosus. XII. In utero effect of indomethacin and sodium salicylate in rats and rabbits. Prostaglandins 9:585, 1975.

Sharpe, G. L., Thalme, B., and Larsson, K. S.: Studies on closure of the ductus arteriosus. XI. Ductal closure in utero by a prostaglandin synthetase inhibitor. Prostaglandins 8:363, 1974.

Shaywitz, B. A.: Fetal alcohol syndrome: an ancient problem rediscovered. Drug Therapy (Hosp.), January 1978, pp. 53–60.

Smith, S. K., and Thompson, D.: The effect of intravenous salbutamol upon plasma and urinary potassium during premature labour. Br. J. Obstet. Gynaecol. 84:344, 1977.

Steer, C. M., and Petrie, R. H.: A comparison of magnesium sulfate and alcohol for the prevention of premature labor. Am. J. Obstet. Gynecol. 129:1, 1977.

Stewart, A.: Follow-up of pre-term infants. In Anderson, A. B. M., et al. (eds.): Proceedings of the Fifth Study Group of the Royal College of Obstetricians and Gynaecologists. London, Royal College of Obstetricians and Gynaecologists, 1977, pp. 372–384.

Stone, S. R., and Pritchard, J. A.: Effect of maternally administered magnesium sulfate on the neonate. Obstet. Gynecol. 35:574, 1970.

Streissguth, A. P., Herman, C. S., and Smith, D. W.: Intelligence, behavior and dysmorphogenesis in the fetal alcohol syndrome: a report on 20 patients. J. Pediatr. 92:363, 1978.

Stuart, M. J., Gross, S. J., Elrad, H., et al.: Effects of acetylsalicylic-acid ingestion on maternal and neonatal homeostasis. N. Engl. J. Med. 307:909, 1982.

Taylor, P. M., and Hall, B. L.: Parent-infant bonding: problems and opportunities in a perinatal center. Semin. Perinatol. 3:73, 1979.

Thomas, D. J. B., Dove, A. F., and Alberti, K. G. M. M.: Metabolic effects of salbutamol infusion during premature labour. Br. J. Obstet. Gynaecol. 84:497, 1977.

Turnbull, A. C.: Aetiology of pre-term labour. In Anderson, A. B. M., et al. (eds.): Proceedings of the Fifth Study Group of the Royal College of Obstetricians and Gynaecologists. London, Royal College of Obstetricians and Gynaecologists, 1977, pp. 56–78.

Wagner, N. N., Butler, J. C., and Sanders, J. P.: Prematurity and orgasmic coitus during pregnancy: data on a small sample. Fertil. Steril. 27:911, 1976.

Wagner, L., Wagner, G., and Guerrero, J.: Effect of alcohol on premature newborn infants. Am. J. Obstet. Gynecol. 108:308, 1970.

Watring, W. G., Benson, W. L., Wiebe, R. A., et al.: Intravenous alcohol—a single blind study in the prevention of premature delivery: a preliminary report. J. Reprod. Med. 16:35, 1976.

Wiqvist, N., Lundstrom, V., and Green, K.: Premature labor and indomethacin. Prostaglandins 10:515, 1975.

Wren, B. G.: Premature labor with renal infections: the action of coliform endotoxin on the pregnant rat uterus. Aust. N.Z. J. Obstet. Gynaecol. 10:211, 1970.

Zervoudakis, I. A., Krauss, A., and Fuchs, F.: Infants of mothers treated with ethanol for premature labor. Am. J. Obstet. Gynecol. 137:713, 1980.

Zlatnick, F. J., and Fuchs, F.: A controlled study of ethanol in threatened premature labor. Am. J. Obstet. Gynecol. 112:610, 1972.

Zuckerman, H., Reiss, U., and Rubinstein, I.: Inhibition of human premature labor by indomethacin. Obstet. Gynecol. 44:787, 1974.

18

PROLONGED PREGNANCY

WINSTON A. CAMPBELL
DAVID J. NOCHIMSON
ANTHONY M. VINTZILEOS

Definition

The gestational period for a developing embryo varies depending on the species. In humans, the duration of gestation (EDC = expected date of confinement) is usually calculated from the first day of the last menstrual period (LMP). The average EDC is 280 ± 14 days (40 ± 2 weeks); an alternative definition is based on the day of ovulation and is 266 ± 14 days (38 ± 2 weeks). A pregnancy is considered prolonged when it has exceeded 294 days from the LMP (42 weeks) or 280 days from the time of ovulation. The majority of pregnant patients (80 percent) will deliver within ±2 weeks of their EDC. Eight percent of pregnancies will deliver preterm (before 36 weeks), and the remaining 12 percent will continue the pregnancy to or beyond 42 weeks. Beyond 42 weeks, there are fewer patients who remain pregnant: Approximately 7 percent continue beyond 42 weeks and only 5 percent beyond 43 weeks.

An obvious weakness in the above definition is that it is based upon the clinical LMP. This is a variable parameter and assumes that each patient has a 28-day menstrual cycle and that ovulation occurs on day 14 of the cycle. Those patients who have longer or shorter menstrual cycles, as well as patients who have irregular menses or who have vague recall of their LMP, can account for a significant number of pregnancies that are incorrectly classified as a prolonged pregnancy (postdates). It has been estimated that approximately 15 to 30 percent of incorrect EDCs are based on some of these factors. A more precise method to determine the duration of gestation would be to use the time of conception, as reflected by the day of ovulation. This information can be obtained from basal body temperature charts; however, since a majority of pregnancies are not so well planned, the obstetrician usually does not have this information available. The usefulness of this technique when such charts are used was indicated in a study of pregnancies in which temperature charts had been kept as an aid to conception; a report on this study showed that pregnancies classified as prolonged by usual clinical means were erroneously classified 70 percent of the time (Boyce et al., 1976).

Significance and Risks

The above discussion suggests that in many cases the classification of a pregnancy as "prolonged" is the result of errors in dating. In such cases, provided there are no other medical or obstetric complications, there should be no increased risk to the fetus. The risk arises when the pregnancy is not only prolonged but there is placental dysfunction as well. Placental dysfunction (placental insufficiency) places the fetus at risk of developing dysmaturity (postmaturity). In fact, prolonged pregnancies not associated with placental insufficiency have a normal outcome in 70 to 80 percent of the cases. The postmaturity syndrome reflects the detrimental effects on the fetus of diminished placental function. Clifford and Vorherr have written extensively about placental dysfunction and the postmaturity

325

syndrome; the reader can refer to these articles for more detail (Clifford, 1954 and 1957; Vorherr, 1975).

Extensive study of placental development and physiology indicates that placental development is complete by the 5th month of gestation. From this point on there are minor modifications to ensure adequate nutritional and oxygen supply to the growing fetus. It appears that peak placental function is achieved at approximately 36 weeks of gestation, after which diminishing function is a normal process. Although the peak function is reached at 36 weeks, there is still fetal and placental growth, but at a slower rate. As depicted in Figure 18–1, an actual plateau of fetal growth and then decrease would not be seen until after 42 weeks of gestation. However, the presence of predisposing factors that can alter placental function may cause abnormalities in fetal growth to appear at an earlier time (Fig. 18–2). This is an important concept, since the postmaturity syndrome has been seen to occur prior to 42 weeks (Fig. 18–3). The difference is in the number of cases that occur. The overall incidence of postmaturity syndrome is estimated at 2 to 6 percent; with an incidence of 3 percent at term compared with 20 to 40 percent when the pregnancy is prolonged. The risk to the fetus is increased perinatal mortality (Fig. 18–4) and morbidity, with rates varying with different reports. At term, the average perinatal mortality rate (PMR)*

---

*PMR (perinatal mortality rate) =
$$\frac{No.\ of\ Stillbirths + No.\ Neonatal\ Deaths}{1000\ Births}$$

is from 1 to 2 percent, versus 5 to 7 percent in cases of prolonged pregnancy. The PMR also varies with maternal age, parity, and sex of the fetus (Vorherr, 1975). The PMR is higher with increasing maternal age, in primigravidas (Fig. 18–4), and in male infants. Compared with term pregnancies there is about a two- to fivefold increase in PMR at 43 weeks, and at 44 weeks a three to sevenfold increase.

As discussed above, placental dysfunction is the factor that complicates a prolonged pregnancy and increases the risk to the fetus. Placental dysfunction occurs in approximately 5 to 12 percent of all pregnancies, and placental pathology is observed in 20 to 40 percent of all perinatal fetal deaths. Depending on the cause of placental insufficiency and the rate at which it develops, one may see a different effect on the infant. If placental dysfunction initially involves a small part of the placenta and then gradually progresses to further placental involvement, chronic placental insufficiency can occur. This can cause nutritional deficiency, as reflected by underweight infants. This form of insufficiency can also cause chronic hypoxia, which can be a significant risk. Chronic hypoxia has been found in some studies to be the cause of 60 to 70 percent of antepartum fetal deaths (Manning et al., 1982). In cases of acute placental dysfunction (e.g., due to abruptio placentae or cord complications), the effect on the fetus is reflected as poor fetal oxygenation manifested as either hypoxia (decreased oxygen concentration) or asphyxia (decreased oxygen and increased carbon dioxide concentra-

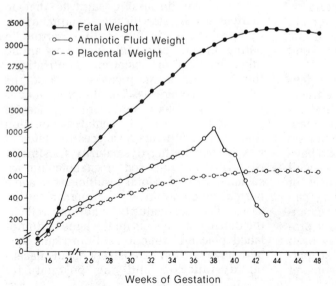

Figure 18–1. Average weights of fetus, placenta, and amniotic fluid throughout human gestation. (From Vorherr, H.: Placental insufficiency in relation to postterm pregnancy and fetal postmaturity. Am. J. Obstet. Gynecol. 123:67, 1975.)

Weeks of Gestation

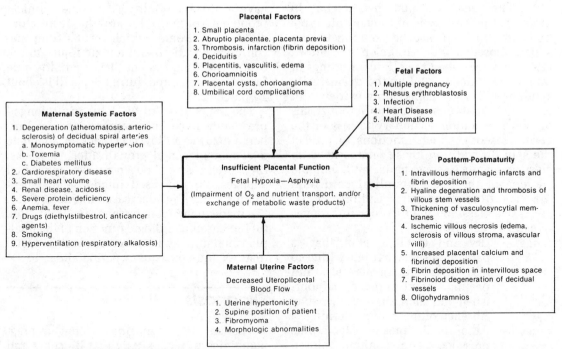

Placental Factors

1. Small placenta
2. Abruptio placentae, placenta previa
3. Thrombosis, infarction (fibrin deposition)
4. Deciduitis
5. Placentitis, vasculitis, edema
6. Chorioamnioitis
7. Placental cysts, chorioangioma
8. Umbilical cord complications

Fetal Factors

1. Multiple pregnancy
2. Rhesus erythroblastosis
3. Infection
4. Heart Disease
5. Malformations

Maternal Systemic Factors

1. Degeneration (atheromatosis, arterio-
   sclerosis) of decidual spiral arteries
   a. Monosymptomatic hypertension
   b. Toxemia
   c. Diabetes mellitus
2. Cardiorespiratory disease
3. Small heart volume
4. Renal disease, acidosis
5. Severe protein deficiency
6. Anemia, fever
7. Drugs (diethylstilbestrol, anticancer
   agents)
8. Smoking
9. Hyperventilation (respiratory alkalosis)

Insufficient Placental Function

Fetal Hypoxia—Asphyxia

(Impairment of O_2 and nutrient transport, and/or
exchange of metabolic waste products)

Postterm-Postmaturity

1. Intravillous hemorrhagic infarcts and
   fibrin deposition
2. Hyaline degeneration and thrombosis of
   villous stem vessels
3. Thickening of vasculosyncytial membranes
4. Ischemic villous necrosis (edema,
   sclerosis of villous stroma, avascular
   villi)
5. Increased placental calcium and
   fibrinoid deposition
6. Fibrin deposition in intervillous space
7. Fibrinoiod degeneration of decidual
   vessels
8. Oligohydramnios

Maternal Uterine Factors

Decreased Uteroplicental
Blood Flow

1. Uterine hypertonicity
2. Supine position of patient
3. Fibromyoma
4. Morphologic abnormalities

Figure 18–2. Abnormal maternal, placental, or fetal conditions. (From Vorherr, H.: Placental insufficiency in relation to postterm pregnancy and fetal postmaturity. Am. J. Obstet. Gynecol. 123:67, 1975.)

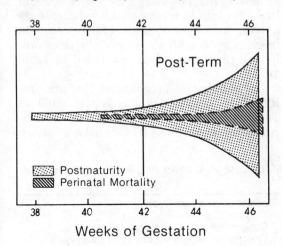

Figure 18–3. Relative incidence of fetal postmaturity syndrome and perinatal mortality. (From Vorherr, H.: Placental insufficiency in relation to postterm pregnancy and fetal postmaturity. Am. J. Obstet. Gynecol. 123:67, 1975.)

Figure 18–4. Preterm, term, and postterm perinatal fetal mortalities in primigravidas and multiparas. (From Vorherr, H.: Placental insufficiency in relation to postterm pregnancy and fetal postmaturity. Am. J. Obstet. Gynecol. 123:67, 1975.)

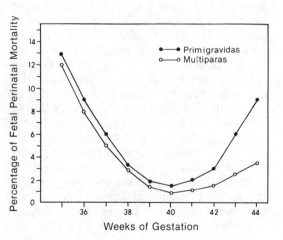

tion). The usual placental insufficiency in prolonged pregnancy is of the chronic type; however, this can also be complicated by superimposed acute insufficiency. Clifford (1954) has described the clinical findings of infants who are affected by the dysmaturity syndrome. These infants show evidence of growth retardation and have different stages of skin maceration secondary to loss of the vernix caseosa, which functions to protect the skin. In addition, these infants have an alert appearance, long nails, and variable staining of the body, umbilical cord, and placenta from meconium. Clifford (1954, 1957) has classified the disorder into stages of severity as follows:

Stage I— Dry and cracking skin that is parchment-like, wrinkled (due to loss of subcutaneous fat), and peeling. Infant appears malnourished but alert or apprehensive. Absence of meconium staining.

Stage II— All of the findings of Stage I, plus presence of meconium colored amniotic fluid and meconium covering the skin. Also green meconium staining of the placental membranes and the umbilical cord.

Stage III—All of the findings of Stages I and II, in addition to which there is bright yellow staining of nails and skin and a yellow-green staining of umbilical cord, membranes, and placenta.

It is felt that the severity of placental dysfunction in Stage II is such that sufficient fetal anoxia exists to cause the passage of meconium. Meconium is a normal product of fetal gastrointestinal function. Its passage in utero is felt to occur when oxygen delivery to the smooth muscle of the gastrointestinal tract is inadequate. This results in relaxation of the anal sphincter and meconium passage. The finding of meconium in Stage II is significant; it represents a severe level of anoxia. According to Clifford (1957), infants in this stage have the highest morbidity and mortality. The overall mortality for infants with dysmaturity syndrome is 36 percent; of those delivered during Stage II, however, two thirds have significant clinical problems and respiratory complications from meconium aspiration, and about 50 percent die. A smaller number may develop intracranial bleeding. Those infants who have survived Stage II and reach Stage III have a lower mortality. The major clinical problems in Stage III are the respiratory distress syndrome, which results from meconium aspiration, and anoxic injury to the central nervous system. The mortality rate for infants delivered during Stage III is about 15 percent.

The major risks to the fetus in prolonged pregnancy have been summarized by Vorherr (1975) as follows: (1) lack of adequate fetal and placental growth after 41 weeks, (2) progressive degenerative placental changes, (3) increased incidence of meconium staining, (4) decreased amniotic fluid, (5) inadequate fetal oxygen and nutrition, (6) increased pathologic function of the fetal-placental unit, and (7) increased rates of fetal distress and consequent perinatal deaths.

Diagnosis

The key to diagnosing prolonged pregnancy lies in recognizing that it occurs and knowing its associated sequelae. With this in mind, the obstetric care providers can look for clues to indicate which patients are at risk. A number of clinical factors seem to be associated with an increased risk of prolonged pregnancy; these are listed in Table 18–1.

The number of pregnancies that are prolonged as a result of the factors cited in Table 18–1 varies with different reports. Also, not all of these factors have a known

Table 18–1. Contributing Factors in Prolonged Pregnancy

Disorder of Menstrual Cycle
  Irregular menses
  Conception during lactation
  Conception with use of oral contraceptives
  Delayed ovulation

Social*
  Parity and age
  Multigravidas—21 to 30 years old.
  Primigravidas—21 to 30 years old.

Race
  Whites more frequently than blacks

Obstetric
  Late registration for prenatal care
  Inadequate prenatal care
  Previous prolonged pregnancy
  First-trimester bleeding
  Sex of fetus (more common with males than with females)
  Congenital anomalies

*See text for details.

associated risk for the pregnancy to be prolonged. Disorders of the menstrual cycle, for example, often result in a pregnancy being diagnosed as prolonged because of difficulty with correct gestational dating. In all likelihood the majority of these cases are term, or even preterm, pregnancies and will probably not be associated with placental insufficiency if there are no complicating medical or obstetric problems.

Although the overall incidence of prolonged pregnancy in multigravidas and primigravidas is essentially the same for the entire reproductive age group (about 20 percent), it varies among specific age groups. There is a tendency for multigravidas to have a lower incidence of prolonged pregnancy. The age groups with the highest incidence for both multigravidas and primigravidas is 21 to 25 years old and 26 to 30 years old. For multigravidas the incidence is 31 percent and 30 percent for the respective age groups. For primigravidas it is 44 percent and 18 percent respectively. Over the age of 30 there is a reversal in the incidence for multigravidas versus primigravidas; by age 35 or more, the incidence for multigravidas is 15 percent versus 4 percent for primigravidas (Vorherr, 1975).

Some of the obstetric factors (late registration or inadequate prenatal care), like disorders of the menstrual cycle, can be a source of gestational dating error. However, it is more likely in these instances that the dating error would lead to a diagnosis of prolonged pregnancy, depending on which parameters are used for dating. A previous history of a prolonged pregnancy carries a 50 percent chance for a repeat occurrence. Some studies have indicated that women pregnant with a male fetus have a higher risk of a prolonged pregnancy than if the fetus were female—8.5 percent versus 4 percent (Vorherr, 1975). This increased incidence with a male fetus is not appreciably changed with parity. Various congenital anomalies (especially anencephaly) have been associated with prolonged pregnancy (about 9 percent of cases).

The foregoing discussion provides guidelines to identify pregnancies at risk, with some being more helpful than others. However, these guidelines do not provide the criteria to make a definitive diagnosis of prolonged pregnancy. The correct diagnosis for true prolonged pregnancy is based on having an accurate gestational age and knowing that the pregnancy has gone beyond 42 weeks from the last menstrual period. There are clinical milestones and diagnostic tests that can help to establish clinical dates. The simplest method is early prenatal care. If a patient seeks prenatal care within 2 weeks after her first missed menses and has a positive urine pregnancy test, this is indicative of a pregnancy of 6 weeks' duration. Alternatively, dating conception by means of a basal body temperature chart with serum testing for hCG* confirmation is also highly accurate. Another clinical milestone is quickening (maternal perception of the first episode of fetal movement), but this is known to vary with maternal parity and placental location. In general, quickening occurs between 18 and 20 weeks of gestation; however, it may occur earlier, and this may be related to placental location. When the placenta is located on the anterior uterine wall, quickening occurs at a mean gestational age of 19 weeks in primigravidas and 17.5 weeks in multiparas. When the placenta is located on the posterior uterine wall, quickening occurs at a mean gestational age of 18 weeks in primigravidas and 16.1 weeks in multiparas (Gillieson et al., 1984). The general guideline for determining the EDC based on quickening is to add 22 weeks for primiparas, and 24 weeks for multiparas, to the date of quickening. The auscultation of fetal heart tones using an unamplified stethoscope occurs at 20 weeks; this tends to correlate with the size of the uterus being enlarged to the level of the umbilicus. Beyond 20 weeks the height of the fundus in centimeters above the symphysis pubis is roughly correlated to gestational age. This commonly accepted measurement is termed McDonald's rule, and is in fact a modification of the rule. In actuality, McDonald's rule states that the height of the fundus in centimeters should be multiplied by a factor of 8/7 to give the gestational age in weeks.†

It must be noted that the milestones discussed above, while useful, are not very accurate. In order to be 90 percent sure of a pregnancy being 38 weeks or more, one needs to be sure that there have been 42 weeks of amenorrhea, unamplified fetal

---

*hCG = human chorionic gonadotropin, a protein hormone produced by the placenta.

†However, the modified method is clinically accepted and used.

heart tones for 21 weeks, and quickening for 25 weeks (Hertz et al., 1978). A more accurate method for confirming or establishing gestational age is diagnostic ultrasound. Many studies have confirmed that the accuracy of ultrasound for dating is most precise in the early part of pregnancy. In the first trimester, crown-rump lengths (in millimeters) are within ±4 days of the EDC; from 16 weeks to 26 weeks, measurement of the fetal biparietal diameter (in centimeters) and fetal femur length (in millimeters) is accurate to within ±1 week of the EDC. After this time the accuracy of ultrasound measurements decreases and predicts the EDC to within only ±2 to 3 weeks. This must be taken into consideration when a patient registers late for prenatal care and an ultrasound exam is obtained to determine gestational age; or when the initial ultrasound exam is obtained late in pregnancy for patients who started early prenatal care.

Management

At this time it is important to state that any pregnancy with a specific complication that in itself carries an increased risk for the fetus (e.g., insulin-dependent diabetes, Rh or other isoimmunization, preeclampsia, chronic hypertension) should not be allowed to progress beyond 40 weeks.

The management schema for prolonged pregnancy can be constructed for two groups of patients: those with a *favorable* cervix for induction, and those with an *unfavorable* cervix. Because of the increased morbidity and mortality that accompany placental insufficiency, induction (if the cervix is favorable) is the best choice. Even when placental function may still be normal, it is safer to deliver rather than to incur the increased risk if placental dysfunction should develop. An important point to consider is that this approach pertains to the *well-established* diagnosis of prolonged pregnancy. If the gestational age is questionably prolonged[*] (> 42 weeks) but the cervix is inducible, pulmonary maturity must be established by amniocentesis prior to initiating induction of labor.

Those patients who do not have a favorable cervix should be entered into a fetal surveillance testing protocol. These protocols will vary depending on the institution. There are a number of clinical parameters that can be evaluated on a weekly basis (Table 18–2) to ensure normal fetal status.

[*]A pregnancy is questionably prolonged when the EDC was calculated by uncertain clinical milestones or by an initial 3rd trimester (≥28 weeks) ultrasound.

Table 18–2. Antepartum Fetal Surveillance in Prolonged Pregnancy

Clinical Finding/Test	Result		
	Normal	*Suspicious*	*Abnormal*
Uterine measurement	Increasing	No change	Decreasing
Maternal weight	Increasing	Decreasing	—
Maternal perception of fetal activity	Unchanged	Decreasing	Cessation
Serum estriol[1] (twice weekly)	Increasing or plateauing	—	Decreasing by 50%
Biophysical profile[2]	≥8	5–7	≤4
Nonstress test (AFHRT)[3]	Reactive	Reactive with variable decelerations	Nonreactive, variable or late decelerations
Fetal movement	Normal[4]	Diminished	None
Fetal tone	Normal[4]	Diminished	Flaccid
Fetal breathing	Normal[4]	Diminished	None or gasping
Amniotic fluid volume	Normal[4]	Diminished	Oligohydramnios
Placental maturation	Grade 0–II	Grade III	—
Fetal growth by ultrasound	Continued growth	Unchanged	Growth retardation
CST	Negative	Equivocal	Positive

[1] Gauthier et al., 1981.
[2] Vintzileos et al., 1983.
[3] AFHRT = antepartum fetal heart rate testing.
[4] See Chapter 3 for normal ranges of biophysical profile.

The testing protocol should be initiated at 41 weeks' gestation.

The initial three clinical findings listed in Table 18–2 should be part of each prenatal exam and easily available to all care providers of obstetric patients. Serum estriol is a measurement of the function of the combined fetoplacental unit. Gauthier and co-workers (1981) have shown that twice-weekly serum unconjugated estriols, starting at 41 weeks' gestation, can identify the infant at risk for a poor outcome. The normal pattern of estriol levels is a progressive rise until term, with a plateau at term followed by a slow decline (12 percent per week) thereafter. Thus it is the patient with a declining estriol pattern who needs further evaluation. These authors also found that a critical level of estriol below 12 mg/ml identified a group of infants that required further evaluation.

In the postdate pregnancy, even if the initial four fetal surveillance factors in Table 18–2 are normal, there should be further evaluation by antepartum fetal heart rate testing (AFHRT) and biophysical profile evaluation (Manning et al., 1982; Vintzileos et al., 1983). AFHRT can reflect the status of fetal oxygenation, and since we are concerned with placental dysfunction and lack of adequate oxygenation, this is a reliable method of evaluation. Studies have shown that AFHRT can identify the fetus at risk and help to prevent stillbirths and neonatal deaths (Thornton et al., 1982). When this test is further coupled with ultrasonic exam to evaluate biophysical parameters of the infant, it allows even better identification of the fetus at risk (Eden et al., 1982; Manning et al., 1982; Vintzileos et al., 1983).

A recent clinical evaluation of different protocols for management of prolonged pregnancy (Eden et al., 1982) demonstrated that the best outcome was achieved when both AFHRT and ultrasonic evaluation (biophysical profile) were used (see also Chapter 3). Most protocols follow a nonreactive nonstress test (NST) by performance of a contraction stress test (CST). However this method does not offer as much information as the ultrasound exam. Ultrasound evaluation allows one to gain more information: Fetal activity (which is governed by levels of oxygenation) can be directly assessed; amniotic fluid volume can be evaluated, with diminished or absent fluid levels being associated with an increased risk of umbilical cord complications (Moya et al., 1985;

Phelan et al., 1985); and lastly, one might identify a congenital anomaly that could alter the obstetric management (Thornton et al., 1982).

Recent observations regarding the NST warrant mention at this time. Although the NST may be reactive, if there are variable decelerations present on the tracing, the test should not be considered normal (Phelan et al., 1982; Phelan and Lewis, 1981). Such findings have been associated with umbilical cord complications (e.g., cord compression associated with oligohydramnios, occult prolapse, and entanglement) in 50 to 95 percent of cases (O'Leary et al., 1980; Phelan et al., 1981). Umbilical cord compression (reflected as variable decelerations on AFHRT) has been associated with antepartum deaths to within 1 week after the test. Umbilical cord compression is not only related to prolonged gestations but is also found with term and preterm pregnancies when there is diminished amniotic fluid. Diminished amniotic fluid can be encountered when the pregnancy is complicated by intrauterine growth retardation or premature ruptured membranes (Pazos et al., 1982; Vintzileos et al., 1985). In our management protocol for the postdate pregnancy, we use the presence of variable decelerations or diminished amniotic fluid as an indication for delivery (Fig. 18–5). Leveno and coworkers (1984) have recently described the importance of oligohydramnios and cord compression as a cause of fetal distress in prolonged pregnancy.

Most protocols recommend that testing be initiated at 42 weeks. Since we are aware that some cases of placental insufficiency exist prior to this time (Fig. 18–3) and in order to obtain baseline information, we initiate our testing at 41 weeks (Fig. 18–5). Abnormalities of the biophysical profile (Fig. 18–5) or evidence of poor fetal growth are indications for delivery. Although the presence of meconium in the amniotic fluid carries an increased risk for the infant, studies show that use of amniocentesis to detect meconium has not been helpful (Green and Paul, 1978; Knox et al., 1979). In such situations, when AFHRT has been normal, intervention based on the finding of meconium did not seem to improve the outcome.

The intrapartum management of prolonged pregnancy should not differ from that for any other complicated pregnancy. Internal monitoring of the fetal heart rate (FHR) should be achieved at the earliest possible

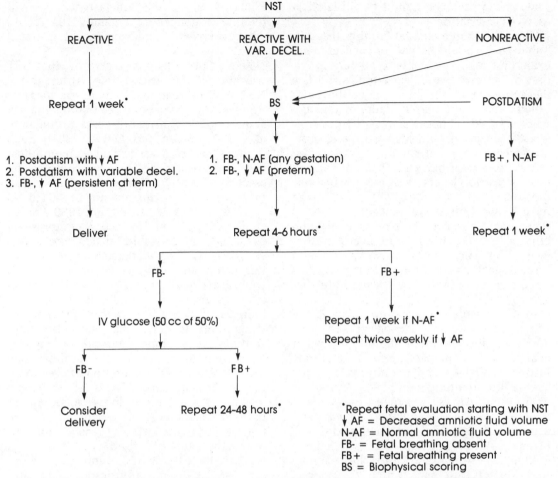

Figure 18–5. Protocol of antepartum fetal evaluation. (Redrawn from Vintzileos, A. M., Campbell, W. A., Ingardia, C. J., et al.: The fetal biophysical profile and its predictive value. Obstet. Gynecol. 62:271, 1983. Reprinted with permission from The American College of Obstetricians and Gynecologists.)

time. A normal FHR assures that the infant is not hypoxic. Since the membranes need to be ruptured for this monitoring technique, one can also evaluate the fluid for meconium. The presence of meconium should serve as a reason for closer surveillance of the FHR tracing, since there may be an increased tendency for these infants to be acidotic if thick meconium is found (Miller and Read, 1981). In cases in which a patient is undergoing oxytocin induction or there is evidence of abnormal fetal heart rate patterns, intrauterine pressures should also be monitored by a catheter. This ensures that uterine stimulation is adequate (not too excessive or insufficient) and allows better classification of the FHR patterns. Fetal scalp blood sampling to assess the fetal acid-base status is done when there are abnormal findings in the FHR tracing. This technique allows one to detect fetuses that may be acidotic and require immediate delivery, as compared with those with an abnormal FHR pattern but without acidosis. In the latter case labor may continue with vigilant monitoring. If meconium is present, the fetal oropharynx and nasopharynx should be suctioned with a DeLee suction as the head is delivered, before the delivery of the chest. Prolonged pregnancy in itself is not an indication for cesarean section; this should be performed only when there are appropriate obstetric indications for doing so (see Chapter 14).

Emotional Aspects

The mother and her family may become very anxious when pregnancy continues past the expected date of confinement. This date is looked forward to with anticipation, and when it comes and goes without a baby, everyone becomes frustrated. Comments from relatives and friends such as "Haven't you had that baby yet?" can add to the mother's frustration. The mother has expected to deliver by her due date, and she is emotionally ready for that date. Also, for mothers who are physically uncomfortable, extension of the pregnancy can seem unbearable.

Therefore, these women and their families will need emotional support and suggestions to try to make them more comfortable. These suggestions could include placing a pillow under her abdomen while resting or sleeping to decrease the pull on her ligaments; raising the head of her bed to aid in breathing and to decrease indigestion; placing a heating pad on her abdomen while she is awake to soothe sore ligaments; elevating her legs to increase circulation; and eating small, frequent meals to aid digestion. If she is physically comfortable, it will help her tolerate waiting for delivery.

The family should be given as much information as possible regarding the timing of delivery, as they will probably be anxious about the fetus's not being delivered. A full explanation of the tests to be done and the circumstances that would call for delivery will be helpful. The mother should also be educated about fetal movements; she can be instructed to count fetal movements for 1 hour, once or twice a day. If there are less than three movements in an hour, she should be instructed to come to the hospital (Rayburn, 1982).

Reassurance during this extended wait is very important to the mother and her family. This reassurance should include information that the baby is well (this can be given during testing) and that she *will* eventually deliver.

Summary

Prolonged pregnancy presents a risk to the fetus when there is associated placental insufficiency. This leads to an inadequate supply of oxygen and nutrients to the fetus and can thus affect growth and central nervous system, cardiac, and respiratory function. Placental dysfunction is a normal occurrence during placental maturation; why some infants are seriously affected and others are not is not well understood. The increased morbidity and mortality associated with this condition can be avoided by attention to history and clinical clues identifying patients with prolonged pregnancy and by using an appropriate antepartum fetal testing protocol to assess the fetus in cases of prolonged pregnancy.

REFERENCES

Boyce, A., Mayaux, M. J., and Schwartz, D.: Classical and "true" gestational postmaturity. Am. J. Obstet. Gynecol. 125:911, 1976.

Clifford, S. H.: Postmaturity—with placental dysfunction. J. Pediatr. 44:1, 1954.

Clifford, S. H.: Postmaturity. Adv. Pediatr. 9:13, 1957.

Eden, R. D., Gergely, R. Z., Schifrin, B. S., et al.: Comparison of antepartum testing schemes for the management of the postdate pregnancy. Am. J. Obstet. Gynecol. 144:683, 1982.

Gauthier, R. J., Griego, B. D., and Goebelsmann, U.: Estriol in pregnancy. VII. Unconjugated plasma estriol in prolonged gestation. Am. J. Obstet. Gynecol. 139:382, 1981.

Gillieson, M., Dunlap, H., Nair, R., et al.: Placental site, parity and date of quickening. Obstet. Gynecol. 64:44, 1984.

Green, J. N., and Paul, R. H.: The value of amniocentesis in prolonged pregnancy. Obstet. Gynecol. 51:293, 1978.

Hertz, R. H., Sokol, R. J., Knoke, J. D., et al.: Clinical estimation of gestational age: rules for avoiding preterm delivery. Am. J. Obstet. Gynecol. 131:395, 1978.

Knox, G. E., Huddleston, J. F., and Flowers, C. E.: Management of prolonged pregnancy: results of a prospective randomized trial. Am. J. Obstet. Gynecol. 134:376, 1979.

Leveno, K. J., Quirk, J. G., Cunningham, F. G., et al.: Prolonged pregnancy. I. Observations concerning the causes of fetal distress. Am. J. Obstet. Gynecol. 150:465, 1984.

Manning, F. A., Morrison, I., Lange, I. R., et al.: Antepartum determination of fetal health: composite biophysical profile scoring. Clin. Perinatol. 9:285, 1982.

Miller, F. C., and Read, J. A.: Intrapartum assessment of the postdate fetus. Am. J. Obstet. Gynecol. 141:516, 1981.

Moya, F., Grannum, P., Pinto, K., et al.: Ultrasound assessment of the postmature pregnancy. Obstet. Gynecol. 65:319, 1985.

O'Leary, J. A., Andrinopoulos, G. C., and Giordano, P. C.: Variable decelerations and the nonstress test: an indication of cord compression. Am. J. Obstet. Gynecol. 137:704, 1980.

Pazos, R., Vuolo, K., Aladjem, S., et al.: Association of spontaneous fetal heart rate decelerations during antepartum nonstress testing and intrauterine growth retardation. Am. J. Obstet. Gynecol. 144:574, 1982.

Phelan, J. P., Cromartie, A. D., and Smith, C. V.: The nonstress test: the false negative test. Am. J. Obstet. Gynecol. 142:293, 1982.

Phelan, J. P., and Lewis, P. E.: Fetal heart rate decelerations during a nonstress test. Obstet. Gynecol. 57:288, 1981.

Phelan, J. P., Platt, L. D., Sze-Ya, Y., et al.: The role of ultrasound assessment of amniotic fluid volume in the management of the postdate pregnancy. Am. J. Obstet. Gynecol. 151:304, 1985.

Rayburn, W. F.: Antepartum fetal assessment. Monitoring fetal activity. Clin. Perinatol. 9:231, 1982.

Thornton, Y. S., Yeh, S. Y., and Petrie, R. H.: Antepartum fetal heart rate testing and the post-term gestation. J. Perinat. Med. 10:196, 1982.

Vintzileos, A. M., Campbell, W. A., Ingardia, C. J., et al.: The fetal biophysical profile and its predictive value. Obstet. Gynecol. 62:271, 1983.

Vintzileos, A. M., Campbell, W. A., Nochimson, D. J., et al.: Degree of oligohydramnios and pregnancy outcome in patients with premature rupture of the membranes. Obstet. Gynecol. 66:162, 1985.

Vorherr, H.: Placental insufficiency in relation to postterm pregnancy and fetal postmaturity. Evaluation of fetoplacental function; management of the postterm gravida. Am. J. Obstet. Gynecol. 123:67, 1975.

19

TWINS AND OTHER MULTIPLE GESTATIONS

JOSE C. SCERBO
PAWAN RATTAN
JOAN E. DRUKKER

Twinning occurs often enough—in approximately 1 of every 80 pregnancies—to constitute a rather important biologic event. Although it has long been known that two different types of twins exist, so-called identical (monozygotic) and fraternal (dizygotic), it was Sir Francis Galton (Charles Darwin's first cousin) who first proposed using twins as a model for the understanding of disease and, by doing so, made twin research an active field.

Predisposing Factors

DIZYGOTIC TWINS

Dizygotic twins make up two thirds of all the twins born yearly in the United States. This type of twinning involves the independent release and subsequent fertilization of two ova. Dizygotic twins are genetically as dissimilar as any other siblings except that they are the same age and are in utero at the same time. They might have different fathers if coitus occurs with two different men within a relatively short period of time.

Familial Inheritance

Dizygotic twinning has a hereditary basis, that is, there is a familial tendency toward multiple ovulation. This phenomenon may be partly due to increased levels of pituitary gonadotropins, which predispose to double ovulations. If such traits are partly inherited (carried and transmitted by both female and male), they can express themselves only in women, because they act through the ovaries exclusively. Women who have given birth to dizygotic twins probably have a twofold increased likelihood, as compared with the general population, of having dizygotic twins in each succeeding pregnancy, although the precise nature of the inheritance remains to be established.

Race

There is a high incidence among blacks in Nigeria, where 1 of every 25 births involves twins. At the other extreme, there is a very low incidence among Asians; in Japan, for example, twinning occurs only once in 150 births.

Age and Parity

For reasons that are poorly understood, the twinning rate is correlated with maternal age: steadily rising from 20 and reaching a maximum between ages 35 and 39, after which the rate falls abruptly (Fig. 19–1). It has been postulated that this increase may be partly due to increasing levels of gonadotropins and a higher incidence of double ovulation. There is also a high correlation between increased numbers of pregnancies and multiple births (Fig. 19–2).

Drugs

The induction of ovulation with clomiphene citrate (Clomid) has been associated

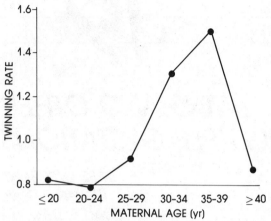

Figure 19–1. Rate of twinning in relation to maternal age, expressed as the ratio of twin births to all births per thousand for comparable ages (at MacDonald House). (From Hendricks, C. H.: Twinning in relation to birth rate, mortality and congenital anomalies. Obstet. Gynecol. 27:48, 1966. Reprinted with permission from The American College of Obstetricians and Gynecologists.)

with a high incidence of multiple gestation, mostly twins, with accumulated national statistics showing an 8 percent rate of multiple births among women who have taken this drug. Kistner (1968) reports a rate of 6 percent, and Hack and coworkers (1972) report 8.4 percent. Speroff and colleagues (1981) state that, in recent years, with a standardization of therapy and doses of about 100 mg/day or less, fewer cases of ovarian hyperstimulation syndrome have been reported, and the incidence of twins has approached that of the normal population.

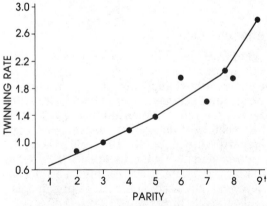

Figure 19–2. Rate of twinning at various parities, expressed as a fraction of the rate in each parity group. (From Hendricks, C. H.: Twinning in relation to birth rate, mortality and congenital anomalies. Obstet Gynecol 27:48, 1966. Reprinted with permission from The American College of Obstetricians and Gynecologists.)

Gonadotropins. Human menopausal gonadotropin, or HMG (Pergonal: one vial contains 75 IU of FSH and 75 IU of LH), in combination with human chorionic gonadotropins, or HCG (one vial contains 10,000 units of LH), is currently being used for induction of ovulation in patients with hypothalamic hypogonadotrophic hypergonadism (primary or secondary amenorrhea and anovulation), and in patients with oligomenorrhea or amenorrhea and anovulation secondary to hypothalamic pituitary dysfunction (i.e., polycystic ovarian syndrome). The effect is dose related.

The most common complication is multiple pregnancy in the range of 18 to 53 percent, owing to the fact that there is a very narrow margin between dosage pregnancy rate and ovarian hyperstimulation with multiple gestation. This incidence may be decreased by several factors, such as (a) proper selection of patients; (b) choice of suitable treatment; and (c) careful monitoring of follicular growth using serial ultrasound and daily estradiol determinations.

Oral Contraceptives. It has been speculated that after cessation of oral contraceptive therapy, pituitary gonadotropin release is increased, possibly leading to an increase in twin conception (Benirschke et al., 1973).

Miscellaneous Factors

The twinning pregnancy rate appears to be greater when a women conceives during the first 3 months after marriage.

In some areas of northern Finland there is a strong seasonal frequency for multiple gestation (peak twin conception is in July); this may be explained by the continuous exposure to light during the summer months, which might result in hypothalamic pituitary stimulation and consequent multiple ovulation.

MONOZYGOTIC TWINS

One third of all twins born in the United States are monozygotic. These twins are derived from a single fertilized ovum that duplicates at any of the preimplantation stages before the embryo has been formed. There are no valid hypotheses that explain monozygotic twinning, and this should probably be considered a teratogenic phenomenon.

The frequency is constant around the world, being roughly about 1 in 250 pregnancies, and is not influenced by race, maternal age, drugs, or any other known factors.

Placentation

MONOZYGOTIC TWINS

There are basically two types of placentas in monozygotic twins:

The first type is *monochorionic* with one single placental disc that might or might not have developed two separate amnia. Monochorionic-monoamniotic or monochorionic-diamniotic twin placentas exist only in monozygotic twins; therefore the newborn are the same sex (Fig. 19–3). The diagnosis can be made readily by examination of the placenta on twins that are born with the same sex (20 percent of all twins in the United States).

Vascular anastomoses between the two fetal circulations in monochorionic placentas are quite common and are of two types: artery-to-artery and arteriovenous. Artery-to-artery anastomoses are very rare, but when they do occur they represent an acute emergency during the delivery because of shifting of blood from one twin to the other. More common are the so-called arteriovenous shunts between the two fetal circulations, which are believed to be the basis of what is known as the *twin transfusion syndrome* (see p. 339).

About 8 percent of all monozygotic twins have *dichorionic-diamniotic* placentas with infants of the same sex, and therefore the zygosity in such a circumstance should be genotypically assessed. This type of placenta can be either fused or separated. Dichorionic-diamniotic placentation is accomplished when splitting of the inner cell mass from the blastocyst occurs before the appearance of the cells that will eventually make the chorion. This phenomenon occurs very early after fertilization, perhaps in the first 60 hours.

In the other extreme, if separation occurs very late after fertilization, conjoined twins will develop as a last possible twinning phenomenon (Fig. 19–4).

DIZYGOTIC TWINS

The number and size of the follicles can now be readily determined by serial sonographic examination of the ovaries during the proliferative phase of the menstrual cycle. Therefore, zygosity of twins can be determined at or before the time of ovulation. All dizygotic twins are derived from two different follicles containing two separate ova and fertilized by two separate spermatozoa.

All dizygotic twins have dichorionic-diamniotic placentas. They might appear as entirely separated organs, or they may be fused if implantation occurred side-by-side. If the infants are different in sex and if pathologic examination of the divided membrane shows four layers (amnion/chorion/

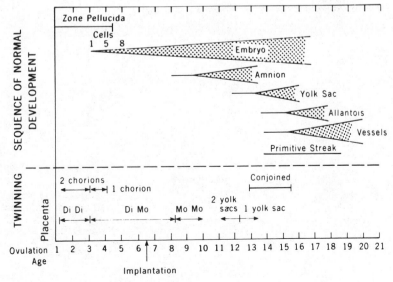

Figure 19–3. Hypothetical scheme of timing of monozygotic placental development. (From Benirschke, K., and Kim, C. K.: Multiple pregnancy. N. Engl. J. Med. 288:1276, 1973. Reprinted by permission of the New England Journal of Medicine.)

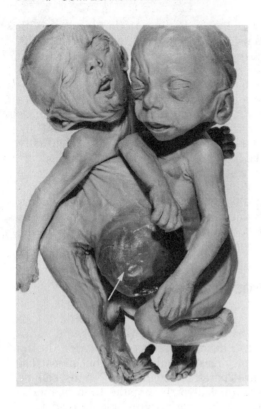

Figure 19–4. Thoraco-omphalopagus twins with omphalocele (arrow)—postmortem appearance. (From Moore, K. L.: The Developing Human: Clinically Oriented Embryology, 3rd ed. Philadelphia, W. B. Saunders Co., 1982.)

Figure 19–5. Incidence and placental development of MZ and DZ twins. (From Iffy, L., and Kaminetzky, H.: Principles and Practice of Obstetrics in Perinatology, Vol. 2. Copyright 1981, John Wiley & Sons, Inc. Reprinted by permission of John Wiley & Sons, Inc.)

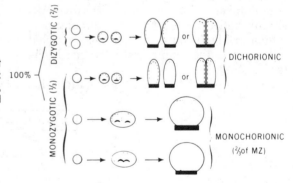

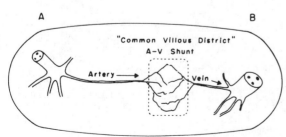

Figure 19–6. Vascular arrangement of the transfusion syndrome. (From Benirschke, K., and Kim, C. K.: N. Engl. J. Med. 288:1276, 1973. Reprinted by permission of the New England Journal of Medicine.)

chorion/amnion), the diagnosis of dizygosity is readily established. This situation accounts for about 35 percent of all the twins born in the United States (Fig. 19–5).

DETERMINATION OF ZYGOSITY

In the United States, about 80 percent of twins are dichorionic and about 20 percent are monochorionic. Pathologic examination of the placenta will detect 20 percent of the monozygotic twins that have monochorionic placentas (same sex). Another 35 percent will have dichorionic placentas, fused or separated, with newborns of different sex, and therefore will be diagnosed as dizygotic. In the remaining 45 percent of the cases, the zygosity must be genotypically established through blood grouping, enzymatic determinations, and HLA typing.

TWIN TRANSFUSION SYNDROME

There are no vascular connections in dichorionic placentas. On the other hand, monochorionic placentas may have a vascular connection between the two fetal circulations (Fig. 19–6). This can be an artery-to-artery connection or, more commonly, an arteriovenous anastomosis within the placental bed. The latter can result in the so-called twin transfusion syndrome (Fig. 19–7), which can cause discordance in twins, as outlined at top of the next column.

Twin Recipient	Twin Donor
1. Twin is usually larger; up to 1000-gram disparity	1. Twin is usually smaller
2. Polycythemia with hemoconcentration thrombosis and disseminated intravascular coagulation (DIC) in the newborn	2. Anemia that can be rather severe
3. Jaundice secondary to hemolysis, occasionally causing kernicterus	3. Hypoglycemia
4. Cardiac hypertrophy	4. Cardiac atrophy
5. Increased muscular mass	5. Decreased muscle mass
6. Polyhydramnios secondary to increased glomerular size and polyuria	6. Oligohydramnios
7. Large congested placenta	7. Small pale placenta
	8. Retarded growth and retarded mental development postnatally
Treatment	*Treatment*
Exchange transfusion with phlebotomy	Blood transfusion

Diagnosis

In cases of multiple gestation—as with any other condition in obstetrics that can cause complications or be potentially harmful to the mother and/or the fetus—early diagnosis is paramount if one wants to achieve a good outcome.

A 1965 study by Barter revealed that up to 50 percent of twin pregnancies were undiagnosed at the time of labor. Farooqui and coworkers (1973) found that the diagnosis of twins was missed before labor in 58 percent of cases, and in about 30 percent of cases the diagnosis was made only after delivery of the first twin.

HISTORY

As mentioned earlier, there is a familial tendency to multiple ovulation. Therefore, a family history of twins should alert the physician to the possibility of multiple gestation.

Women who have been treated with fertility drugs (clomiphene citrate or gonadotropins) or who become pregnant after cessation of oral contraceptive therapy should also be screened for multiple gestation.

CLINICAL EXAMINATION

If the patient is considered to have good dates, the McDonald measurements of the

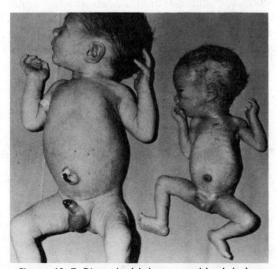

Figure 19–7. Discordant twins caused by twin transfusion syndrome. (From Lubchenco, L. O.: The High Risk Infant. Philadelphia, W. B. Saunders Co., 1976.)

abdomen may be quite helpful in diagnosing multiple gestation. The height of the uterus can be measured with a measuring tape from the symphysis pubis to the fundus. Between 22 and 34 weeks' gestation, the fundal height should equal gestational age in centimeters. Jarvis reported that in 66 out of 94 sets of twins, the initial suspicion of multiple pregnancy arose from finding a large-for-dates uterus. A discrepancy of 4 centimeters or more is highly suggestive of multiple gestation (Fig. 19–8). Palpation of multiple fetal parts through the Leopold maneuver, with the presence of more than two fetal poles, should alert the physician to the possibility of multiple gestation.

The auscultation of more than one fetal heart sound, particularly with a difference of 10 beats per minute, may be another important finding during the physical examination for twin gestation.

Anemia that may not respond to the usual treatment with iron and folic acid (multiple fetuses require extra iron and folic acid), as well as hypertension, especially in a multiparous patient, should also raise the suspicion of multiple gestation.

BIOCHEMICAL TESTS

Indirect biochemical methods are based on the fact that total placental mass and fetal mass are greater in multiple gestations than in singleton pregnancies.

Estriol, HCG, HPL, and AFP levels were measured in an attempt to establish the normal range for twin gestation. The results in the literature are conflicting. AFP, HCG, and HPL were reported in a number of studies to be higher in twin than in singleton preg-

nancies, with an accuracy rate of 80 to 95 percent (Garoff and Seppala, 1973). However, Garoff and Seppala (1973) reported levels of HPL in twin gestations to be similar to those in singleton pregnancies. Persson's group (1979) measured HPL levels in an entire population of pregnant woman in Malmö, Sweden; 16 percent had levels high enough to indicate twin pregnancy but such was not the case, suggesting that other measures, mainly ultrasound, should be used to make a definitive diagnosis.

RADIOGRAPHIC EXAMINATION

Radiography should be used as a last resort for the exceptional situation in which the sonogram was doubtful, especially if more than two fetuses are suspected to be in utero. Another unusual circumstance in which radiographic examination might be used would be for the diagnosis of presentation when the patient arrives in active labor. It must be emphasized, however, that in general, the availability of ultrasound equipment and skillful personnel operational on a 24-hour basis in the labor and delivery area should *obviate* the need to expose the fetus to unnecessary radiation.

ULTRASOUND EXAMINATION

Ultrasound is probably the single most important technologic contribution to obstetrics, equal to what CT scanning has done to radiology. Today the most important reason for increased perinatal morbidity and mortality is still prematurity, and every effort should be made to prevent this. Hawry-

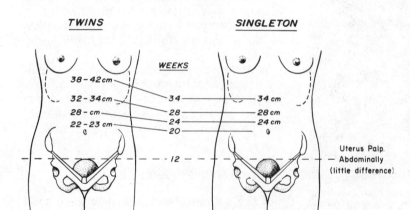

Figure 19–8. Uterine fundal height in twins versus singletons. (From Cetrulo, C. L., Ingardia, C. J., and Sbarra, A. J.: Management of multiple gestation. Clin. Obstet. Gynecol. 23:536, 1980.)

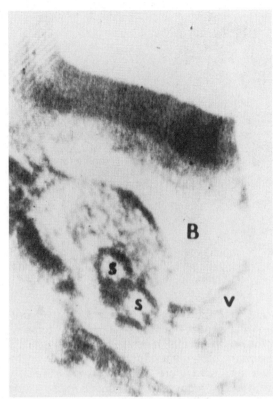

Figure 19–9. Twin pregnancy at about 7 weeks, longitudinal view. B = bladder; V = vaginal vault; S = gestational sacs. (From Sanders, R. C., and James, A. E.: Principles and Practice of Ultrasonography in Obstetrics and Gynecology. East Norwalk, CT, Appleton-Century-Crofts, 1980.)

lyshyn and coworkers (1982) found that 70 percent of the perinatal mortality in twin pregnancies occurred when delivery took place before the 30th week of gestation.

In 1973, routine screening with ultrasound of the entire pregnant population of Malmö, Sweden, was instituted (Persson et al., 1979). The purpose of the study was to improve early diagnosis and therefore prevent preterm labor and allow early diagnosis of complications such as hypertension, anemia, and intrauterine growth retardation in multiple gestation. Studied in the 17th week of gestation, 98 percent of the twins were diagnosed during the first sonographic examination, with no false-positives. In contrast, before routine ultrasound was instituted, the mean gestational age at the time the diagnosis of twin gestation was made was 35 weeks. When sonographic examination was performed routinely in 1973, the mean gestational age at the time of diagnosis was reduced to 30 weeks, and by 1977 it was down to 20 weeks. The diagnosis can be made as early as 6 to 8 weeks by identifying two separate sacs within the uterus (Fig. 19–9). Between 8 and 13 weeks, two sacs with two fetal poles with separate cardiac activity and fetal movements can be clearly identified. From 16 weeks on, different fetal parts can be readily seen, and the measurement of biparietal diameter, femoral length, and abdominal circumference should be attempted serially to assess fetal growth (Figs. 19–10 and 19–11). A strong argument can be made for routine screening with ultrasound of all pregnant patients for early diagnosis of multiple gestation, in an effort to reduce maternal and fetal complications frequently seen in association with this condition.

Figure 19–10. Two fetal bodies—anterior placenta. No dividing membranes. Monozygotic twins. (From Sanders, R. C., and James, A. E.: Principles and Practice of Ultrasonography in Obstetrics and Gynecology. East Norwalk, CT, Appleton-Century-Crofts, 1980.)

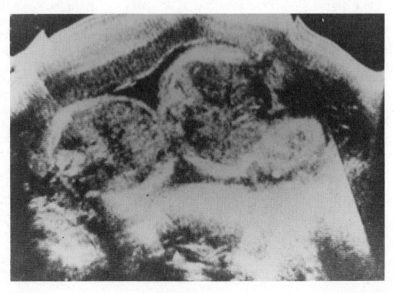

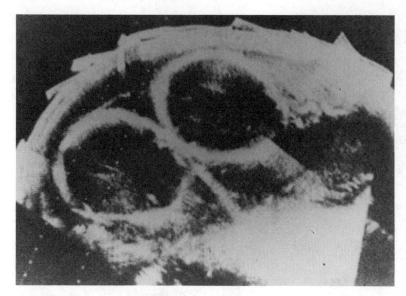

Figure 19–11. Same pregnancy as in Figure 19–10. Both fetal heads are near uterine fundus. (From Sanders, R. C., and James, A. E.: Principles and Practice of Ultrasonography in Obstetrics and Gynecology. East Norwalk, CT, Appleton-Century-Crofts, 1980.)

Antepartum Management

DIET

Increased placental as well as fetal mass in multiple gestation dictates the need for increased caloric intake as well as increased intake of proteins, minerals (iron), vitamins, and folic acid. Dietary intake should be increased to at least 2400 calories per day, which should include a protein intake of 60 grams per day.

Maternal weight gain during a multiple pregnancy frequently ranges from 30 to 40 pounds.

THE BEDREST CONTROVERSY

There are very few studies examining the management of multiple gestation, and bedrest still remains a controversial issue. Nonetheless, the majority of the reports appear to support the view that it has a beneficial effect (Table 19–1).

Powers, in 1973, argued that in England alone, over 88 years of bedrest have been expended on healthy mothers to prolong their twin pregnancies, although the efficacy of bedrest remains unproven.

O'Connor and colleagues (1979) reported on 101 twin pregnancies in which routine bedrest in the hospital was replaced by intensified antenatal care in special "twin clinics." This group of patients clearly benefited from the special care, as evidenced by the fact that there was no increase in the prematurity rate, intrauterine growth retardation, or perinatal mortality. The possibility of psychologic benefit (placebo effect) to the women who were followed very carefully and very frequently was mentioned as one of the contributing factors.

The study by Persson and his colleagues (1979) is probably the most widely quoted. Their approach was as follows: bedrest at home and discontinuance of work as soon as the diagnosis of multiple gestation was made, followed by bedrest in the hospital from 28 to 36 weeks' gestation. The results were impressive: (1) The mean duration of pregnancy was 255 days without the use of tocolytic agents. (2) There was a decreased incidence of twins born with weights below 1500 grams, although no increase in the mean gestational age was found. (3) Decreased incidence of small-for-gestational-age neonates, with all of the twins born after 35 weeks' gestation. (4) The incidence of preterm labor decreased from 33 to 20 percent ($p < 0.01$) as compared with the control group. (5) No twins were born before 33 weeks' gestation. (6) Eighty-five percent of the patients were induced at 38 weeks' gestation because, in Sweden, this has been determined to be the time in pregnancy when twins have the lowest perinatal mortality rate; the incidence of cesarean section in this group was 17 percent. (7) The perinatal mortality in the group on bedrest was 0.6 percent, equal to that of a singleton pregnancy in Sweden.

Table 19–1. Twin Perinatal Mortality and the Effectiveness of Bedrest*

Author	Place	Years	No. of Twins		PND/1000 Live Births		Labor <36 wk (%)	
			Bed	Active	Bed	Active	Bed	Active
Barter et al[4]	Washington	1954–64	25	225	80	217	35	25
Robertson[5]	Scotland	1956–62	152	237	75	206	?	?
Laursen[6]	Denmark	1958–70	79	107	32	85	13	45
Misenhimer et al[7]	Baltimore	1964–75	70	161	7	55	57	48
Jeffrey et al[8]	Denver	1968–73	41	31	61	229		
Jouppila et al[9]	Finland	1971–73	117	161	31	78		
Weekes et al[10]	England	1973–77	60	36	66	55	23	22
Persson et al[1]	Sweden	1973–77	86	24	6	105		

*PND = perinatal deaths; bed = patients treated with bedrest; active = bedrest not instituted.
From Hawrylyshyn, P. A., Barkin, M., Bernstein, A., et al.: Twin pregnancies—a continuing perinatal challenge. Obstet. Gynecol. 59:65, 1982.

In our institution the patient is placed at bedrest on the antepartum floor from 26 to 28 weeks until 32 completed weeks and then discharged home if no other complications are present.

PROGESTERONE

Johnson and coworkers (1975) reported that hydroxyprogesterone caproate administered intramuscularly at a dosage of 250 mg weekly, beginning at 16 to 20 weeks, may be efficacious in the prevention of premature labor. Although this regimen is recommended by some, we have not used this hormonal treatment in our institution.

CERVICAL CERCLAGE

The placement of a prophylactic cervical cerclage in patients with multiple gestation has been suggested. We, in agreement with Dor and colleagues (1982), think that this technique has not proved to be beneficial when it is performed only because of the presence of multiple gestation.

If the diagnosis of incompetent cervix is made on the basis of past obstetric history, or if the cervix is found to be effaced or dilated prior to 20 weeks' gestation, the suture should then be placed around the internal cervical os.

TOCOLYTIC AGENTS

O'Connor and coworkers (1979) conducted a double-blind study using 40 mg daily of ritodrine and showed that prophylactic tocolytic therapy in multiple gestation did not increase birth weight; they were also unable to show any decreased incidence of preterm labor. Cetrulo and colleagues (1980), in a randomized double-blind study at U.S.C., also showed that the use of ritodrine by mouth in a prophylactic fashion was ineffective.

In our institution, preterm labor in the presence of multiple gestation is treated according to established protocols, using either intravenous magnesium sulfate or ritodrine hydrochloride. In addition, betamethasone is currently being used to enhance pulmonary maturity between 28 and 34 weeks' gestation. If intravenous treatment with the tocolytic agent is successful, the patient is then placed on bedrest on the antepartum floor and given either terbutaline or ritodrine by mouth until 34 completed weeks. If there are no further cervical changes or added complications, she is then discharged home.

Antepartum Assessment

NONSTRESS TEST/OXYTOCIN CHALLENGE TEST

In multiple gestations we perform antepartum electronic fetal monitoring on a weekly basis starting at 32 weeks, or at 30 weeks if there is evidence of discordant twins or if any other complications, such as diabetes mellitus, hypertension, or anemia, are present. Nonstress Tests (NSTs) are used as the primary approach in antepartum fetal heart rate evaluation of twin gestation. The criteria for a reactive NST at the University of South Florida is as follows: two accelerations with an amplitude of 20 beats per minute and a duration of 15 seconds occurring within any 10-minute period. Table 19–2 demonstrates the number of patients tested under this protocol and their test results.

If after 20 minutes the fetus has not achieved a reactive test, attempts are made to arouse it by abdominal manipulation, maternal position change, or ambulation. The tracing is continued after 20 minutes. If the NST remains nonreactive at the end of 40 minutes, the NST is repeated either later in the day or the following morning, since most of the fetuses become reactive by that time, eliminating the need for an oxytocin challenge test (OCT). After two consecutive nonreactive NSTs, we proceed with an OCT. Another way to obtain uterine activity would be to stop tocolytic therapy if this had been previously instituted on the patient. A nonreactive NST does not imply immediate fetal jeopardy; rather, it should

Table 19–2. NST/CST in Twins (Spontaneous or Induced)

Total number of patients under protocol	90
Total number of NSTs	281
Range of tests per patient	1 to 12
Mean number of tests per patient	3.1
Total number of nonreactive NSTs	17
Number of patients with positive (+) or equivocal OCTs	8

be viewed as an indication for a need for further evaluation.

Some controversy still exists as to whether an OCT should be performed in cases of twin gestation, since these patients are prone to preterm labor. A report from Braly and Freeman (1977), however, failed to demonstrate an increased incidence of premature labor before 38 weeks' gestation in patients who underwent OCTs, as compared with patients who underwent NSTs prior to 38 weeks. Our data from the University of South Florida would support this. Of 14,215 deliveries between January 1, 1980, and July 1, 1982, a total of 160 sets of twins were delivered. Ninety of these were managed under the protocol. Six patients carrying twins received an OCT. The incidence of premature labor was not increased for this group.

Earlier studies by Freeman (1975) also showed no increased incidence of preterm labor in patients followed by OCTs. Another important point to consider is the fact that spontaneous uterine activity sufficient to meet the requirements of CST is often present in twin gestation, thereby reducing the number of patients who will require oxytocin. The position of the patient and monitoring techniques are similar to those used on patients with singleton pregnancies. However, in twin gestations two monitoring machines and often two operators are needed to perform simultaneous NSTs, although with two distinctive fetal heart rates the tests may be done separately, which makes it easier for one operator to perform.

O'Connor and colleagues (1981) suggested that, in multiple gestation, antepartum fetal heart rate electronic monitoring may be a better predictor of perinatal mortality and morbidity than serial urinary estriol or serial determination of biparietal diameter by sonogram. Research by Devoe and Azor (1981) would support this. In a study of 120 simultaneously recorded NSTs in twin gestations, they noted the following:

1. Synchronous fetal heart rate patterns were associated with twins of similar size, usually supported by monochorionic or fused dichorionic placentas (71 percent).

2. Asynchronous patterns were usually seen in twins with separated placentas (80 percent) and were associated with a greater weight difference between twins.

3. Reactive NSTs (77 percent) were associated with the same prognostically good outcome as those reported for singletons: very low perinatal morbidity and no perinatal deaths.

4. Nonreactive NSTs (23 percent), which predicted fetal outcome less accurately, were associated with two fetal deaths and high perinatal morbidity (28 percent), as indicated by intrapartum fetal distress, neonatal depression, and need for NICU care. The data from the University of South Florida, Tampa General Hospital, substantiated these studies with a 0/1000 fetal mortality rate with our current protocol (Table 19–3) (Knuppel et al., 1985).

Second twins, historically known to be at a higher risk, were responsible for 73 percent of all nonreactive NSTs in our institution and received a CST. Table 19–4 demonstrates that all positive CSTs derived from nonreactive NSTs were on the second twin.

One major unresolved clinical problem is deciding on the proper management when one fetus shows a persistent abnormal pattern, the other one being normal. The decision about timing of delivery in such cases requires careful clinical judgment. Under these circumstances, our recommendation is first to make a careful evaluation of other underlying complications—Rh sensitization, hypertension, diabetes mellitus, vaginal bleeding, premature rupture of the membranes, intrauterine growth retardation, etc.—and then to proceed as follows:

1. If one of the fetuses is "nonreactive" but shows no late decelerations with uterine contractions, pregnancy should be allowed to continue.

2. If one fetus has a persistent nonreacting pattern followed by late decelerations, an amniocentesis should be performed, and if pulmonary maturity has been achieved, de-

Table 19–3. Intrauterine Fetal Death After 32 Weeks—Recent Reports

Author	NST/CST*	IUFDs*/ Total no.	Mortality/ 1000
Bailey et al.	Yes/no	2/101	20
DeVoe et al.	Yes/no	2/48	40
Pritchard and McDonald	No/no	2/288	14
Present report, 1975 to 1979	No/no	6/258	23
Present report, 1980 to 1983	Yes/yes	0/180	0

*NST = nonstress test; CST = contraction stress test; IUFD = intrauterine fetal death.

From Knuppel, R. A., Rattan, P. K., Scerbo, J. C., et al.: Intrauterine fetal death in twins after 32 weeks of gestation. Obstet. Gynecol. 65:172, 1985.

Table 19–4. Six Twin Pregnancies Accounted for Eight Positive or Equivocal CSTs

Case #	Twin	NST	CST	Gestational Age	Apgar Scores	Weight (grams)
1	A	R	Neg	38 weeks	8/10	3416 g
	B	NR	+CST		9/10	2211 g
2	A	NR	Eq	33 weeks	9/9	1644 g
	B	NR	Eq		9/9	1531 g
3	A	NR	Eq	35 weeks	5/8	2268 g
	B	NR	+CST		4/7	2013 g
4	A	R	Neg	32 weeks	7/9	2013 g
	B	NR	+CST		2/4	1899 g
5	A	R	Neg	38 weeks	8/9	3175 g
	B	NR	+CST		5/7	2126 g
6	A	R	Neg	36 weeks	9/9	2268 g
	B	NR	+CST		1/2	1475 g

livery should be accomplished by an expeditious and safe method. If the L/S ratio is below 2, our approach would be to administer betamethasone (12 mg intramuscularly in two doses in 24 hours) and then proceed with the delivery. This is obviously a very difficult decision, since the normal fetus will be electively delivered and might suffer the consequences and complications of prematurity, while the fetus with the abnormal fetal heart rate might demonstrate this pattern because of multiple congenital anomalies incompatible with extrauterine life. The parents as well as the health care team should be actively involved in the decision-making process when confronted with this clinical dilemma, but it is obvious that the optimal management of a nonreactive fetus that has not achieved pulmonary maturity still remains an unresolved problem.

BIOPHYSICAL PROFILE

The continuing search for a more specific and sensitive test that would reduce antepartum stillbirth and neonatal losses led Manning to develop the composite biophysical profile scoring technique (Table 19–5), which he proposed be used as a primary method of fetal surveillance (Manning et al., 1982).

Table 19–5. Technique of Biophysical Profile Scoring

Biophysical Variable	Normal (Score = 2)	Abnormal (Score = 0)
1. Fetal breathing movements	At least 1 episode of at least 30 seconds' duration in 30 minutes' observation	Absent or no episode of ⩾ 30 seconds in 30 minutes
2. Gross body movements	At least 3 discrete body/limb movements in 30 minutes (episodes of active continuous movement considered as a single movement)	Two or fewer episodes of body/limb movements in 30 minutes
3. Fetal tone	At least 1 episode of active extension with return to flexion of fetal limb(s) or trunk. Opening and closing of hand considered normal tone	Either slow extension with return to partial flexion or movement of limb in full extension or absent fetal movement
4. Reactive fetal heart rate	At least 2 episodes of acceleration of ⩾ 15 bpm and at least 15 seconds' duration associated with fetal movement in 30 minutes	Less than 2 accelerations or acceleration <15 bpm in 30 minutes
5. Qualitative amniotic fluid volume	At least 1 pocket of amniotic fluid that measures at least 1 cm in two perpendicular planes	Either no amniotic fluid pockets or a pocket <1 cm in two perpendicular planes

From Manning, F. A., Morrison, I., Lange, I. R., et al.: Antepartum determination of fetal health: composite biophysical profile scoring. Clin. Perinatol. 9:292, 1982.

It is being speculated that fetal biophysical activities are not random events but rather are initiated and regulated by a complex integrated mechanism of the central nervous system (CNS). The presence of a normal response therefore indicates that that portion of the CNS is intact and functioning. A multivariant assessment, such as the biophysical profile, appears to be effective in differentiating the normal sleeping fetus from the asphyxiated fetus, and therefore its use may result in an even greater decrease in the antepartum stillbirth rate.

ASSESSMENT OF FETAL LUNG MATURATION

There are several clinical situations in which amniotic fluid may need to be obtained from each separate sac. These include genetic studies and Rh-sensitized patients.

Spellacy and colleagues (1977) found no significant difference in the L/S ratios obtained from separate sacs in 14 sets of twins. Sims, testing 20 sets of twins, found that the L/S ratio in each pair of sacs was closely related and suggested using L/S ratios of 2.5 or greater to predict functional pulmonary maturity if only one sac is available (Sims et al., 1976). Verduzco reviewed 294 pairs of twins and concluded that the second twin's increased risk of hyaline membrane disease was due to birth asphyxia and not to lung immaturity at birth (Verduzco et al., 1976). Thus, the data available to us seem to indicate that in the majority of cases, the information obtained in one sac is probably a reliable estimate of functional pulmonary maturity for both twins, and even more so if one uses an L/S ratio of 2.5 or above as a lower limit for lung maturation.

An amniocentesis in twin gestation should be performed under careful sonographic examination of the fetuses. The position of the babies, placenta localization, and if possible, the location of the divided membranes should be established. The site for a safe tap should then be chosen, always starting with the easier sac. A 22-gauge needle is introduced and fluid aspirated. After the fluid is withdrawn, 0.5 cc of indigo carmine (blue dye) is instilled into the sac, the needle is removed, and the patient is rescanned to select the site for the second tap. If the fluid on the second tap is clear, the procedure has been successful; if it is blue-stained, how-

ever, the amniocentesis for the second twin must be repeated. Indigo carmine should be used, since Cowett reported hemolysis of fetal red blood cells with methylene blue, which may lead to fetal anemia (Cowett et al., 1974).

Antepartum Complications

SPONTANEOUS ABORTIONS

Spontaneous abortions are more common in twin gestations then in singleton pregnancies. Hellman and coworkers (1973) and Robinson and Caines (1977) reported cases in which there was sonographic evidence of two sacs early in pregnancy, with disappearance and reabsorption of one embryo later on. Schenker and colleagues (1981) state that monozygotic twins are more likely than singleton pregnancies to abort in the 1st trimester. They also found an increased incidence of 2nd-trimester spontaneous abortions in cases of multiple gestation, with the risk increasing according to the number of fetuses. Finally, in cases in which drugs were used to induce ovulation, a *lower incidence* of spontaneous abortion was seen with clomiphene than with HMG-HCG.

Schenker speculates that several factors may account for increased abortion rates (in the vicinity of 20 to 30 percent) in drug-induced pregnancies: (1) faulty ovum as a result of exogenous stimulation with different drugs; (2) a very high level of estradiol, which may increase tubal motility, resulting in early arrival of the conceptus to a very poorly prepared endometrium and therefore poor implantation with subsequent abortion; (3) luteal phase deficiency; (4) earlier diagnostic rate in this very special group of patients on fertility drugs.

ANEMIA

As reported by Pritchard and MacDonald (1980), the mean increment of blood volume in twin gestation is about 50 to 60 percent. As mentioned earlier, multiple gestation causes increased placental as well as fetal mass. These factors predispose to a greater prevalence of maternal anemia. Good nutrition with an increased iron intake as well as supplementation of iron and vitamins with folic acid is recommended.

HYPERTENSIVE DISORDERS

Hypertensive disorders in pregnancies are more common in women with multiple gestation. The development of hypertension in a multiparous patient who had previous otherwise uncomplicated pregnancies should alert the obstetrician to the possibility of twin gestation.

The incidence is being recognized to be 2 to 3 times higher than in singleton pregnancies. This complication not only is more common in twin pregnancies but also tends to develop earlier and to be more severe than in patients with a singleton pregnancy (Pritchard and MacDonald, 1980).

HYDRAMNIOS

The uterus with multiple fetuses may have a volume of 10 liters and weigh over 20 pounds. Rapid accumulation of excessive amounts of amniotic fluid is not unusual, especially in monozygotic twin pregnancies. Approximately 12 percent of all multiple gestations may be complicated with this disorder (Cetrulo et al., 1980). The overdistension of the uterus by excessive amounts of amniotic fluid, in addition to the burden of carrying two or more fetuses, increases the likelihood of premature labor and/or premature rupture of the membranes. Hydramnios has also been associated with increased incidence of gastrointestinal and central nervous system abnormalities in the fetus; therefore, perinatal mortality might be as high as 41 percent when this condition is present in multiple gestation.

ANTEPARTUM HEMORRHAGE

In theory, the condition of large placental mass combined with overdistension of the uterus might lead one to believe that multiple gestations are more commonly complicated with placenta previa and abruptio placentae. Several authors (Farooqui et al., 1973; Cetrulo et al., 1980; O'Connor et al., 1981) have listed antepartum hemorrhage as a complication seen in multiple gestations; however, it is very difficult to assess whether this phenomenon is more common in these cases than in singleton pregnancies.

PREMATURE RUPTURE OF THE MEMBRANES (PROM)

Premature rupture of the chorioamniotic membranes seems to occur more frequently in multiple gestation and obviously can lead to premature labor. It may also be associated with increased incidence of cord prolapse (Cetrulo et al., 1980).

CONGENITAL ANOMALIES

The incidence of congenital anomalies is higher in twin gestations than in singleton pregnancies. In 1195 twins studied in a Collaborative Perinatal Project (Iffy and Kaminetzky, 1981), the incidence of cardiovascular and gastrointestinal tract anomalies in twin gestation was more than twice that for singleton pregnancies. The incidence of central nervous system and skeletal abnormalities was also much higher in multiple gestation. Another study of 2000 twins showed a higher incidence of anencephaly, hydrocephaly, and congenital heart disease in twins of the same sex, suggesting that placental anastomosis may play a role in the etiology of these manifestations (Iffy and Kaminetzky, 1981).

Monozygotic twins have a higher incidence of congenital anomalies than do dizygotic twins, and, as was mentioned earlier in this chapter, the former type of twinning should perhaps be considered a teratologic process. Acardia (absence of the heart) is a malformation confined to only monozygotic twins and occurs once in every 100 cases. Fetuses affected by acardia may differ greatly in appearance and may have different degrees of organogenesis (usually they have an axis, limbs, and frequently a malformed head). They represent probably the ultimate discordance in the development of genetically identical individuals (Benirschke and Kim, 1973).

The anomaly ·of conjoined twins is also more common in monozygotic twins. Most of them are female (70 percent) and are fused by the chest (thoracopagus) (70 percent). The incidence is 1 in 33,000 to 1 in 165,000 births, and the condition is believed to result from separation of the inner cell mass occuring very late on the time scale (13 to 15 days after implantation).

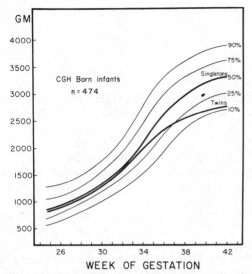

Figure 19–12. Intrauterine growth of twin pregnancies compared with singletons: Weight curve is parallel until approximately 35 weeks, at which time the rate of growth in twin pregnancies slows. (From Lubchenco, L. O.: The High Risk Infant. Philadelphia, W. B. Saunders Co., 1976.)

PERINATAL MORBIDITY AND MORTALITY

Several factors are thought to be of relevance for increased perinatal mortality and morbidity in cases of multiple gestation as compared with singleton pregnancies. Naeye and coworkers (1978) found a perinatal mortality of 13.9 percent for twins, as compared with 3.3 percent for singletons. The reason for this excess in perinatal mortality in most cases is prematurity secondary to preterm labor, with the second most important factor being intrauterine growth retardation (IUGR), especially after 30 weeks' gestation (Figs. 19–12 and 19–13).

Hypertension, anemia, and birth trauma are also mentioned as possible factors for increased perinatal morbidity and mortality in twin gestations. It has been reported that 70 percent of the perinatal mortalities occur before the 30th week of gestation, which is also the period of greatest neonatal morbidity. As the number of fetuses in utero in-

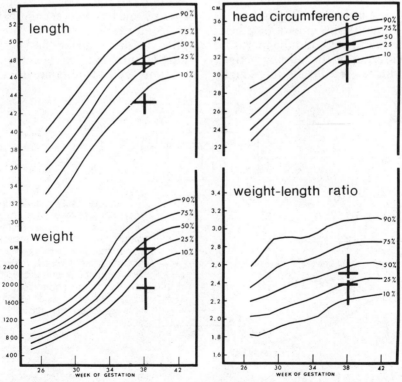

Figure 19–13. Discordant twins with intrauterine growth retardation: comparison of length and weight, head circumference, and weight-length ratio after 35 weeks' gestation. (From Lubchenco, L. O.: The High Risk Infant. Philadelphia, W. B. Saunders Co., 1976.)

creases, both the mean birth weight and the duration of pregnancy decreases.

Dunn (1965) feels that birth trauma occurs in approximately 25 percent of multiple gestations, associated with obstetric interventions such as breech extraction and forceps delivery.

Intrapartum Management

Common intrapartum complications are abnormal presentations, dysfunctional labor, cord prolapse, fetal distress, and abruptio placentae. At the time of labor, several important measures should be implemented to ensure a good outcome in cases of multiple gestation.

VAGINAL DELIVERY FOR VERTEX-VERTEX PRESENTATION

Electronic fetal monitoring has been used successfully to monitor both fetuses simultaneously at the time of labor. When a vaginal delivery is planned, artificial rupture of the membranes should be performed, after which the scalp electrode is applied to the first twin. An intrauterine pressure catheter (IUPC) is then introduced into the uterus for accurate monitoring of the uterine activity (external monitoring of the uterine activity

cannot provide the exact intensity of the contractions nor the resting tone). The internal electrode on the first twin and the IUPC are then attached to a first monitor. The fetal heart tones of the second twin are recorded on a second monitor, externally through ultrasound or phonotransducer technique (Fig. 19–14). A second catheter filled with sterile water is then run between the strain gauges of the first and second monitors (Fig. 19–15). In this way, the tracing from the second twin will also show uterine activity being recorded internally. Several monitor companies now offer an electronic monitor that simultaneously monitors both twins (Figs. 19–16 and 19–17). In some cases, if the same pen traces both fetal heart rates, an accurate assessment of variability is lost. This can be overcome by intermittently allowing only the internal lead to pick up the signal. However, some brands have dual channels so that variability can be assessed from the internal electrode.

As soon as the first twin is delivered, the vertex of the second twin should be guided gently into the pelvis. This can be followed by using ultrasound equipment if this is available in the labor and delivery area. As soon as this has been accomplished, the fetal scalp electrode should be immediately applied to the head of the second fetus. As long as no complications develop, there is no time limit for the delivery of the second

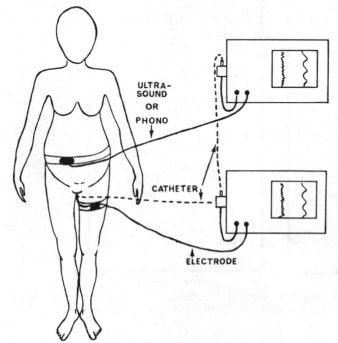

ULTRA-
SOUND
OR
PHONO

CATHETER

ELECTRODE

Figure 19–14. Twin gestation—simultaneous monitoring of intrapartum fetal heart rate and uterine activity. Fetal heart rate on Twin A monitored with internal scalp electrode. Twin B monitored by Doppler ultrasound or phonocardiogram through maternal abdominal wall. Intrauterine pressure catheter is used for uterine activity. (From Cetrulo, C. L., Ingardia, C. J., and Sbarra, A. J.: Management of multiple gestation. Clin. Obstet. Gynecol. 23:536, 1980.)

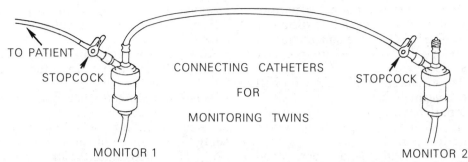

Figure 19–15. Connecting catheters for monitoring twins. (From Paul, R. H., et al.: Fetal Intensive Care. Wallingford, CT, Corometrics Medical Systems, Inc., 1979.)

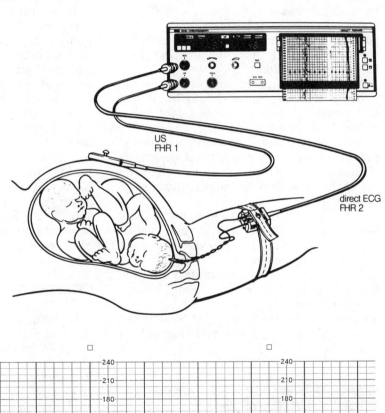

Figure 19–16. The attachment of a single fetal monitor to monitor both twins simultaneously with ultrasound and the internal electrode. (Courtesy of Hewlett-Packard.)

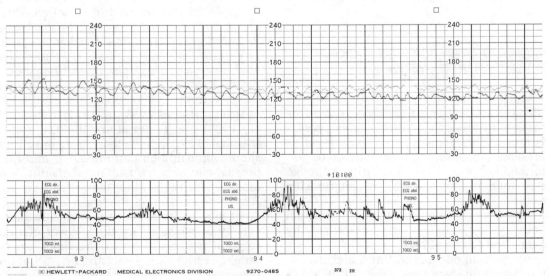

Figure 19–17. Tracing from the monitor that monitors twins simultaneously. The light fetal heart rate line is the internal tracing, and the dark line is the ultrasound tracing. (Courtesy of the Division of Maternal-Fetal Medicine, University of South Florida, College of Medicine, Tampa, FL.)

twin, provided there is a normal pattern of fetal heart rate. We see few contraindications to the use of oxytocin for augmentation of labor, provided both fetuses are properly monitored.

Pudendal anesthesia is probably the best choice for a vaginal delivery.

An appropriately trained obstetrician and an assistant should be available to follow the mother in labor.

On admission to the labor floor, blood should be drawn from the mother, and two units of cross-matched whole blood should be readily available.

An intravenous infusion system with a large bore catheter is mandatory. The delivery area should be immediately operational for emergency surgery.

A neonatal team composed of two neonatologists with assistants should be alerted and present at delivery, since infant resuscitation may be needed.

An anesthesiologist or nurse anesthetist capable of administering general anesthesia should be readily available in case the need for cesarean section or intrauterine manipulations arises.

With this team approach, every patient with a twin gestation and a vertex-vertex presentation should be allowed to progress into labor spontaneously.

If at the onset of labor there is a question about the presentation of one or both fetuses, an ultrasound examination of the uterus (or an x-ray of the abdomen) should immediately be performed to accurately assess fetal position.

VAGINAL DELIVERY FOR PRESENTATIONS OTHER THAN VERTEX-VERTEX

Much controversy still exists in today's literature about vaginal delivery of twin fetuses with other than vertex-vertex presentations. With fetuses in a breech-vertex presentation, cesarean section should be performed because of the possibility, although rare (one in 1000 twins), of interlocking twins.

The risks of a breech infant in a vaginal delivery are meticulously described by Seeds and Cefalo (1982):
- Intrapartum death is 16 times higher.
- Intrapartum asphyxia is 3 to 8 times higher.
- Cord prolapse is 5 to 20 times higher.
- Trauma is 13 times higher.

- Spinal cord injury incidence is 21 percent.
- Hyperextended head incidence is 5 percent.
- Arrest of the aftercoming head is 8 percent.
- Congenital anomalies are in the range of 6 to 18 percent.

Kelsik and Minkoff (1982) suggest that the perinatal mortality is higher for a breech first or second twin in a vaginal delivery (5 percent) than with cesarean section (2.5 percent). The outcome for the first breech twin is no better than that for the second breech twin, and cesarean sections should be done as frequently for breech second as for breech first twins. The indications for cesarean section for breech twins are: (1) prematurity, with an estimated fetal weight between 800 and 2500 grams; (2) footling breech; (3) evidence of contracted pelvis; (4) hyperextension of the fetal head; (5) lack of expertise of the medical staff in vaginal deliveries; (6) fetal distress; and (7) abnormal labor patterns.

It is well known also that twin B may be heavier than twin A (Friedman et al., 1977). In a situation in which twin B is breech and larger than vertex twin A, labor management should be altered (Roberts, 1976) and cesarean section considered to prevent potential birth trauma.

CESAREAN SECTION

Numerous reports in the literature have exposed a recent trend to routinely deliver multiple fetuses by cesarean section. Pritchard quoted that 44 percent of the twins followed at the High-Risk Pregnancy Clinic at Parkland Memorial Hospital were delivered by cesarean section. Table 19–6 shows the cesarean section rate for Tampa General Hospital from 1973 to 1982. After evaluation of several studies by Ware (1971), Cetrulo et al. (1980), and Barter et al. (1965), it seems reasonable to conclude that cesarean section should probably be performed for multiple pregnancies of larger fetal numbers (three or more) or for twins other than vertex-vertex. A vertical incision in the lower uterine segment may be indicated if a fetus lies transversely or when a very thick lower uterine segment is encountered. Indications for cesarean section are fetal distress; abruptio placentae; prolapsed umbilical cord; coexistence of twin gestation with other complications of pregnancy, such as hypertension, diabetes mellitus, or Rh sensitization; evi-

Table 19-6. Cesarean Section in Multifetal Gestation, Tampa General Hospital (University of South Florida), 1973–1982

Year	Total Deliveries	Total C/S Rates	Number of Twin Pregnancies	Cesarean Section in Twins	C/S for Twin B Only (% of Total Cesarean Section Rate in Twins)
1973–74	6889	7.8%	61	10 (16%)	1 (10%)
1975–76	5997	8.5 %	58	13 (22%)	1 (8%)
1977–78	6221	11.1 %	74	27 (36%)	8 (29%)
1979–80	7190	13.0 %	77	34 (44%)	4 (11%)
1981–82	8014	15.7 %	82	51 (62%)	7 (13%)
Total	34,311		352	135	21

dence of discordant twins with intrauterine growth retardation; and perhaps any presentations other than vertex-vertex, in order to avoid birth trauma, the most important labor complication leading to perinatal mortality.

DELIVERY OF THE SECOND TWIN

It has been said that the main problem in delivering twins is the delivery of the second twin. Some authors have stressed that the second twin is at a greater risk of mortality and morbidity than the firstborn. Early reports of cesarean sections done for second twins were mainly in the form of case reports. Evrard and Gold (1981) recently reviewed 4 such cases presented over a 4-year period, and added 5 cases from the recent literature. If one follows the standard of typical textbooks, maternal and perinatal mortality and morbidity undoubtedly would be higher with this mode of delivery. Except when the management protocol includes cesarean section delivery for all twins other than vertex-vertex, this infrequent complication cannot be avoided.

In our institution, in an attempt to define the risks of cesarean section delivery for Twin B after a vaginal delivery of Twin A, we undertook a retrospective review of our last 10 years of experience. As shown in Table 19–7, the indications for cesarean sec-

Table 19-7. Primary Indications for Cesarean Section in Twin B at Tampa General Hospital (University of South Florida), 1973–1982

Indication	Number of Cases (%)
Transverse lie	8 (33%)
Fetal distress	5 (24%)
Contracted cervix	3 (20%)
Prolapsed cord	2 (9%)
Premature breech	2 (9%)
Failed extraction	1 (5%)
Total	21 (100%)

tion for the second twin are prolapse of the cord, abruptio placentae, fetal distress, failed forceps, failed internal podalic version, and probably any presentation other than vertex. One of the concerns regarding cesarean section for the second twin is the risk of infection to the mother when cesarean section is undertaken in these circumstances. Because there is a paucity of literature regarding this subject, some physicians might be reluctant to perform a cesarean section for Twin B when Twin A has been delivered vaginally. On the other hand, some physicians, in order to avoid this infrequent possibility altogether, might use cesarean section for *all* twins. To reduce perinatal mortality and morbidity, cesarean section as a method of choice for delivery of twins has been advised if one or both twins present other than vertex-vertex. We have followed this policy since 1979 (Table 19–8). In our review, we found that 21 of the 352 twin deliveries (6 percent) required cesarean section of Twin B after vaginal delivery of Twin A. This group of 21 cesarean sections made up 15 percent of all the cesarean sections that were performed in our institution for twin gestation. Even with the liberal use of cesarean section in 1979, 11 of the 85 cesarean sections done for twins were done for Twin B after a vaginal delivery of Twin A, and they made up 13 percent of the total number of cesarean sections done in twin pregnancies in this latter period. This compares with 10 cesarean sections for Twin B after vaginal delivery of Twin A, done out of a total of 50 cesarean sections (20 percent) in the 1973 to 1978 period. Failure to diagnose twins continues to be a major factor in the management of twins and often accounts for the need to do a cesarean section for Twin B after vaginal delivery of Twin A. In our review, this factor accounted for about 35 percent of all such cases.

Sometimes a low birth weight becomes apparent only after vaginal delivery of the

Table 19–8. Clinical Features Associated with Cesarean Section for Delivery of the Second Twin (Tampa General Hospital)*

Case No. & Twin	Diagnosis	Position and Presentation	Time Interval	Complication Requiring C/S	Birth Weight	Apgar Score
1A	37 wk; undiagnosed twin	Vertex	54 min	Contracted cervix	2813 g	9/9
1B		Footling breech			2813 g	8/9
2A	35 wk; undiagnosed twin	Vertex	22 min	Fetal distress	1857 g	8/9
2B		Vertex		Abruptio placentae	1775 g	7/8
3A	28 wk; undiagnosed twin	Vertex	89 min	Transverse lie; prematurity	818 g	6/6
3B		Transverse lie			722 g	4/5
4A	36 wk; twins; preeclampsia	Vertex	12 min	Transverse lie; Abruptio placentae	2335 g	9/8
4B		Transverse lie			2225 g	3/8
5A	32 wk; twins	Vertex	15 min	Premature breech	865 g	6/8
5B		Breech			2060 g	2/7
6A	30 wk; PROM over 15 hours	Vertex	12 min	Premature breech	1548 g	6/7
6B		Breech			1520 g	2/8
7A	30 wk; twins	Vertex	10 min	Transverse lie; Prolapsed cord	1885 g	8/9
7B		Transverse lie			1850 g	7/8

*There was only one neonatal death, that of twin 6A, delivered vaginally. This neonate succumbed to overwhelming beta-streptococcal sepsis. All neonates except twins 3A and 3B had Apgar scores of 7 or above at 5 minutes. Twins 3A and 3B had 5-minute Apgar scores of 6 and 5, respectively. Prophylactic antibiotics were used in all cases after cesarean section. Maternal febrile morbidity was zero, and all patients were discharged home on the 5th postoperative day, except patient #4, who was kept in the hospital until postpartum day 7 because of elevated blood pressure.

Table 19–9. Delivery Interval and Apgar Scores of Second Twins

Time Interval (minutes)	Number of Twins	Apgar Scores (below 7 at 5 minutes)
0–10 min	0	—
10–20 min	7	2
21–60 min	9	0
61–120 min	5	1
Total	21	3

first twin, and cesarean section in such a case may be chosen as an optimal route of delivery, as proposed by Barrett (Barrett et al., 1982). In their recent review on this subject, Evrard and Gold had no cases in which cesarean section was done because of prematurity, cord prolapse, or fetal distress, and both perinatal deaths occurred in twins delivered by cesarean section, as compared with our experience, in which both perinatal deaths were in twins delivered vaginally. This might be due to the infrequent occurrence of second twins with a lower birth weight at our institution, or it might reflect a liberal approach to cesarean section rather than internal version.

Since the diagnosis of twin gestation was made only after vaginal delivery of Twin A in 38 percent of the cases, the need for improved antepartum diagnosis to improve outcome in twin gestation is imperative and has been stressed by various authors. In our experience the time interval between vaginally and abdominally delivered twins was not associated with an increase in low Apgar scores for the second twin at 5 minutes, even when delivered after the usual time interval of 15 to 20 minutes suggested to be safe (Table 19–9). Many reports have appeared in the literature regarding post–cesarean section morbidity, with infection being the most important complication in the postpartum period. In our review of cases at Tampa General Hospital, 3 mothers out of 21 (14 percent) experienced extensive febrile morbidity, and all had significant predisposing factors. This review, which covers the largest number of such cases reported, was prepared to address the safety of cesarean section for Twin B only. It supports the view that, whenever indications exist, cesarean section can be performed safely for the delivery of Twin B after vaginal delivery of Twin A. We recognize that indications for cesarean section in twin pregnancy sometimes are controversial; however, in this small number of

patients there was no increase in maternal morbidity when pregnancy was not complicated. There was no increase in neonatal mortality or morbidity resulting from cesarean section for Twin B. This management success reemphasizes the need for anesthesia availability at every twin delivery and continued fetal monitoring for Twin B in the delivery room.

Conclusions Regarding Management

1. The treatment of infertility by the use of drugs for induction of ovulation has increased the overall incidence of multiple gestation.

2. Ultrasound is perhaps the most accurate method of diagnosis. However, whether a sonogram should be done routinely in every pregnancy still remains controversial. The accuracy is about 98 percent. If the diagnosis is still in doubt after ultrasound, or if ultrasound equipment is unavailable, a flat plate of the abdomen is not contraindicated.

3. Since the number 1 problem is prematurity, every attempt should be made to diagnose twin gestations early (between 16 and 20 weeks). Early diagnosis, prolonged bedrest between 26 and 34 weeks' gestation, and the use of tocolytic agents might prolong the pregnancy; maternal administration of glucocorticoids for enhancement of fetal lung maturation may also improve the perinatal outcome. Early diagnosis allows prompt detection and treatment of other complications that frequently are encountered in this clinical situation, such as anemia, hypertension, polyhydramnios, intrauterine growth retardation, and discordance.

4. The patient's diet should be well balanced: 300 kcal/kg/day with at least 1 g of protein per kg of body weight. Supplements of iron and folic acid should be instituted.

5. Malpresentation is a common finding. It is preferable to deliver by cesarean section in these cases, to avoid potential complications. In cases of fetal distress, prolapse of the umbilical cord, or abruptio placentae, the fetuses are probably best served by an abdominal delivery. Avoid birth trauma. Optimal neonatal care requires team effort.

6. Labor and delivery of twins with a vertex-vertex presentation requires intensive electronic fetal monitoring, including the internal pressure catheter. Oxytocin is not

Table 19–10. Patient Care Summary for Multiple Gestations*

	Antepartum			Postpartum
	Outpatient	Inpatient	Intrapartum	
BP, P, R	Each visit	Every 8 hrs (more frequently if hypertensive)	Every 1 hr	On admission; then every 15 min × 4; then every 30 min × 2; then every 1 hr until stable; then every 8 hr on PP (unless also hypertensive, then more frequent BP indicated)
T	Each visit	Every 8 hr	Every 4 hr	On admission to RR; then every 8 hr
FHR	Weekly NST/CST starting 30–32 weeks' gestation in home contraction monitoring	Weekly NST/CST starting 30–32 weeks' gestation	Continuously with electronic fetal monitor (both internal and external). If monitor not available, every 15 min first stage; then every 5 min second stage	—
Contractions	Weekly, with daily home monitoring	Every 8 hr	Continuously with electronic fetal monitor, preferably internal. If monitor not available, every 1 hr by palpation	Fundal checks: every 15 min × 4; then every 30 min × 2; then every 1 hr until stable; then every 8 hr on PP floor
Lochia	—	—	—	Lochia checks: every 15 min × 4; then every 30 min × 2; then every 1 hr until stable; then every 8 hr on PP floor
Laboratory studies				
Hemoglobin	Each visit	Weekly	Admission	First day PR
Hematocrit	Each visit	Weekly	Admission	First day PR
GT (2-hour postprandial)	At 20, 24, 28, 32, and 36 weeks	Same as under outpatient	Admission	First day PR
Sonogram	At least one level II sonogram before 24 weeks to R/O major congenital anomalies	Serial sonogram 2–3 weeks from 28 weeks to R/O discordance; on admission, to check fetal presentations		
Assess fundal heights	Each visit	Each visit		

*Nurse–patient ratio as follows: *antepartum,* 1:6–8; *intrapartum,* 1:1; *at delivery,* 1:1; *postpartum,* 1:1; *postpartum,* 1:6–8.

contraindicated. Local or pudendal block is probably the preferred method of anesthesia. If nuchal cord is encountered, do not cut the cord to deliver Twin A.

7. As soon as the first twin is born, guide the head of the second twin into the pelvis, proceed to rupture the membrane, and apply the scalp electrode. Allow labor under very close surveillance. Oxytocin is not contraindicated. Time between deliveries is not as relevant as it used to be, provided the second twin is monitored properly and labor is well tolerated by the fetus.

8. If delivery is anticipated before 36 weeks, with a birth weight below 2500 grams, the patient is best served by an early transfer in utero to a Level III hospital.

A summary of the management for multiple gestations is presented in Table 19–10 and Figure 19–18.

Psychosocial Considerations

When the diagnosis of a multiple gestation is made, the parents may have many fears concerning the addition of more than one baby to the family. These concerns may include fears of being unable physically and emotionally to care for more than one infant, as well as financial concerns for the cost of caring for more than one baby, which involves doubling items such as clothing, cribs, strollers, etc., as well as increased hospitalization costs for the mother and the infants. These fears may be overwhelming to the new parents, and psychologic and financial counseling should be offered when needed.

The parents will probably recognize that there is a higher risk for prematurity and other maternal and fetal complications, such as anemia, hypertension, increased incidence of congenital anomalies, IUGR, abruptio placentae, prolapse of the cord, placenta previa, and postpartum hemorrhage. The parents should have a clear understanding of these potential complications, which will help them to deal with the stresses that may occur. In some situations the parents may want to tour the neonatal intensive care nursery to prepare for their babies' admittance. They may want to take prepared

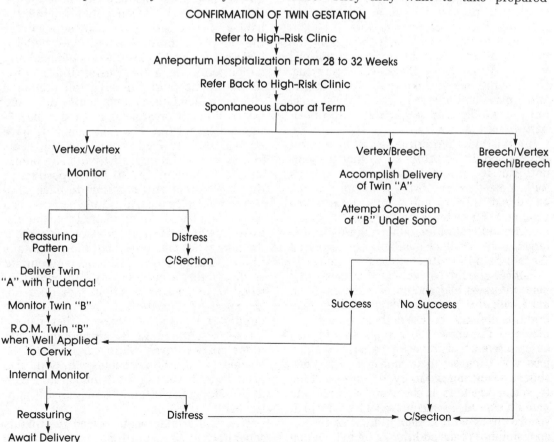

Figure 19–18. Management flow chart for multiple gestations.

childbirth classes earlier, in anticipation of premature labor or restricted activity later in the pregnancy.

Some of the minor discomforts of pregnancy become exaggerated with a larger uterus. Small meals can be helpful to decrease the heartburn caused by the enlargement of the uterus pressing on the stomach. The woman may feel awkward with the size of her uterus. This awkwardness and discomfort may lead to difficulty sleeping. A pillow can be used on her side to support the uterus when she sleeps. A heating pad or hot water bottle can be used while she is awake to soothe aching ligaments. (One of our patients, pregnant with triplets, was so uncomfortable that the physical therapy department devised a harness to help support her uterus.)

These women may also be depressed by their large size and may be anxious over their weight gain; nevertheless, they should be encouraged to maintain their increased caloric intake. Psychologic support is very important.

Home visits to these families can be very helpful in the antepartum period, to help the family prepare for the arrival of more than one baby. The parents should be encouraged to verbalize their concerns to the health care team and to work on solutions for the demands of increased caretaking. Other family members, hired help, or family aides may facilitate the caretaking, at least until schedules can be devised in the postpartum period.

Information on multiple gestation support groups should be provided so that the parents can have contact with other families with more than one baby, who can provide emotional support and "helpful hints" to problems. These hints may include attaching two umbrella strollers rather than using the larger twin strollers available, or allowing the babies to initially sleep in the same crib.

Fathers should be included in these preparatory plans and should be encouraged to help with the caretaking. Some fathers may find this difficult because of their work schedules and demands. The parents should also be counseled that these increased caretaking jobs will decrease their time together. They should be encouraged to try to find some time to spend together. If there are siblings, the parents should be encouraged to try to plan special times with these children, as the responsibilities of the addition of more than one new baby can become all-consuming.

Once the babies have been delivered, the family should be given continued support. Home visits should be maintained and care plans continued and modified as needed in the postpartum period. If the multiple gestation was not identified until the time of delivery, these parents will need additional support and planning in the postpartum period.

Making up a specific schedule for the care for more than one infant may be helpful, at least initially, in getting the family organized. However, the family should also try to remain somewhat flexible, as the schedule will probably be interrupted. *Keeping records* of when each baby was fed, bathed, etc., may be helpful, as fatigue may cause the parents to forget whose turn it is. It should be reinforced that as long as the babies are cleaned well with each diaper change, daily bathing is not necessary. The parents may find it helpful to bathe the babies on the same day, or perhaps to bathe each baby on alternating days.

Initially the sounds of the babies may disturb others in the family, but they will quickly become accustomed to these sounds. Some parents have suggested having the babies share a crib, as the babies may enjoy the closeness and may actually rest better.

Breast-feeding should be encouraged and supported if the mother desires it. Rooming-in in the hospital can give the mother a chance to feed the babies while help and instruction are available. It should be explained to the mother that she will have enough milk to feed more than one baby, i.e., *supply will equal demand.* The family should be encouraged to be supportive, so that the mother will continue to have caretaking help at home. Additional support can be provided with home visits from the visiting nurses, and from contact with other mothers who have breast fed more than one infant. This advice and support is important as the mother's milk supply can be diminished if she becomes fatigued or does not get enough nourishment. With twins, the mother will need to increase her caloric intake to 1100 to 1200 calories above her prepregnancy level. More calories will be needed for additional babies. She will also need to increase her fluid intake, and continue taking her vitamin and mineral supplements.

The mother may want to feed the infants separately at first, until she becomes more comfortable with the babies. Later, with

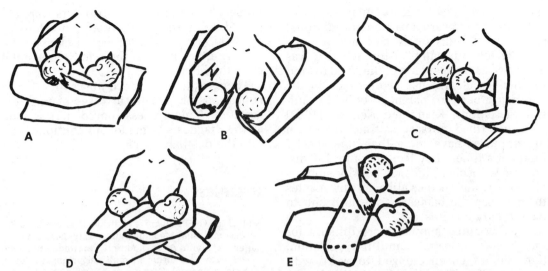

Figure 19–19. Positions for breast-feeding twins. All positions illustrated permit eye-to-eye contact with both infants. For women who have incisional pain from cesarean delivery, position *B* and a modification of *C* are comfortable. In *C*, the infants can be placed on a padded table at the correct height with the mother moving in close to feed them. (From Leonard, L. G.: JOGN Nurs. 11:151, May/June 1982.)

more practice, she may be able to feed both babies simultaneously (Fig. 19–19). It takes less time to feed both babies simultaneously; however, each baby will get more personal attention if fed separately. The mother may also want to express milk so that another family member can feed one of the babies. A combination of feeding the babies separately and together may save time and offer individual attention for each baby.

Mothers should also be prepared for the increased demand of breast-feeding when the babies have growth spurts at about 6 weeks and 3 months. This increased demand from the babies will increase the milk supply for these growth spurts. With two babies suckling, the mother may find she has sore nipples. If the mother is not allergic to wool, lanolin can be applied to the nipples. Milk can be expressed on occasion to rest the sore nipple. Changing the position of the babies when they feed will change the areas of pressure on the nipples. The less hungry baby should be fed on the sorer breast, and the hungrier baby fed from the fuller breast. The mother may also find that a baby may prefer one breast over the other. If the babies have different appetites, the breast will become fuller on the side that supports the hungrier baby.

Attachment and grieving can be much more difficult when dealing with more than one baby. Klaus and Kennell (1982) have described principles that regulate human bonding (Table 19–11). The fact that the mother and father can bond optimally to only one infant at a time has special implications for multiple gestations. Bowlby (1958) used the term "manotropy" to de-

Table 19–11. Crucial Components in the Process of Attachment

1. For later development to be optimal, there is a sensitive period in the first minutes and hours of life during which it is necessary that the mother and father have close contact with their neonate.

2. There appear to be species-specific responses to the infant in the human mother and father that are exhibited when they are first given their infant.

3. The process of the attachment is structured so that the father and mother will become attached optimally to only one infant at a time. Bowlby (1958) earlier presented this principle of the attachment process and termed it *monotropy.*

4. During the process of the mother's attachment to her infant, it is necessary that the infant respond to the mother by some signal such as body or eye movements. We have sometimes described this as "You can't love a dishrag."

5. People who witness the birth process become strongly attached to the infant.

6. For some adults it is difficult simultaneously to go through the processes of attachment and detachment—that is, to develop an attachment to one person while mourning the loss or threatened loss of the same or another person.

7. Some early events have long-lasting effects. Anxieties about the well-being of a baby with a temporary disorder in the first day may result in long-lasting concerns that may cast long shadows and adversely shape the development of the child (Klaus and Kennell, 1982).

scribe a "tendency for instinctual responses to be directed toward a particular individual or group of individuals and not promiscuously toward many." Although this was described as the response of the child toward the mother, it also has significance in the bonding process of parent to child in multiple gestations. Klaus and Kennell (1982) have described nursery settings in which nurses never have more than one special infant at a time. They like the other infants, but one is special. This may be why mothers often dress their babies alike, as this enables them to see the babies as one unit and to take in only one image.

Since bonding may be more difficult for the parents in cases of multiple gestation, they should be encouraged to work with each child individually, especially in the initial "getting acquainted" period. The nurse can help the parents to relate to each child as an individual, not as a unit, and to identify the unique characteristics of each child. The individual reactions of each baby to the parents should be pointed out as part of each baby's uniqueness. Early contacts with the babies, which might include rooming-in, will help the mother to gain confidence in caretaking as well as get her acquainted with her babies. Antepartum ultrasound can also help the parents to recognize more than one baby and to start the bonding process even before delivery.

Evans further investigated the problems of this difficult simultaneous bonding, and found that not only the process of attachment but also that of detachment cannot easily occur simultaneously (Evans et al., 1972). He found that if one baby dies, it is difficult to completely mourn that child while at the same time attach to the survivor. (This same phenomenon can be seen if a mother quickly becomes pregnant after the loss of a neonate.) Evans also found that one third of infants with failure-to-thrive that was not organic had parents who had recently suffered the loss of a close family member. He concluded that while they were grieving the loss, the parents could not adequately care for their newborns.

This also has implications when one of the babies is sick, or has congenital anomalies, and the other is well. The parents do not have enough energy to mourn for the less-than-perfect child. Klaus and Kennell (1982) found that when one twin was sent home and the other was left to grow in the nursery, more mothering disorders were observed with the latter twin. Therefore, if possible, twins should be discharged together, either back to the referring hospital or to the home.

There is a great need for support and education for parents in cases of multiple gestation. This process should start as soon as the diagnosis is made and continue well into the postpartum period.

REFERENCES

Andreassi, G.: Problemi e considerazioni sulla graficanza multipla. Medicus Vatican City 3:41, 1947.

Bailey, D., Flynn, A. M., and Kelly, J.: Antepartum fetal heart rate monitoring in multiple pregnancy. Br. J. Obstet. Gynaecol. Commonw. 87:561, 1980.

Barrett, J. M., Staggs, S. M., van Hooydonk, J. E., et al.: The effect of type of delivery upon neonatal outcome in premature twins. Am. J. Obstet. Gynecol. 143:360, 1982.

Barter, R. H., Hsu, I., Ekkenbech, R. V., et al.: The prevention of prematurity in multiple pregnancy. Am. J. Obstet. Gynecol. 91:787, 1965.

Benirschke, K., and Kim, J.: Multiple pregnancy. N. Engl. J. Med. 288:1276, 1973.

Bowlby, J.: The nature of the child's tie to his mother. Int. J. Psychoanal. 39:350, 1958.

Braly, P., and Freeman, R. K.: The significance of fetal heart rate reactivity with a positive oxytocin challenge test. Obstet. Gynecol. 50:689, 1977.

Cetrulo, C. L., Ingardia, C. J., and Sbarra, A. J.: Management of multiple gestation. Clin. Obstet. Gynecol. 23:536, 1980.

Clausen, J., Flook, M. H., Ford, B., et al.: Maternity Nursing Today. New York, McGraw-Hill, 1973.

Cowett, R. M., Hakanson, D. O., and Kocon, R. W.: Untoward neonatal effect of intra-amniotic administration of methylene blue. Obstet. Gynecol. 43(Suppl):74, 1974.

Devoe, L. D., and Azor, H.: Simultaneous nonstress fetal heart rate testing in twin pregnancy. Obstet. Gynecol. 58:450, 1981.

Dickerson, P. S.: Early postpartum separation and maternal attachment to twins. JOGN Nurs. 10:120, 1981.

Dor, J., Shalev, S., Mashiach, J., et al.: Elective cervical suture of twin pregnancies diagnosed ultrasonically in the first trimester following induced ovulation. Gynecol. Obstet. Invest. 13:55, 1982.

Duncan, S. L. B., Ginz, B., and Wahab, H.: Use of ultrasound and hormone assays in the diagnosis, management and outcome of twin pregnancies. Obstet. Gynecol. 53:367, 1979.

Dunn, P. M.: Some perinatal observations on twins. Dev. Med. Child. Neurol. 7:121, 1965.

Evans, S., Reinhart, J. B., and Succop, R. A.: A study of 45 children and their families. J. Am. Acad. Child Psychiatry 11:440, 1972.

Evrard, J. R., and Gold, E. M.: Cesarean section for the delivery of the second twin. Obstet. Gynecol. 57:581, 1981.

Farooqui, M. O., Grossman, J. H., III, and Shannon, R. A.: A review of twin pregnancies. Obstet. Gynecol. Surv. 28:144, 1973.

Freeman, R. K.: The use of oxytocin challenge test for antepartum clinical evalution of uteroplacental respiratory function. Am. J. Obstet. Gynecol. 121:481, 1975.

Friedman, E. A., and Sachtleben, M. R.: Relative birth weights of twins. Obstet. Gynecol. 49:717, 1977.

Galton, F.: The history of twins as a criterion of relative powers of nature and nurture. Inst. Gr. Br. Irel. 5:391, 1876.

Garoff, L., and Seppala, M.: Alpha fetoprotein and human placental lactogen levels in maternal serum in multiple pregnancies. J. Obstet. Gynaecol. Br. Commonw. 80:695, 1973.

Hack, M., Brish, M., Serr, D. M., et al.: Outcome of pregnancy after induced ovulation. Follow-up of pregnancies and children after clomiphene therapy. JAMA 220:1329, 1972.

Hawrylyshyn, P. A., Barkin, M., Bernstein, A., et al.: Twin pregnancies—a continuing perinatal challenge. Obstet. Gynecol. 59:463, 1982.

Hellman, L. M., Koboyashi, M., and Cromb, E.: Ultrasonic diagnosis of embryonic malformations. Am. J. Obstet. Gynecol. 115:615, 1973.

Hendricks, C. H.: Twinning in relation to birth weight, mortality and congenital anomalies. Obstet. Gynecol. 27:47, 1966.

Ho, S., and Wu, P.: Perinatal factors and neonatal morbidity in twin pregnancy. Am. J. Obstet. Gynecol. 122:979, 1975.

Iffy, L., and Kaminetzky, H.: Principles and Practice of Obstetrics and Perinatology, Vol. 2. New York, John Wiley & Sons, 1981, p. 1172.

Jarvis, G. J.: Diagnosis of multiple pregnancy. Br. Med. J. 2:593, 1979.

Johnson, J. W. C., Hustink, L., Jones, G. S., et al.: Efficacy of 17-alphahydroxyprogesterone caproate in the prevention of premature labor. N. Engl. J. Med. 293:675, 1975.

Keegan, K. A., and Paul, R. H.: Antepartum fetal heart rate testing. V. The nonstress test: an outpatient approach. Am. J. Obstet. Gynecol. 136:81, 1980.

Keegan, K. A., and Paul, R. H.: Antepartum fetal heart rate testing. IV. The nonstress test: a primary approach. Am. J. Obstet. Gynecol. 136:75, 1980.

Kelsik, F., and Minkoff, H.: Management of breech second twin. Am. J. Obstet. Gynecol. 144:783, 1982.

Kistner, K. W.: Induction of ovulation with clomiphene citrate. In Bertram, S. J., and Kistner, K. W. (eds.): Progress in Infertility. Boston, Little, Brown & Co., 1968, pp. 407–453.

Klaus, M. H., and Kennell, J. H.: Parent-Infant Bonding, 2nd ed. St. Louis, C. V. Mosby Co., 1982.

Knuppel, R. A., Rattan, P. K., Scerbo, J. C., et al.: Intrauterine fetal death in twins after 32 weeks of gestation. Obstet. Gynecol. 65:172, 1985.

Lemburg, P.: Nursing My Twins. Franklin Park, IL, La Leche League International, Inc., 1979.

Leonard, L. G.: Twin pregnancy: maternal fetal nutrition. JOGN Nurs. 11:139, 1982.

Leonard, L. G.: Breastfeeding twins. JOGN Nurs. 11:148, 1982.

Manning, F. A., Morrison, I., Lange, I. R., et al.: Antepartum determination of fetal health: composite biophysical profile scoring. Clin. Perinatol. 9:285, 1982.

Moore, M. L.: Realities in Childbearing. Philadelphia, W. B. Saunders Co., 1983.

Naeye, R. L., Tafari, N., Judge, D., et al.: Twins: causes of perinatal death in 12 United States cities and one African city. Am. J. Obstet. Gynecol. 31:267, 1978.

O'Connor, M. C., Arias, E., and Royston, J. P.: The merits of special antenatal care for twin pregnancies. Br. J. Obstet. Gynecol. 88:222, 1981.

O'Connor, M. C., Murphy, H., and Dalrymple, I. J.: Double blind trial of ritodrine and placebo in twin pregnancy. Br. J. Obstet. Gynaecol. 86:706, 1979.

Paul, H. P., and Petrie, R. H.: Fetal Intensive Care. USC School of Medicine; distributed by Corometrics Medical Systems, Inc., 1981.

Persson, P. H., Grennert, L., Gennser, G., et al.: On improved outcome of twin pregnancies. Acta Obstet. Gynecol. Scand. 58:3, 1979.

Pritchard, J. A., and MacDonald, P. C. (eds.): Multifetal pregnancy. In Williams Obstetrics, 16th ed. New York, Appleton-Century-Crofts, 1980, pp. 639–663.

Powers, W. F.: Bedrest in twin pregnancy: identification of a critical period. Obstet. Gynecol. 42:795, 1973.

Roberts, R. B.: Infant weights in multiple births. Obstet. Gynecol. 47:382, 1976.

Robinson, H. P., and Caines, J. S.: Sonar evidence of early pregnancy and failure in patients with twin conceptions. Br. J. Obstet. Gynecol. 84:22, 1977.

Rothman, K. J.: Fetal loss, twinning and birth weight after oral contraceptive use. N. Engl. J. Med. 297:468, 1977.

Schenker, J. G., Yarkoni, S., and Gronat, M.: Multiple pregnancy following induction of ovulation. Fertil. Steril. 35:105, 1981.

Seeds, J. W., and Cefalo, R. C.: Malpresentations. Clin. Obstet. Gynecol. 25:145, 1982.

Sims, C. D., Cowan, D. B., and Parkinson, C. E.: The lecithin/sphingomyelin (L/S) ratio in twin pregnancies. Br. J. Obstet. Gynaecol. 83:447, 1976.

Spellacy, W. H., Cruz, A. C., Buhi, W. C., et al.: Amniotic fluid L-S ratio in twin gestation. Obstet. Gynecol. 50:68, 1977.

Speroff, L., Glass, R. H., and Kaso, N. G.: Clinical Gynecological Endocrinology and Infertility, 2nd ed. Baltimore, Williams & Wilkins, 1981.

Verduzco, R., Rosario, R., and Rigatto, H.: Hyaline membrane disease in twins. Am. J. Obstet. Gynecol. 125:668, 1976.

Ware, H. H.: The second twin. Am. J. Obstet. Gynecol. 110:865, 1971.

20

HYPERTENSION IN PREGNANCY

ROBERT A. KNUPPEL
JOAN E. DRUKKER

The term toxemia of pregnancy was formerly applied to a number of conditions manifesting vascular derangements that arise either during pregnancy or during the early peurperal period. These conditions were characterized by hypertension and other signs. Unfortunately, the term toxemia was all-inclusive; thus, discrepancies in statistical reporting occurred, making it extremely difficult to evaluate the results obtained with different treatment programs. This highlights only a few of the controversies surrounding the data supporting the empirical management of preeclampsia-eclampsia and chronic hypertension. Despite 40 years of intensive research, the etiology of preeclampsia-eclampsia is still unknown, and epidemiologic surveys remain clouded in the shroud of confounding variables (Friedman, 1976, and Chesley, 1978). This chapter will discuss preeclampsia, eclampsia, chronic hypertension, and chronic hypertension with superimposed preeclampsia.

Terminology

In 1972, the Committee on Terminology of the American College of Obstetricians and Gynecologists, after careful consideration and consultation with authorities in the field, suggested a classification for the group of conditions hitherto loosely referred to as "toxemias of pregnancy"; this is shown in Table 20–1 (Page and Christianson, 1976).

The term toxemia has been in widespread use for so long that probably the best we can hope for is the adoption of one inclusive term, with "preeclampsia" and "eclampsia" used to designate the two clinical phases of the same disorder. A recent modification in terminology suggests the overall designation gestational edema–proteinuria hypertensive disorders (GEPH), with the recommendation that no preeclampsia be considered "mild." Hypertension complicated by pregnancy (HCP) is basically synonymous with the "chronic hypertensive" state, which is quite different from the elevated blood pressure in GEPH.

This chapter will use the terms preeclampsia, eclampsia, chronic hypertension, and superimposed preeclampsia, as referred to in the 1972 terminology report mentioned above and defined in Table 20–1.

Preeclampsia-Eclampsia

THE CLASSIC TRIAD: HYPERTENSION, EDEMA, AND PROTEINURIA

Hypertension

Hypertension is a measurable sign of preeclampsia. Hypertension is a rise in the systolic blood pressure of at least 30 mm Hg, or a rise in the diastolic pressure of at least 15 mm Hg, or a diastolic pressure of at least 90 mm Hg. A blood pressure of 140/90 mm Hg represents a mean arterial pressure (MAP) of 107 mm Hg. The MAP is an indicator of cardiac work, for it measures the resistance against which the heart works. The mean arterial pressure is calculated by adding the diastolic pressure to one third of the pulse pressure:

Table 20–1. Classification of "Toxemias of Pregnancy"

Gestational Edema	The occurrence of a general and excessive accumulation of fluid in the tissues of greater than 1+ pitting edema after 12 hours in bed, or of a weight gain of 5 lb or more in 1 week due to the influence of pregnancy.
Gestational Proteinuria	The presence of proteinuria during or under the influence of pregnancy, in the absence of hypertension, edema, renal infection, or known intrinsic renovascular disease.
Gestational Hypertension	The development of hypertension during pregnancy, or within the first 24 hours post partum, in a previously normotensive woman. No other evidence of preeclampsia or hypertensive vascular disease is present. The blood pressure returns to normotensive levels within 10 days following parturition. Some patients with gestation hypertension may in fact have preeclampsia or hypertensive vascular disease, but they do not satisfy the criteria for either of these diagnoses.
Preeclampsia	The development of hypertension with proteinuria, edema, or both, due to pregnancy or the influence of a recent pregnancy. It occurs after the 20th week of gestation, but it may develop before this time in the presence of trophoblastic disease and isoimmunization. Preeclampsia is predominantly a disorder of primigravidas.
Eclampsia	The occurrence of one or more convulsions, not attributable to other cerebral conditions such as epilepsy or cerebral hemorrhage, in a patient with preeclampsia.
Superimposed Preeclampsia or Eclampsia	The development of preeclampsia or eclampsia in a patient with chronic hypertensive vascular or renal disease. Occurs when the hypertension antedates the pregnancy, as established by previous blood pressure readings, or when there is a rise in the systolic pressure of 30 mm Hg and/or a rise in the diastolic pressure of 15 mm Hg, and the development of proteinuria or edema, or both.
Chronic Hypertensive Disease	The presence of persistent hypertension, from whatever cause, before pregnancy or before the 20th week of gestation, or persistent hypertension beyond the 42nd postpartum day.
Unclassified Hypertensive Disorders	Those in which information is insufficient for classification. They should compose a minority of the hypertensive disorders of pregnancy.

$$\text{MAP} = \text{DP} + \frac{[(\text{SP} - \text{DP})]}{3}.$$

Page and Christianson (1976) feel that a rise of 20 mm Hg in the MAP is ominous and that an MAP of 100 is "abnormal." An MAP of 105 definitely indicates hypertension. The blood pressures cited above must be manifested on two occasions at least 6 hours apart and should be judged on the basis of *previously known blood pressure levels*. Ideally, baseline blood pressures should be established early in the first trimester.

Attempts to standardize techniques for obtaining blood pressure levels have been unsuccessful. Patients in a supine poistion can develop the supine hypotensive syndrome, resulting in falsely low values. Standardization of position for recording a blood pressure should be maintained from the outpatient to the inpatient departments. Ideally, patients who have hypertension as outpatients should have their blood pressures checked in the hospital in a similar standardized fashion. There continues to be a controversy about whether Korotkoff's 5th phase (the disappearance of sound) correlates better with the true diastolic pressure than does the 4th phase (muffling). Most American authorities use the 5th phase, whereas many investigators and some clinicians use the 4th phase because the complete disappearance of sound fails to occur in many pregnant women. However, it is much more difficult to educate observers to record the 4th phase, and this difficulty is reflected in a large variance of 4th phase pressure readings; thus, this chapter will refer to the 5th phase method. Furthermore, the physiologic reduction in the mean arterial pressure during weeks 8 to 30 of gestation underlines the importance of having an accurate record of 1st-trimester blood pressure evaluations. The cuff of the sphygmomanometer can be another confounding variable in epidemiologic evaluation. The cuff must be wide enough and long enough for the blood pressure to be assessed accurately. Many other studies have called into question the sensitivity and specificity of single measurements.

Data from over 50,000 pregnancies reported by Friedman in 1976 have shown that a maternal blood pressure as low as 125/75 mm Hg is ominous if it occurs before the 32nd week of gestation or exceeds 84 mm Hg thereafter (Friedman, 1976). However, each case must be individualized, because a blood pressure level of 140/90 mm Hg in a patient whose pressure is usually 134/84 is less significant than is a pressure 140/90 mm Hg in a patient whose usual level is 110/70 mm Hg. The *degree of elevation* is more important than the absolute value.

An important feature of severe preeclampsia is the variance of *nocturnal hypertension* (Redman et al., 1976). During pregnancy there appears to be a reversal of the normal diurnal-nocturnal pattern. Normally, in the nonpregnant state, the lowest blood pressures are found during sleep; however, since in pregnancy the reverse is true, any regimen of hypotensive therapy in preeclampsia should be scheduled to have the maximum effect during the nocturnal hours of sleep, when the blood pressure is higher.

The critical blood pressure at which an individual will develop permanent vascular damage is unknown. Although direct evidence is lacking, it has been found experimentally that arterial damage can occur rapidly. In women with severe preeclampsia, examination of the optic fundi reveals segmental arteriolar constriction and dilatation that are indistinguishable from the changes observed in experimental hypertensive encephalopathy. Hypotensive agents may prevent this damage. Blood pressure levels of 170 to 180 over 110 to 120 mm Hg (mean arterial pressure of 130 to 140 mm Hg) are similar to those at which acute vascular damage occurs experimentally. A blood pressure of 160/110 is the critical level at which antihypertensive agents are needed for the urgent reduction of the blood pressure.

Unfortunately, at the present time it is not known whether suppression of hypertension ameliorates the underlying disorder; thus, the disease may progress despite antihypertensive treatment and bedrest. Therefore, even if apparent control of blood pressure has been achieved, the fetus must be monitored for uteroplacental insufficiency and the mother must continually be observed for disseminated intravascular coagulation, excessive weight gain, renal failure, and central nervous system irritability.

Edema

Edema has traditionally been described as the earliest sign of developing preeclampsia. However, edema by itself is a common concomitant of pregnancy. Edema is a general and excessive accumulation of fluid in the tissues, generally demonstrated by the swelling of the extremities and face. The fluid may be intracellular or extracellular, and edema is not usually demonstrated until there is a weight gain of 10 percent from the prepregnancy weight. Edema is usually physiologic, but when it occurs in association with hypertension and/or proteinuria, the perinatal mortality rate is increased. Edema might be a protective mechanism against the development of preeclampsia. Approximately 85 percent of patients who develop generalized edema have normal pregnancies; only about 15 percent develop preeclampsia. Edema is thus a very rough clinical parameter and can reflect changes that are nonpathologic. The Perinatal Task Force on Preeclampsia demonstrated a relatively greater incidence of edema among white (39.8 percent) than among black gravidas (23.3 percent). The perinatal mortality rate of 25.4:1000 for offspring of mothers who manifested edema alone was significantly lower than the rate of 32.8:1000 among those without edema. This relationship was observed both in white and in black gravidas. Moreover, edema and high blood pressure were unrelated in white nulliparas (Fig. 20–1). In the light of these considerations we should reassess our previous commitment to the traditional but purely arbitrary standards. Perhaps edema should be deleted from the clinical triad of preeclampsia. It is important, however, not to confuse edema with excessive weight gain (Fig. 20–2).

The concept that treating edema will prevent toxemia is invalid. In fact, the use of diuretics may be harmful. They reduce the metabolic clearance rate of dehydroisoandrosterone sulfate (MCRds) in relation to maternal weight loss. Because diuretics decrease plasma volume, the decrease in the MCRds probably reflects reduced placental perfusion (Gant et al., 1975). Both of these factors (i.e., decreased plasma volume and

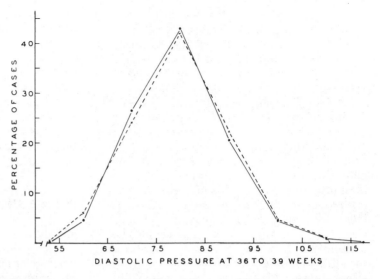

Figure 20–1. Frequency distribution of diastolic blood pressures recorded between 36 and 39 weeks in white nulliparas without proteinuria. Continuous line indicates women with edema, and broken line women without edema. (From Chesley, L. C.: Classification. *In* Friedman, E. A. (ed.): Blood Pressure, Edema and Proteinuria in Pregnancy. New York, A. R. Liss, 1976.)

reduced uteroplacental perfusion) are thought to be important in the pathogenesis of preeclampsia-eclampsia, so that administration of diuretics may actually predispose the patients to the disease. These considerations and others generally contraindicate the use of diuretics in pregnancy unless there are other compelling reasons for their use or if future research suggests benefit.

Proteinuria

Proteinuria is usually the last of the triad to appear. Proteinuria is the presence of urinary protein in concentrations greater than 300 mg/liter in a 24-hour collection, or in a concentration greater than 1+ or 2+ by standard turbidimetric methods (dipstick) on two or more occasions at least 6 hours apart. The urine must be a clean-voided midstream specimen or one obtained by catheterization. Proteinuria may be the most ominous sign of preeclampsia. A combination of 2+ proteinuria (1 g/liter) and hypertension at least doubles the perinatal mortality rate (deAlvarez, 1976). Edema with proteinuria also increases perinatal risks (Vosburgh, 1976). In the absence of contamination of the specimen, 1+ proteinuria (300 mg/liter) should be considered significant, particularly with a diastolic blood pressure of 85 mm Hg or higher.

Proteinuria may help to differentiate preeclampsia from other disorders of pregnancy. Also, quantitative and qualitative urinalyses may help to differentiate preeclampsia and eclampsia from other disorders in which proteinuria may occur. In

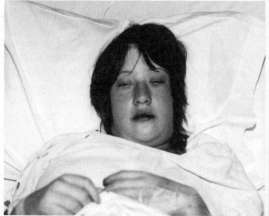
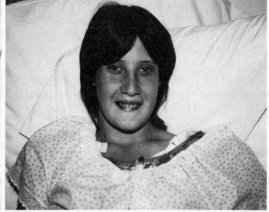

Figure 20–2. The patient (left) developed severe preeclampsia at 34 weeks' gestation. She gained 10 pounds during the week previous to her admission. She developed central edema, and shortly after this photograph was taken had a respiratory arrest. Her appearance changed markedly by her fourth day post partum (right). (Photographs courtesy of Dr. Gary Cohen, University of South Florida College of Medicine, Tampa, FL.)

orthostatic proteinuria, the commonly used 24-hour sample demonstrates 1 or 2 g per 24-hour collection, whereas the nephrotic syndrome is indicated by a loss of 10 to 15 g/day. The usual protein content in a 24-hour specimen is 0.3 to 2 g in mild preeclampsia. The greatest proteinuria occurs during the most severe episodes of the process. Proteinuria reduces the concentrations of the various serum proteins. In fractionation of the proteinuria in severe toxemia, albumin accounts for 50 to 60 percent of the total protein excreted. This may also account for hypoalbuminemia consistently below the level for a normal pregnancy of the same duration. DeAlvarez has suggested that, because of the increased loss of α_2-globulin in the urine at the height of preeclampsia, angiotensinase is lost at a greater rate than with a normal pregnancy (deAlvarez, 1976), thus supporting the vasospastic influence of angiotensin II.

INCIDENCE AND IMPORTANCE

Approximately 10 percent of Americans have hypertension. Hypertensive patients have a 25 percent chance of experiencing superimposed preeclampsia. In the United States preeclampsia complicates about 1.5 percent of pregnancies among women receiving care from private physicians. However, there is a 15 percent incidence among patients of low socioeconomic status giving birth in public and teaching hospitals. Thus, the overall rate of occurrence in the United States is approximately 5 percent. In general, preeclampsia is a disease of the first pregnancy and tends to beset women who are pregnant for the first time after the age of 25. The diagnosis may be complicated by the fact that the mean blood pressure tends to rise with increasing age. If the prepregnancy blood pressure is unknown, the differential diagnosis between preeclampsia and preeclampsia superimposed upon chronic hypertension cannot be made with certainty. Preeclampsia-eclampsia has its highest incidence among groups of women who have a high predilection for hypertension. Thus, the incidence of preeclampsia and eclampsia is always higher among blacks than among whites. Few studies, however, have corrected for the higher prevalence of essential hypertension in the black population.

Preeclampsia-eclampsia is an important entity for several reasons:
1. It is a major cause of perinatal mortality.
2. It is the second leading cause of maternal deaths in the United States.
3. It is often associated with intrauterine fetal growth retardation.
4. It is associated with an increased tendency toward mental retardation in surviving offspring.

ETIOLOGY AND PATHOGENESIS

Study of the etiology and pathogenesis of preeclampsia-eclampsia has focused on six major factors:
1. *Immunologic phenomena:* Interest in this aspect has been lacking until recently, when immunofluorescent studies identified immunoglobulins in the tissues of women with preeclampsia-eclampsia. This is the most promising research frontier for finding the etiology of preeclampsia.
2. *Dietary factors:* The geographic distribution of eclampsia suggests that diet plays an important part in the etiology. Various dietary factors have been incriminated, including deficiencies of protein, thiamine, calcium, iron, and vitamins, and excesses of carbohydrate and sodium.
3. *Endocrine dysfunction:* During normal pregnancy, enlargement of the anterior pituitary, adrenal, thyroid, and parathyroid glands occurs. Interference with hormonal activity or metabolism by the developing placenta has also been noted.
4. *Toxic manifestations:* Water intoxication and other miscellaneous agents have been incriminated.
5. *Hemodynamic hypotheses:* Preeclampsia and placenta previa rarely coexist. It has been suggested that when the placenta is implanted in the upper uterine segment, much of the venous blood returns to the heart via the ovarian veins. In traversing this route, the additional blood volume encourages congestion of the renal, hepatic, and cerebral venous systems, resulting in hypoxic changes. Another hemodynamic theory is that the cause of toxemia is hypovolemia, which leads to a hypoperfusion syndrome.

The weight of evidence suggests that hypovolemia, like disseminated intravascular coagulation (DIC), plays an important part in pathogenesis but is not the primary cause of preeclampsia-eclampsia.

6. *Uterine stretch reflex:* It has been suggested that the resistance of the myometrium to stretching initiates a uterorenal reflex and results in renal cortical ischemia. This, in turn, has been said to result in generalized vasoconstriction, with hypertension, proteinuria, and edema as the major clinical manifestations. Although this theory is appealing, because of the association between toxemia and such factors as multiple pregnancy, the weight of experimental evidence of pathogenesis is against it.

Preeclampsia has a geographic distribution that is not entirely related to the quality of obstetric care and is sometimes seen de novo in the immediate postpartum period. Misenhimer et al. reported on an experimental model of chronically impaired uterine artery flow in the rhesus monkey (Misenhimer et al., 1970). These workers did not measure blood pressure, but angiographic studies showed a marked reduction in intervillous space inflow in some animals; the fetal mortality rate was 60 percent, with all deaths occurring near the beginning of the 3rd trimester of pregnancy.

If the uteroplacental blood flow is decreased, the uterine renin-angiotensin system is activated. There is some evidence that plasma-renin levels are higher in the uterine vein than in the peripheral circulation in preeclampsia. Thus, the release of angiotensin II from the uterus, stimulated by a de-crease in uteroplacental blood flow, may possibly explain the apparent paradox of low renin-angiotensin levels in this condition.

Between 1968 and 1984, Cavanagh et al. (1974, 1977) conducted a multidisciplinary program with the aim of developing a "toxemia model" in a subhuman primate. The baboon was used in these studies because the reproductive physiology of baboons is remarkably similar to that of human subjects. When the ovarian arteries were transected in pregnant animals, hypertension, proteinuria, and reduced renal artery flow followed. The same sequelae were observed in those animals whose uterine arteries had been partially occluded by metal clips prior to conception. Subsequently, 50 percent occlusion of aortic blood flow produced the same changes. In addition, fibrin-fibrinogen deposits were detected in pregnant study animals by immunofluorescence, although no evidence of DIC could be found in those baboons whose coagulation profiles were studied. Investigations by light microscopy, electron microscopy, and immunofluorescence revealed the renal lesions in the toxemic baboon to be indistinguishable from those in women with preeclampsia-eclampsia.

In the light of present knowledge, it appears that uteroplacental ischemia is the "trigger mechanism" for initiating "toxemia," not only in the rabbit and dog but also in the primate experimental model. Im-

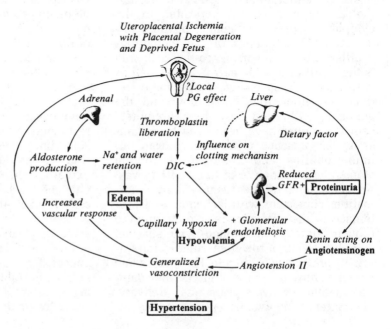

Figure 20–3. The presumed pathologic mechanism of eclamptogenic toxemia. (From Cavanagh, D., Woods, R. E., and O'Connor, T. C. F.: Obstetric Emergencies, 3rd ed. New York, Harper & Row, 1982.)

Table 20–2. Important Observations in Preeclampsia

- The trophoblast plays a role. When abundant trophoblast is present (mole, twins), there is an increased incidence of preeclampsia.
- When the placenta is removed, the disease abates.
- There is an increased risk in preexisting vascular disease.
- There is a genetic or familial predisposition.

munologic mechanisms may play a critical role. If blocking antibodies develop against antigenic sites on the placenta, the risk of pregnancy-induced hypertension is increased. Present evidence suggests that a different "mate" may make a multigravid patient react as a primigravida in regard to the risk of preeclampsia (Scott and Freeney, 1980).

Some important features in the pathogenesis of preeclampsia are presented in Figure 20–3 and Table 20–2.

PATHOLOGY

Donnelly and Lock (1954) investigated the cause of death in 533 women with toxemia of pregnancy and found that death was directly attributable to the disease in 393 cases. The most common causes of death were cerebral vascular accidents, cardiopulmonary insufficiency, and acute renal failure.

The characteristic lesion in preeclampsia-eclampsia is a renal glomerular endotheliosis. The endothelial cells are swollen, and the amorphous material deposited in the cytoplasm causes enlargement of the capillary tufts. The lumens of the glomerular capillaries become narrow, so that ischemia is the result of organic narrowing as well as vasospasm. These changes presumably reduce the glomerular blood flow and the glomerular filtration rate. Immunofluorescent techniques have been used to demonstrate the presence of fibrin-fibrinogen immunoglobulins and complement in the glomerular mesangium of the capillary vessel walls. Renal tubules usually show abnormalities consistent with ischemia, and proteinaceous material often is noted within the tubular lumens. In women who survive, complete repair of the glomerular lesion following pregnancy is the rule. However, some patients show evidence of glomerular damage months or even years after delivery. Severe renal involvement may produce ex-

tensive arterial thrombosis resulting in bilateral renal cortical necrosis. This is especially likely to occur in patients with preeclampsia-eclampsia complicated by abruptio placentae.

Significant liver damage may occur in pregnancy-induced hypertension. In eclampsia, about 75 percent of the patients show some evidence of hepatic dysfunction, but permanent damage is rare. The most common hepatic lesion in the eclamptic patient is periportal hemorrhagic necrosis; this may extend toward the center of the hepatic lobule. The surrounding blood sinuses may be compressed. In some areas, extravasation may occur and fibrin clots may form, especially at the bases of the liver cell columns. These changes are believed to result from thrombosis in the hepatic arterioles. Hemorrhage under the capsule of the liver may occur in severe preeclampsia-eclampsia, and the associated intraabdominal bleeding presents an acute surgical emergency.

In 1976, Arias and Mancilla-Jimenez reported immunofluorescent evidence of fibrin-fibrinogen, immunoglobulins, and complement in the livers of patients with preeclampsia-eclampsia. Fibrin-fibrinogen deposits of immunoglobulins G and M (IgG, IgM) and of the heat-stable component of complement (C3) are found in areas of necrosis. These investigators postulated that changes in the liver and kidneys in patients with toxemia were due to generalized vasospasm. They pointed out that the increased vasospasm, in the presence of systemic blood hypercoagulability, would create adequate local conditions for the precipitation of fibrin-fibrinogen.

In patients who die of eclampsia, there is almost always evidence of pulmonary edema and diffuse hemorrhagic bronchopneumonia. In the mycoardium, subendothelial hemorrhages, fibrin thrombi, and focal necroses may be found. The latter changes are sometimes so severe as to cause discoloration in the heart. This damage helps to explain the related pathophysiologic changes, such as impaired cardiac reserve, arrhythmias, and rapid pulse.

Histologic changes in the placenta reveal signs of premature aging, syncytial degeneration, and congestion of the intervillous spaces. Degeneration and thrombosis of the spiral arterioles in the decidua indicate an acute atheroma. Red infarction is a typical gross lesion in the placenta, being present in about 60 percent of the cases. The spiral arteries undergo hyperplasia and hypertrophy, as do all major uterine vessels during pregnancy. These histologic and physiologic changes allow normal development for the majority of fetuses whose mothers suffer from preeclampsia. It has been hypothesized that in this condition the implantation, for some unknown reason, is superficial and not interstitial as in normal pregnancy, and this leads to defective development of the placental vascular bed (Brosens et al., 1967).

MANAGEMENT

The obstetric team always treats two patients: the mother and the fetus. The most definitive treatment for preeclampsia-eclampsia is termination of the pregnancy. All other treatment is supportive, the main objective being to ensure maternal and fetal well-being.

The rate of maternal mortality in preeclampsia is low. However, the risks of maternal death from eclampsia are appreciable, especially when cerebral hemorrhage, pulmonary edema, or repeated seizures occur. Long-term follow-up studies have failed to implicate preeclampsia and eclampsia as significant factors in the development of subsequent cardiovascular or renal disease.

Naeye and Friedman, reviewing information from the Collaborative Perinatal Project, found a twofold increase in perinatal mortality rates among women with hypertension and proteinuria (diastolic blood pressure higher than 85 mm Hg and proteinuria of 1 + or more) as compared with normotensive patients without proteinuria (Naeye and Friedman, 1979). The excessive perinatal mortality rate was due to placental infarcts, placental growth retardation, and abruption

of the placenta. These data emphasize the need for continuous assessment of the fetal reserve and the evaluation of abrupt changes in maternal status.

Often preeclampsia cannot be prevented, but it is possible to select groups of patients who are particularly prone to develop it and to monitor those patients carefully for predisposing factors and early signs of the disease. Table 20–3 lists those conditions that predispose to preeclampsia.

OUTPATIENT ANTEPARTUM CARE

The blood pressure should be checked at each prenatal visit with the patient in the sitting position. The systolic and 4th and 5th phases of Korotkoff should be recorded. A significant rise in blood pressure usually indicates developing preeclampsia. A mean arterial pressure in excess of 92 mm Hg during the second trimester is a good indicator that the patient will subsequently develop preeclampsia. However, in many patients the mean arterial pressure does not attain this level in the second trimester, and hypertension may develop rapidly without premonitory symptoms. The need for a test to detect patients who will develop preeclampsia is obvious. The "roll-over test," or a modification of the same, may serve this need (Table 20–4). The roll-over test has not met with universal application, primarily because of its difficult requisites.

Gant and coworkers (1974) found that patients in whom the roll-over test was positive were very sensitive to angiotensin infusion. They also found that 98 percent of these patients subsequently developed preeclampsia, whereas 91 percent of the patients in whom the test was negative did not become hypertensive. Gusdon and colleagues (1977), however, were more conservative in their assessment of the test. They found that only

Table 20–3. Conditions That Predispose to Preeclampsia*

Nulliparity
Multiple pregnancy
Hydatidiform mole
Chronic hypertension
Chronic renal disease
Diabetes mellitus
Hydrops fetalis
Malnutrition

*The first three factors are beyond the control of the obstetrician, but meticulous control of the remaining ones, with frequent hospitalization when necessary, will help to decrease the adverse effects of this disease.

Table 20–4. Roll-Over Test

Procedure
1. Measure blood pressure in the lateral recumbent position until stable
2. Roll patient to supine position
3. Measure blood pressure immediately
4. Repeat blood pressure in 5 minutes

Positive test—An increase of 20 mm Hg or more in the diastolic pressure at the 5-minute reading

Negative test—Less than a 20 mm Hg rise in diastolic blood pressure at the 5-minute reading

a negative test was accurate in predicting the failure to develop preeclampsia. Pregnancy-induced hypertension is insidious, and its subtle changes are often missed. However, progression to the severe forms of the disease should be preventable. Good prenatal observation is necessary for the success of the treatment of pregnancy-induced hypertension. It is important for the nurse and physician to observe subtle changes and to screen for patients with a potential for this disease. Any patient of greater than 20 weeks' gestation with the predisposing criteria should be seen once or twice a week, and a roll-over test should be performed between the 28th and 32nd week of gestation (Zuspan, 1980; O'Shaughnessy and Zuspan, 1981).

Some authors have suggested that once the diagnosis of preeclampsia has been made, the patient should be hospitalized (Zuspan, 1980; Cavanagh and Knuppel, 1982). Others have suggested that *selected* patients could be managed on an outpatient basis (Pritchard, 1980; Zuspan, 1980). Patients managed on an outpatient basis must maintain a diastolic blood pressure no greater than 85 mm Hg and have a good knowledge of the signs and symptoms of their disease, a home environment conducive to bedrest, and the opportunity to be examined twice a week. However, hospitalization is recommended for most of these patients.

If the patient can be examined only once a week, a visiting nurse could observe the patient at home during the week. These patients should follow a good diet with increased protein and no added salt (salt restriction is not necessary [Zuspan, 1980]), and should rest at mid-day for 1½ hours. If the roll-over test is positive, the bedrest should be increased, even if the patient is asymptomatic. Once the diagnosis of pregnancy-induced hypertension has been made, the patient should be examined weekly or twice a week for signs of the following:

1. Increased blood pressure (when increased, the blood pressure should be taken again in 15 minutes and both the high and low readings should be recorded).
2. Proteinuria.
3. Increased deep tendon reflexes.
4. Increased weight.
5. Increased edema.
6. Increased hematocrit and hemoglobin.
7. Visual changes.
8. Reduced fundal growth.

Weekly nonstress testing (NST)/contraction stress testing (CST) should be started at 30 to 32 weeks' gestation to observe for fetal compromise. A sonogram should be performed every 4 weeks to serially measure fetal growth, and an amniocentesis should be carried out at 33 weeks for an L/S ratio to assess fetal maturity in case delivery is indicated. An oral glucose tolerance test should be performed, as diabetic patients have a higher incidence of preeclampsia than does the normal population.

Since decreased peripheral resistance during pregnancy lowers the blood pressure, it is important that serial blood pressure with baseline values be established. Also, it is imperative to have good gestational dating through the use of early pregnancy testing, early ultrasound, auscultation of the fetal heart sounds with a DeLee stethoscope at 18 to 20 weeks, documentation of quickening, and a good menstrual history. The patient must also realize that although she may feel better, the disease will only be controlled, not cured, with this home regimen. The regimen should be continued despite abatement of symptoms. Strict bedrest in the left lateral position and good nutrition are necessary for outpatient management. However, with clinical improvement, allowance of some patient activity to encourage compliance has been suggested.

If the patient is noncompliant, is not stable on the home management program, or if a proper surveillance program does not exist, she should be hospitalized. We recommend hospitalization for the vast majority of our patients.

INPATIENT ANTEPARTUM CARE

The patient should be hospitalized if she demonstrates *any* of the following signs or symptoms:

1) A blood pressure of 140/90 mm Hg on two readings, 6 hours apart (home blood pressure monitoring can help).
2) A systolic increase of 30 mm Hg; on two readings, 6 hours apart at bedrest.
3) A diastolic increase of 15 mm Hg on two readings, 6 hours apart at bedrest.
4) Proteinuria of 3 g/liter in a 24-hour urine collection, or 1 g/liter in at least two random samples, 6 hours apart (5 grams of protein demonstrates severe preeclampsia, or 3+ or 4+ proteinuria on a dipstick).

Expectant management is appropriate in mild cases of preeclampsia when it may permit further fetal development. Most obstetric centers in the United States prefer to hospitalize all patients with diagnosed preeclampsia. Immediate evaluation for assessment of fetal maturity is performed on admission if the patient is of greater than 33 weeks' gestational age. If the preeclampsia worsens, the liberal use of magnesium sulfate is instituted to prevent convulsion, and delivery is initiated.

Once hospitalized, the patient is put on bedrest with bathroom privileges. The lateral recumbent position is advisable because it avoids compression of the vena cava and aorta and improves renal function by increasing the cardiac output. This increases the glomerular filtration rate and should increase urinary output. Bedrest is also beneficial to the fetus by increasing uterine profusion. The patient's room should be arranged to enhance maintenance of this positioning. For example, facing the wall could become boring, whereas facing the television or visitors will result in better patient compliance. The patient should be kept in a quiet, dimly lit private room, or a well-selected semiprivate room. A semiprivate room allows availability of another person to call for a nurse if the patient should have a seizure. The blood pressure should be taken at least twice during an 8-hour shift. To be most effective, the width of the blood pressure cuff should be 20 percent greater than the diameter of the limb, and the length of the cuff should be 1.2 times the limb diameter. Since there are standard cuff sizes, choose the one closest to the above dimensions. A cuff that is too small may give a falsely high reading (Wheeler and Jones, 1981). Do not measure blood pressure while the patient is in the supine position.

Daily weights should be performed in the hospital, as this is a good indicator of fluid retention. An increase of 1 to 1½ pounds per day may indicate fluid retention. For a more accurate measurement, the patient should be weighed at the same time daily, using the same scale. The patient will usually have physiologic diuresis within 36 to 48 hours following hospitalization with bedrest. The weight can decrease as much as 4 to 9 lb during the next 3- to 5-day period.

Serial weekly hematocrits should be obtained and compared to any hematocrits obtained early in pregnancy. An increase in the hematocrit indicates that more fluid has moved from the blood vessels to the interstitial tissue as edema (indicating worsening of the disease). A decrease in the hematocrit shows fluid moving from the tissues back into the bloodstream, thereby diluting the red blood cells, which indicates an improvement in the disease. A complete blood chemistry should be done for proper assessment, including a DIC screen and liver enzyme evaluations.

Intake and output should be measured every 8 hours. Oliguria occurs as pregnancy-induced hypertension worsens. The excess fluid is not excreted. This overloads the vascular system and further stresses the heart. The fluid may move from the circulation into the interstitial space (Wheeler and Jones, 1981).

A urine specimen should be tested daily for protein, and if it is greater than 1+ with a dipstick, a 24-hour collection should be obtained. If the 24-hour urine collection shows more than 300 mg of protein, it should be repeated within the next 24 hours. Contamination of the urine with amniotic fluid and blood will increase the protein content. If this presents a problem, a catheterized specimen is recommended. No casts or cells should be seen on microscopic examination of the urine. The normal plasma uric acid should be within normal limits (3.5 to 7 mg/100 ml).

A 24-hour urine collection for creatinine clearance, to test renal function, should be done weekly (normal = 150 cc/min). However, a serum creatinine may be a more sensitive test and is more easily obtained. A 24-hour urine collection should begin at a specific time and continue to that same time the following day, e.g., 6 AM to 6 AM. The first void at 6 AM should be discarded, and the last void at 6 AM the following day should be collected. The urine for a creatinine clearance must be refrigerated or cooled on ice during the collection.

Deep tendon reflexes and vital signs should be checked every 4 to 8 hours while the patient is in the hospital. If the patient is stable, the midnight to early morning vital signs can be eliminated, to allow the patient more rest. When the nurse checks the patient's vital signs, assessment should be made for the patient's general appearance, alertness, condition of skin, edema (especially of the face, hands, and feet), and reflexes.

The patient is kept on a regular diet with

good protein and caloric intake. (This may be a definite improvement from outpatient care.) Salt and fluids should neither be encouraged nor restricted.

Brewer has written extensively on the importance of good nutrition in reducing the tendency to hypovolemia and a hypoperfusion state (Brewer, 1970, 1975, 1976). In a group of 7000 underprivileged patients in whom particular attention was paid to nutrition, he reported a toxemia rate of 0.55 percent, with no cases of eclampsia. A nutritionist is an integral part of the team.

Patients are not kept on large doses of sedatives, as it is hard to evaluate the patient's condition when she is heavily sedated. Moreover, sedatives do not adequately prevent seizure activity. The oversedated patient may not be able to control her bodily functions, clear her airway, or verbalize pain, visual disturbances, contractions, and so forth. Since the sedatives cross the placenta, the fetus, who might already be stressed, may also be oversedated. A nonreactive nonstress test may result.

Since strict bedrest may improve urine output and decrease the edema, the blood pressure may decline and the patient's general condition and circulatory status may improve. It is a widely accepted policy, therefore, to avoid induction of labor during the first 24 to 36 hours, even in relatively severe cases, if fetal immaturity exists. When the preeclampsia is mild and the improvement is sustained, it is reasonable to postpone induction of labor until fetal lung maturity has occurred. In such cases, amniocentesis may need to be performed to determine fetal lung maturity, as measured by (1) an L/S ratio greater than 2.0, and (2) presence of phosphatidylglycerol.

Under these conditions, the pregnancy may be continued if the maternal status remains improved, the fetoplacental function is stable, and the fetus has not reached the stage of lung maturity. However, worsening of the clinical signs (Table 20–5) warrants intervention irrespective of the stage of fetal maturity.

Bioelectric monitoring of the fetal reserve is accomplished with an NST. Any change in maternal status requires prompt reevaluation of the fetus. If the maternal status is satisfactory and there is evidence of fetal reactivity, the test may be repeated once a week. However, if the nonstress test is not reassuring, a contraction stress test is indi-

Table 20–5. Signs and Symptoms of Worsening Pregnancy-Induced Hypertension

Increased edema (weight gain)
Headache
Epigastric pain
Visual disturbance
Increased hematocrit
Decreased urinary output
Increased blood pressure
Increased proteinuria
Decreased creatinine clearance
Increased serum creatinine

cated. If the NST is nonreactive and the CST is positive, induction still may be attempted if the condition of the cervix and the station of the vertex permit rupturing of the membranes and the application of a scalp electrode without difficulty. In the presence of a nonreactive NST and a positive CST, in cases in which it is not possible to evaluate the fetus by direct bioelectric monitoring, cesarean section should be strongly considered.

Prior to the days of cost-containment, the experience of academic and public institutions, as well as that of Armed Forces dependents' units, supported without question the use of hospitalization with limited activity as the primary component of the care of the preeclamptic patient. These experiences certainly raise doubts as to the validity and effectiveness of using sophisticated techniques for evaluating fetal or placental reserve. The data of Parkland Hospital (Hauth et al., 1976) confirm the value of hospitalization among their 346 hypertensive gravidas, 50 percent of whom showed edema, with only 14 percent demonstrating proteinuria. These patients received a normal diet without sedation, antihypertensive therapy, or the use of diuretics. They were allowed free ambulation. Eighty-one percent of these patients became normotensive before delivery.

The perinatal mortality rate was 9:1000, as compared with 129:1000 for those who left the hospital against medical advice. No patient with any of the following symptoms was ever admitted directly to this unit: diastolic blood pressure of 110 mm Hg or greater, significant proteinuria (2 + or more), headaches, scotomas, and epigastric pain. These patients were managed as severe preeclamptics (see below).

The same group (Gilstrap et al., 1978) reported equally satisfactory results among 576 nulliparous gestational hypertensive patients with single pregnancies. The blood pressure was taken 4 times daily, urine dipsticks and weight were checked 3 times weekly, and creatinine clearance and fetal growth (sonography) were monitored weekly. The investigators measured the L/S ratio of the amniotic fluid but performed no bioelectric fetal assessment. Spontaneous labor and delivery at term were permitted unless there was evidence of deterioration of the patient's condition at bedrest. The earlier experiences, as well as these and other recent reports (Fleigner, 1976), raise serious questions as to whether prompt delivery of the mild preeclamptic patient offers the best solution for the mother and the fetus. Certainly, the conservative management described above reduces the rate of prematurity and its associated high incidence of neonatal mortality.

Severe preeclampsia should not be managed expectantly. These patients should be placed at bedrest and given hydralazine intravenously to maintain the diastolic pressure at approximately 100 mm Hg. Magnesium sulfate should be used liberally. While the preeclamptic patient is being observed closely for signs of neuromuscular hyperexcitability, the fetus should also be evaluated for loss of fetal reserve (NST or CST). After the condition of the severe preeclamptic patient has been stabilized in the hospital, termination of pregnancy is indicated in the interest of both the mother and the fetus. A Foley catheter is inserted to determine hourly urine excretion for an accurate record of intake and output.

INTRAPARTUM CARE

When fetal maturity has been reached, further procrastination serves no useful purpose, unless the patient has been stable for a prolonged period of time (Knuppel and Montenegro, 1985). The mode of delivery will be established by the condition of the patient, her cervix, and the fetal-placental unit. If the cervix is favorable for induction and the mother and fetus are stable, induction is preferable, with use of oxytocin and (circumstances permitting) artificial rupture of the membranes. With an uninducible cervix, or with a very premature or distressed fetus, a cesarean section is advisable. This approach is particularly desirable when the estimated fetal weight is less than 1500

grams. When the blood pressure cannot be controlled, or the weight gain continues at bedrest, or proteinuria increases, the patient is delivered regardless of fetal age or lung maturity (Table 20–6). This approach is justifiable even when the gravida is less than 30 weeks pregnant, because it is in this group of patients that ominous maternal sequelae are particularly prone to occur.

MEDICATIONS

The medications that may be used for treatment of preeclampsia-eclampsia are summarized in Table 20–15, at the end of this chapter. The most frequently used medications are highlighted here.

Hydralazine (Apresoline) acts by causing arteriolar vasodilatation. It also increases cardiac output and renal blood flow; appreciable blood pressure reduction usually occurs with an oral dose of 100 mg/day in 4 divided doses. A recent observation suggests that the administration of the same daily dose in 2 doses is equally effective for blood pressure control in many patients. Hydralazine is completely absorbed after oral administration; peak serum concentrations are obtained within 1 to 2 hours. Intravenous injections reach a peak effectiveness in 15 to 20 minutes. Therefore, adequate reduction

Table 20–6. Hospitalized Patients: Indications for Delivery Despite Fetal Prematurity

Rapid weight gain at bedrest
Blood pressure progressively elevates at bedrest
Premonitory symptoms of eclampsia
Increasing proteinuria
IUGR diagnosed with lung maturity
Impaired liver function
Thrombocytopenia

Management Schema

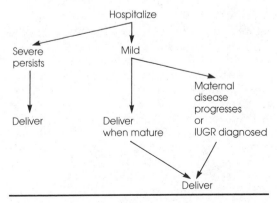

of high diastolic blood pressures should be achieved by repeating the appropriate dose every 10 to 15 minutes. One may prefer a 5-mg initial IV bolus and repeat it in 15 to 20 minutes if there is no response. Alternatively, hydralazine may be given slowly by continuous intravenous infusion: 20 to 40 mg in 1000 ml 5 percent dextrose with 0.45 percent saline. The rate of infusion of the intravenous fluid should be titrated to the patient's blood pressure. The latter should be stabilized at a level consistent with an adequate urinary output (100 to 110 mm Hg diastolic). The fetal heart rate should be monitored carefully during administration of hydralazine, since a sudden fall in blood pressure may cause severe fetal hypoxia. The most common side effect is tachycardia, which may be severe and may occasionally progress to arrhythmias; this effect may be abolished by the intravenous administration of propranolol. Hydralazine is a very valuable drug for the treatment of hypertension associated with toxemia, but chronic administration in doses exceeding 200 mg/day can lead to an acute rheumatoid state, which, when fully developed, gives rise to a syndrome resembling disseminated lupus erythematosus.

Diazoxide (Hyperstat), administered IV as a 300-mg dose, is effective in treating acute hypertensive states. However, since it may cause sudden and irreversible hypotension, which can produce severe fetal hypoxia, it is not the treatment of choice (Neuman et al., 1979). Maternal death has occurred from the administration of 5 mg per kilogram of body weight.

Magnesium sulfate ($MgSO_4 \cdot 7\ H_2O$) has for over 50 years been the cornerstone of treatment for severe preeclampsia. Its main effect is at the neuromuscular junction. It is administered when preeclampsia displays a progressive tendency.

To prevent seizures, $MgSO_4$ can be administered intravenously or intramuscularly. Intravenous administration is preferable because of the rapid achievement of appropriate magnesium levels in the blood and for patient comfort. When $MgSO_4$ is given intravenously, usually a 4-g loading dose is administered over 15 minutes, followed by 1 to 2 g per hour (Gant, 1980), administered by a constant infusion pump in a "piggyback" fashion. Usually 1 g is given per 100 cc of D5W. If the dose is kept constant at 2 g/hour, the concentration of $MgSO_4$ should

be increased, not the fluid volume. If the nursing staff is unable to monitor the patient and the IV infusion adequately, it is beneficial to give the $MgSO_4$ intramuscularly, as described in the next paragraph.

Deep intramuscular injection of $MgSO_4$ is given "Z-track" in the upper outer quadrant of the buttocks with a 3-inch, 20-gauge needle. It is very painful, and 1 ml of lidocaine may be added to the syringe after the $MgSO_4$ (Gant and Worley, 1980). One-half cc of air should be at the end of the plunger to ensure that the needle is cleared of all medication when injected. The patient should be alerted to the pain of the injection so that she is not startled, which could lead to seizure activity. The intramuscular loading dose is 10 g; 5 g injected into each buttocks, then 5 g every 4 hours, alternating hips. If the dose lapses for more than 6 hours, the loading dose should be given again (Gant and Worley, 1980). With the initial loading dose of $MgSO_4$, the patient may experience nausea and vomiting. She may also feel flushed and state that she "feels hot all over."

Chesley demonstrated that after an initial IV dose of 3 mg magnesium sulfate followed by 10 mg IM, the average peak serum level at 60 minutes was 4.5 mEq/liter, and that at the end of 4 hours the accumulative renal excretions ranged from 38 to 53 percent of the injected dose (Chesley, 1979). The conclusion from this study was that the initial dose is safe even in anuric patients. However, repeated doses may not be safe.

Constant supervision, with a minimum 1:2 nurse–patient ratio, should be provided for the preeclamptic patient receiving $MgSO_4$. These patients should be given the same care as patients in any other intensive care unit, since pregnancy-induced hypertension is associated with high maternal and perinatal mortality rates (Wheeler and Jones, 1981). Mild preeclampsia warrants at least a 1:2 nurse–patient ratio; severe preeclampsia requires a 1:1 nurse–patient ratio.

The dose of $MgSO_4$ should be withheld if the patient's reflexes are absent, if the respiratory rate is depressed (lower than 10–14/min), or if the urinary output is less than 30 cc/hour, or 100 cc in 4 hours (Chesley, 1979). This assessment must be made prior to each dose of $MgSO_4$. Since the standard intravenous dose is 1 g per hour, assessment should be done every hour.

$MgSO_4$ is used to control seizures—it is

not an antihypertensive. However, there may be a transient decrease in the blood pressure for the first 60 minutes, owing to the vaso-dilatation and relaxation of the smooth muscle. $MgSO_4$ may increase cerebral blood flow, urinary output, and the uterine blood flow by decreasing the spasms of the vessels to the uterus and intervillous space. $MgSO_4$ may also cause uterine activity to decrease, and labor augmentation may be necessary.

$MgSO_4$ is excreted through the kidneys. If the patient has an increase in output, an increase in the dose of $MgSO_4$ may be necessary. If the output decreases, a lower dose may be necessary. Impaired renal function may also necessitate a lower dose of $MgSO_4$.

Rarely does a patient convulse if she has received therapeutic levels of magnesium sulfate as described above. Experimental studies have failed to conclusively demonstrate the primary nervous system effect of parenterally administered magnesium. This has resulted in the controversial speculation that the anticonvulsant effect of magnesium is merely masking the clinical convulsions by neuromuscular blockade. Borges and Gucer determined the effects of intravenously infused magnesium sulfate on the epileptic neuroactivity induced by the topical application of penicillin in anesthetized cats and dogs and in awake, undrugged primates (Borges and Gucer, 1978). Magnesium sulfate was able to suppress directly neuronal burst firing and electroencephalographic spike generation at serum levels below those producing paralysis. There was a direct relation between serum-magnesium concentrations and suppression of spike generation. The effect was reversible.

Although newer anticonvulsants have been introduced for the management of convulsive disorders, magnesium sulfate has remained the medication of choice for the prevention and treatment of eclamptic convulsions. As the levels of $MgSO_4$ reach their therapeutic dose of 6 to 7 mEq/liter, the deep tendon reflexes decrease at 4 mEq/liter, and may be absent when levels approach 10 mEq/liter. At 5 mEq/liter, cardiac conduction is prolonged, as measured by the P-R interval and the QRS restoration. Occasional instances of complete heart block have been reported at levels below 10 mEq/liter. Excessive levels of magnesium will block muscular transmission by decreasing the amount of acetylcholine released in response to nerve action potential. Calcium antagonizes this effect. At a level above 10 mEq/liter, an additional hazard is respiratory paralysis, which can be counterbalanced by the administration of calcium salts. Magnesium poisoning is characterized by a sharp drop in blood pressure and by respiratory paralysis. Artificial respiration should be administered until calcium salts can be injected intravenously.

As an antagonist to $MgSO_4$, 1 g of calcium gluconate is administered intravenously over 3 minutes (10 ml of a 10 percent solution) (Gant and Worley, 1980). There is usually a good response to the calcium unless the reaction is severe enough to cause cardiac arrest.

Hypermagnesemia in the newborn has not been correlated with maternal or fetal magnesium levels. In normal pregnancy the maternal and cord serum levels of magnesium are identical. Pritchard has shown that after parenteral administration of magnesium sulfate to normal and preeclamptic women, there is delayed increase in the concentration of fetal magnesium. Chesley and Tepper reported that, using usual doses, the fetal level reaches 90 percent of maternal concentrations in 3 hours (Chesley and Tepper, 1957).

Barbiturates act as sedatives and anticonvulsants. They cross the placenta rapidly and should not be given if delivery is imminent. Phenobarbital does not prevent convulsions. After an isolated seizure, 0.25 to 0.5 g amylbarbitol (sodium amytal) is effective when given by slow intravenous injection; however, $MgSO_4$ may be the drug of choice in the emergency situation, as sodium amytal must be reconstituted to use.

Diazepam (Valium) possesses an anticonvulsant effect when given intravenously; it stops convulsions quickly, but its effect may last only 20 minutes. Convulsions in adults usually stop after one or two 5-mg injections, but 20 mg or more may be required. Since the drug crosses the placenta and the neonate cannot excrete the drug readily, toxic levels have been detected in the infant as long as 3 weeks after delivery. Twelve minutes after maternal intravenous injection of diazepam, concentrations of the drug in the umbilical cord and the maternal plasma are equal. Valium is primarily recommended for postpartum eclampsia.

Mannitol may cause a fluid overload. The role of diuretics should be limited to patients with proved pulmonary edema. Acute pulmonary edema is a common cause of death and should be handled as a very serious medical emergency in an intensive care unit. The treatment involves the administration of oxygen, morphine, and digitalis (digoxin).

Furosemide (Lasix) is very useful in treating pulmonary edema; however, theoretical objections have been raised to its use in preeclampsia-eclampsia–induced pulmonary edema, since increased peripheral resistance and systemic hypertension may lead to left ventricular failure and pulmonary edema. Therefore, under ideal circumstances the use of furosemide and the infusion of colloid or crystallized solutions should be governed by the pulmonary artery wedge pressure.

Digitalization should be considered if signs of congestive heart failure develop. Electrocardiography (ECG) should be performed to determine whether any contraindication to its use exists. Initially, 0.6 mg lanatoside C is given intravenously for tachycardia above 120. Digitalization is maintained with 0.25 to 0.5 mg digoxin daily. Maintenance of a patent airway may require an endotracheal tube. Tracheostomy may be necessary in case of laryngeal obstruction.

PATIENT MANAGEMENT

Persistently symptomatic patients, particularly those with severe preeclampsia demonstrating a diastolic pressure of 110 mm Hg or greater, severe proteinuria (3 +), oliguria, pulmonary edema, and cyanosis, should be cared for in a quiet, darkened room with a 1:1 nurse–patient ratio (Table 20–7). A supportive person should attend the patient; however, visitors should be limited. All observations must be recorded carefully on flow sheets. Observe for signs and symptoms of impending eclampsia (Table 20–8).

Table 20–8. Signs and Symptoms of Impending Eclampsia

Scotomata or blurred vision
Epigastric pain
Persistent or severe headache
Vomiting
Neurologic hyperactivity
Pulmonary edema or cyanosis

fully on flow sheets. Observe for signs and symptoms of impending eclampsia (Table 20–8).

Vital signs, including respirations, pulse, blood pressure, and fetal heart rate, should be monitored every 15 minutes while the patient is receiving $MgSO_4$. The fetal heart rate should be monitored closely. Since uterine perfusion is already compromised, persistent late decelerations and fetal acidosis can be anticipated. Abrupt changes in the fetal heart rate have been demonstrated during convulsions (Vink et al., 1980). Uterine activity should be documented with an intrauterine pressure catheter and assessed every hour. If oxytocin is administered, assessment should be made every 15 minutes (Wheeler and Jones, 1981; Butts, 1965). Since these patients will be NPO and will be mouth breathing during labor, they should have good mouth care.

Fetal monitoring should be started, preferably with an internal monitor. If fetal monitoring is not available, the fetal heart rate should be assessed every 15 minutes during the first stage of labor, and every 5 to 15 minutes during the second stage. The fetal heart rate should be listened to during the last half of the contraction and for 30 seconds after the end of the contraction (Wheeler and Jones, 1981). If the patient has severe preeclampsia, a Swan-Ganz pulmonary artery catheter should be used to accurately assess blood pressure, volume, and cardiac output. However, a central venous pressure (CVP) catheter is most commonly used to assess fluid replacement and intravascular volume. A urinary catheter with a urimeter should be inserted to measure hourly output. Fluid intake should also be monitored hourly. The patient's fluid intake should be limited, but if hypovolemia occurs, it requires careful correction. Aggressive fluid infusion may produce circulatory overload, since in eclampsia the intravascular compartment is reduced significantly. The fluid intake for 24 hours should not exceed 1000 ml plus the amount of urinary output of the preceding 24 hours. If the

Table 20–7. Patient Management Basics When Maternal Disease or Severe Preeclampsia Persists

1. 1:1 nurse–patient ratio
2. $MgSO_4$ administered to prevent convulsions
3. Hydralazine given to keep diastolic blood pressure <110 mm Hg
4. Type and cross-match and CBC
5. DIC profile
6. Fetal monitoring
7. Urimeter
8. CVP line if indicated
9. Intake and output (hourly)
10. Blood pressure every 15 to 30 minutes
11. Liver enzymes
12. Eclampsia tray at bedside

patient is severely hypovolemic and in shock, when proved with monitoring of the circulatory pressure by the CVP line or Swan-Ganz catheter, additional fluid is recommended. Blood replacement (packed red blood cells), if required, should be initiated early in eclamptic patients. However, precautions should be observed to prevent overloading of the cardiovascular system. Oliguria is a common consequence of eclampsia and indicates the need for prompt termination of pregnancy. Diuretics may mask the intensity of the hypovolemia and oliguria.

The urine should have a specific gravity of at least 1.018 and should be yellow. Zuspan (1980) has noted that "severe preeclampsia occasionally causes hemolysis manifested by either jaundice or dark-colored urine, which probably represents hepatocellular damage and red blood cell destruction." This is usually an ominous sign. Sometimes hematuria is found with the administration of $MgSO_4$. The etiology is unknown.

An eclampsia tray (Table 20–9) should be kept at the *bedside* during the antepartum hospitalization, the intrapartum period, and in the recovery room. It should include: needles, syringes, an airway, and a padded tongue blade to be carefully inserted between the jaws to protect the tongue. Calcium gluconate should be included in case of $MgSO_4$ overdose. Sodium amylbarbital can be included to stop seizures. Since $MgSO_4$ potentiates it, the dose should be less than 0.25 to 0.5 g (Cavanagh and Knuppel, 1982). However, sodium amylbarbital must be reconstituted. In an emergency $MgSO_4$ is more readily available. From 4 to 6 g should be administered slowly by the intravenous route over 3 to 4 minutes (Cavanagh and Knuppel, 1982).

Because of the use of $MgSO_4$, and also depending on the fetal condition, a pediatrician or neonatologist should attend the birth of the baby of a preeclamptic or eclamptic mother.

Table 20–9. Items for a Preeclampsia Tray

Needles
Syringes
An airway
Padded tongue blade
Calcium gluconate—two 1-cc vials
Sodium amylbarbital—two 1-cc vials
$MgSO_4$
Suction and O_2 should be available

ECLAMPSIA

Eclampsia represents the convulsive phase of preeclampsia. Eclampsia is more prevalent among patients who had inadequate antenatal care and in those who have had unsuspected deterioration of the maternal status during the early puerperium. Approximately 5 percent of preeclamptic patients will become eclamptic. Earlier diagnosis, skillful prenatal care, and careful management of preeclampsia are capable of reducing the incidence of eclampsia and, thus, the accompanying maternal and perinatal risks. The worldwide perinatal mortality rate associated with eclampsia may be as high as 30 to 35 percent. Eclampsia is seldom encountered in patients who have received appropriate antenatal care and were hospitalized promptly when preeclampsia first became evident.

Assessment should be made when seizures occur, with notation of the onset of the seizure, the progress of the seizure, the body involvement, and the length of the convulsion. Usually the convulsion begins with facial twitching, and then the head turns to one side, with the neck tense and the eyes staring. During the seizure the patient should be protected from injury. Tongue blades should be used to protect the tongue. Padding of the side rails of the bed has also been recommended. To break the seizure, 4 g of $MgSO_4$ is administered over 5 minutes. Sodium amylbarbital has also been used; however, this requires reconstitution, which may be difficult at the time of an emergency.

During a convulsion there may be fetal bradycardia. If possible, allow the mother and fetus to recover before delivery. This stress may decrease the length of labor and precipitate delivery (Pritchard, 1980). It is important to give constant nursing care (1:1 nurse–patient ratio) to assess fetal and maternal status and to avoid precipitous delivery, which has a risk of laceration and increased bleeding.

After the seizure, routine observations are imperative. The maternal lungs are checked frequently, as acute pulmonary edema is common in eclamptic patients. A detailed intake and output chart must be available, with the amounts recorded hourly. Blood should be obtained immediately for typing and cross-matching with a baseline hematocrit.

It may be necessary to establish a patent airway and administer oxygen. A nasogastric tube may be used to empty the patient's stomach and instill 30 cc of antacid. After delivery, coughing, turning, deep breathing, and IPPB treatments may be needed to prevent aspiration pneumonia. If the patient's electrolytes are abnormal, the IV may have to be changed to a more physiologic solution, perhaps D5/normal saline. Monitor the vital signs every 5 minutes until stable, and then every 15 minutes, observing lab work and $MgSO_4$ as before. The patient should be encouraged to stay on her left side, to increase urinary excretion and uterine perfusion and to prevent aspiration of saliva and nasopharyngeal secretions.

To decrease the patient's agitation and confusion, a family member should be at the bedside as she regains consciousness. Continue to avoid bright lights, noises, and numerous people at the bedside. Also try to organize care to avoid frequent disturbances.

The number of convulsions may vary from 1 or two to as many as 10 or 20. "The duration of coma after the seizure is variable. When the convulsions are infrequent, the woman usually recovers some degree of consciousness after each seizure. As the woman arouses, a semiconscious combative state may ensue. In severe cases, the coma persists from one convulsion to another, and death may result before the mother awakens"(Pritchard and MacDonald, 1980).

The most dreaded maternal complication is cerebral hemorrhage, which occurs when the blood pressure is not controlled. Loss of vision from edema or hemorrhage may be a sign of impending cerebrovascular accident, although usually this loss of vision is temporary (Zuspan, 1980). To control the blood pressure, hydralazine is given.

Pritchard has reported excellent success in treating 154 consecutive eclamptics over a 20-year period (Pritchard, 1975). Approximately three fourths of the patients in whom eclampsia developed were delivered vaginally. Steps were initiated to effect delivery as soon as the patient regained consciousness.

The latent period between induction of labor and/or cesarean section is quite variable. Procrastination is unwise, and the patient should be delivered soon after stabilization is achieved. It is better to deliver a low-birth-weight infant by cesarean section if the cervix is not inducible or if the fetus is not in vertex presentation.

When cesarean section is performed for patients with preeclampsia-eclampsia, anesthesia with sodium thiopental (Pentothal), nitrous oxide, and a muscle relaxant has many advantages. The primary advantage is the low incidence of hypotension. However, with adequate preliminary hydration with Ringer's lactate, prior to the administration of epidural anesthesia, hypotension may be obviated. Fluid overload must be prevented. Since hypotension from regional anesthesia may result in death for the fetus with a minimal reserve, regional anesthesia is generally contraindicated in severe preeclampsia.

Oxytocin is used for induction; however, assessment of the antidiuretic effect in these patients is imperative. At 45 mU/min, the antidiuretic effect is at its maximum (Chesley, 1979). Any woman on oxytocin is at an increased risk for water intoxication, and thus fluid intake and output should be monitored closely. The patient with pregnancy-induced hypertension is at an even greater risk, and thus a continuous infusion pump should be used to control intravenous fluid intake. This risk of water intoxication is the result of a combination of factors: The patient may already have spontaneous oliguria; oxytocin has an antidiuretic effect; the patient may lie on her back, which decreases urinary blood flow; and antihypertensive drugs decrease urinary output. These combined processes inhibit the excretion of water while increasing the patient's circulating volume and diluting the electrolytes (Chesley, 1979). Thus, keep intake low. If the oxytocin has to be increased, increase the concentration, rather than continuing to increase the total fluid volume.

If the patient has a seizure, it may be due to water intoxication rather than to eclampsia or vasoconstriction alone. In water intoxication seizures, there is muscle weakness and cramping, and a decrease in respiration. However, the best way to diagnose the cause of the seizure is to look at the intake and output. A decreased sodium level in the plasma, usually 115 to 125 mEq/liter, is found in patients having seizures due to water intoxication (Chesley, 1979).

The patient with eclampsia may be very sensitive to oxytocin. Be alert for hyperstimulation and precipitous delivery. An intrauterine catheter is advisable to measure uterine tone. Chesley (1979) has reported that most patients with eclampsia can be delivered by oxytocin induction. Zuspan (1980) reports that most eclamptic patients are delivered within 18 hours.

If the eclamptic patient is being transported to a regional center, $MgSO_4$ should be initiated during transport. The patient should be accompanied by a person trained to use a preeclamptic tray and who understands the use and side effects of $MgSO_4$.

Placental abruption is a complication of pregnancy-induced hypertension. As a result of the vasospasm there is a decrease in the perfusion of the intervillous space, which seems to increase the risk of abruption. Observe for severe sustained pain with a rigid abdomen. The resting tone on the contraction channel of the internal fetal monitor usually increases significantly. There can be vaginal bleeding; however, in some cases the blood may accumulate behind the placenta during abruption, with no vaginal bleeding.

POSTPARTUM CARE

Once the fetus has been delivered, preeclampsia commonly abates within 24 hours. We maintain $MgSO_4$ for 24 hours after delivery. However, there are some patients who will continue to be preeclamptic for up to 5 weeks after delivery. It is important to recognize that the salutary effects of delivery result from delivery of the *placenta* rather than of the fetus. Eclampsia has been reported in several instances after intrauterine fetal death. Although most women become normotensive within a day or two after delivery, their blood pressures occasionally remain elevated for a few weeks rather than a few days. On our service, if the hypertension remains severe with a diastolic pressure of 110 mm Hg or greater, we reassess the patient to be sure that a detectable cause of hypertension has not been overlooked. If the patient does not demonstrate a diastolic blood pressure of greater than 110 mm Hg and there are no complications, we usually discharge the patient without instituting antihypertensive medication. We do so only after arranging for the patient to return weekly to our office, so that we can continue to monitor her blood pressure.

Immediately post partum, the patient should be placed under close observation for 24 hours, since about one third of the patients will have seizures during the first 24 hours. The patient should be continued on $MgSO_4$ for 24 hours at a minimum, or

Table 20–10. Signs and Symptoms of Pulmonary Edema

Rales
Tachycardia
Increased CVP (normal: 9–11 cm H_2O)
Shortness of breath
Distended neck veins

until the blood pressure has returned to normal with normal reflexes for two 4-hour consecutive periods. During the administration of $MgSO_4$, either intramuscularly or intravenously, the patient should remain in the recovery room.

While in the recovery room, vital signs should be monitored every 15 minutes until stable. Because of the toxemic state and the administration of $MgSO_4$, vital signs should be continued every 15 to 30 minutes while the patient is on $MgSO_4$. Remember that the patient with preeclampsia-eclampsia is very sensitive to blood loss, because of a decreased intravascular compartment. Even a moderate amount of bleeding after delivery may cause serious hypovolemia, with resulting oliguria. Thus, a decreased blood pressure may be a sign of hypovolemia, rather than relief of the vasospasm.

Since output is an indicator of blood volume, hourly intake and output should be continued while the patient receives $MgSO_4$. Oliguria of less than 30 cc/hr may signify a worsening of the disease; however, if the oliguria is accompanied by normal blood pressure and normal reflexes, it may indicate hypovolemia. Patients with normal output and normal blood pressures may have relief of their vasospasm. The bladder should be kept empty to avoid uterine relaxation. This should be easy to accomplish, since a Foley catheter should already be in place.

During this initial period, as in the antepartum and intrapartum periods, the patient should be observed for signs of pulmonary edema (Table 20–10), cardiac failure (Table 20–11), and disseminated intravascular coagulation (DIC) (Table 20–12).

Table 20–11. Signs and Symptoms of Cardiac Failure

Cyanosis
Increased pulse rate
Decreased blood pressure
Tachypnea and rales
Distended neck veins
Increased central venous pressure

Table 20–12. Signs and Symptoms of DIC

Oozing from IV suture sites, bleeding gums, etc.
Clotting studies—While awaiting lab results, set aside a tube of blood and see how long it takes for it to clot; without DIC, blood should clot in 6 to 7 minutes
PT: 10.6–13.3 sec
PTT: 27.8–38 sec
Fibrinogen: 400 mg/100 sec
FSP: None
Platelets: 200,000–500,000

While the patient is in the recovery room, she should be allowed visitors for short periods of time. She should be allowed to visit with her new baby as much as her condition allows. Breast-feeding should not be discouraged, even with the MgSO₄ therapy. If the fetus has died, grief counseling can be initiated at this time.

The magnesium sulfate should be continued for 24 hours after delivery. After that, once the blood pressure is stable and the reflexes are normal for two 4-hour consecutive periods, the MgSO₄ can be discontinued. The patient can then be transferred to the postpartum floor. She should have her blood pressure and pulse observed and recorded every 4 hours, and a hematocrit should be obtained daily. The patient usually remains in the hospital for 3 to 5 days after delivery, depending on her clinical course.

After discharge, the patient should be seen in 1 week. If the blood pressure is still elevated, the patient should be seen weekly until the hypertension is resolved (Zuspan, 1980). If the patient's blood pressure is still elevated at the 6-week checkup, she should be sent for a hypertensive workup. The management for these patients is summarized in Table 20–13.

In regard to counseling the patient for further pregnancies, Zuspan has stated that pregnancy-induced hypertension does not increase the incidence of hypertension in later life (Zuspan, 1980). Furthermore, Chesley has indicated that pregnancy-induced hypertension does not lead to residual hypertension. Nonetheless, most women with recurrent preeclampsia ultimately do become hypertensive. However, in regard to residual hypertension and recurrence of preeclampsia-eclampsia, the incidence is unlear because of the poor definition of pregnancy-induced hypertension, particularly preeclampsia (Chesley, 1979).

Because the fetus of a mother with preeclampsia-eclampsia is at high risk, a pediatrician should be in attendance at delivery.

The baby may be growth-retarded (Fig. 20–4) and have the problems associated with this condition, i.e., hypoglycemia, hypocalcemia, asphyxia at birth due to decreased placental function, meconium aspiration, polycythemia, pulmonary hemorrhage, and an increased risk of infection. The baby may also be depressed as a result of hypermagnesemia. If the baby is hypotonic, he or she can be treated with calcium; however, this rarely occurs.

Intrauterine growth retardation (IUGR) is associated with preeclampsia. Accelerated aging of the placenta has been documented and can be visualized by the use of ultrasonography. The obstetrician and the pediatrician must work together closely in order to provide optimum care to both the mother and the neonate. A physician skilled in cardiopulmonary resuscitation must be in the delivery room, since premature or growth-retarded newborns often suffer from poor thermal regulation, hyperviscosity, and episodes of hypoglycemia. The IUGR infant is generally asymmetric, its head appears disproportionately large for its height and weight, and the paucity of subcutaneous fat causes it to have the appearance of an old man (Fig. 20–4). Quirk and coworkers (1979) suggest that atraumatic delivery of the low-birth-weight infant may reduce the incidence of respiratory distress syndrome (RDS). Bowes has demonstrated that deliv-

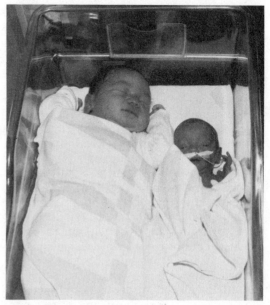

Figure 20–4. IUGR infant (*right*) compared with normal newborn (*left*). (Photograph courtesy of Dr. Gary Cohen, University of South Florida College of Medicine, Tampa, FL.)

Table 20–13. Patient Care Summary for Preeclampsia-Eclampsia*

	Antepartum		Intrapartum	Postpartum
	Outpatient	*Inpatient*		
BP	1–2 times/week	q 4 hr	q 15 min	q 15 min until stable; then q 15–30 min while on $MgSO_4$; then q 1 hr × 2 then q 4 hr
P, R	Weekly	q 4 hr	q 15 min	As above
T	Weekly	q shift	q 4 hr	q 4 hr
Bedrest	Yes	Yes	Yes	While on $MgSO_4$
Weight	Weekly	Daily	—	—
Edema	Weekly	Daily	On admission	—
Urinalysis for protein	Weekly	Daily	On admission; then q 4 hr	—
24-hr collection	Weekly	Weekly	—	—
Retinal changes	Weekly	Daily	On admission	—
Hematocrit	Weekly	Weekly	On admission	On admission to RR; then prn
Serum creatinine and/or creatinine clearance	Weekly	Weekly	—	—
DTR	Weekly	q shift	q 1 hr while on $MgSO_4$	q 1 hr while on $MgSO_4$
I & O	—	q shift	q 1 hr	q 1 hr while on $MgSO_4$
Fetal heart rate	NST-CST weekly, starting at 30–32 weeks' gestation	NST-CST weekly q shift FHR	Continuous during labor, preferably internal. If no monitor available, q 15 min in first stage and q 5 min in second stage, listening through 2–3 contractions	—
Contractions Frequency Duration Quality Resting tone	Weekly	q 8 hr	Continuously with electronic fetal monitor. If no monitor available, q 15 min in first stage	Fundal checks: q 15 min × 4; then q 30 min × 2; then q 1 hr until stable; then q 4 hr Lochia: Same as above
Estriols Urinary Plasma	qd qod	qd qod	— —	— —
Sonogram	q 4 weeks	q 4 weeks	—	—
Amniocentesis (for L/S ratio)	Weekly after 33–34 weeks until mature		—	—
Laboratory values; analysis with: DIC screen Liver enzymes Magnesium levels	—	Weekly	On admission	After delivery
Sexual counseling	No restrictions	—	—	—

*Nurse–patient ratios: *antepartum,* 1:6–8; *intrapartum,* 1:1; *recovery room,* 1:2–4, *postpartum* 1:6–8.

ery by cesarean section, or atraumatic vaginal delivery, may reduce neonatal problems and the probability of RDS (Bowes, 1977).

Chronic Hypertension

Occasionally the patient is first seen with chronic hypertension. If seen after the 20th week of gestation, the differential diagnosis may be difficult, because of the well-documented decrease in blood pressure that occurs during the second trimester in normotensive as well as in most chronically hypertensive women. It is important to have historical evidence documenting previous hypertension. Typically as pregnancy progresses, the patient's blood pressure often returns to the previous hypertensive reading, requiring an increase in the antihypertensive medication, or the dilemma of deciding whether the patient has preeclampsia and/or chronic hypertension persists. The diagnostic problem for the physician is to differentiate between the chronic hypertensive state and acute preeclampsia-eclampsia. Chronic hypertensive disease is suggested by the following:

1. Hemorrhages and exudates seen in the optic fundi.
2. Plasma creatinine concentrations greater than 1 mg/dl.
3. Plasma urea nitrogen concentrations greater than 20 mg/dl.
4. The presence of chronic diseases such as diabetes mellitus with nephropathy, and connective tissue disease.

The uric acid level in the maternal serum may also help to differentiate the chronic hypertensive from the patient with acute pregnancy-induced hypertension.

The patient with chronic hypertension may have an underlying condition predisposing to the hypertension, the two most common being hypertensive disease and renal and urinary tract disease. In addition to these, there are numerous other conditions that may cause or underlie chronic hypertension complicating pregnancy. The obstetric team should search for evidence of such conditions when evaluating the women with pregnancy-associated hypertension. During the physical examination, one can appropriately record blood pressure in both the upper and lower extremities. In addition, the thorax should be auscultated and the femoral pulses palpated to rule out coarcta-

tion of the aorta. Auscultation of the flank may identify the bruit of unilteral renovascular stenosis. The urinary metanephrine spot test will detect the presence of a pheochromocytoma. A search for antinuclear antibodies or the anti-DNA antibody, a glucose intolerance test, and measurement of the BUN and creatinine, as well as creatinine clearance and quantitative protein excretion determinations, are all part of a reasonable evaluation of the patient.

MANAGEMENT (Table 20–14)

Antepartum Care

The outpatient care for the pregnant patient with chronic hypertension is essentially the same as in a routine case of hypertension, with medications regulated according to the patient's blood pressure response. These patients should be seen weekly for blood pressure checks. In addition, a weekly NST-CST should be performed starting at 30 to 32 weeks, to assess fetal reserve. Observation should be made for IUGR, as these babies are at risk because of uteroplacental insufficiency. Examinations should include fundal heights and sonograms every 3 weeks.

The patient with chronic hypertension usually can be managed on an outpatient basis as long as her blood pressure remains under control. Occasionally our patients are hospitalized so that their medications can be regulated for good blood pressure control. If they are maintained at home, a visiting nurse may be used between weekly visits to take blood pressure measurements and assess the patient. A summary of the medications used for treatment is presented in Table 20–15, at the end of the chapter.

Intrapartum Care

These patients are managed under normal protocols for labor and delivery, with vital signs taken every hour and intake/output recorded every shift. More frequent monitoring would be required if the blood pressure remained high during labor and delivery.

Postpartum Care

Routine vital signs can be observed in the recovery room. The blood pressure should be monitored twice a shift on the postpartum

Table 20–14. Patient Care Summary for Chronic Hypertension*

	Antepartum		Intrapartum	Postpartum
	Outpatient	*Inpatient*		
BP, P, R	Weekly	q 4 hr	q 1 hr if normotensive q 15 min with ↑ BP	On admission to RR; then q 15 min × 4; then q 30 min × 2; then q 1 hr until stable; then q 4 hr on PP floor
T	Weekly	q 4 hr	q 4 hr	On admission to RR; then q 4 hr
Fetal heart rate	NST-CST weekly starting at 32 weeks' gestation	NST-CST weekly starting at 32 weeks' gestation	Continuous electronic fetal monitoring, preferably internal If no monitor available, q 15 min in first stage and q 5 min in second stage, listening through 2–3 contractions	—
Contractions Frequency Duration Quality Resting tone	Weekly	q 8 hrs	Continous electronic fetal monitoring If no monitor available, q 1 hr by palpation	Fundal checks: q 15 min × 4; then q 30 min × 2; then q 1 hr until stable; then q 4 hr Lochia: Same as above
Sonogram	q 3 weeks	q 3 weeks	—	—
Amniocentesis	Weekly after 33–34 weeks if patient not stable or IUGR is present		—	—

*Nurse–patient ratios: *antepartum,* 1:6–8; *intrapartum,* 1:2.

floor. All other vital signs can be taken per routine.

The patient may be taking antihypertensive medications to control her blood pressure. Most of these are safe to take while the mother is breast-feeding (Table 20–15).

Chronic Hypertension with Superimposed Preeclampsia

Approximately 25 percent of patients who have been identified as chronic hypertensive are predisposed to superimposed preeclampsia. It is imperative that the medical team identify preexisting chronic hypertension, either historically or before the 20th week of gestation. The hypertension of preeclampsia superimposed on chronic hypertension is often severe. In such cases, we maintain the patient on her previous chronic hypertensive medicine and place her in the hospital for observation. If signs of a worsening of the hypertension, proteinuria, or weight gain develop while the patient is on bedrest in the hospital, we seriously consider intervention. Management would continue as for the preeclamptic-eclamptic patient (see Table 20–13).

Patient Education

The patient and her family should be fully informed about her treatment regimen and about the severity of pregnancy-induced hypertension, especially since these patients usually do not feel or appear sick. However, severe facial edema or seizures may cause grave concern. If the patient has a seizure while family members are present, provide dignity and support to the patient and her family. The patient will need a great deal of support in dealing with a disease that may be life-threatening to her and her fetus. Offer information and show the patient the positive results of her being maintained at bedrest, such as decreased blood pressure, weight loss, and decreased facial, head, and leg edema. Blood pressure and weight charts can be helpful to show the patient her progress or the reason for hospitalization (Fig.

20–5). The patient should be instructed to observe for headaches, visual disturbances, epigastic pain, right upper quadrant pain (liver pain), continued abdominal pain or rigidity, tremors, and increased facial or other edema. If she is at home, she should be instructed to come to the hospital if any of these conditions occur. If she is hospitalized, she should alert the nursing staff.

Long-term hospitalization may be necessary. This would provide a good opportunity for individual or group teaching, since the patient may have had no prenatal classes, or her classes may have been interrupted by her hospitalization. Classes or group sessions can be arranged for all of the antepartum patients, to discuss prenatal care; high-risk factors, including equipment to be used and procedures to be completed; and attitude toward hospitalization, including fears, family relationships, and expectations for hospitalization. Our patients are given graphs to chart the progress of their blood pressure. These charts seem to help the patients better understand their disease. Information on induction of labor and cesarean section should be given, as well as an estimate of when she can expect to deliver. Patients admitted for long-term hospitalization also should be informed that they will stay in the hospital until they deliver, al-though in some situations in which the patient's condition has stabilized, short out-of-the-hospital passes may be beneficial. Patients who have been transported to the hospital from out of town may have additional needs and fears because of being separated from their families.

The family may also have trouble adjusting to the absence of the mother from the home. Social agencies may be able to provide a homemaker, babysitting services, and other supportive personnel in these cases. Children should be encouraged to visit whenever possible, and family resources such as the church or synagogue should be utilized.

If the patient convulses, she may not remember coming into the hospital for her delivery. It will be important to go over this information with the patient beforehand, to help her deal with her delivery and her new infant in the event that this occurs.

The patient with pregnancy-induced hypertension has many concerns and physical problems. This potentially serious disease should be controllable by good available prenatal care, good nutrition, and good patient education (Zuspan, 1980). The general management scheme for care of the pre-eclamptic patient is summarized in Table 20–15.

Text continued on page 396

Blood Pressure Graph

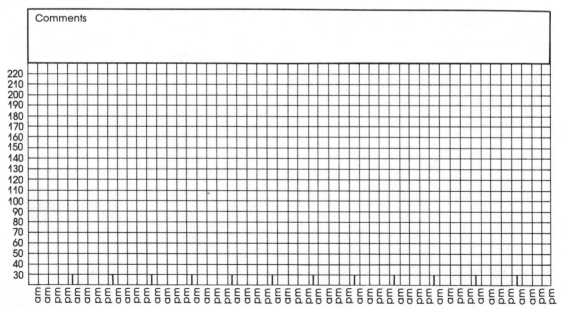

Figure 20–5. Blood pressure graph. (Courtesy of Marian Lake and Tom Johnson, University of South Florida College of Medicine, Tampa, FL.)

Table 20–15. Medication Summary for Preeclampsia-Eclampsia

Medication	Action	Route	Dose	Pregnancy Precautions	Maternal Side Effects	Nursing Considerations	Fetal/Neonatal Considerations	Breast-Feeding
				Anticonvulsants				
Magnesium sulfate	To control CNS irritability through action at the neuromuscular junction	IV with constant infusion pump	*Loading dose:* 4 g over 15 min *Maintenance dose:* 1–2 g/hr, to be continued 12–72 hours after delivery For seizures: 4 g over 5 min	Should not be used on digitalis patients because of danger of arrhythmias	Hypotension, flushing, circulatory collapse, depressed cardiac function, heart block, respiratory paralysis, hypocalcemia	Keep IV calcium gluconate available to reverse MgSO$_4$ Monitor vital signs q 15 min when administered IV in a specialized care setting I & O	Occasional hypermagnesemia	Excreted in breast milk but not absolute contraindication to breast-feeding
		IM	*Loading dose:* 10 g; 5 g into each buttock *Maintenance dose:* 5 g/4 hr, alternating hips, to be continued 12–72 hours after delivery (If more than 6 hours elapse between doses, the loading dose should be repeated)			IM Z-track Add 1 cc lidocaine to 5-g dose Allow ½ cc of air to clear 3" needle		
Diazepam (Valium)	Anticonvulsant	IV	5 mg over 60 sec; may repeat (20 mg or more may be required)	Not recommended for obstetric use Associated with congenital malformations when taken during the first trimester Fetal toxicity	Fatigue, drowsiness, ataxia, dizziness, headache, dysarthria, slurred speech, tremor, hypotension, bradycardia, cardiovascular collapse, blurred vision, nausea	Vital signs q 5 min Do not mix with other IV drugs Do not infuse through plastic tubing or store in plastic syringe Do not inject into small veins	Crosses placenta and is not excreted well by fetus Toxic levels have been detected 3 weeks after maternal administration in the neonate Hypothermia	Excreted in breast milk; because of long-acting metabolities, diazepam should be avoided during breast-feeding

Table continued on following page

Table 20–15. Medication Summary for Preeclampsia-Eclampsia *Continued*

Medication	Action	Route	Dose	Pregnancy Precautions	Maternal Side Effects	Nursing Considerations	Fetal/Neonatal Considerations	Breast-Feeding
				Magnesium Antagonist				
Calcium gluconate	Reverses magnesium intoxication	IV only	1 g over 3 min (10 ml of a 10% solution)		Tingling sensation, sense of oppression or heat waves, mild decrease in blood pressure, hypercalcemia, polyuria with rapid administration, syncope, vasodilation, bradycardia, cardiac arrhythmias, and cardiac arrest	Continue to monitor vital signs closely	No data available	No data available
				Barbiturates				
Barbiturates	Sedative	Dependent on medication		Not helpful in preventing eclampsia, but IV amylbarbital useful in eclampsia	Drowsiness, lethargy, hangover, nausea and vomiting, rash	May mask symptoms of toxemia if patient is too sedated	Crosses placenta rapidly and should not be given if delivery is imminent	Excreted in breast milk (shortacting preferred, as smaller amounts appear in the milk)
				Antihypertensives				
Aldomet (Methyldopa)	Central-acting adrenergic inhibitor	Oral	500–2000 mg/day, usually given in divided doses twice daily	None (safe for use in pregnancy)	Hemolytic anemia, reversible granulocytopenia, thrombocytopenia, sedation, headache, asthenia, weakness, dizziness, decreased mental activity, psychic disturbances, depression, bradycardia, orthostatic hypotension, dry mouth, nasal stuffiness, diarrhea	Monitor BP and potassium frequently Daily weight	None reported	Observe carefully; appears to be secreted in significant amounts

Drug	Action	Route	Dosage	Precautions	Contraindications/Side effects	Nursing implications	Effects on fetus/neonate	Breast-feeding/Comments
Reserpine	Peripheral-acting adrenergic antagonist	Oral	0.05–0.25 mg/day	None	Contraindicated in patients with a history of mental depression; use with caution in patients with history of peptic ulcer	Patient may be lethargic	Causes nasal obstruction in newborn	No data available
Propranolol hydrochloride (Inderal)	β-adrenergic inhibitor	Oral	40–480 mg/day, usually given in divided doses twice daily	Exercise/activity must be monitored by physician. Use with caution in patients with heart disease. Drug is associated with IUGR, prolonged bradycardia, and hypoglycemia	Fatigue, lethargy, vivid dreams, hallucinations, bradycardia, hypotension, peripheral vascular disease, nausea and vomiting, diarrhea, hypoglycemia without tachycardia rash	Check apical heart rate before administration. Monitor BP frequently. May mask common signs of shock and hypoglycemia. Give with meals	Associated with hypoglycemia, bradycardia, intrauterine growth retardation. Respiratory depression has been reported in neonates when propranolol has been administered to the mother by IV immediately before cesarean section	No adverse effects reported. Observe infant for hypoglycemia and cardiovascular effects. Amounts in breast milk too small to produce adverse effects in normal infants; however, caution should be used in premature or sick infants. Propranolol appears to provide the greatest margin of safety of all the beta-adrenergic drugs studied

Antihypertensives
Arteriolar Dilators

Drug	Action	Route	Dosage	Precautions	Contraindications/Side effects	Nursing implications	Effects on fetus/neonate	Breast-feeding/Comments
Hydralazine (Apresoline)	Arteriolar vasodilation	Oral, IV, or IM	50–300 mg/day, usually given in divided doses twice daily. Maximum effect 3–4 hr; duration of action 6 hr; 5% of dose excreted unchanged in urine		Flushing, headache, tachycardia, palpitations, angina pectoris, lupus syndrome	Vital signs: with IV check q 1 min for 5 min, then q 5 min for 30 min; with IM check q 5 min for 30 min. Watch for signs of SLE-like syndrome	None reported with long-term use; fetal heart rate changes when given acutely at term	No data available

Table continued on following page

Table 20–15. Medication Summary for Preeclampsia-Eclampsia *Continued*

Medication	Action	Route	Dose	Pregnancy Precautions	Maternal Side Effects	Nursing Considerations	Fetal/Neonatal Considerations	Breast-Feeding
Antihypertensives Continued								
Arteriolar Dilators								
Papaverine* (Pavabid)	Relief of cerebral and peripheral ischemia associated with arterial spasm and myocardial ischemia	Oral	100–450 mg/day	Exercise/activity must be monitored by physician	Cardiac arrhythmias, tachycardia, palpitations, nausea, and sweating	Monitor blood pressure, heart rate and rhythm, especially in cardiac disease. Most effective if given early in the disease process. FDA has announced this drug may not be effective for disease states indicated	No data available	No data available
Prazosin (Minipress)	Peripheral-acting α₁-adrenergic blocker	Oral	1–20 mg/day; peak action in 2 hr	Exercise/activity should be monitored by physician	Tachycardia, palpitations, dizziness, postural hypotension, weakness, headache, syncope	Use cautiously in patients receiving other hypertensive drugs. Monitor blood pressure frequently. Severe syncope with loss of consciousness may develop with an initial dose greater than 1 mg	No data available	No data available
Nitroprusside (Nipride)	To lower BP quickly in hypertensive emergencies	IV in D5W Do not inject	50 mg/liter Start at 0.2–0.5 ml/min Immediate effect; works only during IV infusion, which should be less than 24 hr in duration; carefully controlled with an intravenous pump	The safety of nitroprusside in women who are pregnant or who may become pregnant has not been established; hence, the drug should be given only when the po-	Nausea, diaphoresis, apprehension, cyanide poisoning	Use cautiously with hypothyroidism or hepatic or renal disease, or if patient is receiving other hypertensives. Wrap IV in foil because of light sensitivity; tubing not necessary to cover	Associated with case reports of intrauterine fetal death	No data available

*In 1986, not commonly used in pregnancy.

Drug	Action	Route	Dose	Effect on fetus	Maternal side effects	Comments	Effect on neonate	Effect on breast milk
(continued)					...tential benefits outweigh the hazards to mother and child	Fresh solution should have a slight brownish tint; Discard after 4 hr. Check BP q 5 min ×6 at start of infusion, then q 15 min. Needs intraarterial line. Use constant infusion pump. Best run piggyback with no other medications. Check serum thiocyanate levels q 72 hr	No data available	No data available
Minoxidil, guanacydine (Lonitem)	Vasodilator	Oral	5–100 mg/day Single daily dose is longacting.	None known	Hirsutism, edema, tachycardia, pericardial effusion and tamponade, congestive heart failure, breast tenderness	Contraindicated in patients with pheochromocytoma. Use only when other vasodilators have failed. Usually prescribed with a beta-blocking drug to control tachycardia	No data available	
Osmotic Diuretics								
Mannitol	Increases blood volume and GFR; reduces cerebral edema	IV	12.5 gm	None known	May worsen status in circulatory failure, water intoxication, cellular dehydration	Contraindicated in anuria, severe severe pulmonary congestion, frank pulmonary edema, severe congestive heart disease, severe dehydration, metabolic edema, progressive renal disease or dysfunction	Diuretics apparently have no adverse side effects in the neonate	Can cause a decrease in the production of milk

Table continued on following page

Table 20–15. Medication Summary for Preeclampsia-Eclampsia *Continued*

Medication	Action	Route	Dose	Pregnancy Precautions	Maternal Side Effects	Nursing Considerations	Fetal/Neonatal Considerations	Breast-Feeding
Osmotic Diuretics Continued								
Mannitol *(Continued)*						Monitor vital signs at least q hr If solution crystallizes, warm bottle in hot water bath, shake vigorously Use IV in-line filter Use catheter to measure I & O		
Urea*	Reduces intracranial or intraocular pressure	IV	30%, 1–1.5 g/kg	Use with caution in pregnancy	Headache, tachycardia, volume expansion, nausea and vomiting, sodium and potassium depletion	Contraindicated in severely impaired renal function, marked dehydration, frank hepatic failure, active intracranial bleeding Use cautiously in pregnancy, lactation, cardiac disease, hepatic impairment, or sickle cell with CNS involvement Do not administer through the same tubing as blood Avoid rapid IV infusion; may cause hemolysis or increased capillary bleeding Use within minutes of reconstitution Use catheter to measure I & O	None known	No data available

*In 1986, not commonly used in pregnancy.

Acid-Forming Salts

Drug	Action	Route	Dose	Contraindications	Side Effects		
NH₄Cl*	Creates renal acidosis for 2–3 hr	Oral	8–12 mg/day	None noted	GI irritation, acidosis, renal functional impairment	No data available	No data available

Mercurials

| Meralluride* | Diuresis in 2–3 hr; ceases at 12–24 hr | | | None noted | Allergic reactions, fatal and nonfatal; GI irritation, electrolyte depletion, Hg poisoning | No data available | No data available |
| Mercurophyllin* Mersalyl* Others* | | IM | 0.5–2.0 mg | None noted | | | |

Carbonic Anhydrase Inhibitors

| Acetazolamide* | Anticonvulsant | Oral | 25.5 g/day | None noted | Drowsiness, paresthesias, hepatic cirrhosis, disorientation, calculus formation, hypersensitivity | Contraindicated in sulfonamide sensitivity, chronic pulmonary disease, renal or hepatic dysfunction, hyponatremia, hypocalcemia, hyperchloremic acidosis. Use cautiously in patients with diabetes, gout, or respiratory acidosis. CBC & serum electrolytes q 3 months. Reconstitute 500-mg vial with 5-ml sterile water; refrigerate reconstituted solution; discard after 24 hr. May cause hyperglycemia in prediabetics or diabetics on insulin. Decreases motor excitability | No data available |

*In 1986, not commonly used in pregnancy.

Table continued on following page

Table 20–15. Medication Summary for Preeclampsia-Eclampsia *Continued*

Medication	Action	Route	Dose	Pregnancy Precautions	Maternal Side Effects	Nursing Considerations	Fetal/Neonatal Considerations	Breast-Feeding
			Carbonic Anhydrase Inhibitors Continued					
Acetazolamide* (*Continued*)						Contraindicated in hepatic insufficiency, renal failure, adrenocortical insufficiency, hyperchloremic acidosis, depressed sodium or potassium levels, severe pulmonary obstruction with inability to increase alveolar ventilation, Addison's disease Monitor electrolytes May cause positive results in urine protein tests Contraindicated in severe glaucoma, patients with depressed sodium or potassium serum levels, renal and hepatic disease, adrenal gland dysfunction, hyperchloremic acidosis, emphysema, chronic pulmonary disease Monitor I & O, weight, and serum electrolytes frequently May cause false-positive urine protein tests	No data available	No data available

*In 1986, not commonly used in pregnancy.

Aldosterone Antagonists

Drug	Classification	Route	Dosage	Comments	Side Effects	Nursing Considerations	Placental/Fetal	Lactation
Spironolactone (Aldactone)	Potassium-sparing diuretic	Oral	50–100 mg/day	Diuretics can cause a decrease in maternal intramuscular volume and consequently diminish uteroplacental perfusion. These agents *do not prevent development of toxemia*	Nausea, vomiting, leg cramps, dizziness	Contraindicated in anuria; occasional acute or progressive renal inefficiency, hyperkalemia	None known	Excreted in breast milk (short-acting preferred, as smaller amounts appear in the milk)
Triamterene (Dyazide)	Potassium-sparing diuretic	Oral	50–100 mg/day			Monitor serum potassium levels, electrolytes, I & O, weight, BP. Protect drug from light. Give with meals to enhance absorption	No data available	

Thiazides

Drug	Classification	Route	Dosage	Comments	Side Effects	Nursing Considerations	Placental/Fetal	Lactation
Benzothiadiazides	Increased urinary excretion of sodium and water by inhibition of sodium readsorption	Oral	250–500 mg/day	Diuretics can cause a decrease in maternal intravascular volume and consequently diminish uteroplacental perfusion. These agents *do not prevent development of toxemia*	Electrolyte depletion, hyperglycemia, gout, thrombocytopenia, hypersensitivity reactions, hemorrhagic pancreatitis	Contraindicated in anuria. Use cautiously in severe renal disease, impaired renal function, progressive hepatic function. Monitor I & O, weight & serum potassium levels. May cause hyperglycemia. Give in AM to prevent nocturia	Crosses placenta. Thrombocytopenia	Excreted in breast milk. Decreases lactation. No absolute contraindications to breast-feeding
Hydrochlorothiazide		Oral	25–50 mg/day					
Chlorothiazide (Diuril)		Oral	250–500 mg/day					
Flumethiazide		Oral	25–50 mg/day					
Hydroflumethiazide		Oral	25–50 mg/day					
Bendroflumethiazide		Oral	25–50 mg/day. Effect within 1 hr of oral dose; excreted in 3–6 hr					

Miscellaneous Antihypertensives

Drug	Classification	Route	Dosage	Comments	Side Effects	Nursing Considerations	Placental/Fetal	Lactation
Veratrium alkaloids (Protoveratrine A & B)*	Antihypertensive	IV	0.15–0.5 mcg/min	Exercise/activity must be monitored under physician surveillance	Hypotension, loss of reflexes, respiratory paralysis	Monitor blood pressure closely	No data available	No data available
Cryptenamine acetate (Unitensen)	Antihypertensive	Oral, IM	4–12 mg/day, 0.25–0.5 mg. Length of action: 12 hr		Same as above plus cardiac Irritability	Contraindicated in patients with pheochromocytoma. Use cautiously in patients with angina, cerebrovascular disease, bronchial asthma, renal insufficiency, or those taking other antihypertensives	No data available	No data available

*In 1986, not commonly used in pregnancy.

Table continued on following page

Table 20–15. Medication Summary for Preeclampsia-Eclampsia *Continued*

Medication	Action	Route	Dose	Pregnancy Precautions	Maternal Side Effects	Nursing Considerations	Fetal/Neonatal Considerations	Breast-Feeding
Miscellaneous Antihypertensives Continued								
Cryptenamine acetate *(Continued)*						Monitor BP and P closely Range between therapeutic and toxic dose is narrow		
Thiocyanate*	Anion effect on Na and K			Exercise/activity must be monitored by physician	Weakness, nausea, vomiting, palpitations, diarrhea, facial edema, nephrosis, hepatic necrosis, anemia, depressed thyroid function	Monitor blood pressure closely Watch for side effects	No data available	No data available
Mebutamate*		Oral	600–2400 mg/day In the meprobamate family; lasts 12–48 hr	Exercise/activity must be monitored by physician	Drowsiness, sedation		Crosses placenta	Excreted in the breast milk
Ethacrynic Acid—Lasix								
Furosemide (Lasix)	For treatment of pulmonary edema	Oral	40–200 mg/day	Safety in pregnancy has not been established	Hyponatremia, paresthesias, rash, GI irritability, thrombocytopenia, neutropenia, tinnitus, deafness Patients may have allergic reactions Will need increased potassium May cause hyperglycemia in diabetic patients Store tablets in light-resistant container to prevent discoloration (does not effect potency); store in refrigerator	Use cautiously in cardiogenic shock complicated by pulmonary edema, anuria, hepatic coma, or electrolyte imbalance Monitor BP and P_1 potassium levels Sulfonamide-sensitive		Diuretics can cause a decrease in milk production and have been known to suppress postpartum lactation
		IV	20–40 mg/day Diuretic response immediately with IV; in 30 min when given orally; bound to plasma proteins; also produces renal vasodilatation	Diuretics can cause a decrease in maternal intravascular volume and consequently diminish uteroplacental perfusion These agents do *not prevent development of toxemia*				

*In 1986, not commonly used in pregnancy.

Ganglionic Blocking Agents

| Trimethaphan (Arfonad Ampules) | To decrease BP quickly in hypertensive emergencies | 0.3–6 ml/min | IV titered
Oral intake incomplete, erratic, unpredictable
Parenteral dose excreted unchanged; tolerance develops | None noted | Dilated pupils, extreme weakness, severe orthostatic hypotension, tachycardia, anorexia, nausea, vomiting, dry mouth, urinary retention, respiratory depression | Contraindicated in patients with anemia, respiratory insufficiency
Use cautiously in patients with cardiac, hepatic, or renal disease, and in patients receiving glucocorticoids and other antihypertensives
Monitor vital signs frequently
Use constant infusion IV pump
Use oxygen therapy during administration of this drug
Do not use discolored (yellow) injectable
Use prepared solution within 24 hr | Meconium ileus | No data available |

REFERENCES

Abitbol, M. M., Pirani, C. L., Ober, W. B., et al.: Production of experimental toxemia in the pregnant dog. Obstet. Gynecol. 48:537, 1976.

Abitbol, M. M., Gallo, G. R., Pirani, C. L., et al.: Production of experimental toxemia in the pregnant rabbit. Am. J. Obstet. Gynecol. 124:460, 1976.

Abitbol, M. M., Driscoll, S. G., and Ober, W. B.: Placental lesions in experimental toxemia in the rabbit. Am. J. Obstet. Gynecol. 125:942, 1976.

Anderson, P. O.: Drugs and pregnancy. Drug Intelligence Clin. Pharm. 1:208, 1977.

Arias, F., and Mancilla-Jimenez, R.: Hepatic fibrinogen deposits in pre-eclampsia: immunofluorescent evidence. N. Engl. J. Med. 295:578, 1976.

Assali, N. S., Vergon, J. M., Tada, Y., et al.: Studies on autonomic blockade. VI. The mechanisms regulating the hemodynamic changes in the pregnant woman and their relation to the hypertension of toxemia of pregnancy. Am. J. Obstet. Gynecol. 63:978, 1952.

Bartholomew, R. A., Colvin, E. D., Grimes, W. H., Jr., et al.: Facts pertinent to the etiology of eclamptogenic toxemia: a summation of previous observations (1930–1955). Am. J. Obstet. Gynecol. 74:64, 1957.

Beecham, J. B., Watson, W., and Klapp, J. F.: Eclampsia, pre-eclampsia and disseminated intravascular coagulation. Obstet. Gynecol. 18:368, 1929.

Beker, J. C.: The effects of pregnancy on blood circulation in their relation to so-called toxemia. Am. J. Obstet. Gynecol. 18:368, 1929.

Berger, M., and Cavanagh, D.: Toxemia of pregnancy—the hypertensive effect of acute experimental placental ischemia. Am. J. Obstet. Gynecol. 87:293, 1963.

Berkowitz, R. L., Coustan, D. R., and Mockizuki, T. K.: Handbook for Prescribing Medications During Pregnancy. Boston, Little, Brown & Co., 1981.

Bonnar, J., McNicol, G. P., and Douglas, A. S.: Coagulation and fibrinolytic systems in pre-eclampsia and eclampsia. Br. Med. J. 2:12, 1971.

Borges, L. F., and Gucer, G.: Effects of magnesium on epileptic foci. Epilepsia 19:81, 1978.

Bowes, W.: Results of the intensive perinatal management of very low birth weight infants (150–1500 gms). Proceedings of the Fifth Study Group of Royal College of Obstetricians and Gynaecologists. London, 1977, p. 331.

Brewer, T. H.: Human pregnancy nutrition: an examination of traditional assumptions. Aust. NZJ Obstet. Gynaecol. 10:87, 1970.

Brewer, T. H.: Consequences of malnutrition in human pregnancy. Ciba Review: Perinatal Medicine, Vol. 13, p. 175. Basel, Ciba-Geigy, 1975.

Brewer, T. H.: Letter: Role of malnutrition in pre-eclampsia and eclampsia. Am. J. Obstet. Gynecol. 125:281, 1976.

Brosens, J., Robertson, W. B., and Dixon, H. G.: The physiological response of the vessels of the placental bed to normal pregnancy. J. Pathol. Bacteriol. 93:569, 1967.

Brown, G. J., Curtis, J. R., Lever, A. F., et al.: Plasma renin concentration at the control of blood pressure in patients on maintenance haemodialysis. Nephron 6:329, 1969.

Browne, F. J.: Aetiology of pre-eclamptic toxaemia and eclampsia. Lancet 1:115, 1958.

Browne, J., and Veall, N.: The maternal placental blood flow in normotensive and hypertensive women. J. Obstet. Gynecol. Br. Commonw. 60:141, 1953.

Burke, T. F., Spalding, C. T., and Jones, V. D.: Influence of sodium and potassium content on arterial responsiveness. Circ. Res. 29:525, 1971.

Butts, P.: Magnesium sulfate in the treatment of toxemia. Am. J. Nurs. 77:1294, 1977.

Cavanagh, D., and Knuppel, R. A.: Preeclampsia and eclampsia. *In* Cavanagh, D., et al. (eds.): Obstetric Emergencies. Philadelphia, J. B. Lippincott, 1982, pp. 107–132.

Cavanagh, D., Rao, P. S., Tung, K. S. K., et al.: Eclamptogenic toxemia: the development of an experimental model in the subhuman primate. Am. J. Obstet. Gynecol. 120:183, 1974.

Cavanagh, D., Rao, P. S., O'Connor, T. C. F., et al.: Experimental hypertension in the pregnant primate. Am. J. Obstet. Gynecol. 128:75, 1977.

Chesley, L. C., and Tepper, I.: Plasma levels of magnesium attained in magnesium sulfate therapy for pre-eclampsia and eclampsia. Surg. Clin. North Am. 37:353, 1957.

Chesley, L. C.: The renin-angiotensin system in pregnancy. J. Reprod. Med. 15:173, 1975.

Chesley, L. C.: Hypertensive Disorders in Pregnancy. New York, Appleton-Century-Crofts, 1978.

Chesley, L. C.: Parenteral magnesium sulfate and the distribution, plasma levels, and excretion of magnesium. Am. J. Obstet. Gynecol. 133:1, 1979.

Common errors in blood pressure measurements. Am. J. Nurs. 65:133, 1965.

deAlvarez, R. R.: Proteinuria relationships. *In* Friedman, E. A. (ed.): Blood Pressure, Edema and Proteinuria in Pregnancy. New York, A. R. Liss, 1976.

Demers, L. M., and Gabbe, S. G.: Placental prostaglandin levels in pre-eclampsia. Am. J. Obstet. Gynecol. 126:137, 1976.

DeWolf, F., Robertson, W. B., and Rosen, I.: The ultrastructure of acute atherosis in hypertensive pregnancy. Am. J. Obstet. Gynecol. 123:164, 1975.

Dieckmann, W. J.: The Toxemias of Pregnancy. St. Louis, C. V. Mosby Co., 1952.

Donnelly, J. F., and Lock, F. R.: Causes of death in 533 fatal cases of toxemia of pregnancy. Am. J. Obstet. Gynecol. 68:184, 1954.

Fliegner, J. R. H.: Placental function and renal tract studies in preeclampsia and long term maternal consequences. Am. J. Obstet. Gynecol. 126:211, 1976.

Franklin, G. O., Dowd, A. J., Caldwell, B. V., et al.: The effect of angiotensin II intravenous infusion on plasma renin activity and prostaglandins A, E, and F levels in the uterine vein of the pregnant monkey. Prostaglandins 6:271, 1974.

Friedman, E. A. (ed.): Blood Pressure, Edema and Proteinuria in Pregnancy. New York, A. R. Liss, 1976.

Gant, N. F., Daley, G. L., Chand, S., et al.: A study of angiotensin II pressor response throughout primigravid pregnancy. J. Clin. Invest. 52:2683, 1973.

Gant, N. F., Chand, S., Worley, R. J., et al.: A clinical test useful for predicting the development of acute hypertension in pregnancy. Am. J. Obstet. Gynecol. 120:1, 1974.

Gant, N. F., Madden, J. D., Siiteri, P. K., et al.: The metabolic clearance rate of dehydroisoandrosterone sulfate. III. The effect of thiazide diuretics in normal and future pre-eclamptic pregnancies. Am. J. Obstet. Gynecol. 123:159, 1975.

Gant, N. F., and Worley, R.: Hypertension in Pregnancy: Concepts and Management. New York, Appleton-Century-Crofts, 1980.

Gilstrap, L. C., Cunningham, F. G., and Whaley, P. S.: Management of pregnancy-induced hypertension in the nulliparous patient remote from term. Semin. Perinatol. 2:75, 1978.

Goldblatt, H., Kahn, J. R., and Hanzal, R. F.: Studies on experimental hypertension. Effect on blood pressure of constriction of abdominal aorta above and below site of origin of both main renal arteries. J. Exp. Med. 69:649, 1939.

Goldby, F. S., and Beilin, L. J.: Relationship between arterial pressure and the permeability of arterioles to carbon particles in the rat. Cardiovasc. Res. 6:384, 1972.

Goldby, F. S., and Beilin, L. J.: How an acute rise in arterial pressure damages arterioles. Electron microscopic changes during angiotensin infusion. Cardiovasc. Res. 6:569, 1972.

Grannum, P. A. T., Berkowitz, R. L., and Hobbins, J. C.: The ultrasonic changes in the maturing placenta and their relation to fetal pulmonic maturity. Am. J. Obstet. Gynecol. 133:915, 1979.

Gusdon, J. P., Anderson, S. G., and May, W. J.: A clinical evaluation of the "roll-over" test for pregnancy-induced hypertension. Am. J. Obstet. Gynecol. 127:1, 1977.

Gyongyossy, A., and Kelentey, B.: An experimental study of the effect of ischemia of the pregnant uterus on the blood pressure. J. Obstet. Gynaecol. Br. Commonw. 65:617, 1958.

Hauth, J. C., Cunningham, F. G., and Whaley, P. J.: Management of pregnancy-induced hypertension in the nullipara. Obstet. Gynecol. 48:254, 1976.

Hodgkinson, C. P., Hodari, A. A., and Bumpus, F. M.: Experimental hypertensive disease of pregnancy. Obstet. Gynecol. 30:371, 1969.

Hunter, C. A., Jr., and Howard, W. F.: Amelioration of the hypertension of toxemia by post-partum curettage. Am. J. Obstet. Gynecol. 81:441, 1961.

Ikedif, D.: Eclampsia in multiparity. Br. Med. J. 280:985, 1980.

Iles, A., Collinge, D. A., McNaulty, H., et al.: Drugs excreted in mother's milk. Patient Care, June, 1980, pp. 2–11.

Knuppel, R. A., and Montenegro, R.: Preeclampsia–eclampsia: an overview. J. Fla. Med. Assoc. 70:741, 1983.

Kumar, D.: Chronic placental ischemia in relation to toxemia of pregnancy—a preliminary report. Am. J. Obstet. Gynecol. 84:1323, 1962.

Magara, M.: On the pathogenic power of a placental extract. An experimental and clinical study of the etiology of toxemia of pregnancy. Gynecol. Obstet. 59:478, 1960.

McCubbin, J. H., Siabi, B. M., Ardella, T. W., et al.: Cardiopulmonary arrest due to acute maternal hypermagnesium. Lancet, 1:1058, 1981.

McKay, D. G., Merrill, S. J., Weiner, A. E., et al.: The pathologic anatomy of eclampsia, bilateral renal cortical necrosis, pituitary necrosis, and other acute fatal complications of pregnancy, and its possible relationship to the generalized Shwartzman phenomenon. Am. J. Obstet. Gynecol. 66:507, 1953.

McKay, D. G., and Wong, T. C.: Studies of the generalized Shwartzman reaction produced by diet. J. Exp. Med. 115:1117, 1962.

McKay, D. G.: Clinical significance of the pathology of toxemia of pregnancy. Circulation 30(Suppl II):66, 1964.

McKay, D. G.: Cryofibrinogenemia in toxemia of pregnancy. Obstet. Gynecol. 23:508, 1964.

McKay, D. G.: Disseminated Intravascular Coagulation: An Intermediary Mechanism of Disease. New York, Hoeber, 1965.

McKay, D. G., Goldenberg, V., Kaunitz, H., et al.: Experimental eclampsia—an electron microscope study and review. Arch. Pathol. 84:557, 1967.

McKay, D. G.: Hematologic evidence of disseminated intravascular coagulation in eclampsia. Obstet. Gynecol. Surv. 27:399, 1972.

Misenhimer, H. R., Ramsey, E. M., Martin, C. B., et al.: Chronically impaired uterine artery blood flow. Obstet. Gynecol. 36:415, 1970.

Morris, N., Osborn, S. R., Wright, H. P., et al.: Effective uterine blood flow during exercise in normal and preeclamptic pregnancies. Lancet 2:481, 1956.

Nadjii, P., and Sommers, S. C.: Lesions of toxemia in first trimester pregnancies. Am. J. Clin. Pathol. 59:344, 1973.

Naeye, R. L., and Friedman, E. A.: Causes of perinatal death associated with gestatinal hypertension and proteinuria. Am. J. Obstet. Gynecol. 133:8, 1979.

Newman, J., Weiss, B., Rabello, Y., et al.: Diazoxide for the acute control of severe hypertension complicating pregnancy: a pilot study. Obstet. Gynecol. 53:505, 1979.

Neuweiler, W., Berger, M., and Widmer, J.: Second World Cong. Int. Fed. Gynecol. Obstet. Montreal, June, 22–28, 1958. Kongressband: Tendances actuelles en gynécologie et obstétrique, p. 398. Montreal, Librairie Beachemin Limitée, 1959.

Ogden, E., Hildebrand, O. J., and Page, E. W.: Rise in blood pressure during ischemia of the gravid uterus. Proc. Soc. Exp. Biol. Med. 43:49, 1940.

Olds, S. B.: Obstetric Nursing. Reading, MA, Addison-Wesley, 1980, pp. 262–267.

O'Shaughnessy, R., and Zuspan, F. P.: Managing acute pregnancy hypertension. Contemp. Ob/Gyn 18:85, 1981.

Page, E. W.: Placental dysfunction in eclamptogenic toxemia. Obstet. Gynecol. Surv. 3:615, 1948.

Page, E. W., and Christianson, R.: Influence of blood pressure changes with and without proteinuria upon the outcome of pregnancy. Am. J. Obstet. Gynecol. 126:821, 1976.

Perez, R. H.: Protocols for Perinatal Nursing Practice. St. Louis, C. V. Mosby Co., 1981, pp. 134–148.

Pritchard, J. A.: Management of preeclampsia and eclampsia. Kidney Int. 18:259, 1980.

Pritchard, J. A.: Standardized treatment of 154 consecutive cases of eclampsia. Am. J. Obstet. Gynecol. 123:543, 1975.

Pritchard, J. A., Cunningham, F. G., and Mason, R. A.: Coagulation changes in eclampsia: frequency and pathogenesis. Am. J. Obstet. Gynecol. 125:855, 1976.

Pritchard, J. A., and MacDonald, P. C. (eds.): Williams Obstetrics. New York, Appleton-Century-Crofts, 1980, pp. 665–700.

Quirk, J. G., Raker, R. K., Petrie, R. H., et al.: The role of glucocorticoids, unstressful labor, and atraumatic delivery in the prevention of respiratory distress syndrome. Am. J. Obstet. Gynecol. 134:768, 1979.

Redman, W. G., Beilin, L. J., and Bonnar, J.: Variability of blood pressure in normal and abnormal pregnancy. In Lundheimer, M. D., Katz, A. I., and Zuspan, F. P. (eds.): Hypertension in Pregnancy. New York, John Wiley & Sons, 1976.

Reeder, S. J.: Maternity Nursing. Philadelphia, J. B. Lippincott Co., 1980, pp. 516–528.

Roberts, J. M., and May, W. J.: Consumptive coagulation in severe pre-eclampsia. Obstet. Gynecol. 48:163, 1976.

Rubenstein, A.: Ueber das toxische Prinsip in der placenta bei schwangerschafts toxaemie. Thesis, Berne, 1962.

Scott, J., and Freeney, J. G.: Preeclampsia and eclampsia and change of paternity. Br. Med. J. 281:565, 1980.

Sophian, J.: Discussion on the pathological features of cortical necrosis of the kidney and allied conditions associated with pregnancy. Proc. R. Soc. Med. 42:387, 1949.

Sophian, J.: Toxaemias of Pregnancy. London, Butterworths, 1953.

Sophian, J.: Myometrial resistance to stretch: the cause of preeclampsia. J. Obstet. Gynaecol. Br. Commonw. 62:37, 1955.

Sophian, J.: Letter to the Editor: Pregnancy toxemia. Lancet 1:48, 1957.

Sophian, J.: Letter to the Editor: Etiology of pre-eclamptic toxemia and eclampsia. Lancet 1:434, 1958.

Sophian, J.: Correspondence: Toxemia of pregnancy. Am. J. Obstet. Gynecol. 78:688, 1959.

Sophian, J.: Correspondence: Hypertension of pregnancy. Br. Med. J. 2:1501, 1961.

Sophian, J.: Proceedings of the Third World Cong. Int. Fed. Gynecol. Obstet., Vienna, September 3–9, 1961.

Speroff, L.: Toxemia of pregnancy. Mechanism and therapeutic management. Am. J. Cardiol. 32:582, 1973.

Spiegelberg, O.: Lehrbuch der Geburtshilfe fuer Aerzte und Studierende Lahr. Verlage M. Schauenburg, 1878.

Talledo, O. E., Chesley, L. C., and Zuspan, F. P.: Renin-angiotensin system in normal and toxemic pregnancies. III. Differential sensitivity to angiotensin II and norepinephrine in toxemia of pregnancy. Am. J. Obstet. Gynecol. 100:218, 1968.

Terragno, N. A., Terragno, D. A., and Pacholczk, D., et al.: Prostaglandins and the regulation of uterine blood flow in pregnancy. Nature 249:57, 1974.

Thompson, R. H. S., and Tickner, A.: Observations on the mono-amine oxidase activity of placenta and uterus. Biochem. J. 45:125, 1949.

Trolle, D., Bock, J. E., and Gaeda, P.: The prognostic and diagnostic value of total estriol in urine and in serum and of human placental lactogen hormone in serum in the last part of pregnancy. Am. J. Obstet. Gynecol. 126:834, 1976.

van Bouwdijk Bastiaanse, M. A.: Etiological aspects in the problem of toxemia in pregnancy. Am. J. Obstet. Gynecol. 68:515, 1964.

Vane, R. R.: The dynamics of the renin-angiotensin system. Proc. R. Soc. Lond. (Biol.) 173:339, 1969.

Vink, G. J., Moodley, J., and Philpott, R. H.: Effect of dihydralazine on the fetus in the treatment of maternal hypertension. Obstet. Gynecol. 55:519, 1980.

Vosburgh, G. J.: Edema relationships. In Friedman, E. A. (ed.): Blood Pressure. Edema and Proteinuria in Pregnancy. New York, A. R. Liss, 1976, p. 155.

Wheeler, L., and Jones, M. B.: Pregnancy-induced hypertension. JOGN Nurs. 10:212, 1981.

Young, J.: The aetiology of eclampsia and albuminuria and their relation to accidental hemorrhage: an anatomical and experimental investigation. J. Obstet. Gynaecol. Br. Empire 26:1, 1914.

Zuspan, F. P.: Acute hypertension. In Queenan, J. T. (ed.): Management of High Risk Pregnancy. Oradell, NJ, Medical Economics Co., 1980, p. 441.

Zuspan, F. P.: Hypertension: chronic and pregnancy-induced—a symposium. In Queenan, J. T. (ed.): Management of High Risk Pregnancy. Oradell, NJ, Medical Economics Co., 1980, p. 375.

Zuspan, F. P.: Hypertension in pregnancy. In Quilligan, E. J., and Kretchmer, N. (eds.): Fetal and Maternal Medicine. New York, Wiley Medical, 1980, pp. 547–568.

Zuspan, F. P.: Problems encountered in the treatment of pregnancy-induced hypertension. Am. J. Obstet. Gynecol. 131:591, 1978.

Zuspan, F. P., and Talledo, O. E.: Factors affecting delivery in eclampsia: conditions of the cervix and uterine activity. Am. J. Obstet. Gynecol. 100:672, 1968.

Zuspan, F. P., and Zuspan, K.: Strategies for controlling eclampsia. In Queenan, J. T. (ed.): Managing Ob/Gyn Emergencies. Oradell, NJ, Medical Economics Co., 1981, pp. 99–105.

DIABETES MELLITUS IN PREGNANCY

JANE L. BERRY
STEVEN G. GABBE

Remarkable improvement has been made in the prognosis for the 2 to 3 percent of pregnancies complicated by diabetes mellitus. Excluding deaths due to major congenital malformations, the perinatal mortality rate of infants of diabetic women receiving optimal care is as low as that observed in normal gestations. Such care demands the collaborative efforts of a health care team that should include a perinatologist, nurse specialist, nutritionist, and neonatologist.

This chapter will review the pathophysiology of diabetes mellitus in pregnancy, emphasizing those changes that lead to perinatal morbidity and mortality. The important objectives of therapy, especially the need to maintain maternal glucose levels within physiologic limits throughout gestation, will be outlined.

Carbohydrate Metabolism In Pregnancy

During gestation, significant metabolic changes occur that must be understood for the successful management of the pregnancy complicated by diabetes (Table 21–1). The fetus depends upon the maternal compartment for an uninterrupted supply of fuel. Several maternal adaptations are normally made to meet these fetal needs. Pregnancy is characterized by maternal hyperinsulinemia associated with insulin resistance, changes that are most marked late in gestation (Kalkhoff et al., 1978). There is also an increased likelihood of ketosis developing during maternal food deprivation, a state of

"accelerated starvation" related to the limited availability of gluconeogenic precursors (Metzger and Freinkel, 1978). Metzger has observed that normal pregnant women who are fasted after dinner and skip breakfast demonstrate a significant fall in glucose levels (Metzger et al., 1982). After meals, a state of "facilitated anabolism" characterized by greater carbohydrate-induced hypertriglyceridemia and enhanced suppression of glucagon has been described. Placental syncytiotrophoblast is the source of human placental lactogen (HPL), a growth hormone–like glycoprotein that produces insulin resistance and augments maternal lipolysis. With increased maternal utilization of fats for energy, glucose is spared for fetal consumption. Levels of HPL are directly related to placental mass, increasing as pregnancy progresses and heightening the *"diabetogenic stress."* Other hormones that also produce this state of insulin resistance include

Table 21–1. Metabolism in Pregnancy

	Early	Late
Fasting glucose	↓	↓
Oral GTT	Normal	Deteriorates
Intravenous GTT	Improved	Normal
Fasting insulin	↑	↑ ↑
Postprandial insulin	↑	↑ ↑ ↑
Free fatty acids	Normal	↑
Triglycerides	↑	↑ ↑ ↑
Body fat	↑	
Liver glycogen	↑	Normal
Lean muscle	?	?

Data from Kalkhoff, R. K., Kissebah, A. H., and Kim, H. J.: Carbohydrate and lipid metabolism during normal pregnancy: relationship to gestational hormone action. Semin. Perinatol. 2:291, 1978.

free cortisol and possibly prolactin. Estrogen and progesterone directly alter maternal islet cell function, producing beta cell hyperplasia and hyperinsulinemia (Kalkhoff et al., 1978).

The "diabetogenic stress" of pregnancy demands increased insulin production by the maternal pancreas. In most pregnancies, the patient's pancreas can increase insulin secretion several-fold and preserve maternal glucose homeostasis. Glucose crosses the placenta by carrier-mediated facilitated diffusion. The rate of glucose transfer from mother to fetus is limited largely by these transport characteristics as well as by the glucose consumption rate of the placenta (Simmons et al., 1979). Insulin does not cross the placenta, however, and although the fetus receives a continuous supply of maternal glucose, it will not be affected by maternal insulin. During pregnancy, periods of maternal hyperglycemia will produce fetal hyperglycemia. Late in pregnancy, elevated levels of glucose in the fetus stimulate the fetal pancreas, resulting in fetal beta cell hyperplasia and hyperinsulinemia (Van Assche, 1975). This combination of fetal hyperglycemia and hyperinsulinemia contributes to much of the morbidity and mortality observed in the infant of the diabetic mother.

Maternal Morbidity and Mortality

Patients with vascular and/or unstable diabetes are at greatest risk for morbidity and mortality during pregnancy. Although there is no evidence that pregnancy shortens the life expectancy of women with diabetes, and maternal mortality is rare, women with diabetes who have coronary artery disease may suffer an increased mortality in pregnancy (Silfen et al., 1980). Pregnancy will not produce a permanent deterioration of renal function in women with diabetic *nephropathy* (Kitzmiller et al., 1981). Carstensen observed no difference in the prevalence or severity of *retinopathy, nephropathy,* or *neuropathy* in patients who had been pregnant when compared with those who had never been pregnant (Carstensen et al., 1982). Nevertheless, there does remain uncertainty concerning the course of diabetic retinopathy during gestation. Benign reti-

nopathy may worsen as the pregnancy advances, but will usually regress after delivery. Dibble has recently reported that women who demonstrate neovascularization that has not been treated with laser therapy before pregnancy may be at great risk for deterioration of their vision (Dibble et al., 1982).

Much of the maternal morbidity observed in pregnancies complicated by diabetes can be attributed to the changes in maternal metabolism reviewed above, which cause deterioration of glycemic control. A review of maternal mortality in diabetic patients showed that 7 of 24 deaths could be directly attributed to the metabolic complications of diabetes (Gabbe et al., 1976). Before the utilization of home glucose monitoring techniques, severe *hypoglycemic reactions* requiring hospitalization occurred in approximately 10 percent of insulin-dependent patients (Roversi et al., 1979). Early in gestation, estrogen increases the sensitivity of adipose tissue and skeletal muscle to insulin (Kalkhoff et al., 1978). Therefore, deaths due to hypoglycemia were observed in the 1st trimester. Nausea and vomiting, common problems early in pregnancy, may also necessitate a reduction in insulin dosage. After delivery, the contrainsulin effects of HPL are lost, and hypoglycemia may again result. Insulin-dependent diabetics usually require only a small dose of insulin or no insulin replacement at all during the first days after delivery.

Ketoacidosis most often occurs during the 2nd and 3rd trimesters, when the "diabetogenic stress" of pregnancy is greatest. The recently diagnosed diabetic who becomes pregnant is most likely to develop ketoacidosis, because she fails to appreciate its causes and symptoms. Ketoacidosis has been associated with a maternal mortality rate of 5 to 15 percent and a perinatal mortality rate as high as 90 percent (Kitzmiller, 1982).

Perinatal Morbidity and Mortality

Fetal hyperglycemia and hyperinsulinemia produce most of the perinatal complications observed in the pregnancy complicated by diabetes. Insulin is an important fetal growth hormone. Cord blood and amniotic fluid levels of C-peptide, which reflect endogenous insulin secretion, correlate well with birth weight (Lin et al., 1981). The combination of excess glucose plus excess insulin leads to excessive fetal growth. Susa has demonstrated such changes in fetal rhesus monkeys exposed to sustained insulin infusions (Susa et al., 1979). Fetal *macrosomia* may be associated with a 15 percent incidence of traumatic complications during vaginal delivery (Horger et al., 1975). If shoulder dystocia results, perinatal asphyxia as well as injuries to the brachial plexus may occur. Ultrasound has been used with some success to assess fetal size at term. Recent studies show an approximate 80 percent accuracy rate. Nevertheless, the decision of whether to deliver the fetus vaginally should not be based on ultrasound alone (Reece and Hobbins, 1984).

After 36 weeks' gestation, the frequency of *fetal deaths* in pregnancies complicated by diabetes is increased tenfold (Hagbard, 1956). Although the etiology for these intrauterine deaths remains unknown, data from the animal laboratory indicate that fetal hyperglycemia and hyperinsulinemia play important roles. Insulin infusions in fetal sheep will increase the oxidative metabolism of glucose and reduce fetal arterial oxygen content (Carson et al., 1980). Patients who are poorly controlled, who have suffered a prior stillbirth, or who have pregnancy-induced hypertension and/or vasculopathy are also at greater risk for an intrauterine death.

In the past, obstetricians terminated the pregnancies of diabetic patients between 35 and 38 weeks' gestation, to prevent intrauterine deaths. However, premature delivery may result in increased fetal morbidity and mortality from *respiratory distress syndrome*. Robert and her colleagues have demonstrated that at any gestational age, the infant of the diabetic is 5 to 6 times more likely to develop respiratory distress syndrome (Robert et al., 1976). Recent experimental studies by Smith have proved that fetal hyperinsulinemia impairs cortisol-stimulated lung surfactant synthesis in vitro (Smith et al., 1975).

Improved understanding of maternal metabolism and of the need to carefully regulate maternal glycemia, together with the development of reliable techniques for fetal surveillance and improved neonatal care, have markedly reduced perinatal mortality arising from intrauterine deaths, trauma, and respiratory distress syndrome. At the present time, the most frequent cause of perinatal loss in pregnancies complicated by insulin-dependent diabetes is the fatal *congenital malformation*. Infants of diabetic mothers have a two- to threefold greater frequency of severe malformations involving many organ systems (Gabbe, 1977). Whereas the incidence of major malformations in normal pregnancies may be 2 to 3 percent, the frequency observed in the offspring of insulin-dependent diabetic patients is 6 to 8 percent (Mills, 1982). The caudal regression syndrome and cardiac, renal, and central nervous system anomalies are the most common defects. Such anomalies must occur during the first 7 weeks of development, long before most diabetic patients seek prenatal care (Mills et al., 1979).

There is increasing evidence that these malformations, which today account for 30 to 50 percent of all deaths in infants of diabetic mothers, may be attributed to hyperglycemia during the early weeks of pregnancy. Hemoglobin A_{1c} levels reflect glycemic control in previous weeks and months. The incidence of major anomalies is significantly higher in pregnancies of diabetic mothers who have elevated hemoglobin A_{1c} concentrations during the 1st trimester (Miller et al., 1981). Baker has recently demonstrated that the increased incidence of lumbosacral skeletal defects observed in fetuses of diabetic rat mothers can be reduced to control levels by aggressive insulin treatment (Baker et al., 1981). Eriksson has confirmed these findings in a similar study (Eriksson et al., 1982). Hypoglycemia itself has not been established as a fetal teratogen.

After delivery, considerable neonatal morbidity has been reported in the offspring of diabetic women. The characteristic triad of hypoglycemia, hypocalcemia, and hyperbilirubinemia may be seen in as many as 25 percent of these offspring (Soler et al., 1978). The incidence of macrosomia and hypoglycemia can be related to cord blood C-peptide levels (Sosenko et al., 1979). Infants of diabetic mothers have recently been observed to demonstrate a cardiomyopathy associated with septal hypertrophy, polycythemia with hyperviscosity, and the small left colon syndrome. The long-term prognosis for infants of diabetic mothers remains to be determined. The incidence of subsequent insulin-dependent diabetes in the infants of those women who themselves have insulin-dependent diabetes is approximately 1.5 percent (Kobberling and Bruggeboes, 1980).

Detection of Diabetes in Pregnancy

Gestational diabetes constitutes 90 percent of all diabetes in pregnancy, occurring in approximately 30,000 to 90,000 women in the United States each year (Freinkel, 1980). Using a rat model, Aerts and Van Assche (1979) have observed that the female offspring of rats mildly diabetic during pregnancy are at an increased risk to develop gestational diabetes when they become pregnant. They have suggested that, therefore, gestational diabetes is an inherited disorder.

Gestational diabetes has been characterized as a state restricted to pregnant women in whom the onset or recognition of diabetes or impaired glucose tolerance occurs during pregnancy. It is a result of an inadequate pancreatic reserve in response to the "diabetogenic stress" of pregnancy and is, therefore, most often encountered in late pregnancy. These patients are diagnosed by means of a 100-gram oral glucose tolerance test (Table 21–2). A well-organized *screening program* must be established to detect this abnormality. In the past, screening was based upon recognized historical or clinical clues, including a family history of diabetes; delivery of a macrosomic infant, an infant with a malformation, or an unexplained stillborn; and maternal obesity, hypertension, and glycosuria (Gabbe et al., 1977). O'Sullivan has emphasized that screening patients by such means is inadequate, as up to 50 percent of women who go on to develop gestational diabetes fail to manifest these clues (O'Sullivan et al., 1973). Furthermore, glycosuria is extremely common in pregnancy as a result of a physiologic increase in glomerular filtration rate. O'Sullivan has recommended that all pregnant patients be screened after fasting, using a 50-gram oral glucose load followed by a glucose determination 1 hour later. This screening test has a sensitivity of 79 percent and a specificity of 87 percent when compared with subsequent glucose tolerance test results (O'Sullivan et al., 1973). If one uses this approach, Lavin has calculated that the estimated costs per patient screened and per

Table 21–2. Detection of Diabetes in Pregnancy (Upper Limits of Normal)

	Whole Blood[1] (mg/dl)	Plasma[2] (mg/dl)
Screening Test		
50 g, 1 hr	130	150
Oral GTT*		
Fasting	90	105
1 hr	165	190
2 hr	145	165
3 hr	125	145

[1]Soler et al., 1978.
[2]Lavin et al., 1981.
*Diagnosis of gestational diabetes is made when any two values are exceeded. These values may differ from one hospital to another.

case of gestational diabetes detected are $4.75 and $328.96 respectively (Lavin et al., 1981).

Approximately 10 to 15 percent of all gestational diabetics demonstrate significant fasting or postprandial hyperglycemia and will require a program of care identical to that used for the pregestational diabetic (Gabbe et al., 1977). As many as 35 to 50 percent of patients who exhibit gestational diabetes will show further deterioration of carbohydrate metabolism during the next 15 years of life (O'Sullivan, 1975). Diabetes is most likely to occur in the obese woman who has carbohydrate intolerance during pregnancy (O'Sullivan, 1982). Patients who have been diagnosed as gestational diabetics should not subsequently take oral contraceptive agents, as these hormones may produce the derangements in carbohydrate metabolism observed during pregnancy (Kalkhoff, 1975). Recently, Skouby observed no significant changes in glucose tolerance in women with a history of gestational diabetes treated with a low-dose (30 µg ethinyl estradiol) combination oral contraceptive (Skouby et al., 1982).

Management of the Diabetic Pregnant Patient
(Table 21–3)

RISK ASSESSMENT

A program of patient care may be best developed when the risks to the patient and her infant are first considered. Pregnancies complicated by diabetes mellitus may be

Table 21–3. Patient Care Summary in Diabetes*

	Antepartum		Intrapartum	Postpartum
	Outpatient	*Inpatient*		
BP, P, R	Weekly	q shift except while sleeping (if stable); may be more frequent	q 15 min	On admission; then q 15 min × 4; then q 30 min × 2; then on discharge to PP floor; then q 8 hr
T	Weekly (optional per discretion of physician)	q shift; more frequently if infection present	q 1 hr	On admission; then q 4 hr; then on discharge to PP floor; then q 8 hr
Bedrest	No	No (May be indicated with vasculopathy)	Yes	—
Fetal monitor	Class A patients not usually tested unless they go post dates All Class B, C, D, and R patients, and Class A patients with a previous stillbirth, PIH, chronic hypertension, or fetal growth retardation are given weekly (or twice weekly) NSTs beginning at 28 weeks; OCT only if NST is nonreactive Diabetics with vascular disease (e.g., Class F) are tested more frequently (even daily), at discretion of physician		Continuously during labor, preferably with internal monitor	
Contractions	—	—	Continuously during labor, preferably with internal monitor	—
I & O		q shift	q 1 hr	While in RR note first void
Amniocentesis	37–38 weeks (or as clinically indicated)	37–38 weeks (or as clinically indicated)		
Sonogram	Class B–R q 4 weeks	Class B–R q 4 weeks	—	—
Blood sugar	Glucose oxidase strips or glucose meter daily, fasting and before each meal, and prn	Same as for outpatient	On admission; then prn	q 4 hr
Ophthalmologic examination	At first visit; with return visits based on initial findings and with any visual changes			

*Nurse–patient ratio = 1:2; with IV insulin (intrapartum), 1:1.

divided into two groups: (1) those women with pregestational diabetes, including patients with vascularized complications; and (2) those women with gestational diabetes.

The most widely applied risk assessment system has been that of Dr. Priscilla White. She observed that the age of onset of diabetes, its duration, and the presence of maternal vascular disease, factors that could be determined in the pre-pregnant state, would all have an important impact on pregnancy outcome (White, 1949) (Table 21–4). In general, the earlier the onset of diabetes, the longer its duration; and the greater the degree of vasculopathy, the worse the prognosis in pregnancy. Of course, the quality of

maternal glucose control must also be considered in assessing perinatal risk. When women have gestational diabetes but maintain a normal fasting glucose, intrauterine deaths rarely occur (Gabbe et al., 1977). Hare and White (1980) have recently stressed that Class A diabetes is not synonymous with gestational diabetes. Rather, Class A includes women treated with diet alone in whom diabetes antedated pregnancy.

Pedersen noted that *prognostically bad signs of pregnancy*, specifically ketoacidosis, pyelonephritis, pregnancy-induced hypertension, poor clinic attendance, and self-neglect, were associated with an unfavorable outcome (Pederson et al., 1974).

Table 21–4. White Classification of Diabetes in Pregnancy

Class	Age of Onset (yr)		Duration (yr)	Vascular Disease	Insulin
A	Any		Any	0	Diet only
B	>20		<10	0	+
C	10–19	or	10–19	0	+
D	<10	or	>20	Benign retinopathy	+
F	Any		Any	Nephropathy	+
R	Any		Any	Proliferative retinopathy	+
H	Any		Any	Heart disease	+

THE INSULIN-DEPENDENT PATIENT

Care of the insulin-dependent patient should begin prior to gestation (Table 21–5) (Steel et al., 1982; Graber et al., 1978). The patient must be assessed as to her suitability for pregnancy. Does she have active and untreated proliferative retinopathy or significant nephropathy and hypertension? The patient and her family should be advised of the financial demands of pregnancy. In addition, a program of contraception must be established (Table 21–6) (Steel and Duncan, 1980). The increased risk of thromboembolic disease precludes the use of combined estrogen/progestogen oral contraceptive preparations, and the efficacy of copper-containing intrauterine devices has recently been questioned (Gosden et al., 1982). Therefore, patients may be offered a progestogen-only pill or a mechanical method. Sterilization should be discussed after the diabetic woman has completed her family.

With increasing evidence indicating that congenital malformations are related to hyperglycemia during early embryogenesis, insulin-dependent patients should be in optimum control at the time of conception and throughout the 1st trimester of pregnancy. In normal pregnancies, maternal plasma glucose levels rarely exceed 100 mg/dl with excursions between fasting levels of 60 mg/dl and postprandial levels of 120 mg/dl. Mean plasma glucose concentrations during the 3rd trimester are 86 mg/dl (Gillmer et al., 1975; Cousins et al., 1980).

The benefits of careful regulation have been recognized for many years. More than a decade has passed since Karlsson and Kjellmer observed a perinatal mortality of 38 per 1000 when mean maternal blood glucose levels were maintained below 100 mg/dl during the 3rd trimester (Karlsson and Kjellmer, 1972). If mean glucose levels exceeded 150 mg/dl, perinatal mortality rose almost sixfold. In several recent series in which maternal fasting plasma glucoses have been maintained between 100 and 150 mg/dl, perinatal mortality rates of 30 to 50 per 1000 were reported (Roversi et al., 1979; Gabbe et al., 1977). The frequency of neonatal macrosomia was 11 to 22 percent, and hypoglycemia occurred in 28 to 49 percent of neonates in association with this degree of control. However, in a treatment program

Table 21–5. Pre-pregnancy Care for the Diabetic Patient

1. Assess patient's fitness for pregnancy, especially vasculopathy
2. Establish contraceptive program
3. Identify and treat infertility and gynecologic problems
4. Emphasize need for cooperation of patient and her partner
5. Educate both the patient and her partner
6. Obtain optimum glycemic control before conception
7. Check immune status against rubella

Adapted from Steel, J. M., Johnstone, F. D., Smith, A. F., et al.: Five years' experience of a "prepregnancy clinic for insulin-dependent diabetes. Br. Med. J. 285:353, 1982.

Table 21–6. Contraception for the Diabetic Patient

Combination Oral Contraceptives
    Increased risk of vascular complications in insulin-dependent patients
    Deterioration of carbohydrate tolerance in gestational diabetics
Progestogen-only Pills
    Acceptable for insulin-dependent patients
Intrauterine Device (IUD)
    Possibly less effective in insulin-dependent patients
Mechanical or Barrier Methods
    Less effective than oral contraceptives or IUD
Sterilization
    When family has been completed
    Especially for patients with serious vasculopathy

in which physiologic glucose levels were achieved, Jovanovic and her colleagues have essentially eliminated macrosomia and neonatal morbidity (Jovanovic et al., 1981). The perinatal risks associated with maternal hypoglycemia have not been well documented.

Maintenance of physiologic glucose levels in the pregnant insulin-dependent diabetic usually requires two to three injections of insulin daily as well as careful adjustment of dietary intake. Most patients require a mixture of intermediate acting (NPH) and rapid acting (regular) insulin in the morning. As a general guideline, the amount of NPH exceeds that of regular insulin by a 2 to 1 ratio (Jovanovic and Peterson, 1982). In the evening, equal amounts of NPH and regular insulin are employed. Patients usually receive two thirds of their total insulin dose at breakfast and the remaining third at suppertime. A profile of glucose levels in the fasting state and before lunch, dinner, and bedtime should initially be monitored each day. If these levels remain elevated, the corresponding insulin dose is increased by 20 percent. Jovanovic and Peterson (1982) have found that the administration of separate injections of regular insulin at dinnertime and NPH at bedtime may reduce the occurrence of nocturnal hypoglycemia. The latter is likely to occur during the night when the patient is in a relative fasting state and placental and fetal glucose consumption continue.

Cohen has recently evaluated the effectiveness of a continuous subcutaneous insulin infusion pump in controlling maternal glycemia during the 3rd trimester (Cohen et al., 1982). In an effort to mimic normal pancreatic function, a basal dosage is administered and additional boluses are given preprandially. Although a trend toward a decrease in glycemic excursions was observed with continuous infusion therapy, no significant improvement over standard insulin therapy was noted. Rudolf has demonstrated the efficacy and safety of outpatient pump therapy in pregnant diabetic women (Rudolf et al., 1981). Such therapy remains investigational and demands intensive surveillance. Ketoacidosis and fetal deaths have occurred in association with pump failure (Gardner, 1982). Serious hypoglycemic reactions have also been reported (Lock and Rigg, 1981).

Diabetic control must be assessed regularly. This surveillance should be achieved at home, with the use of glucose oxidase reagent strips (Tattersall and Gale, 1981; Schneider et al., 1980). In the past, control was assessed primarily by reviewing the results of double-voided urine specimens tested for glucose and acetone and by weekly surveys of a 24-hour glucose profile. The physiologic glycosuria of pregnancy limits the value of urine tests. Patients should, therefore, be instructed to use glucose oxidase–impregnated strips with a color chart or a glucose reflectance meter. In this way, they may assess their control 4 to 6 times each day while following their usual diet and program of exercise. Hospitalization for diabetic control will rarely be required if such a program is employed.

Hemoglobin A_{1c} determinations are of limited value in the management of the pregnant insulin-dependent diabetic patient. However, this determination may be made at the patient's first visit, to provide rapid assessment of the patient's prior diabetic regulation (Schwartz et al., 1976).

Early in gestation, hospitalization may be required to assess diabetic management and educate the patient. The initial hospitalization also provides an opportunity to assess the patient's vascular status with an ophthalmologic consultation, to determine baseline creatinine clearance and protein excretion, and to take an electrocardiogram. Screening for fetal neural tube defects by maternal serum alpha-fetoprotein assessment must be considered (Milunsky et al., 1982). An initial urine culture is also obtained and then repeated every 4 to 6 weeks.

Antepartum Management

Hospitalization for Initial Evaluation and Management

In recent years, larger hospitals and teaching centers have developed specialized units to meet the needs of the high-risk obstetric patient. For *optimal* care of the pregnant diabetic, admission to such a unit is preferable. If a specific care plan is devised and implemented early in the 1st trimester, these patients can be brought to term successfully.

Upon the patient's admission to the hospital for initial evaluation and management, a complete assessment should be made, including response to hypo- or hyperglycemia, her dietary habits, and her feelings concerning the pregnancy. Educational needs will vary for every patient, and do not necessarily correlate with the age of onset or the severity of diabetes.

A discussion of hospital routine and procedures is appropriate at this time, to allow the patient the opportunity to ask questions and to facilitate total patient involvement in the plan of care. If possible, the family and/or significant others should be present at the initial interview.

The standard regimen that is initiated upon admission to the hospital involves four aspects of care:

1. *Blood/urine glucose evaluation*
2. *Insulin administration*
3. *Fetal and maternal assessment*
4. *Dietary management*

Blood glucose evaluation should be performed before meals and at bedtime. Ideally, the patient will be instructed in the use of a glucose meter. She is then encouraged to perform self-testing and to report all results to her primary nurse. The patient may experience difficulty in adapting to lower blood glucose levels and frequent adjustments in insulin dosages. Patience and understanding on the part of the nursing staff will assist her in coping with these stress factors.

Insulin is prescribed by the physician based on the daily glucose profiles. A medication summary is provided in Table 21–7. All patients should be encouraged to administer their own insulin. Therefore, they must be assessed for proficiency regarding injection technique, mixing of insulins, and rotation of injection sites. Class B gestational diabetes as well as recently diagnosed adult-onset diabetics may require additional supervision until they are able to demonstrate adequate skill and confidence.

Patients with visual impairment may benefit from the use of specially adapted syringes. These syringes have larger numbers or presetting devices and are commercially available.

In order to allow the patient total participation in her care, it is important that she understand the rationale for all diagnostic tests. Consequently, a thorough explanation regarding ultrasonography and baseline renal function studies is essential. The nurse can be instrumental in assuring that the patient is kept appropriately informed.

A nutritionist should be scheduled to meet with the patient on the day of admission to the hospital. At this time, a dietary history is obtained, caloric requirements are determined, and a modified carbohydrate diet is prescribed.

In the average diet for a pregnant insulin-dependent diabetic patient, 20 percent of the calories are derived from protein, 35 percent from fats, and 45 percent from carbohydrates (Ney and Hollingsworth, 1981). In terms of caloric distribution, 25 percent of the calories are provided with breakfast, 30 percent with lunch, 30 percent with dinner, and 15 percent with a bedtime snack. In addition, it must be taken into account that some patients are more prone to hypoglycemia and may require snacks in mid-morning and/or mid-afternoon. In such cases, 5 percent of the calories are subtracted from breakfast and lunch respectively. The average daily caloric intake for the pregnant diabetic woman ranges from 2200 to 2400 calories. Those patients who are restricted in activity or who demonstrate early excessive weight gain may require a lower caloric prescription. Obese patients are not encouraged to lose weight during pregnancy; however, they should be counseled not to overeat. Ideally, all patients should be provided with an exchange list and meal pattern. The nutritionist will then visit the patient on a regular basis during this hospitalization, to assess her knowledge base and level of understanding. Caloric adjustments are made as needed, varying from one patient to another.

Following discharge, the patient should continue to consult with the nutritionist at the time of each prenatal visit, in order to discuss any changes in her dietary regimen. In the event that a nutritionist is not available for routine follow-up, the role of nutrition consultant will, in all probability, be taken on by the patient's nurse.

Subsequent Antepartum Outpatient Care

In most cases, glucose control can be stabilized within 1 week after admission to the hospital. Prior to discharge, arrangements should be made for continued home glucose monitoring. Although a glucose meter is preferable, visual assessments of test strips may also be used. A record should be kept of all test results and reviewed by the physician at each office visit. The patient should also be instructed to see the physician about glucose levels that are too high or too low.

At these visits, the patient may be asked to perform a glucose measurement so that her technique can be evaluated.

Prior to 28 weeks, the patient will be assessed by the physician at 1- to 2-week intervals, depending on the complexity of the diabetes. However, after 28 weeks, weekly appointments are the rule. At this time, further tests to evaluate fetal well-being are initiated. The patient will require instruction regarding antepartum heart rate testing, fetal activity assessment, and estriol determinations.

The stable and compliant diabetic patient may continue as an outpatient until 34 to 36 weeks. However, factors such as infection, changes in activity, emotional stress, hypertension, and other complications of pregnancy may alter the control, thereby necessitating more frequent or long-term hospitalization. If benign retinopathy has been detected early in gestation, repeat ophthalmologic examinations should be obtained in the 2nd and 3rd trimesters. Proliferative retinopathy requires more intensive follow-up.

During the 3rd trimester, when sudden intrauterine deaths are most likely to occur, a program of daily *fetal surveillance* is initiated, using both biophysical and biochemical methods. Although many biochemical assays have been applied in the evaluation of diabetic pregnancies, *estriol* analyses are the most helpful. Goebelsmann has stressed that the results of estriol assays must be available on a daily basis (Goebelsmann et al., 1973). He has observed that the day-to-day variation in urinary estriol is greater in diabetic gravidas than in normal pregnant patients. Errors in urine collection can be corrected by calculating an estriol/creatinine ratio. Goebelsmann noted that a rising estriol/creatinine ratio in 24-hour urine collections was rarely associated with an intrauterine death. On the other hand, he observed that a 35 percent *fall* in estriol excretion from the mean of the three highest consecutive values or levels that were consistently two standard deviations below the expected mean for gestational age could reflect fetal jeopardy. However, urinary estriol assays are associated with significant false-positive results. Furthermore, the 24-hour urine collection involves considerable delay in obtaining information about fetal status. In the past year (1984–1985), the majority of high-risk perinatal centers have ceased utilization of estriol evaluation in the management of pregnant diabetics.

The *contraction stress test* (CST) has proved to be an extremely valuable tool for fetal evaluation (Gabbe et al., 1977). Many studies have demonstrated that in a metabolically stable diabetic patient, a negative CST predicts fetal survival for 1 week (Gabbe et al., 1977). Positive CSTs have been observed in approximately 10 percent of insulin-dependent diabetic patients and are more frequently associated with perinatal death, fetal stress during labor, and neonatal depression. However, the CST does have a significant false-positive rate of up to 60 percent (Gabbe et al., 1977). Most recently, the *nonstress test* (NST) has been used in the assessment of the diabetic pregnancy. If the initial NST is nonreactive, a CST must then be undertaken. Whittle has recently reported his experience monitoring 70 consecutive diabetic patients with daily unconjugated plasma estriol assays and weekly NSTs (Whittle et al., 1979). No perinatal deaths occurred. In 2 patients, significant estriol drops occurred 2 days and 6 days after a reactive NST. After these falls in estriol, the NST was repeated and found to be nonreactive, and the CSTs were positive. Whittle concluded that daily unconjugated plasma estriol assays represent a reliable first-line test of fetal status in diabetic pregnancies. He emphasized that, if antepartum fetal heart rate testing alone is to be used, it must be done daily. These data support the view that biophysical and biochemical testing should be combined, both to eliminate the need for unnecessary premature intervention and to detect fetal distress. Insulin-dependent patients who maintain glucose levels within the physiologic range exhibit a low incidence of antepartum fetal distress. In these cases, antepartum fetal testing enables the perinatologist to delay delivery safely and allow further fetal maturity (Jorge et al., 1981).

A simple and practical approach to the evaluation of fetal condition has been maternal assessment of *fetal activity*. Although this technique has not been applied to a large group of diabetic patients, several authors have reported its value in the monitoring of high-risk pregnancies (Pearson and Weaver, 1976; Liston et al., 1982). Fetal activity assessment provides information

Table 21-7. Medication Summary for Diabetes

Medication	Action	Route	Dose* (Individualized per Patient)
Note: Insulin is necessary for the efficient transport of glucose to tissues other than those of the central nervous system, renal medulla, pancreatic beta cells, and gut epithelium. It also favors hepatic glycogen synthesis and storage of glucose in adipose tissue as triglycerides. Insulin facilitates the transport of ingested amino acids into cells, thus increasing protein synthesis. It inhibits lipolysis and is therefore antiketogenic. Exogenous insulin can reverse the symptoms of diabetes.			

Regular insulin
  Beef
  Pork
  Concentrated
	Peaks in 1–2 hr with a duration of 5–6 hr	Subcutaneous; may be given IV for control, especially during labor
		Subcutaneous; do not give IV
			Sliding scale dose to try to keep the patient "euglycemic"
			Fasting values of 60–100 mg/dl and below 120 mg/dl the rest of the day
			If a combination of an intermediate and short-acting insulin is given, it is usually in a ratio of 2:1 in AM and 1:1 before dinner; AM dose is twice the evening dose

Prompt insulin zinc suspension (Semilente)	Peaks at 2–8 hr with a duration of 12–16 hr	Subcutaneous; do not give IV	
NPH (Isophane insulin suspension)	Peaks at 6–12 hr with a duration of 24–48 hr	Subcutaneous; do not give IV	
Insulin zinc suspension (Lente)	Peaks at 6–12 hr with a duration of 24–28 hr	Subcutaneous in a ratio of 2:1 in the AM and 1:1 prior to dinner The AM dose is twice the PM dose	
Globin zinc	Same as for insulin zinc	Same as for insulin zinc	
Protamine zinc insulin suspension (PZI)	Same as for insulin zinc	Same as for insulin zinc	
Extended insulin zinc suspension	Same as for insulin zinc	Same as for insulin zinc	

*During pregnancy a sliding scale dose is used based on careful blood glucose monitoring. Some of the purified insulins, such as Actrapid, Monotard, Velosulin, and Insulatard, have been useful in treating brittle patients. Patients may respond to a change in type of insulin (e.g., beef vs. pork) when a previously used type causes the patient to be unresponsive.

Table 21–7. Medication Summary for Diabetes *Continued*

Pregnancy Precautions	Maternal Side Effects	Nursing Considerations	Fetal/Neonatal Considerations	Breast-Feeding
Insulin requirements may decrease slightly during the first third to half of pregnancy During second half of pregnancy, requirements may increase to 2–3 times that of the pre-pregnancy dose Immediately post partum, insulin requirements drop drastically, sometimes to below the pre-pregnancy dose (insulin may not even be needed the first 24–48 hours after delivery)	Overdose may cause hypoglycemia Allergic reactions to *beef* are commonly reported	With regular insulin, a deep secondary hypoglycemic reaction may occur 18–24 hours after injection Dosage is expressed in USP units. Strength is U-100 (for very large dose U-500 is available; store in separate area) Regular, intermediate, and long-acting insulins may be mixed; all insulins should be in the same concentration	The use of low doses of regular insulin in mild gestational diabetics has been found effective in reducing macrosomia in the fetus (even though the mother may not require the insulin to remain "euglycemic") Neonates should be observed for hypoglycemia, especially if the mothers has had high blood sugars	Patients may breast-feed their infants while on insulin
All suspensions: same as for regular insulin (above)	All suspensions: same as for regular insulin (above)	With all suspensions, gently agitate so that the contents are mixed uniformly; suspension should appear white and cloudy after mixture		
		Store in a cool area; refrigeration is desirable but not essential except for regular insulin concentrated Do not use insulin that has changed color Check expiration date before administration Press, do not rub injection site. Rotate injection sites. Have patient chart sites to avoid overuse of one area. *However,* unstable patients may achieve better control if injection site is rotated within the same anatomic region	Does not cross the placenta	

Table continued on following page

Table 21-7. Medication Summary for Diabetes *Continued*

Medication	Action	Route	Dose* (Individualized per Patient)
Note: Insulin is necessary for the efficient transport of glucose to tissues other than those of the central nervous system, renal medulla, pancreatic beta cells, and gut epithelium. It also favors hepatic glycogen synthesis and storage of glucose in adipose tissue as triglycerides. Insulin facilitates the transport of ingested amino acids into cells, thus increasing protein synthesis. It inhibits lipolysis and is therefore antiketogenic. Human insulin, like the exogenous types, can reverse the symptoms of diabetes.			
Human Insulins†			
Actrapid	Effect begins in approximately ½ hour; peaks between 2½ and 5 hours; terminates after 8 hours	Subcutaneous	U-100 pork; sliding scale
Velosulin	Effect begins in approximately ½ hour; peaks between 1st and 3rd hour; terminates after 8 hours	Subcutaneous	U-100 pork; sliding scale
Monotard	Effect begins after 2½ hours; peaks between 7 and 15 hours; terminates at approximately 24 hours	Subcutaneous	U-100 pork; sliding scale
Insulatard (NPH)	Effect begins at 1½ hours; peaks between 4th and 12th hour; terminates at approximately 24 hours	Subcutaneous	U-100 pork; sliding scale

*During pregnancy a sliding scale dose is used based on careful blood glucose monitoring. Some of the purified insulins, such as Actrapid, Monotard, Velosulin, and Insulatard, have been useful in treating brittle patients. Patients may respond to a change in type of insulin (e.g., beef vs. pork) when a previously used type causes the patient to be unresponsive.

Patients may react differently to the human insulins than to the beef and pork varieties and must be observed carefully.

†*Humulin* is a more recently developed human insulin, now used frequently in the United States.

that is quite comparable to the NST and may be more sensitive than estriol analyses. Patients are instructed to record fetal activity over a 12-hour period extending from 9 o'clock in the morning until 9 o'clock in the evening. If they observe fewer than 10 movements during this period, or if it takes progressively longer before the 10 movements are appreciated, further evaluation of fetal status is indicated. This daily assessment of fetal activity may be begun as early as 30 weeks of gestation.

Ultrasound studies have permitted the assessment of fetal growth as well as the detection of hydramnios. A sonogram should first be performed at 20 to 26 weeks of gestation as a baseline and then repeated at 4- to 6-week intervals. Elliott has used ultrasonography to predict the risk for shoulder dystocia in macrosomic infants at term (Elliott et al., 1982).

Hospitalization versus Outpatient Care in Late Pregnancy

As the diabetic gravida approaches the final month of gestation, hospitalization may be required. Such a policy was considered an important part of successful treatment programs established in the past. Many of the centers following this regimen dealt with large indigent populations, patients who were unable to maintain good diabetic control at home and who could not come to the

Table 21–7. Medication Summary for Diabetes *Continued*

Pregnancy Precautions	Maternal Side Effects	Nursing Considerations	Fetal/Neonatal Considerations	Breast-Feeding
Same as for regular insulin (above)	Same as for regular insulin (above)	Same as for regular insulin (above)	Same as for regular insulin (above)	Same as for regular insulin (above)
Same as for regular insulin (above)	Same as for regular insulin (above)	Store in refrigerator	Same as for regular insulin (above)	Same as for regular insulin (above)
Same as for regular insulin (above)	Same as for regular insulin (above)	See notes for suspensions, above (Prompt insulin zinc suspension)	Same as for regular insulin (above)	Same as for regular insulin (above)
Same as for regular insulin (above)	Same as for regular insulin (above)	See notes for suspensions, above (Prompt insulin zinc suspension) Avoid heavy foam Do not use if contents remain clear after shaking Do not use if you see lumps that float or stick to the sides	Same as for regular insulin (above)	Same as for regular insulin (above)

hospital for daily estriol assays. For these reasons, a liberal policy of hospitalization was employed. Physicians have now become more comfortable in treating selected diabetic gravidas as outpatients. At-home assessment of maternal glycemia by means of the glucose reflectance meter, the availability of unconjugated plasma estriols, and the use of outpatient nonstress testing have reduced the need for hospitalization. Many centers are now reporting comparable reductions in perinatal mortality with such an outpatient approach. However, for the patient who has had poor diabetic control throughout pregnancy or who has been unable to make adequate ·arrangements for daily antepartum surveillance, hospitalization still remains an important part of the treatment program.

ANTEPARTUM HOSPITALIZATION FOR FINAL EVALUATION AND MANAGEMENT

As the time of delivery approaches, the patient's anxiety level will increase. Frequently, there is uncertainty regarding the method of delivery. The primigravida as well as those patients who have experienced previous fetal losses may require extra attention and support. Since diabetic patients are more likely to require an operative delivery, their childbirth classes should place as much emphasis on cesarean section as on vaginal delivery.

It is often reassuring for the patient and her support person to visit the labor and delivery suite and nursery facilities prior to delivery. This process may alleviate anxiety and will allow the patient the opportunity to orient herself to these unfamiliar environments. Infants of diabetic mothers are frequently admitted to the intensive care nursery for observation. Although the majority of infants will require only regular assessment of glucose levels and prompt treatment of hypoglycemia, some may require respiratory assistance and cardiac monitoring. The mother will be less likely to panic if she is familiar with the monitors and ventilators used in her infant's care.

The patient will also benefit from a visit by the obstetric anesthesiologist, neonatologist, and primary nursery nurse prior to delivery. Her questions can be answered and she will be further reassured.

Intrapartum Management

Timing of Delivery

If the patient has been maintained in excellent glycemic control and all parameters of antepartum surveillance have remained normal, delivery should be safely delayed until fetal maturation has been achieved. Elective delivery should be planned at a gestational age of 38 weeks if amniotic fluid analysis reveals evidence of completed *pulmonary maturation* as documented by a lecithin/sphingomyelin (L/S) ratio of 2.0 or greater and the presence of the acidic phospholipid phosphatidylglycerol (PG) (Cunningham et al., 1962; Kulovich and Gluck, 1979). Diabetes in pregnancy is an unstable metabolic state, and a well-controlled patient who develops an upper respiratory tract infection or pyelonephritis may rapidly become ketoacidotic. Thus, despite careful antepartum management, allowing a patient to continue her pregnancy after full fetal maturation has been attained is accompanied by continued risk. For patients at highest risk, i.e., those who have been in poor control, who have had a previous stillbirth, or who have not been compliant, delivery at 38 weeks should be undertaken if fetal pulmonary maturation can be confirmed. If the pregnant diabetic patient develops pregnancy-induced hypertension, progressive proliferative retinopathy, hydramnios, or evidence of fetal distress on antepartum fetal testing, delivery prior to 38 weeks may be indicated. It has been suggested that pregnancy-induced hypertension, nephropathy, and proliferative retinopathy are associated with acceleration of fetal lung maturation (Kulovich and Gluck, 1979).

However, if an immature L/S ratio and absence of PG are noted on amniotic fluid evaluation, betamethasone or dexamethasone may be used to induce pulmonary maturation. Corticosteroids will cause hyperglycemia and can precipitate ketoacidosis (Kitzmiller et al., 1978). Therefore, if steroids are given prior to delivery, glycemic control must be carefully assessed by obtaining blood sugar levels every 2 to 4 hours. Repeated injections of regular insulin or a continuous insulin infusion may be required.

When fetal compromise is suggested by antepartum testing, immediate delivery must be considered. *In the presence of an L/S ratio of 2.0 or greater, delivery should be accomplished.* Few infants with an L/S ratio of 2.0 or more will develop severe respiratory distress despite the absence of PG (Cunningham et al., 1982). If the L/S ratio is immature, clinical management must be individualized.

Premature labor may occur in pregnancies complicated by diabetes, especially when hydramnios is present. Combined therapy with corticosteroids and tocolytic drugs has been used to accelerate fetal lung maturation and halt uterine contractions. However, such treatment may lead to rapid decompensation of diabetic control, and requires intensive glucose monitoring (Schilthuis and Aarnoudse, 1980).

Selection of the Route of Delivery

Once the decision to deliver the diabetic patient has been made, the route of delivery must be selected. Approximately 50 percent of insulin-dependent diabetics will be delivered by cesarean section (Gabbe et al., 1977; Kitzmiller et al., 1978). (In about 10 percent of cases there is a trial of labor first.) If antepartum testing suggests intrauterine fetal distress, cesarean section is indicated. In patients at 38 weeks' gestation with documented fetal lung maturation who are suspected to be at increased risk for an intrauterine death because of poor glycemic control or a history of a previous stillbirth, elective cesarean section is also undertaken if the cervix is not favorable for induction.

During induction of labor, electronic fetal heart rate and contraction monitoring is mandatory. Labor should be allowed to progress as long as cervical dilatation and descent follow the established normal labor curve. Any evidence of an arrest pattern should alert the physician to the possibility of cephalopelvic disproportion and fetal macrosomia. The incidence of shoulder dystocia in macrosomic infants after a prolonged second stage approaches 25 percent (Benedetti and Gabbe, 1981). The timing of any delivery must be coordinated with the neonatologists who are to be present. If adequate neonatal care cannot be provided, the pregnant diabetic should be transferred to a hospital with an appropriately equipped nursery.

Intrapartum Glucose Control

Delivery produces a rapid change in the hormonal milieu that has produced the "diabetogenic stress" of pregnancy. The fall in HPL levels after the placenta has been removed causes a marked decrease in the insulin replacement required to maintain glycemic control. Thus, management of the patient's blood sugars during labor, delivery, and post partum is a most challenging and important clinical problem (Cohen and Gabbe, 1981). The incidence of neonatal hypoglycemia can be related to the level of maternal glycemia maintained during labor as well as the degree of antepartum control. If the mean maternal blood sugar exceeds 90 mg/dl, the frequency of neonatal hypoglycemia in infants of diabetic mothers increases significantly (Soler et al., 1978).

Several approaches have been employed to maintain normal maternal blood sugar levels during labor while preventing hypoglycemia after delivery (Table 21–8). White has used one third to one half of the prepregnancy dosage of insulin (White, 1965). NPH insulin is given subcutaneously on the morning of induction or after delivery by cesarean section. Blood glucose values are

Table 21–8. Intrapartum Diabetic Management

Subcutaneous Insulin Administration
Method of White (1965)
1. One third to one half of total pre-pregnancy insulin dose as NPH on the morning of induction or after baby has been delivered by cesarean section
Method of Jovanovic and Peterson (1980)
1. Night prior to induction—one sixth of total daily insulin dose as NPH
2. Repeat dose of NPH on morning of induction
3. Determine blood glucose every hour using a glucose reflectance meter
Continuous Insulin Infusion
Method of Steel et al. (1977)
1. Give 1 unit insulin/hr or 10 units regular insulin/1000 ml D5W solution infused at 100 ml/hr

determined every 2 to 4 hours, and supplemental regular insulin is given to maintain good glycemic control. In studies using an artificial pancreas, the Biostator, Jovanovic has observed that no insulin is required during active labor and that glucosed utilization is approximately 2.5 mg/kg/min (Jovanovic and Peterson, 1980). By administering one sixth of the total dose of insulin as NPH on the morning of delivery and adjusting the intravenous glucose infusion according to hourly blood sugar values, excellent glycemic control has been achieved during labor.

A continuous intravenous infusion of both insulin and glucose has also been used during labor and delivery. Five units of regular insulin may be added to 500 ml of D5W, which is mixed with 5 ml of 25 percent albumin (Yeast et al., 1978). Albumin decreases insulin binding to glass and plastic surfaces. The mixture is given at an infusion rate of 100 ml per hour. Steel has further simplified the continuous insulin infusion regimen (Steel et al., 1977). He adds 10 units of regular insulin to 1000 ml of D5W without albumin. In most patients, regardless of their antepartum insulin requirements, this combination infused at 100 ml per hour (1 unit per 100 cc) will usually result in good glycemic control.

If an elective cesarean section is performed, the patient is maintained NPO the night before delivery, and her morning insulin dose is withheld. The cesarean section should be scheduled in the early morning. Epidural anesthesia will allow the anesthesiologist to continually evaluate the mental status of the patient and detect early signs of hypoglycemia. However, regional anesthesia must be carefully administered, as maternal hypotension has been associated with more profound fetal acidosis in pregnancies complicated by diabetes (Datta and Kitzmiller, 1982). To avoid maternal hyperglycemia with resultant fetal hyperglycemia, dextrose infusions should be limited to no more than 6 g/hr (Kenepp et al., 1982). After the operation has been completed, blood sugars should be monitored every 2 to 4 hours and an intravenous solution containing 5 percent dextrose continued, at a rate of 100 to 125 cc/hr. No insulin may be required for the remainder of the operative day. Cesarean section may also be required if the elective induction of labor is unsuccessful. It has been generally recommended that a patient who is not progressing adequately after 6 to 8 hours of oxytocin stimulation be delivered by cesarean section.

Intrapartum Emotional Support

Emotional support for the patient and her family is essential during the intrapartum period, as fears regarding the condition of the infant are heightened prior to delivery. If possible, a member of the antepartum nursing team should visit the patient during labor and be present at delivery, thereby providing support and continuity of care for the patient and family. The mother should be permitted to see and touch the infant as soon as possible after delivery. This will eradicate any doubts that the infant is *normal*. On the other hand, if there are complications such as respiratory distress syndrome or unexpected congenital anomalies, additional support and encouragement will be required. The antepartum and labor and delivery nursing teams must work together to meet these needs.

Postpartum Management

In the postpartum period, the patient's insulin requirements are usually significantly lower than were her pre-pregnancy requirements (Lev-Ran, 1974). The antepartum objective of physiologic glycemic control is relaxed during this period, and blood sugars of 150 to 200 mg/dl are satisfactory. The patient who has delivered vaginally and is able to eat can be given one half of her pre-pregnancy dosage of insulin as NPH on the first postpartum day. Glucose levels should be monitored at least 4 times daily and regular insulin given for glucose levels greater than 200 mg/dl. The following day, additional NPH insulin is given in the morning to equal two thirds of the supplemental regular insulin required on the previous day. Using this method, one can stabilize the patient within several days after delivery.

In addition to the usual postpartum measures of assessing fundal tone, evaluating fluid balance, and providing for comfort, close monitoring of blood glucose levels is necessary. Following a vaginal delivery, hourly glucose evaluations are obtained in the recovery room, using a glucose meter. Once the patient has been transferred to the postpartum unit, a fasting glucose as well as measurements before meals and bedtime is usually needed. If the patient remains NPO, the glucose levels should be ascertained every 2 hours. Intravenous fluids are maintained, and regular insulin is prescribed as needed. When glucose levels are stabilized, the frequency of assessment may be decreased to once every 4 hours until a regular meal pattern is resumed.

After delivery, the insulin dose required is usually less than that needed pre-pregnancy. The safety of insulin for breast-feeding mothers should be emphasized. *Lactation* or *infection* may increase insulin requirements, and this should be explained to the patient, to reassure her that fluctuations in glucose levels are expected and thus avoid any unnecessary concern. The postpartum nurse must be particularly observant for the sudden onset of hypoglycemic reactions, which may occur despite reductions of the insulin dose.

The patient who has been delivered by cesarean section often requires no additional insulin on the day of delivery. During the first several postoperative days, while her diet is being adjusted, the patient should be given one third of her pre-pregnancy dosage of insulin as NPH. More insulin will be required each day as her diet is advanced. Patients should be encouraged to breast-feed, working closely with a nutritionist and with close observation of blood glucose levels.

Prior to discharge, an assessment should be made concerning the need for family planning and further nutritional counseling.

THE PATIENT WITH GESTATIONAL DIABETES

Women with gestational diabetes are usually identified late in pregnancy. Once this diagnosis has been established by glucose tolerance testing, these patients are started on a dietary program of approximately 2000 to 2500 calories daily, with the exclusion of simple sugars (Gabbe et al., 1977). Their fasting and postprandial glucose levels should be evaluated at 2-week intervals until delivery. If fasting plasma glucose levels reach 105 mg/dl and postprandial glucose values exceed 120 mg/dl, insulin treatment should be considered. Insulin therapy has been associated with a reduction in macrosomia and therefore a reduction in traumatic delivery (Coustan and Imarah, 1982). However, at the present time, routine insulin therapy in cases of gestational diabetes cannot be advocated (Conference on Gestational Diabetes, 1980). Recent studies suggest that diets high in soluble fiber may be helpful in controlling postprandial hyperglycemia (Gabbe et al., 1982).

Gestational diabetic patients may be safely followed until 40 weeks, as long as fasting glucose levels remain normal. If labor cannot be induced at 40 weeks, fetal surveillance should be initiated with twice weekly estriol determinations and nonstress testing. The risk of intrauterine death is greater in those gestational diabetics who have had a prior stillbirth or who develop pregnancy-induced hypertension. In these patients, therefore, a program of fetal surveillance using estriol analyses and heart rate testing should be initiated at 32 weeks' gestation.

Psychosocial Considerations

ANXIETY AND CONFLICT

It is conceivable for the diabetic patient to have been told that with careful control of diet and blood glucose levels a "normal" life is possible. Nevertheless, the diabetic woman may have also been advised against becoming pregnant because of the potential risk to both her and the fetus. For most women, pregnancy and childbirth is considered to be a natural and normal part of life. Thus, to be denied this experience is to give up that right to be a "whole" woman. Consequently, when the diabetic does become pregnant, the customary anxieties are exacerbated by the conflict concerning her own health versus her desire for motherhood. It is not uncommon for the patient to experience deep concern regarding possible congenital anomalies in the infant. Others are apprehensive because of previous fetal loss. While these fears are often justified, recent advances in perinatal and nursing management have significantly improved the chances for a successful outcome. Taking these facts into consideration will assist the health care providers to more appropriately assess the patient's emotional needs and to initiate an individualized plan of care.

It is essential to recognize that despite similarities in diagnosis and/or history, *no two patients have the same needs.* Consequently, the importance of *individualized care* cannot be overemphasized. Single mothers and patients whose homes are far from the referral center are but two examples of patients facing particular hardship when hospitalization is required. Concern over family welfare, financial status, or the lack of support systems often leads to conflict regarding the need for hospitalization. Women with these concerns are literally torn between acknowledging their need to remain in the hospital for their own well-being and that of the fetus and agonizing over the problems that this separation from their family will cause.

Additional stress factors must also be considered in the management of the pregnant diabetic. The unpredictable fluctuations in glucose levels and the frequent readjustments in insulin dosages are often sources of frustration for the patient. Also, stress may make "physiologic" glucose control more difficult to achieve. Constant reassurance by the nursing staff that such control can be attained will assist the patient in coping with the situation. Superimposed complications, e.g., hypertension, premature labor, proliferative retinopathy, and nephropathy, bring added anxiety. Since the treatment for such conditions frequently involves prolonged periods of hospitalization, restrictions in activity, and early delivery, these patients will require consistent therapeutic intervention and emotional support (Barglow et al., 1981).

Regularly scheduled rounds for the entire high-risk team may be established to provide more effective and holistic implementation of the care plan. Quite often the patient will benefit from the sharing of her experiences with other diabetic patients, either on a one-to-one basis or in an organized group. If such is the case, interaction on this level should be encouraged and provided for whenever possible. For example, women with diabetes who have delivered can be asked to return to the unit for a luncheon with antepartum patients.

UNMET EXPECTATIONS

Unfortunately, not all diabetic pregnancies will have a successful outcome. Fetal loss may occur, or the infant may be born with congenital anomalies. The mother's hopes are dashed and her worst fears are realized.

Regardless of the circumstances, the grief process will be experienced to one degree or another. The shock, suffering, and recovery phases may vary for each individual. Nevertheless, each stage is essential and must be dealt with before resolution will occur and plans for the future can begin. There will usually be an element of guilt interspersed with feelings of grief and anger. This too must be understood and worked through for the patient and her partner.

During the initial crisis period, the physicians and nursing staff, in collaboration with the social worker, psychiatric liaison service, and the clergy, can provide valuable support to the patient and her family. Prior to discharge, information should be provided regarding available support groups in the community (e.g., *Compassionate Friends, Unite, Share, Resolve*) that can assist her with the long-term process of resolution and adaptation.

Conclusion

Pregnancy presents a special health care opportunity in the life of a woman with diabetes mellitus. The patient is highly motivated to do whatever may be necessary to assure a good perinatal outcome. The physician and nurse must work with the patient, stressing that the knowledge gained and the habits developed during pregnancy be maintained in years to come.

REFERENCES AND RECOMMENDED READING

Aerts, L., and Van Assche, F.A.: Is gestational diabetes an acquired condition? J. Dev. Physiol. 1:219, 1979.

Baker, L., Egler, J. M., Klein, S. H., et al.: Meticulous control of diabetes during organogenesis prevents congenital lumbosacral defects in rats. Diabetes 30:955, 1981.

Barglow, P., Hatcher, R., Wolston, J., et al.: Psychiatric risk factors in the pregnant diabetic patient. Am. J. Obstet. Gynecol. 140:46, 1981.

Benedetti, T. J., and Gabbe, S. G.: Shoulder dystocia: a complication of fetal macrosomia and prolonged second stage of labor with midpelvic delivery. Obstet. Gynecol. 52:526, 1978.

Borg, S., and Lasker, J.: When Pregnancy Fails. Boston, Beacon Press, 1981.

Carson, B. S., Philipps, A. F., Simmons, M. A., et al.: Effects of a sustained insulin infusion upon glucose uptake and oxygenation of the ovine fetus. Pediatr. Res. 14:147, 1980.

Carstensen, L. L., Frost-Larsen, K., Fugleberg, S., et al.: Does pregnancy influence the prognosis of uncomplicated insulin-dependent diabetes mellitus? Diabetes Care 5:1, 1982.

Cohen, A. W., and Gabbe, S. G.: Intrapartum management of the diabetic patient. Clin. Perinatol. 8:165, 1981.

Cohen, A. W., Liston, R. M., Mennuti, M. T., and Gabbe, S. G.: Glycemic control in pregnant diabetic women using a continuous subcutaneous insulin infusion pump. J. Reprod. Med. 27:651, 1982.

Conference on Gestational Diabetes, Diabetes Care 3:501, 1980.

Cousins, L., Rigg, L., Hollingsworth, D., et al.: The 24 hour excursion and diurnal rhythm of glucose, insulin, and C-peptide in normal pregnancy. Am. J. Obstet. Gynecol. 136:483, 1980.

Coustan, D. R., and Imarah, J. E.: Insulin treatment of class A diabetes can reduce operative deliveries and birth trauma. Diabetes 30(Suppl. 1):78A, 1982.

Cunningham, M. D., McKean, H. E., Gillispie, D. H., et al.: Improved prediction of fetal lung maturity in diabetic pregnancies: a comparison of chromatographic methods. Am. J. Obstet. Gynecol. 142:197, 1982.

Datta, S., and Kitzmiller, J. L.: Anesthetic and obstetric management of diabetic pregnant women. Clin. Perinatol. 9:153, 1982.

Dibble, C. M., Kochenour, N. K., Worley, R. J., et al.: Effect of pregnancy on diabetic retinopathy. Obstet. Gynecol. 59, 699, 1982.

Distler, W., Gabbe, S. G., Freeman, R. K., et al.: Estriol in pregnancy. V. Unconjugated and total plasma estriol in the management of diabetic pregnancies. Am. J. Obstet. Gynecol. 130:424, 1978.

Elliott, J. P., Garite, T. J., Freeman, R. K., et al.: Ultrasonic prediction of fetal macrosomia in diabetic patients. Obstet. Gynecol. 60:159, 1982.

Eriksson, U., Dahlstrom, E., Larsson, K. S., et al.: Increased incidence of congenital malformations in the offspring of diabetic rats and their prevention by maternal insulin therapy. Diabetes 30:1, 1982.

Evertson, L. R., Gauthier, R. J., and Collea, J. V.: Fetal demise following negative contraction stress tests. Obstet. Gynecol. 51:671, 1978.

Freinkel, N.: Gestational diabetes 1979: philosophical and practical aspects of a major health problem. Diabetes Care 3:399, 1980.

Gabbe, S. G.: Congenital malformations in infants of diabetic mothers. Obstet. Gynecol. Surv. 32:125, 1977.

Gabbe, S. G., Cohen, A. W., Herman, G. O., et al.: Effect of dietary fiber on the oral glucose tolerance test in pregnancy. Am. J. Obstet. Gynecol. 143:514, 1982.

Gabbe, S. G., Mestman, J. H., Freeman, R. K., et al.: Management and outcome of class A diabetes mellitus. Am. J. Obstet. Gynecol. 127:465, 1977.

Gabbe, S. G., Mestman, J. H., Freeman, R. K., et al.: Management and outcome of diabetes mellitus, Classes B–R. Am. J. Obstet. Gynecol. 129:723, 1977.

Gabbe, S. G., Mestman, J. H., and Hibbard, L. T.: Maternal mortality in diabetes mellitus. Obstet. Gynecol. 48:549, 1976.

Gardner, D. G.: More vigilance is needed during pregnancy. Diabetes Care 5:349, 1982.

Gillmer, M. D. G., Beard, R. W., Brooke, F. M., et al.: Carbohydrate metabolism in pregnancy. I. Diurnal plasma glucose profile in normal and diabetic women. Br. Med. J. 3:399, 1975.

Goebelsmann, U., Freeman, R. K., Mestman, J. H., et al.: Estriol in pregnancy. II. Daily urinary estriol in the management of the pregnant diabetic woman. Am. J. Obstet. Gynecol. 115:795, 1973.

Gosden, C., Ross, A., Steel, J., et al.: Intrauterine contraceptive devices in diabetic women. Lancet 1:530, 1982.

Graber, A. L., Christman, B., and Boehm, F. H.: Planning for sex, marriage, contraception, and pregnancy. Diabetes Care 1:202, 1978.

Hagbard, L.: Pregnancy and diabetes mellitus. Acta Obstet. Gynecol. Scand. 35(Suppl. 1):50, 1956.

Hare, J. W., and White, P.: Gestational diabetes and the White classification. Diabetes Care 3:394, 1980.

Horger, E. O., III, Miller, M. C., III, and Conner, E. D.: Relation of large birthweight to maternal diabetes mellitus. Obstet. Gynecol. 45:150, 1975.

Jorge, C. S., Artal, R., Paul, R. H., et al.: Antepartum fetal surveillance in diabetic pregnant patients. Am. J. Obstet. Gynecol. 141:641, 1981.

Jovanovic, L., Druzin, M., and Peterson, C. M.: Effect of euglycemia on the outcome of pregnancy in insulin-dependent diabetic women as compared with normal control subjects. Am. J. Med. 71:921, 1981.

Jovanovic, L., and Peterson, C. M.: Management of the pregnant, insulin-dependent diabetic woman. Diabetes Care 3:63, 1980.

Jovanovic, L., and Peterson, C. M.: Optimal insulin delivery for the pregnant diabetic patient. Diabetes Care 5(Suppl. 1):24, 1982.

Kalkhoff, R. J.: Effects of oral contraceptive agents on carbohydrate metabolism. J. Steroid Biochem. 6:949, 1975.

Kalkhoff, R. K., Kissebah, A. H., and Kim, H. J.: Carbohydrate and lipid metabolism during normal pregnancy: relationship to gestational hormone action. Semin. Perinatol. 2:291, 1978.

Karlsson, K., and Kjellmer, I.: The outcome of diabetic pregnancies in relation to the mother's blood sugar level. Am. J. Obstet. Gynecol. 112:213, 1972.

Kenepp, N. B., Shelley, W. C., Gabbe, S. G., et al.: Fetal and neonatal hazards of maternal hydration with 5% dextrose before caesarean section. Lancet 1:1150, 1982.

Kennel, J. H., and Trause, M. A.: Helping parents cope with perinatal death. Contemp. Ob/Gyn 12:53, 1978.

Kitzmiller, J. L.: Diabetic ketoacidosis and pregnancy. Contemp. Obstet. Gynecol. 20:141, 1982.

Kitzmiller, J. L., Brown, E. R., Phillippe, M., et al.: Diabetic nephropathy and perinatal outcome. Am. J. Obstet. Gynecol. 141:741, 1981.

Kitzmiller, J. L., Cloherty, J. P., Younger, M. D., et al.: Diabetic pregnancy and perinatal morbidity. Am. J. Obstet. Gynecol. 131:560, 1978.

Kobberling, J., and Bruggeboes, B.: Prevalence of diabetes among children of insulin-dependent diabetic mothers. Diabetologia 18:459, 1980.

Kowalski, K.: Helping mothers of stillborn infants to grieve. *MCH*, January 1977, pp. 29–32.

Kulovich, M. V., and Gluck, L.: The lung profile. II. Complicated pregnancy. Am. J. Obstet. Gynecol. 135:64, 1979.

Lavin, J. P., Barden, T. P., and Miodovnik, M.: Clinical experience with a screening program for gestational diabetes. Am. J. Obstet. Gynecol. 141:491, 1981.

Lev-Ran, A.: Sharp temporary drop in insulin requirement after cesarean section in diabetic patients. Am. J. Obstet. Gynecol. 120:905, 1974.

Lin, C.-C., Moawad, A. H., River, P., et al.: Amniotic fluid C-peptide as an index for intrauterine fetal growth. Am. J. Obstet. Gynecol. 139:390, 1981.

Liston, R. M., Cohen, A. W., Mennuti, M. T., et al.: Antepartum fetal evaluation by maternal perception of fetal movement. Obstet. Gynecol. 60:424, 1982.

Lock, D. R., and Rigg, L. A.: Hypoglycemic coma associated with subcutaneous insulin infusion by portable pump. Diabetes Care 4:389, 1981.

Metzger, B. E., and Freinkel, N.: Effects of diabetes mellitus on endocrinologic and metabolic adaptations of gestation. Semin. Perinatol. 2:309, 1978.

Metzger, B. E., Vileisis, R. A., Ravnikar, V., et al.: "Accelerated starvation" and the skipped breakfast in late normal pregnancy. Lancet 1:588, 1982.

Miller, E., Hare, J. W., Cloherty, J. P., et al.: Elevated maternal hemoglobin A1$_c$ in early pregnancy and major congenital anomalies in infants of diabetic mothers. N. Engl. J. Med. 304:1331, 1981.

Mills, J. L.: Malformations in infants of diabetic mothers. Teratology 25:385, 1982.

Mills, J. L., Baker, L., and Goldman, A. S.: Malformations in infants of diabetic mothers occur before the seventh gestational week: implications for treatment. Diabetes 28:292, 1979.

Milunsky, A., Alpert, E., Kitzmiller, J. L., et al.: Prenatal diagnosis of neural tube defects VIII. The importance of serum alpha-fetoprotein screening in diabetic pregnant women. Am. J. Obstet. Gynecol. 142:1030, 1982.

Ney, D., and Hollingsworth, D. R.: Nutritional management of pregnancy complicated by diabetes: historical perspective. Diabetes Care 4:647, 1981.

Olds, S. B., London, M. L., Ladewig, P. A., et al.: Obstetric Nursing. Menlo Park, CA, Addison-Wesley, 1980.

O'Sullivan, J. B.: Body weight and subsequent diabetes mellitus. JAMA 248:949, 1982.

O'Sullivan, J. B.: Prospective study of gestational diabetes and its treatment. *In* Sutherland, H. W., and Stowers, J. M. (eds.): Carbohydrate Metabolism in Pregnancy and the Newborn. Edinburgh, Churchill Livingstone, 1975, p. 195.

O'Sullivan, J. B., Mahan, C. M., Charles, D., et al.: Screening criteria for high-risk gestational diabetic patients. Am. J. Obstet. Gynecol. 116:895, 1973.

Pearson, J. F., and Weaver, J. B.: Foetal activity and foetal well-being: an evaluation. Br. Med. J. 1:1305, 1976.

Pedersen, J., Pedersen, L. M., and Anderson, B.: Assessors of fetal perinatal mortality in diabetic pregnancy. Diabetes 23:302, 1974.

Penticuff, J. H.: Psychologic implications in high-risk pregnancy. Nurs. Clin. North Am. 17; No. 1, March, 1982, 69–78.

Peppers, L., and Knapp, R. J.: Motherhood and Mourning. New York, Praeger Publishers, 1980.

Perez, R. H.: Protocols for Perinatal Nursing Practice. The C. V. Mosby Co., 1981, St. Louis, pp. 70–88.

Rancilio, N.: When a pregnant woman is diabetic: postpartal care. Am. J. Nurs., 79:453, 1979.

Reece, E. A., and Hobbins, J. C.: Ultrasound's role in diabetic pregnancies. Contemp. Ob/Gyn 23:87, 1984.

Robert, M. F., Neff, R. K., Hubbell, J. P., et al.: Maternal Diabetes and the Respiratory Distress Syndrome. N. Engl. J. Med. 294:357, 1976.

Roversi, G. D., Gargiulo, M., Nicolini, U., et al.: A new approach to the treatment of diabetic pregnant women. Am. J. Obstet. Gynecol. 135:567, 1979.

Rudolf, M. C. J., Coustan, D. R., Sherwin, R. S., et al.: Efficacy of the insulin pump in the home treatment of pregnant diabetics. Diabetes 30:891, 1981.

Saylor, D. E.: Nursing response to mothers of stillborn infants. JOGN Nurs. 6:39, 1977.

Schiff, H. S.: The Bereaved Parent. New York, Penguin Books, 1977.

Schilthuis, M. S., and Aarnoudse, J. G.: Fetal death associated with severe ritodrine induced ketoacidosis. Lancet 1:1145, 1980.

Schneider, J. M., Huddleston, J. F., Curet, L. B., et al.: Pregnancy complicating ambulatory patient management of diabetes. Diabetes Care 3:77, 1980.

Schuler, K.: When a pregnant woman is diabetic: antepartal care. Am. J. Nurs. 79:448, 1979.

Schulman, P. K.: Diabetes in pregnancy: Nutritional aspects of care. J. Am. Dietetic Assoc., 76:585–88, 1980.

Schwartz, H. C., King, K. C., Schwartz, A. L., et al.: Effects of pregnancy on hemoglobin A_{1c} in normal, gestational diabetic, and diabetic women. Diabetes 25:1118, 1976.

Silfen, S. L., Wapner, R. J., and Gabbe, S. G.: Maternal outcome in Class H diabetes mellitus. Obstet. Gynecol. 55:749, 1980.

Simmons, M. A., Battaglia, F. C., and Meschia, G.: Placental transfer of glucose. J. Dev. Physiol. 1:227, 1979.

Skouby, S. O., Molsted-Pedersen, L., and Kuhl, C.: Low dosage oral contraception in women with previous gestational diabetes. Obstet. Gynecol. 59:325, 1982.

Smith, B. T., Giroud, C. J. P., Robert, M., et al.: Insulin antagonism of cortisol action on lecithin synthesis by cultured fetal lung cells. J. Pediatr. 87:953, 1975.

Soler, N. G., Soler, S. M., and Malins, J. M.: Neonatal morbidity among infants of diabetic mothers. Diabetes Care 1:340, 1978.

Sosenko, I. R., Kitzmiller, J. L., Loo, S. W., et al.: The infant of the diabetic mother. Correlation of increased cord C-peptide levels with macrosomia and hypoglycemia. N. Engl. J. Med. 301:859, 1979.

Steel, J. M., and Duncan, L. J. P.: Contraception for the insulin-dependent diabetic woman: the view from one clinic. Diabetes Care 3:557, 1980.

Steel, J. M., Duncan, L. J. P., and Clarke, B. F.: Letter. Br. Med. J. 1:1536, 1977.

Steel, J. M., Johnstone, F. D., Smith, A. F., et al.: Five years' experience of a "prepregnancy" clinic for insulin-dependent diabetics. Br. Med. J. 285:353, 1982.

Susa, J. B., McCormick, K. L., Widness, J. A., et al.: Chronic hyperinsulinemia in the fetal rhesus monkey: effects on fetal growth and composition. Diabetes 28:1058, 1979.

Tattersall, R., and Gale, E.: Patient self-monitoring of blood glucose and refinements of conventional insulin treatment. Am. J. Med. 70:177, 1981.

Van Assche, F. A.: The fetal endocrine pancreas. *In* Sutherland, H. W., and Stowers, J. M. (eds.): Carbohydrate metabolism in pregnancy and the newborn. Edinburgh, Churchill Livingstone, 1975, pp. 68–82.

White, P.: Pregnancy and diabetes: medical aspects. Med. Clin. North Am. 49:1015, 1965.

White, P.: Pregnancy complicating diabetes. Am. J. Med. 7:609, 1949.

Whittle, M. J., Anderson, D., Lowensohn, R. I., et al.: Estriol in pregnancy. VI. Experience with unconjugated plasma estriol assays and antepartum fetal heart rate testing in diabetic pregnancies. Am. J. Obstet. Gynecol. 135:764, 1979.

Wimberley, D.: When a pregnant woman is diabetic: intrapartal care. Am. J. Nurs. March, 1979, pp. 451–52.

Yeast, J. D., Porreco, R. P., and Ginsberg, H. A.: The use of continuous insulin infusion for the peripartum management of the diabetic pregnancy. Am. J. Obstet. Gynecol. 131:861, 1978.

22

BLEEDING IN PREGNANCY

ROBERT H. HAYASHI
MARIA S. CASTILLO

Bleeding or hemorrhage in pregnancy is one of the most frequent contributors to maternal mortality, along with toxemia and infection. Significant blood loss poses a threat to the well-being of both the mother and her fetus. In this chapter we will discuss the clinical entities in pregnancy associated with vaginal bleeding. The entities will be grouped according to their occurrence in either early or late pregnancy, during labor, or in the postpartum period. The discussion will include the description, pathophysiology, and management principles of each clinical entity.

Bleeding in Early Pregnancy

Vaginal bleeding in the first two trimesters is seen in 16 to 21 percent of pregnancies. In most of these instances, the bleeding occurs from the 9th to the 12th weeks of pregnancy. Most of the time the cause of the bleeding remains undetermined; about 10 to 15 percent of pregnancies in which there is bleeding at this time will terminate in a spontaneous abortion. The frequency of occurrence of abortion increases as maternal age increases and as the number of previous abortions increases. Also, patients treated with infertility drugs have a higher frequency of abortions (Joupilla, 1980).

The etiology of spontaneous abortion is still not well understood. The role of exogenous factors, such as viral, bacterial, chemical, and traumatic, is small. Most often, spontaneous abortion is attributed to chromosomal or embryonic defects incompatible with life. Clinical signs and symptoms for all types of abortion are outlined in Table 22–1.

THREATENED ABORTION

Threatened abortion may occur at any time during the first half of pregnancy. The diagnosis is presumed when vaginal bleeding ensues with or without cramping in the presence of a live fetus. The bleeding is usually slight and may last a few days or even weeks. It may be fresh bright red bleeding or vary according to the amount of mucus mixed with the blood, or it may be a dark brown when it is old blood. The presence of a live fetus can be documented by real-time ultrasonography. After 5 weeks of gestation, a fetus can be seen, and fetal movement as well as fetal cardiac activity can be documented. Also, the diameter of the gestational sac can be measured serially to document an intact growing fetus. In threatened abortion, the cervical os will remain closed, although the bleeding may continue, and there will be no evidence of the passage of tissue into the vagina.

Some bleeding about the time of the expected menses is physiologic. Implantation of the blastocyst may cause bleeding about a week prior to the expected menses, resulting in vaginal spotting. The luteoplacental shift of the hormonal support of pregnancy occurs at about 8 weeks and is thought by some to cause vaginal bleeding. Cervical polyps or cervical erosion can also cause bleeding. These could easily be ascertained by a vaginal speculum examination of the cervix.

The usual treatment for threatened abortion is bedrest for 48 hours following each

419

Table 22–1. Clinical Signs and Symptoms of Abortions

Type of Abortion	Fever	Abdominal Cramps	Bleeding	Passage of Tissue	Internal Os Dilatation
Threatened	No	Slight cramps (may or may not be present)	Slight	No	None
Inevitable	No	Moderate	Moderate	No	Open
Complete	No	None	Small	Complete placenta with fetus	Partially open with tissue in vagina
Incomplete	No	Severe	Severe	Fetal or placental tissue	Open with tissue in cervix
Missed	No	None No FHT with Doppler or heart motion on sonar	None to severe if coagulopathy	None	None
Septic	Yes	Severe	Mild to severe	Possibly; foul smelling discharge	Closed or open with or without tissue

incident of vaginal bleeding. The patient is instructed to count the number of perineal pads used, to note the quantity and color of the blood on the pads, and to look for evidence of the passage of tissues. She should also abstain from coitus, since increased uterine contractions occur during orgasm. The above treatment program is instituted because the exact etiology of the vaginal bleeding is not known. The patient should call her physician if excessive bleeding or pain occurs or if there is rupture of the membranes. At this point a threatened abortion has progressed to an inevitable abortion.

INEVITABLE ABORTION

Inevitable abortion is the presence of cervical dilatation and/or spontaneous rupture of membranes in addition to vaginal bleeding. Given these conditions, abortion is almost certain to occur. The fetus is generally not viable at this time. The uterine contractility will be manifested by painful low abdominal cramps and will continue until expulsion of the products of conception occurs. The treatment of this condition is initially expectant, to allow a natural evacuation of the uterine contents. If bleeding is excessive or the process appears to be prolonged or incomplete, a dilatation and curettage (D & C) under anesthesia is carried out by the physician.

COMPLETE ABORTION

An abortion occurring before the 10th week of pregnancy will usually result in the complete expulsion of the products of conception. This is because the gestational sac has a sufficient amount of decidual tissue surrounding it (decidua capsularis) and the placenta is not too firmly attached to the uterine wall. A careful examination of the tissues passed per vagina will confirm a complete abortion. If the uterus is firmly contracted and there is no further active bleeding, the patient may be discharged. She should rest and be cautioned to watch for further bleeding, pain, or fever; a follow-up visit with her doctor should be scheduled.

INCOMPLETE ABORTION

An abortion occurring after the 10th week of pregnancy will usually result in the incomplete expulsion of the products of conception. After the 10th week, there is less decidua between the fetal membranes and the endometrium and they are therefore more adherent; the placenta is also more adherent, and the basal plate of the placenta is incompletely formed. Once this basal layer (Nitabuch's layer) is formed, the placenta tends to separate cleanly. Incomplete evacuation of the uterine contents results in continued bleeding, which is the main sign of an incomplete abortion. The retained tissue interferes with myometrial contractility, thereby preventing sufficient constriction around the spiral arteries of the placental site to control bleeding. The amount of bleeding can reach alarming proportions over a period of time. A D & C is now necessary for complete removal of all placental tissues, to allow normal control of placental site bleeding.

In any situation in which an abortion has occurred, the practitioners should be cognizant of the emotional aspect involved in the patient's ability to cope with the pregnancy loss. During the bleeding episodes preceding the abortion, the expectant couple may feel vulnerable and helpless. The thought of hospitalization may be frightening to them. For the woman, the fear of more pain may be predominant in her mind, and heavy vaginal bleeding will compound her fear. A simple and brief explanation of what has occurred and what is being or will be done to help them should be provided. Answering questions for the patient also provides support.

The couple should be permitted to remain together as much as possible. By sharing in the experience, they may provide emotional support to each other immediately and later on. The husband may feel awkward and unsure. He should be reassured that these feelings are normal and that his presence and support to his wife are essential and very important (Pizer and Palinski, 1980).

Anger, disappointment, and guilt are some of the normal emotions a woman may feel after a pregnancy loss. Of these, guilt is usually the strongest. For this reason, it is imperative that she be informed early in the bleeding episode that she may still abort in spite of bedrest and all other precautions. Once the abortion has occurred it should be reemphasized that the abortion occurred as a result of some abnormality in the developing embryo. Perhaps an illustration of what an embryo looks like will help to allay their guilt. If they choose and if possible, allow the couple to see the products of conception, but prepare them for the experience beforehand. Encourage the couple to communicate openly, as they will each experience the loss differently. Another source of emotional support may be for them to talk with another woman who has had a previous pregnancy loss. If there are children in the family, help provide the parents with an explanation that is appropriate for the children's age. Sharing the experience with the entire family can add additional support to the grieving parents (Pizer and Palinski, 1980).

MISSED ABORTION

Prolonged retention of the products of conception after embryonic or fetal demise is known as missed abortion. The usual clinical picture is that of a patient who ceases to experience the physiologic changes of pregnancy (such as morning sickness, fatigue, and breast enlargement) following an episode of vaginal bleeding or even without a bleeding history. After fetal death the hormonal production by the placenta gradually diminishes. The uterus and breasts regress in size. Some patients may present with persistent amenorrhea. Patients with a missed abortion may be amenorrheic for prolonged periods of time. They may eventually resume menses after almost total resorption of the products of conception or they may eventually bleed and pass the tissues spontaneously.

Sonography, urinalysis, and serum pregnancy tests are helpful in making the diagnosis. Real-time sonography will demonstrate the absence of fetal life signs (heart action or fetal movements). This sign is very reliable by the 6th week of gestation. Serial pregnancy tests should indicate a decline in placental hormone production. Once the diagnosis of a missed abortion is made or confirmed, a D & C can be performed at once or after a waiting period, since 93 percent will spontaneously abort within 3 weeks of fetal death (Tricomi and Kohl, 1957). Because of the slow absorption of thromboplastin material in the amniotic fluid into the maternal circulation, about 20 percent of women carrying a dead fetus for longer than 5 weeks may have the manifestations of a consumptive coagulopathy. These patients will have bleeding from the gums and nose and from slight trauma. Patients who are at risk for coagulopathy (over 5 weeks after fetal death) should be followed by weekly serum fibrinogen levels. Evacuation of the uterine contents is indicated if the fibrinogen level begins to decrease. If the level is at or below 100 mg/dl, the patient should be anticoagulated with heparin until the fibrinogen level rises to normal (usually 48 hours) before evacuation of the uterine contents is performed. An occasional patient will develop an infection of the dead products of conception. This will be manifested by crampy abdominal pain, foul vaginal discharge, and spiking fevers. Cervical and blood cultures should be taken, and systemic broad-spectrum antibiotics should be started and the uterus evacuated.

The usual management of a missed abortion once the diagnosis is confirmed is to wait for spontaneous resolution over 3 to 5 weeks if the patient is emotionally stable or to induce labor to evacuate the uterine contents using ecbolic agents. Currently the use of prostaglandin E_2 vaginal suppositories (20 mg) given repetitively (every 3 hours) has met with good results. The process may take from 6 to 18 hours, and the patient may suffer side effects of the prostaglandin such as nausea, vomiting, diarrhea, and fever, which can be treated palliatively.

SEPTIC ABORTION

When an illegal abortion is performed it is often a D & C done under unsterile conditions and it is often an incomplete evacuation of the uterine contents. This results in a serious intrauterine infection that if left untreated will cause serious sequelae or even the death of the patient. (In fact, before abortions were legalized in the United States, the death rate attributable to illegal abortions contributed significantly to maternal mortality statistics.) The patient usually presents to the hospital emergency room in a septic condition (high fever, tachycardia, and shocky), complaining of abdominal pain and vaginal bleeding. A history of an illegal abortion can usually be elicited.

The patient's condition should be rapidly stabilized with intravenous fluids and blood transfusions. Blood, cervical, and uterine cultures for both aerobic and anaerobic organisms should be obtained. A Gram stain of the uterine discharge should be examined for Clostridia, and high-dose, multiple-regimen parenteral antibiotics begun. When the patient is stable, a D & C with preparations for a possible total hysterectomy should be carried out.

A supportive rather than interrogative atmosphere should be provided for the patient. She may have guilt feelings as well as a fear of persecution because of the illegal abortion. She has already suffered psychological and physical trauma. She will need a sympathetic ear and emotional support through her recovery.

HABITUAL ABORTION

Habitual abortion is defined as three or more consecutive spontaneous abortions. Various studies indicate that women who have had a spontaneous abortion are at greater risk for another; thus, the greater the number of previous abortions, the higher the risk (Goldzieher and Benigno, 1958; Warburton and Fraser, 1961).

A specific cause can be found in about two thirds of habitual aborters, usually based on genetic, hormonal, anatomic, immunologic, or infectious factors, or on a chronic systemic illness (Tho et al., 1979).

Genetic factors are the cause of about 25 percent of recurrent abortions, with 13 percent of the cases being due to multifactorial gene abnormalities and 12 percent due to chromosomal abnormalities. The most common chromosomal abnormality is trisomy, with X monosomy with polyploidy being next in frequency. Chromosomal translocations account for 5 to 10 percent of habitual abortions. Paternal factors implicated in recurrent abortion include balanced translocation and polyspermia secondary to hyperspermia (MacLeod and Gold, 1957).

Hormonal causes of recurrent abortion include luteal phase (or progesterone) deficiency. Insufficient corpus luteum function can be related to hyperprolactinemia or a hyperandrogen state, but for the most part its pathophysiology is poorly understood.

Anatomic abnormalities of the reproductive tract associated with habitual abortion include developmental anomalies of the müllerian duct, such as bicornuate, unicornuate, or subseptate uterus; uterine cavity distortion secondary to myomas, and incompetent cervix.

Chronic systemic illnesses associated with recurrent abortion include lupus erythematosus, advanced diabetes mellitus, and renal and cardiac diseases.

Immunologic factors include maternal levels of sperm-agglutinating or immobilizing antibodies and possibly HLA-related suppression of maternal immunologic response to paternal antigens (Moghissi, 1982).

Finally, chronic reproductive tract infections have been implicated in recurrent abortions. Pathogens so incriminated are *Toxoplasma gondii*, *Listeria monocytogenes*, *Chlamydia trachomatis*, *Ureaplasma urealyticum* (T-mycoplasma), and herpesvirus (Moghissi, 1982).

When a patient has a recurrent abortion, the medical personnel should make every effort to determine the cause. Carefully collected samples of the products of conception should be sent for genetic analysis. Appropriately collected samples for culture of pathogens should be sent. A thorough pelvic examination, including an intrauterine cavity exploration, should be performed. Finally, a detailed history of the events and factors surrounding the abortion should be recorded. Only by doing the above can the physician arrive at an etiology and counsel the couple regarding future pregnancy attempts.

ECTOPIC PREGNANCY

Ectopic pregnancy is defined as the implantation of the blastocyst at any site other than the endometrium. The vast majority (95 percent) of ectopic pregnancies are located in the fallopian tubes, within which the four most common sites are (in order of frequency) the ampullary, isthmic, fimbrial, and interstitial portions of the tube (Cavanagh and Woods, 1982). (See Fig. 22–1.) Besides the fallopian tubes, other, much less frequent sites include the cervix, ovary, and

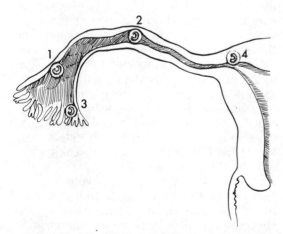

Figure 22–1. Location of ectopic pregnancy in the fallopian tube. *1*, Ampullar. *2*, Isthmic. *3*, Fimbrial. *4*, Interstitial. (Locations listed in order of frequency of occurrence.)

peritoneal cavity. The incidence of ectopic pregnancy varies widely across the United States, with reports of its occurrence in from 1 in 90 to 1 in 200 pregnancies (Cavanagh and Woods). Etiologic factors that predispose to ectopic pregnancy are any conditions that prevent or retard the passage of the fertilized ovum into the uterus, such as chronic salpingitis, congenital tubal abnormalities, tubal endometriosis, and pelvic adhesions. Patients wearing an intrauterine device appear to have a higher incidence of ectopic pregnancy. In an ectopic implantation, the trophoblastic cells of the blastocyst will proliferate and penetrate the tubal wall and arterial vessels, resulting in internal hemorrhage. The insufficient hormonal production by this faulty placenta will at first stimulate the endometrium to grow; then, as the hormone level fluctuates, the hormonal support for the endometrium fails and vaginal bleeding ensues. There is a wide variation of signs and symptoms, depending on the location of the ectopic pregnancy. Signs and symptoms associated with tubal pregnancy will begin with a missed or delayed menses followed by an episode of vaginal bleeding. As the tubal pregnancy begins to rupture, the patient will experience unilateral lower abdominal pain progressing to diffuse lower abdominal pain and vasomotor disturbances (e.g., fainting). The abdomen becomes exquisitely tender upon palpation, and a pelvic mass develops as the blood collects in the cul-de-sac. There will be exquisite unilateral adnexal pain elicited during pelvic exam. In about 50 percent of cases, referred right shoulder pain occurs, resulting from blood irritating the subdiaphragmatic phrenic nerve when the patient is supine. (See Table 22–2 for clinical signs and symptoms of ectopic pregnancy.) Culdocentesis is a most helpful diagnostic tool in establishing a high enough index of suspicion to operate. If a positive tap (free-flowing blood without clots) is obtained, prompt surgical intervention is mandatory.

The patient should be advised about her condition and impending surgical procedures, one of which may be hysterectomy. If possible, she should be queried regarding her desire for future fertility or any history of infertility. This information may influence the type of surgery chosen. Blood (crossmatched) and intravenous fluids are started, but if the patient is in shock no time should be wasted in stabilizing her, since prompt

Table 22–2. Clinical Signs and Symptoms of Ectopic Pregnancy

History	Abdomen	Temperature	Pelvic Exam	Uterus
Missed or delayed period; irregular bleeding; unilateral lower abdominal pain progressing to diffuse lower abdomen pain; shoulder pain; fainting	Abdominal distention; lower abdominal pain; rebound tenderness	Subnormal (98.4) or mild elevation (99.4)	Adnexal mass or mass in cul-de-sac; culdo-centesis yields unclotted blood	Normal or slightly enlarged

surgical intervention is required to control the bleeding. Complete excision of the affected tube is the treatment of choice, to prevent a recurrence of an ectopic pregnancy. However, if the patient has another previously damaged tube besides the tube containing the ectopic pregnancy and she desires fertility, one may elect to perform conservative tubal surgery. A linear salpingostomy is done to evacuate the ectopic pregnancy tissues, the bleeding is carefully controlled, and that tube is conserved. On the other hand, a hysterectomy may be performed if the ectopic pregnancy is in the portion of the tube within the uterine wall (interstitial), or if the only remaining tube contains the ectopic pregnancy, provided the patient desires sterility and her condition permits more extensive surgery.

In cases of ectopic pregnancy or abortion, an Rh-negative, unsensitized patient (negative indirect Coombs test) should receive hyperimmune gamma globulin (RhoGAM) injection before discharge.

HYDATIDIFORM MOLE

Hydatidiform mole is an abnormal development of the placenta resulting in the formation of grapelike vesicles as the fetal part of the pregnancy fails to develop. Unlike the usual abortion that occurs with an abnormal fetus, a mole placenta continues to grow at a very rapid pace to eventually outgrow its own blood supply and degenerate into grapelike vesicles. The incidence in the United States is 1 in 2000 pregnancies. In Orientals, the incidence may be as high as 1 in 200 pregnancies. The patient usually experiences exaggerated nausea and vomiting, and she may have intermittent to continuous brownish vaginal discharge associated with frank bleeding by the 12th week. Many times

the patient is more anemic than her bleeding history might indicate. There is a disproportionate rapid growth of the uterus in 50 percent of the cases. There is absence of fetal movement or fetal heart sounds. The uterus is usually tender and boggy because of overstretching of the lower uterine segment. Signs of preeclampsia appear before the 24th week of gestation in some of these patients. Finally, the passage of grapelike vesicles is diagnostic of the condition. The diagnosis is corroborated by persistently higher than normal titers of human chorionic gonadotropin (HCG) (> 20,000 IU/24 hr). Ultrasonography is the most efficacious and reliable test to identify a molar pregnancy. A sonogram demonstrating a large uterus filled with multiple small echoes (vesicles) with the absence of any fetal parts is pathognomonic of a mole pregnancy.

Evacuation of the mole by suction curettage is the treatment of choice. Occasionally a hysterectomy is required if the molar pregnancy is far advanced (> 20 week uterine size) or if the patient is older, since these two factors increase the risk of malignant degeneration. After the uterine evacuation, continuous follow-up of the patient is needed to detect any malignant changes of the remaining trophoblastic tissues, since choriocarcinoma is reported to occur in 0.5 to 9.5 percent of all patients with hydatidiform mole. Apparently, small groups of the trophoblastic tissues are disseminated in the bloodstream at evacuation and may degenerate into choriocarcinoma. To detect this, serum HCG titers are measured weekly for 6 months, and then every 6 months for the next year. The patient should avoid conception during this follow-up period of a year to 24 months, since an increase in titer suggests the development of choriocarcinoma.

Table 22–3 summarizes the clinical signs and symptoms of hydatidiform mole.

Table 22–3. Clinical Signs and Symptoms of Hydatidiform Mole

History	Diagnostic Signs	Conclusive Diagnostic Signs	Uterus
Hyperemesis; brownish discharge and bleeding by 12th week	Signs of preeclampsia before the 24th week Passage of grapelike vesicles	Persistent HCG > 20,000 IU/24 hr Ultrasonogram reveals large uterus filled with multiple small echoes (vesicles) and absence of fetal parts	Large for dates; tender and boggy

Bleeding in Late Pregnancy

ANTEPARTUM BLEEDING

The incidence of significant vaginal bleeding in the last half of pregnancy is approximately 3 percent. Several of the conditions that produce vaginal bleeding carry significant risk for the mother and fetus. Over half of these instances are associated with abnormal conditions of the placenta, i.e., placenta previa and abruptio placentae.

Significant vaginal bleeding is bright red blood not mixed with mucus, as in a "bloody show," and equivalent in amount to that which occurs with menstrual bleeding or more. Hemorrhage that is severe enough to lower maternal cardiac output can impair placental blood flow and place the fetus in jeopardy. A patient in this condition should quickly have her circulating volume expanded by intravenous fluids and blood. Once stable, the patient should have a careful and limited vaginal speculum examination to determine the cause of the bleeding, e.g., cervical or vaginal trauma, cervicitis, cervical cancer or polyps, or bleeding from cervical, vaginal, or labial venous varicosities. A digital examination is not to be done at this time. If the uterine bleeding is not associated with pain, the presumptive diagnosis is placenta previa. The diagnosis can be confirmed by sonography.

PLACENTA PREVIA

Placenta previa is the implantation of the placenta low in the uterus, either overlying or reaching the vicinity of the cervical os. The placenta's position near or over the cervix predisposes to hemorrhage as the placenta separates upon cervical dilatation or during the development of the lower uterine segment in late pregnancy. This serious obstetric complication occurs in 0.5 percent of cases, or 1 in 200 pregnancies. The incidence increases with increasing age (3 times more common in women over 35) and parity of the patient. If the patient has a past history of low segment cesarean section or placenta previa, there is a 12 times higher rate of recurrence. Defective vascularization of the decidua appears to be a major contributing factor to the development of placenta previa. Patients with a history of puerperal endometritis, lower uterine scar, or myomectomy and well-worn uterus (high parity) are at risk. Large low-lying placentas occurring in twin gestation or erythroblastosis may also encroach on the internal cervical os (Hellman and Pritchard, 1971).

The classification of placenta previa (Fig. 22–2) is as follows (Cavanagh and Woods, 1982):

Type I—Low placental implantation but the lower edge does not reach the internal cervical os.

Type II—The lower placental edge reaches the internal cervical os but does not cover it.

Type III—The placenta completely covers the internal os when the cervix is closed, but only partially covers the internal os when the cervix is dilated.

Type IV—The placenta covers the internal cervical os when the cervix is either closed or dilated.

The classic symptom of placenta previa is painless vaginal bleeding that usually occurs after the 28th week of gestation. This symptom is reported by 80 percent of patients. Ten percent will report bleeding and uterine contractions, and the remaining 10 per cent will be diagnosed incidentally before symptoms appear. This latter situation is becoming more common as ultrasound screening increases (Huff, 1982). However, the majority of unsymptomatic "ultrasound-diag-

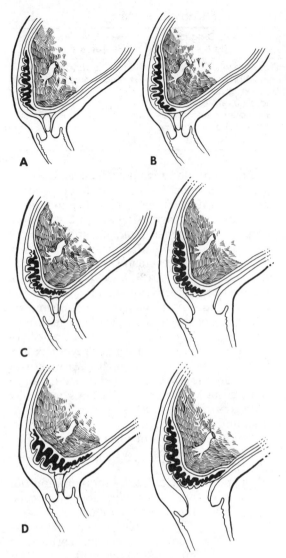

Figure 22–2. The classification of placenta previa. *A,* Class I. *B,* Class II. *C,* Class III with closed and partially open cervix. *D,* Class IV with closed and partially open cervix.

nosed placenta previas" in the mid-trimester will move up and away from the internal cervical os as the lower uterine segment develops from cervical tissue late in the 3rd trimester (Korducki, 1979). Joupilla points out that this is especially true if the ultrasound diagnosis of placenta previa is made in early pregnancy (Joupilla, 1979).

The first bleeding episode is generally characterized by occurring while the patient is asleep and is rarely fatal. The bleeding generally ceases only to reoccur without warning. The earlier in pregnancy the bleeding episodes occur, the more serious the type of placenta previa (type IV). Fifty percent of patients with type IV placenta previa will have episodic bleeding before the 30th week of gestation (Cavanagh and Woods, 1982). A type I or type II placenta previa may not bleed until the onset of labor. Approximately 90 percent of patients with placenta previa will experience at least one episode of bleeding, and 10 to 25 percent will develop hypovolemic shock during the course of their pregnancies (Cavanagh and Woods, 1982).

A presumptive diagnosis of placenta previa should be made with any episode of painless 3rd-trimester vaginal bleeding. The diagnosis can be confirmed by the use of ultrasound, which has over 95 percent accuracy in cases of placenta previa. Many hospitals have ultrasound capabilities; however, other methods such as soft tissue radiography, radioactive tracer concentration, and radioangiography may be used if ultrasound is unavailable.

Several studies have indicated that placenta previa can account for intrauterine fetal growth retardation. Bjerre and Bjerre (1976) reported that in their series the most common cause of low-birth-weight infants was placenta previa. Neri and coworkers (1980) demonstrated fetal growth retardation in 129 cases of placenta previa. In 1973, Varma reported a study indicating that placental insufficiency and fetal growth retardation may be a common problem in patients with placenta previa who experience recurrent bleeding episodes (Varma, 1973).

Any patient suspected of having a placenta previa should be initially hospitalized at bedrest. Initial management should be directed at ascertaining how much bleeding (per hour) the patient had and is having, i.e., light (50 cc), moderate (100 cc), or profuse (500 cc). Upon admission, blood should be drawn for blood count and type and cross-match for blood and Rh factor. If the bleeding is continuous and significant in amount, an intravenous infusion should be started. The amount of bleeding after the patient is placed in bed should be noted by frequently changing and counting (weighing) the disposable pads under the patient. Periodically the maternal abdomen should be palpated for uterine activity or rigidity. Expectant management is usually carried out in the hospital. While at bedrest the patient should be instructed to notify the nurses immediately if she feels fluid escaping from the vagina. External fetal monitoring (NST/CST) should be done weekly and in conjunction with any bleeding episode, to assess fetal well-being. A hematocrit above 30 is maintained by hematinics or blood transfusions, if necessary. Until the patient is stabilized, vital signs should be taken every 15 minutes with external fetal monitoring, and hourly intake and output determinations should be made. Once the patient is stable, the taking of vital signs can be reduced to hourly. Once the patient is on the antepartum floor, vital signs with fetal heart tones can be taken every 4 hours, and intake and output determinations and pad counts can be made on every shift. Once the bleeding has subsided, an occasional patient may be managed at home, provided that the following criteria are met:

1. The patient is intelligent, reliable, and fully understands the nature of her condition and that she must remain at bedrest and avoid coitus (see Chapter 10).

2. She should have round-the-clock transportation and communication available and live within 20 to 30 minutes' driving distance from the hospital.

3. She must have a hematocrit above 30, to allow some reserve in the face of significant bleeding.

4. She must be followed closely (i.e., sonography repeated at 3-week intervals and weekly antepartum fetal testing [NST-CST]) for fetal growth and fetal well-being.

The expectant management program requires that the patient remain at bedrest until one of the following occurs to terminate the program:

1. The patient goes into labor.

2. The fetus is mature (most reliable indicator is the L/S ratio) or the gestational age reaches 37 weeks.

3. The fetus expires.

4. An intrauterine infection develops.

5. The membranes rupture.

6. The amount of bleeding is excessive or life-threatening.

Usually about one third of patients with placenta previa can be managed expectantly as above, since over half of the patients are at term when they bleed for the first time. The remainder go into labor or have excessive bleeding.

Determining the Route of Delivery

The diagnosis of placenta previa usually means delivery by cesarean section. However, under certain circumstances, i.e., when there is only partial placental covering of the cervical os or a low-lying placenta, a vaginal delivery may be allowed. Although the placenta can be localized in the lower uterus accurately by ultrasound, the exact relationship of the lower placental edge to the cervical os is less accurate. Also, during the interval of expectant management, the lower uterine segment develops progressively from cervical tissue. Thus, an accurate assessment of the relationship of the lower edge of the placenta to the cervical os must be made to determine the route of delivery. The most definitive method by which to do this is digital palpation. This should be done only after termination of the expectant management program (see above) and under "double set-up" conditions—that is, do the examination in the operating room with blood ready, IV's going, anesthesia standing by, and all preparations completed for an immediate cesarean section. The palpation of placental tissue covering the cervical os or part of it mandates proceeding to cesarean section. Occasionally this palpation of the placenta can evoke profuse bleeding. It should be done with caution and care, yet firmly enough to make a diagnosis. If no placental tissue is palpated over the cervical os, the examining finger is inserted through the cervical os; if several centimeters of the lower uterine segment can be palpated, diagnosis of a low-lying or marginal placenta previa is made. A posterior low-lying or marginal placenta will usually warrant a cesarean delivery, because this situation is often associated with a significant incidence of intrapartum fetal asphyxia due to cord or placental compression against the sacrum by the presenting part; it is also associated with soft tissue dystocia. On the other hand, a trial of labor may be allowed with an anterior low-lying placenta. The goal of the "double set-up" examination is to determine the route of delivery only. If a trial of vaginal delivery is to be allowed, induction of labor (amniotomy) should be dictated by the ripeness of the cervix.

The type of cesarean section preferred will depend largely on the conditions at hand. A low cervical transverse incision is preferred; however, in the case of an anterior placenta previa, a vertical incision may be required to avoid incising the placenta, which may increase maternal and fetal blood loss. An occasional placenta previa is complicated by varying degrees of placenta accreta—placental tissue growing right into the myometrial layer of the placental attachment site. This usually occurs when there is a previous low cervical cesarean section scar. When the separation of the placenta is difficult and it is hard to control bleeding by conservative measures, a hysterectomy is usually required for control of hemorrhage.

Other Management Concerns

Maternal death from placenta previa is rare, but the perinatal mortality is still over 5 percent. A pediatrician must attend the delivery, and if a trial of labor is allowed, internal fetal monitoring is recommended. Extreme care must be exercised when placing the intrauterine catheter and scalp electrode. While the patient is undergoing the expectant management program, it is advisable to assign the same nurse personnel to this patient, to alleviate anxiety generated in having to relate to different nurses. During labor and delivery a 1:1 nurse–patient ratio is recommended because of the possibility of bleeding and emergency surgery. Also, vital signs with fetal heart tones and hourly intake and output determinations should be initiated. Throughout hospitalization the patient should be encouraged to verbalize her concerns and questions. By the time the second bleeding episode occurs, the patient should know and understand the medical and surgical intervention that may be required (Kilker and Wilkerson, 1973). She should understand the principle of expectant management and the reason for the "double set-up" examination. She should understand that she is at risk for postpartum hemorrhage, because the lower uterine segment does not have the same contractile strength as the upper uterine segment, and

that hysterectomy may be necessary because of the placenta's attachment to the thin lower uterine segment.

If the baby is born prematurely, the parents should be encouraged to visit their baby in the NICU and partake in his or her care as often as possible (Klaus and Kennell, 1976). If the mother wants to breast-feed her baby she should be encouraged to do so. Prematurity is not a deterrent to breast-feeding. She can use the breast pump to supply milk for the baby until the baby is able to feed at her breasts. Breast-feeding will also encourage uterine contractility.

ABRUPTIO PLACENTAE

Abruptio placentae is premature separation of a normally implanted placenta that results in retroplacental bleeding after the 20th week of gestation and before the fetus is delivered.

Two main types of abruptio placentae occur: that in which the hemorrhage is concealed (20 percent) and that with external hemorrhage (80 percent). The concealed type of hemorrhage is the more dangerous, as bleeding is confined to the uterine cavity and the complications may be severe. In the external type of abruptio placentae, there is vaginal bleeding and complications are fewer and less severe. The most common classification of abruptio placentae is as follows (see also Fig. 22–3 for illustration of types of abruptio placentae):

Grade 0—Asymptomatic. Diagnosed after delivery when a small retroplacental clot is discovered. Rupture of a marginal sinus is also included in this category.

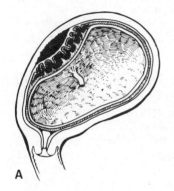 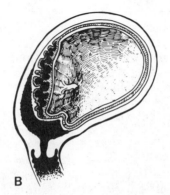 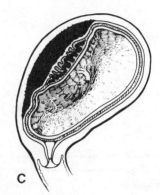

Figure 22–3. Types of abruptio placentae. *A*, Mild abruption with some concealed hemorrhage. *B*, Severe abruption with external hemorrhage. *C*, Severe abruption with concealed hemorrhage.

Grade 1—Vaginal bleeding. Uterine tetany and tenderness may be present. There are no signs of maternal shock or fetal distress.

Grade 2—External vaginal bleeding may or may not be present. Uterine tenderness and tetany are present. There are no signs of maternal shock. Signs of fetal distress are present.

Grade 3—External bleeding may or may not be present. There is marked uterine tetany, yielding a board-like consistency on palpation. Persistent abdominal pain, maternal shock, and fetal demise are present. Coagulopathy may become evident in 30 percent of the cases.

Abruptio placentae in general is reported to occur in about 1 in 250 to 1 in 155 pregnancies. The incidence of severe or Grade 3 abruptio placentae is 1 in 500 pregnancies. In about half of the cases, abruptio placentae occurs after the 36th week of gestation. Maternal mortality is about 2 percent if Grade 0 is excluded. In the more severe cases associated with fetal demise, maternal mortality increases to 10 percent. The incidence of abruptio placentae is increased with higher parity and previous abruption but not with advanced maternal age.

The exact cause of abruptio placentae is unknown; however, the following conditions seem to be predisposing factors: trauma to the abdomen, short umbilical cord, polyhydramnios, sudden decompression of the uterus, leiomyomas, uterine anomalies, compression or occlusion of the inferior vena cava, circumvallate placenta, and hypertensive disorders. Hypertensive disease in pregnancy is by far the most common predisposing condition. The severity of abruptio placentae increases with parity; and furthermore, the woman with a history of abruptio placentae has a risk of reoccurrence of about 1 in 12 (Pritchard and Brekken, 1967). Some have contended that folic acid deficiency has an etiologic role; however, further studies have failed to substantiate this theory. Naeye demonstrated a correlation between placental abruption and cigarette smoking and poor maternal weight gain (Naeye et al., 1977). He suggested that poor maternal nutrition during pregnancy may contribute to the development of abruptio placentae. It is believed that placental abruption is caused by degenerative changes in the small arteries that supply the intervillous space, resulting in thrombosis, decidual degeneration, and rupture of vessels, causing a retroplacental hematoma (Page et al., 1981). The continued arterial pumping will cause further separation of the placenta from its decidual attachment; thus, in the most severe cases complete separation can occur. If half or more of the placental surface is separated, fetal death is inevitable (Page et al., 1981). A Couvelaire uterus (retroplacental apoplexy) results in cases of concealed hemorrhage with blood infiltration into the myometrium. The condition was once believed to decrease uterine contractility sufficiently to produce postpartum hemorrhage by disrupting the myometrial bundles; however, the Couvelaire uterus is not an indication for hysterectomy (Hellman and Pritchard, 1971).

The clinical picture of a severe abruptio placentae usually includes some vaginal bleeding, uterine tetany, uterine tenderness, absence of fetal heart tones, and hypovolemic shock (Table 22–4). With a severe abruption the patient can lose up to one half of her blood volume (250 ml). The thromboplastin material in the amniotic fluid can find its way into the maternal bloodstream to initiate an acute disseminated intravascular coagulopathy.

Signs of shock may be out of proportion to the amount of hemorrhage evident in concealed hemorrhage; however, uterine rigidity and tenderness will be marked. Oliguria due to inadequate renal perfusion before treatment of hypovolemia may also be observed.

In the less severe grades of abruptio placentae (less than half placental separation), fetal distress may be manifested by fetal heart rate patterns of late decelerations, decreased short- and long-term variability, and tachycardia. Internal uterine pressure mon-

Table 22–4. Clinical Signs and Symptoms of Abruptio Placentae

1. Vaginal bleeding may or may not be present
2. Port-wine-colored amniotic fluid
3. ↓ BP, ↑ pulse, dyspnea, pallor, oliguria
4. Symptoms of shock may be out of proportion to the amount of bleeding seen
5. Severe and/or sudden pain (retroplacental separation) or painless (marginal separation)
6. Uterus with boardlike tone; rigidity or tenderness

itoring will usually demonstrate an increased resting presure (> 16 mm Hg) and polysystole (Fig. 22–4).

Although the more severe cases of abruptio placentae are usually heralded by the classic signs and symptoms, the mildest form (Grade 0) usually goes unrecognized until after delivery. Thus, in the presence of vaginal bleeding in the 3rd trimester, it is necessary to rule out previa and other causes of vaginal bleeding by clinical inspection and ultrasound evaluation.

Management of a patient with abruptio placentae requires adherence to the following basic tenets:

1. Rule of 30's. Maintenance of a minimum urine output of 30 ml/hr and a hematocrit of 30 volume percent at all times by intravenous infusion of crystalloid solutions or blood as required.

2. Delivery as quickly as possible. The goal is a vaginal delivery if the fetus is healthy or dead. A cesarean section may be required if fetal distress is present. The use of oxytocin is not contraindicated, although it is rarely necessary.

3. Early amniotomy to decrease the amnioinfusion into the maternal bloodstream.

4. Intensive maternal and fetal monitoring of vital signs every 15 minutes and of circulating volume status (I & O) every hour. The nurse–patient ratio should be 1:1 because of hemorrhage, assessment of fetal distress, possible emergency surgery, and the need to provide emotional support for this emergency situation.

Any patient diagnosed as having an abruption (even if it is of a lower grade, since it may progress) should have a reliable, large-bore intravenous line established (two or more in cases of severe abruption), have 6 or more units of blood cross-matched, have bladder drainage by an indwelling catheter,

have an amniotomy, have internal fetal monitoring with a live fetus, and have blood coagulation studies performed. A central venous pressure line or a Swan-Ganz balloon flotation catheter may help in the fluid management of a patient in shock. A peripheral venous blood sample placed in a red-top tube taped to the wall and checked in 7 to 10 minutes will indicate the coagulation status of the patient. If the clot is not formed or is fragile, the patient has a coagulopathy. If vaginal delivery is anticipated, correction of the coagulopathy is not necessary and will not alter the outcome (Hellman and Pritchard, 1971). However, careful hemostasis for an episiotomy will be required. The coagulopathy will usually be present when the patient first enters the hospital, but will be restored to normal 12 to 24 hours post partum by a normally functioning liver. If the patient requires an abdominal delivery for obstetric indications (e.g., transverse lie, no progress in labor), the coagulopathy will have to be corrected with fresh frozen plasma and cryoprecipitate (15 to 20 bags will increase fibrinogen 100 mg/dl). At the time of laparotomy one may encounter a bruised-appearing uterus (Couvelaire uterus). This appearance of the uterus should not belie its ability to contract sufficiently to control bleeding after delivery. A coagulopathy developing with a live fetus would be quite unusual, but a blood sample should be checked for clotting ability before surgery as a precaution.

By maintaining an adequate circulating volume (rule of 30's) during labor in a patient with an abruption, the incidence of the not uncommon sequelae of the past of renal damage, adult pulmonary distress syndrome, and Sheehan's syndrome can be minimized.

The perinatal mortality of abruptio placen-

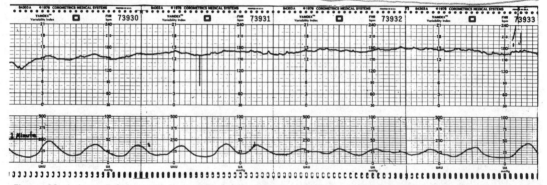

Figure 22–4. A cardiotocograph in a patient with abruption. Note the presence of frequent uterine contractions and elevated baseline tone in the bottom panel. Note the presence of "late decelerations" in the upper panel. (From Paul, R. H., et al.: Fetal Intensive Care. Wallingford, CT, Corometrics Medical Systems, Inc., 1979.)

Table 22–5. Clinical Signs and Symptoms of the Complications of Abruptio Placentae

1. Clinical signs of shock
   a. Hypothermia
   b. Tachycardia with weak and thready pulse
   c. Rapid shallow respirations; hypotension with reduced pulse pressure; pale mottled or cyanotic skin; cold, clammy skin
   d. Cerebral manifestation of inadequate perfusion: patient complains of thirst, anxiety, confusion, restlessness
2. Increased bleeding with signs of hypovolemia
3. Decreased urine output (< 30 cc/hr)
4. CVP readings (↓ hypovolemia < 2 cm; ↑ hypervolemia; cardiac failure; or fluid overload > 10 cm)
5. Bleeding from puncture sites (coagulopathy)

tae is over 50 percent, and the maternal mortality is 1 percent or less.

Continuous fetal and maternal monitoring is *imperative* for the woman who is allowed to labor with a live fetus. Vital signs at least every 15 minutes, accurate hourly I & O, CVP readings, and continuous fetal electronic monitoring will keep the medical team abreast of the maternal and fetal conditions. Observe for signs of shock, hypofibrinogenemia, and acute renal failure. (See Table 22–5.)

At all times be prepared for emergency cesarean section or precipitous delivery. To encourage the best placental perfusion, instruct the mother to labor in the lateral position.

Intrapartum Bleeding

Significant bleeding during the intrapartum period not associated with placental abruption is rare. Cervical trauma can cause bleeding but is usually not enough to cause problems. There are two causes of intrapartum bleeding that pose a threat to the well-being of the fetus and mother: vasa previa and uterine rupture.

VASA PREVIA

A vasa previa may occur when there is a velamentous insertion of the umbilical cord into a low-lying placenta. In this condition the cord vessels begin to separate as the cord nears the placental surface, like fingers spreading apart. These single vessels no longer have the gelatinous rubbery protective surrounding as they do in the intact cord, and they often traverse across part of the amniotic membrane to the placental surface. A vasa previa occurs when the vessel in the amniotic membranes is draped across

the cervix ahead of the presenting part. When amniotomy is performed, the fetal vessels are torn and fetal bleeding commences. The incidence of this condition is low. Recognition of it requires a high index of suspicion when bleeding follows amniotomy. The determination of a fetal bleed requires the ability to quickly differentiate between fetal and maternal blood (which can result from cervical trauma during the amniotomy procedure), as the baby can die within 1 to 2 minutes if a vessel in the umbilical cord is ruptured. An Apt test can do this (Apt and Downey, 1955). This test is based on the physiologic principle that fetal hemoglobin is alkaline-stable whereas adult hemoglobin is not. (See methodology for Apt test in Table 22–6.) If fetal blood is documented, the baby should be rapidly delivered. Usually a cesarean section is required. During the assessment and diagnosis of this emergency situation, a 2:1 nurse–patient ratio should be maintained.

UTERINE RUPTURE

The major cause of uterine rupture is previous cesarean section, and the second most common cause is overstimulation with oxytocin (Pritchard, 1985). (See Chapter 14.) Spontaneous rupture of the uterus is a devastating complication of labor, carrying a very high maternal and perinatal mortality. It tends to occur in older, multiparous

Table 22–6. The Apt Test Method

1. Collect bloody specimen in a lavender-top tube.
2. Concurrently, obtain two controls:
   a. Maternal blood sample
   b. Fetal blood sample—e.g., use cord blood from recent delivery (nursery lab always has a control available)
   c. Sample in question
3. Place 0.2 ml of each sample in a separate test tube (use pipette or tuberculin syringe).
4. Add 2 ml of tap water or distilled water to each test tube (10:1 dilution). This will lyse the red cells and produce a pink supernatant in all tubes.
5. Centrifuge the tubes for approximately 2 minutes. This step will intensify the color of the supernatant as the sediment falls to the bottom of the tube.
6. Add 1 ml of 0.25 normal (1%) NaOH solution to each tube.
7. Read the color change in 2 minutes. If the test solution is adult hemoglobin, its color will change from pink to yellow-brown. If the solution is fetal hemoglobin, its color will remain predominantly pink. It is essential to compare the color change of the test solution with that of the control specimens.
8. If there is any question about the interpretation of the test, and time permits, request the laboratory to perform a Kleihauer-Betke test or hemoglobin electrophoresis.

women, and cephalopelvic disproportion is a significant factor. It occurs once in 1000 to 1500 births and is responsible for at least 5 percent of all maternal deaths. At the height of a uterine contraction the patient will complain of sudden sharp shooting abdominal pain. She frequently states that "something has given way" inside her. Uterine contractions cease to bother the patient, and vaginal bleeding is noted. Abdominal palpation reveals tenderness, the presenting part has receded, and two large round objects (one the contracted empty uterus and the other the fetus) can be palpated in the lower abdomen. Shortly thereafter the patient becomes shocky. A vaginal examination sometimes reveals a rent in the lower uterine segment. The treatment is immediate laparotomy and frequently hysterectomy after rapid stabilization of the patient's hypovolemic state. Perinatal mortality is virtually 100 percent. During this obstetric emergency, at least a 1:1 nurse–patient ratio is recommended. With both vasa previa and uterine rupture, maternal vital signs should be taken at least every 15 minutes with continuous fetal heart rate monitoring.

Postpartum Hemorrhage

Postpartum hemorrhage is a significant contributor to maternal mortality today. Most textbooks define it as the occurrence of more than 500 ml of blood loss during and after delivery. However, Pritchard and others have demonstrated that actual blood loss from a normal vaginal delivery exceeds 500 ml (Pritchard et al., 1962; Newton, 1966). Nonetheless, in most large clinical obstetric services, estimates of more than the usual amount of blood loss at delivery and immediately post partum have been noted in around 4 percent of deliveries. Postpartum hemorrhage severe enough to cause signs and symptoms of hypovolemic shock has an incidence of less than 0.5 percent.

The majority of cases of postpartum hemorrhage are due to uterine atony (75 to 80 percent). Other causes include genital tract trauma during delivery, and rarely placenta accreta, uterine inversion, and coagulopathies.

UTERINE ATONY

Predisposing factors for uterine atony in the order of their frequency include the following: (1) precipitous labor, (2) $MgSO_4$ treatment in preeclamptic patients, (3) chorioamnionitis, (4) macrosomia ($>$4000 mg) or multiple gestations, and (5) prolonged labor (Hayashi et al., 1984). Also, patients with a previous history of a postpartum hemorrhage due to uterine atony are likely to repeat that performance. We have found that the majority of patients who experienced a serious postpartum hemorrhage were delivered by cesarean section.

When excessive uterine bleeding occurs and the uterus is atonic, the physician will usually manually explore the uterus and remove any retained placental fragments or membranes, administer dilute oxytocin intravenously (40 to 60 units added to a liter IV bottle), and give methyl ergonovine, 0.2 mg IM (if the patient is not hypertensive). The uterus is manually massaged to increase uterine muscle tone. If bleeding continues despite these standard therapies, the physician is forced to perform an emergency laparotomy to control the hemorrhage by surgical intervention. Recently, the use of prostaglandin has been reported to successfully increase uterine tone and abate hemorrhage. Prostaglandin $F_2\alpha$ given by the intramyometrial route (Takagi et al., 1972; Jacobs and Arias, 1980), prostaglandin E_2 by vaginal suppository (Hertz et al., 1980), and recently a 15 methyl analogue of prostaglandin $F_2\alpha$ that is 10 times as potent, has a longer duration of action, and is given by the intramuscular route have been reported to be very successful in preliminary studies (Toppozada et al., 1981; Hayashi et al., 1981). Side effects of prostaglandin treatments have been reported to be mild fever, diarrhea, and vomiting (Hayashi et al., 1981). However, prostaglandins do not affect breast-feeding. Especially with cesarean section patients, prophylactic antinausea and antidiarrhea medications should be initiated with the prostaglandins. The use of prostaglandins would follow failure of the standard therapies mentioned above. Failing all else, the physician may have to ligate the uterine arteries or the hypogastric arteries, or even perform a hysterectomy to control the hemorrhage. The nurse will be required to recognize when there is a need for rapid volume expansion, to type and cross-match for many units of blood, and to anticipate the pharmacologic therapy required and have the appropriate agents at hand for immediate use. Fibrinogen must also be on hand in every delivery room. It must be

Table 22–7. Management of Postpartum Hemorrhage Due to Uterine Atony (in Order of Procession)

1. Standard therapies
   a. Uterine exploration and massage
   b. IV oxytocin (dilute)
   c. IM methylergonovine (*never* IV)
2. Prostaglandin therapy
   a. Prostin 15M, 250 mcg IM or intramyometrial injection
   b. Prostin $F_{2\alpha}$, 1.0 mg by intramyometrial injection
   c. Prostin E_2, 20-mg vaginal suppository
3. Surgical therapies
   a. Uterine artery ligation
   b. Hypogastric artery ligation
   c. Hysterectomy

remembered to never inject a bolus of oxytocin directly intravenously or into the IV line, as this practice has been associated with acute hypotension and cardiac arrest. See Table 22–7 for a summary of the above therapies for postpartum hemorrhage. During these therapies the nurse–patient ratio should be 1:1. Vital signs should be taken at a minimum of every 15 minutes, and an accurate I & O should be done.

GENITAL TRACT TRAUMA

Lacerations of the cervix and vagina occur with spontaneous as well as with instrumented vaginal deliveries. Any patient with excessive postpartum bleeding should be carefully inspected for cervical and vaginal lacerations, even in the face of atony, to rule out a combined source of bleeding. Genital tract trauma can cause significant blood loss through continuous nonalarming bleeding or bleeding into a dead space to form a large retroperitoneal hematoma over hours.

A careful exploration of the vaginal vault, looking for vaginal and cervical lacerations, should follow every delivery, particularly operative deliveries. Vaginal lacerations are likely to occur over the perineal body and the periurethral area and over the ischial spines in the posterior-lateral aspects of the vaginal vault. Repair of vaginal lacerations requires good exposure and lighting and utilizes the principle of tissue approximation without leaving any dead space. Most important is placing the first suture well above the apex of the laceration. Cervical lacerations are likely to occur at 9 or 3 o'clock and do not need suturing unless they are bleeding. Vaginal and labial hematomas are usually just carefully observed, unless they are large or rapidly enlarging, in which case the hematoma should be excised. If no bleeding vessel is identified (as is common), just pack the area with pressure gauze and observe carefully. Astute observation of the perineal area is mandatory during the postpartum period, especially with any of these lacerations or hematomas. Initially ice can help to decrease swelling and reduce pain. Later warm compresses, heat lamps, and analgesic spray can be useful to decrease discomfort.

UTERINE INVERSION

Uterine inversion is the "turning inside out" of the uterus in the third stage of labor. The uterus is usually atonic, the cervix open, and the placenta attached. As the fundus of the uterus moves through the vagina, the tugging on the peritoneal structures elicits a strong vasovagal response, leading to hypotension. If the placenta is completely or partially separated, bleeding will be excessive. Thus, this condition unless quickly corrected is life-threatening. Its spontaneous occurrence is quite rare (1 in 20,000 pregnancies). Improper management of the third stage of labor may increase the risk of its occurrence, particularly when there is fundal placentation, incomplete separation, or an atonic uterus, and a health care provider exerts fundal pressure with his or her fingers, producing traction on the cord (Watson et al., 1980).

Management of a uterine inversion requires quick thinking and action. The diagnosis is readily apparent when one recognizes a shaggy ball with the placenta attached to it protruding from the vaginal opening. The patient will show signs of hypovolemic shock, so that rapidly increasing intravenous fluids should be instituted and help obtained from other personnel, especially anesthesia standby. (The increased IV fluids should not contain oxytocin.) The placenta should be manually removed. The physician then institutes a gradual but continuous replacement of the inverted uterus, using the palm of the hand to elevate the uterine fundus through the vagina and into the peritoneal cavity. Once the uterus is replaced, agents are given to increase uterine tone and to control the bleeding at the placental site.

PLACENTA ACCRETA

Placenta accreta is an abnormal condition in which the placenta villi grow into the myometrium owing to defective formation of decidua. The placenta is adherent to the myometrium and will usually be removed in pieces manually. The result is postpartum hemorrhage. Its occurrence is quite rare, but it is more likely to occur in a patient with a placenta previa over a previous low cervical transverse cesarean section scar. The usual treatment is immediate hysterectomy.

COAGULOPATHIES

These entities are well covered in Chapter 23.

Summary

When bleeding occurs in pregnancy, the outcome is potentially disastrous. In early pregnancy, the loss of the fetus will require the nurse to be supportive and aware of the grieving process. An understanding of the pathophysiologic processes of abortions, ectopic pregnancy, and hydatidiform mole will result in more effective nurse intervention. In late pregnancy, quick thinking and action, as well as the organizational ability of the nurse, are essential in dealing with the life-threatening hemorrhage seen with placenta previa, abruptio placentae, and postpartum conditions such as uterine inversion. The subtleties of the diagnosis of bleeding during
Text continued on page 439

Table 22–8. Patient Care Summary in Bleeding Management*

	Antepartum			
	Outpatient	*Inpatient*	*Intrapartum*	*Postpartum*
ABORTIONS (Nurse–Patient Ratio = 1:2)				
BP†	—	On admission; then q 1 hr	q 1 hr	q 15 min × 4; then q 30 min × 2; then q 1 hr until stable; then on discharge to PP floor
P, R†	—	On admission; then q 1 hr	—	q 15 min × 4; then q 30 min × 2; then q 1 hr until stable; then on discharge to PP floor
T†	—	On admission; then q 4 hr	q 4 hr	On admission; then q 4 hr; then on discharge to PP floor
Observe for bleeding and tissue passage	Frequently	On admission; then q 30 min	q 30 min	On admission; then q 1 hr till stable; then q 4 hr; then on discharge to PP floor
Ultrasound	Gestational dating	—	—	—
Sexual limitations	Two weeks' abstention, or until vaginal discharge ceases		—	—
Bedrest	With bathroom privileges	With bathroom privileges	Yes	
ECTOPIC PREGNANCY (Nurse-Patient Ratio = 2:1)				
BP†	—	On admission; then q 1 hr	q 15 min during surgery	q 15 min × 4; then q 30 min × 2; then q 1 hr until stable; then on discharge from RR
P, R†	—	On admission; then q 1 hour	As above	q 15 min × 4; then q 30 min × 2; then q 1 hr until stable; then on discharge from RR
T†	—	On admission; then q 4 hr	—	q 4 hr
Fetal heart rate	q 1 hr		—	—
Check for:				
Vaginal bleeding	q 1 hr		—	q 15 min × 4; then q 30 min × 2; then q 1 hr
Tender abdomen		On admission		until stable; then on discharge from RR
Right shoulder pain		On admission	—	—
Culdocentesis	—	On admission	—	—

Table continued on opposite page

Table 22–8. Patient Care Summary in Bleeding Management *Continued*

	Antepartum		Intrapartum	Postpartum
	Outpatient	*Inpatient*		
HYDATIDIFORM MOLE (Nurse–Patient Ratio = 2:1)				
Ultrasound to confirm diagnosis	Performed on all patients suspected of having hydatidiform mole		—	—
BP	—	On admission; then q 1 hr	q 15 min during surgery	On admission; then q 15 min × 4; then q 30 min × 2; then q 1 hr until stable; then on discharge from RR
R, P	—	On admission; then q 1 hr	q 15 min during surgery	On admission; then q 15 min × 4; then q 30 min × 2; then q 1 hr until stable; then on discharge from RR
T	—	On admission; then q 4 hr	—	On admision to RR; then q 4 hr
Check for bleeding	—	On admission; then q 30 min	—	On admission to RR; then q 4 hr
Fetal heart rate	—	On admission	—	On admission; then q 15 min × 4; then q 30 min × 2; then q 1 hr; then on discharge from RR
HCG titers	—	Follow up for 6–12 months and instruct patient to avoid conception during this time		
PLACENTA PREVIA—NO BLEEDING (Nurse–Patient Ratio = 1:6–8 antepartum, 1:2 intrapartum)				
Ultrasound for placental location and to rule out IUGR	—	q 2 weeks	On admission	—
BP	—	On admission; then q 4 hr	Per C/S routine if allowed to labor same as normal	On admission; then q 15 min × 4; then q 30 min × 2; then on discharge to PP floor
R, P	—	On admission; then q 4 hr	Per C/S routine if allowed to labor same as normal	On admission; then q 15 min × 4; then q 30 min × 2; then on discharge to PP floor
T	—	On admission, then q 4 hr	q 4 hr	On admission; then q 4 hr; then on discharge to PP floor
Check bleeding (pad count)	Count pads at home	q 8 hr, prn	q 1 hr	On admission; then q 4 hr; then on discharge to PP floor
I & O		q 8 hr	q 8 hr (q hr with active bleeding)	q shift in RR
Bedrest	With bathroom privileges	With bathroom privileges	Yes	Yes
Fetal heart rate monitoring	—	On admission; then q 8 hr	Record q 1 hr with continuous monitoring, preferably internal. Without monitor, q 15 min continuously through 2–3 contractions	—
Contractions Frequency Duration Quality Resting tone	—	q shift	Continuous	—
Lochia	—	—	—	On admission; then q 15 min × 4; then q 30 min × 2; if stable, then q 4 hr

Table continued on following page

Table 22–8. Patient Care Summary in Bleeding Management *Continued*

	Antepartum			
	Outpatient	*Inpatient*	Intrapartum	Postpartum
PLACENTA PREVIA—NO BLEEDING *Continued*				
NST-CST	Weekly, unless significant bleeding—then repeat immediately	On admission; then weekly unless significant bleeding—then repeat immediately	—	—
H & H	Weekly	On admission; then weekly	Admission	Morning after delivery
Type & cross-match	—	Keep current	Keep current	—
Sexual activity	None	None	—	—
PLACENTA PREVIA WITH BLEEDING (Nurse–Patient Ratio = 2:1)				
Fetal heart rate	—	Continuous external monitor	prn while reading for C/S	—
BP, P, R	—	On admission; then q 15 min	C/S per anesthesia	q 15 min × 4; then q 30 min × 2; then q 1 hr until stable; then q 4 hr
T	—	On admission; then q 4 hr	C/S	On admission to RR; then q 4 hr; then on discharge to PP floor
I & O	—	Initiate on admission q 1 hr while bleeding	—	Hourly while in RR; then q 8 hr till stable
Check bleeding (lochia)	—	Constantly	Constantly until C/S	q 15 min × 4; then q 30 min × 2; then q 1 hr until stable; then q 4 hr
H & H	—	On admission	On admission to OR	On admission to RR; morning after delivery
Clotting studies	—	On admission	—	—
Type & cross-match	—	On admission Keep current	Keep current	—
Bedrest		Yes	Yes	Yes
Prepare for C/S if unable to stop bleeding				
ABRUPTIO PLACENTAE—SEVERE (Nurse–Patient Ratio = 2:1)				
BP, P, R	—	—	q 15 min	On admission; then q 15 min × 4; then q 30 min × 2; then q 1 hr until stable; then on discharge to PP floor
T			On admission	On admission to RR; then q 4 hr; then on discharge to PP floor
Fetal heart rate monitoring	—	—	Continuously during labor, preferably internal Without monitor, q 15 min listening through 2–3 contractions	—
Contractions Frequency Duration Quality Resting tone	—	—	Continuously during labor, preferably internal Without monitor, q 15 min	—
I & O	—	—	q 1 hr	q shift
H & H	—	—	Stat	On admission to RR
Type & cross-match	—	—	On admission Keep current	

Table continued on opposite page

Table 22–8. Patient Care Summary in Bleeding Management *Continued*

	Antepartum		Intrapartum	Postpartum
	Outpatient	*Inpatient*		
ABRUPTIO PLACENTAE—MILD (Nurse–Patient Ratio = 1:6–8 antepartum, 1:2 intrapartum)				
BP, P, R	—	q 4 hr	q 15 min	On admission; then q 15 min × 4; then q 30 min × 2; then q 1 hr until stable; then on discharge to PP floor
T	—	On admission; then q 4 hr	q 4 hr	On admission to RR; then q 4 hr; then on discharge to PP floor
Fetal heart rate monitoring	—	NST-CST weekly starting 32 weeks FHR q shift	Continuously during labor, preferably internal Without monitor, q 15 min listening through 2–3 contractions	—
Contractions Frequency Duration Quality Resting Tone	—	FHR q shift	Continuously during labor, preferably internal Without monitor, q 30 min	—
I & O	—	q shift	q shift	q shift
H & H	—	Daily	—	Morning after delivery
Type & cross-match	—	Keep current	Keep current	—
VASA PREVIA (Nurse–Patient Ratio = 2:1)				
Immediate emergency Prepare for cesarean section				
Fetal heart rate monitoring			Continue until start of cesarean section, if possible with internal monitor Without monitor, q 5 min	
Contractions			Continuously during labor, preferably internal Without monitor, q 30 min	
BP, R, P			Taken by anesthetist q 15 min before cesarean section	
I & O			q 1 hr	
UTERINE RUPTURE (Nurse–Patient Ratio = 2:1)				
Immediate emergency Prepare for cesarean section (C/S)			—	—
				—
Fetal heart rate monitoring			Continuously until start of C/S, preferably internal Without monitor, q 5 min	—

Table continued on following page

Table 22–8. Patient Care Summary in Bleeding Management *Continued*

| | Antepartum | | | |
	Outpatient	Inpatient	Intrapartum	Postpartum
UTERINE RUPTURE *Continued*				
Contractions			Continuously until start of C/S, preferably internal Without monitor, q 15 min	On admission to RR
Lochia assessment				q 15 min × 4; then q 30–60 min until stable; then q 4–8 hr
BP, R, P			Per C/S routine	q 15 min × 4; then q 30 min × 2; then q 1 hr until stable; then on discharge to PP floor
T			q 4 hr	On admission; then q 4 hr; then on discharge to PP floor
I & O			q 1 hour	q 1 hr in RR; then q 8 hr till stable
POSTPARTUM HEMORRHAGE (Nurse–Patient Ratio = 1:1)				
BP, P, R				q 15 min until stable
T				q 1 hr if receiving blood q 4 hr if not receiving blood
I & O				q 1 hr
H & H				Yes
Type & cross-match				Yes
Lochia assessments				q 15 min minimum
Administer prostaglandins				As needed
Perineal assessment				q 15 min
Ice compresses				Continuously with trauma
UTERINE INVERSION (Nurse–Patient Ratio = 1:2)				
BP, P, R				q 15 min during emergency; then q 15 min × 4; then q 30 min × 2; then q 1 hr until stable; then on discharge to PP floor
I & O				Continuously
Laboratory values				Serial H & H after acute phase

*This table lists *minimal* requirements for taking BP, P, R, and T; presence of excessive bleeding or infection may require more frequent readings.

†This is minimal; excessive bleeding or infection may require more frequent BP, T, P, and R.

labor are important and must not be overlooked. Once recognized, these emergency conditions demand continuous nursing vigilance, which usually dictates a 1:1 nurse–patient ratio. Table 22–8 summarizes patient care procedures in the management of various forms of pregnancy-associated bleeding.

REFERENCES

Apt, L., and Downey, W. S.: Melena neonatorum, the swallowed blood syndrome. J. Pediatr. 47:6, 1955.

Bjerre, B., and Bjerre, I.: Significance of obstetrical factors in prognosis of low birth weight children. Acta Paediatr. Scand. 65:577, 1976.

Cavanagh, D., and Woods, R.: Hemorrhage in early pregnancy. In Cavannagh, D., et al. (ed): Obstetric Emergencies. Philadelphia, Harper & Row, 1982, p. 133.

Goldzieher, J. W., and Benigno, B. B.: The treatment of threatened and recurrent abortion: a critical review. Am. J. Obstet. Gynecol. 75:1202, 1958.

Hayashi, R., Castillo, M. S., and Noah, M. L.: Management of severe postpartum hemorrhage due to uterine atony using an analogue of prostaglandin $F_2\alpha$. Obstet. Gynecol. 58:426, 1981.

Hayashi, R., Castillo, M. S., and Noah, M. L.: Three year experience using Prostin 15M in the management of severe postpartum hemorrhage. Obstet. Gynecol. 63:806, 1984.

Hellman, L. M., and Pritchard., J. A. (eds.): Williams Obstetrics, 14th ed. New York, Appleton-Century-Crofts, 1971.

Hertz, R. H., Sokol, R. J., and Dierker, L. J.: Treatment of postpartum uterine atony with prostaglandin E_2 vaginal suppositories. Obstet. Gynecol. 56:129, 1980.

Huff, R. W.: Third trimester bleeding. Contemp. Obstet. Gynecol. 20:40, 1982.

Jacobs, M. M., and Arias, F.: Intramyometrial prostaglandin $F_{2\alpha}$ in the treatment of severe postpartum hemorrhage. Obstet. Gynecol. 55:665, 1980.

Jensen, M., and Bobak, T.: Handbook of Maternity Care. St. Louis, C. V. Mosby Co., 1980, p. 189.

Joupilla, P.: The evaluation of prognosis in threatened early pregnancy. J. Perinat. Med. 8:3, 1980.

Joupilla, P.: Vaginal bleeding in the last two trimesters of pregnancy: a clinical and ultrasonic study. Acta Obstet. Gynecol. Scand. 58:461, 1979.

Kilker, R., and Wilkerson, B.: Nursing care in placenta previa and abruptio placentae. Nurs. Clin. North Am. 8:479, 1973.

Klaus, M., and Kennell, J.: Maternal-Infant Bonding. St Louis, C. V. Mosby Co., 1976, p. 122.

Korducki, S.: Bleeding late in pregnancy. Wis. Med. J. 78:35, 1979.

MacLeod, J., and Gold, R. Z.: The male factor in fertility and sterility. Fertil. Steril. 8:36, 1957.

Moghissi, K. S.: What causes habitual abortion. Contemp. Obstet. Gynecol. 20:45, 1982.

Naeye, R. L., Harkness, W. L., and Utts, J.: Abruptio placentae and perinatal death: a prospective study. Am. J. Obstet. Gynecol. 128:740, 1977.

Neri, A., Goradesky, I., Bahary, C., et al.: Impact of placenta previa on intrauterine fetal growth. Isr. J. Med. Sci. 16:6, 1980.

Newton, M.: Postpartum hemorrhage. Am. J. Obstet. Gynecol. 94:711, 1966.

Page, E., Villee, C., and Villee, D.: Human Reproduction: Essentials of Reproductive Medicine, 3rd ed. Philadelphia, W. B. Saunders Co., 1981, p. 408.

Pizer, H., and Palinski, O.: Coping with a Miscarriage. New York, Plume Books, 1980, p. 106.

Pritchard, J. A., Baldwin, R. M., Dickey, J. C., et al.: Blood volume changes in pregnancy and the puerperium. II. Red blood cell loss and changes in apparent blood volume during and following vaginal delivery, cesarean section and cesarean section plus total hysterectomy. Am. J. Obstet. Gynecol. 84:1271, 1962.

Pritchard, J., and Brekken, A.: Clinical and laboratory studies on severe abruptio placentae. Am. J. Obstet. Gynecol. 97:681, 1967.

Pritchard, J. A., and MacDonald, P. C.: Williams' Obstetrics. New York, Appleton-Century-Crofts, 1985.

Takagi, S., Yoshida, T., Togo, Y., et al.: The effects of intramyometrial injection of prostaglandin $F_2\alpha$ on severe postpartum hemorrhage. Prostaglandins, 12:565, 1976.

Tho T. P., Byrd, J. R., and McDonough, P. G.: Etiologies and subsequent reproductive performance of 100 couples with recurrent abortion. Fertil. Steril. 32:389, 1979.

Toppozada, M., El Bassaty, M., El Rahmin, H. A., et al.: Control of intractable atonic postpartum hemorrhage by 15 methyl prostaglandin $F_2\alpha$. Obstet. Gynecol. 58:327, 1981.

Tricomi, V., and Kohl, S. C.: Fetal death in utero. Am. J. Obstet. Gynecol. 4:1092, 1957.

Varma, T.: Fetal growth and placental function in patients with placenta previa. J. Obstet. Gynaecol. Br. Commonw. 80:311, 1973.

Warburton, D., and Fraser, F. C.: On the probability that a woman who has had a spontaneous abortion will abort with subsequent pregnancies. J. Obstet. Gynaecol. Br. Commonw. 68:784, 1961.

Watson, P., Besch, N., and Bowes, W.: Management of acute and subacute puerperal inversion of the uterus. Obstet. Gynecol. 55:12, 1980.

23

DISSEMINATED INTRAVASCULAR COAGULATION, IDIOPATHIC THROMBOCYTOPENIC PURPURA, AND HEMOGLOBINOPATHIES

MARCELLA L. McKAY
JAMES N. MARTIN, JR.
JOHN C. MORRISON

Disseminated Intravascular Coagulation

Disseminated intravascular coagulation (DIC) is a pathologic syndrome resulting from an inappropriate activation of the clotting process. DIC is characterized by a disruption of hemostatic mechanisms due to an underlying disease process that causes intravascular consumption of plasma clotting factors and platelets (Fig. 23–1).

DIC is not a primary disease but occurs instead as a consequence of other disease processes. As clotting occurs throughout the microcirculation, fibrin is deposited in small vessels, producing mechanical injury to red blood cells. This activates the fibrinolytic process, which attempts to dissolve the fibrin clots. Secondary to clot lysis there is an anticoagulant effect that results in erythrocyte fragmentation, hemorrhage, tissue ischemia, and anemia. A paradoxic positive feedback system ensues in which clotting is the primary problem, although hemorrhage is the predominant physical finding. DIC is referred to as *consumptive coagulopathy* or *defibrination syndrome* owing to the acute consumption of large amounts of fibrinogen, platelets, and clotting factors (especially factors II, V, and VIII) as the body attempts to regain its hemostatic mechanisms (Abildgaard, 1968; Perez, 1981).

INCIDENCE

The incidence of DIC in obstetric patients is difficult to ascertain owing to the wide variation of precipitating events and the exceedingly complex range of clinical manifestations. DIC may range from a mild chronic disease state to a fulminating syndrome with some fatal results. This syndrome of imbalance between the coagulation and fibrinolytic systems may occur in association with a wide variety of obstetric complications including pregnancy-induced hypertension, abruptio placentae, intrauterine fetal death, retained placenta, amniotic fluid embolism, intraamniotic injection of saline, hemorrhagic shock, and sepsis. Secondary to such

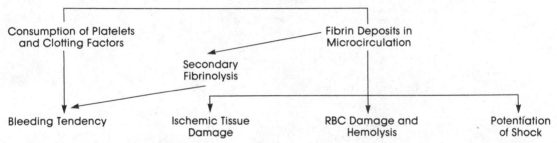

Figure 23–1. The disease process of DIC. (From Perez, R. H.: Protocols for Perinatal Nursing Practice. St. Louis, C. V. Mosby Co., 1981, p. 356. (Adapted from original in Williams, W. J.: Hematology. New York, McGraw-Hill, 1972.)

a precipitating event or stress, paradoxic coagulation and fibrinolysis occur. To further complicate the situation, the incidence of underlying precipitating events varies according to the population under study. Obstetrics is one specialty in which DIC is encountered very frequently, averaging 1 per 500 deliveries for the severe type and more commonly for milder forms.

PATHOPHYSIOLOGY

In order to understand the pathophysiology of DIC, one must consider three background components: (1) changes in hemostasis related to pregnancy; (2) normal blood coagulation; and (3) the fibrinolytic system.

Hemostasis in Pregnancy

In a normal pregnancy the components of coagulation and blood volume are altered to facilitate hemostasis. Blood volume of the normal woman late in pregnancy expands approximately 1500 ml. Factors I (fibrinogen), VII, VIII, IX, and X are elevated but the platelet count does not change considerably. Throughout the antepartum period, plasminogen levels are elevated, although plasmin activity is relatively normal. When stress, such as hemorrhage, occurs, plasminogen to plasmin conversion is stimulated; thus, coagulation and fibrinolysis are initiated. The greater amounts of available clotting factors may be initiated whenever physiologic insult occurs (Lavery, 1982; Pritchard and MacDonald, 1980).

Normal Blood Coagulation

The most widely accepted theory of blood coagulation is the Ratnoff and Bennett (1972) cascade theory, which divides the blood coagulation system into two components: the intrinsic system and the extrinsic system (Bennett, 1972). Common regulatory mechanisms work through the clotting system, and a common convergent pathway brings the intrinsic and extrinsic systems together for the final stages of clot formation.

The intrinsic pathway is so named because its activation is dependent upon a substance found in the plasma. When stimulated by pathologic events, factor XII converts factor XI (plasma thromboplastin antecedent) to its activated form. This disruption involves the release of collagen or subendothelial substances, which trigger the intrinsic system. Activated factor XI in the presence of Ca^{++} causes activation of factor IX (Christmas factor); in turn, activated factor IX in the presence of Ca^{++}, phospholipid, and thrombin-modified factor VIII) causes activation of factor X (Stuart-Prower factor) (Bennett, 1972; Davie and Ratnoff, 1964) (Fig. 23–2).

Tissue thromboplastin released with tissue injury activates the extrinsic pathway. In this system factor VII and Ca^{++} activate factor X (Stuart-Prower factor), a necessary step in association with calcium to convert prothrombin to thrombin (Fig. 23–3). At this point in the clotting mechanism the extrinsic and intrinsic systems merge into a common pathway for completion of clot formation. Thrombin from the extrinsic pathway acts upon fibrinogen A and B chains to split off fibrinopeptides A and B, resulting in the formation of fibrin monomers. Fibrin monomer formation is the initiating event of the formation of a fibrin clot. By linking end-to-end and side-to-side, fibrin monomers form an insoluble network, which, when stabilized by thrombin-activated factor XIII, is the basis for clot formation (Perez, 1981; Stefanini, 1974; Talbert and Blatt, 1979).

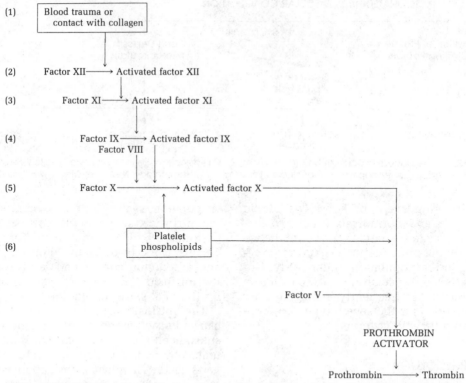

Figure 23–2. Clotting mechanism—intrinsic pathway. (From Guyton, A. C.: Physiology of the Human Body. Philadelphia, W. B. Saunders Co., 1979, p.72.)

To a large extent the coagulation cascade is controlled by the regulatory activities of the serine antiproteinases. Antithrombin III (AT III) is one of the most important of these proteins. By neutralizing the enzymatic reaction sites of serine proteinases, antithrombin III effectively and progressively acts as

an important regulatory mechanism for the control of normal clotting by actively neutralizing thrombin, plastin, and activated forms of factors XII, XI, IV, and VII (Gambino and Altman, 1979; Ogston, 1977; Talbert and Blatt, 1979).

Guyton simplifies the basic pathways of

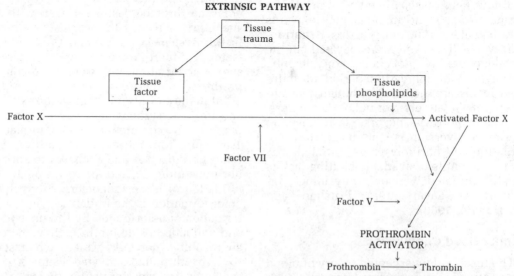

Figure 23–3. Clotting mechanism—extrinsic pathway. (From Guyton, A. C.: Physiology of the Human Body. Philadelphia, W. B. Saunders Co., 1979, p. 72.)

the overall clotting mechanism by pointing out that the extrinsic pathway is explosive in nature. It is initiated within moments following an inciting event. The rapidity of its activation and the magnitude of its effects are limited only by the quantity of tissue factors and tissue phospholipids released from the trauma site and by the amount of factors X, VII, and V available in the blood for consumption. In contrast, the intrinsic pathway by its very nature is much slower and more susceptible to the proteolytic action of plasmin against fibrin, fiberinogen, and factors V and VIII (Guyton, 1976).

Fibrinolytic System

The fibrinolytic system, sometimes referred to as the plasminogen-plasmin system, is the system that is activated in DIC to effect the breakdown of fibrin into soluble fibrin split products (Fig. 23–4). Activation of the fibrinolytic system occurs when plasminogen is converted into circulating plasmin (Guyton, 1976). Plasmin is a potent proteolytic enzyme that not only acts on fibrin but also effectively lyses fibrinogen and factors V and VIII. As fibrinogen and fibrin are lysed, fibrin degradation products (FDP) are created. The degradation products are known as X, Y, D, and E fragments and have a profoundly negative effect on hemostatic mechanisms (Wiman and Collen, 1978). Fibrin degradation products act to inhibit the action of thrombin and render platelets dysfunctional by coating their surfaces. As DIC progresses, fibrin polymerization becomes incomplete and leads to the presence of nonpolymerized fibrin monomers in the peripheral circulation. Fibrin degradation fragments X, Y, D, and E bind with these nonpolymerized fibrin monomers to create the soluble fibrin monomers, which are characteristic of DIC and which can be measured by the protamine sulfate test (Gambino and Altman, 1979; Kaplan et al., 1978; Lavery, 1982; McNichol and Davis, 1973).

DIAGNOSIS

In its most acute, fulminating form DIC is a disease process that is usually not difficult to diagnose. In its chronic or milder forms, however, it may pose significant challenges to the practicing physician. Diagnosis of DIC is generally dependent upon a sound understanding of predisposing factors, clinical manifestations, and laboratory findings.

Predisposing Factors

DIC should be suspected in obstetric patients with abruptio placentae, a retained dead fetus for longer than 4 weeks, amniotic fluid embolism, saline-induced abortion, sepsis, hydatidiform mole, pregnancy-induced hypertension, hemorrhagic shock, and liver disease (Pritchard, 1959, 1967; Roberts and Hay, 1976; Talbert and Blatt, 1979).

Clinical Manifestations

The clinical manifestations of DIC relate primarily to hemorrhage, anemia, and is-

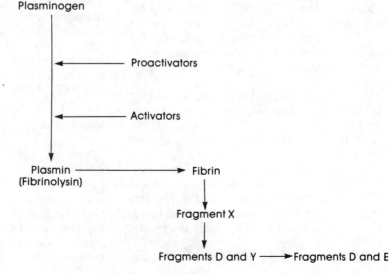

Figure 23–4. Fibrinolytic system.

Plasminogen

← Proactivators

← Activators

Plasmin (Fibrinolysin) ⟶ Fibrin

Fragment X

Fragments D and Y ⟶ Fragments D and E

chemia (Ziegel, 1978). Patients generally have frank bleeding or a tendency to bleed from mucous membranes, intravenous line sites, injection sites, and surgical incisions. Abnormal bruising, purpura, petechiae, and ecchymoses frequently are noted. Occult blood usually is present in stool, with frank hematemesis, hematuria, and vaginal bleeding noted fairly often in severe cases. The quantity and character of bleeding are directly related to the severity and explosiveness of the disease process (McGillick, 1982; O'Brian and Woods, 1978). Certainly in an acute, uncontrolled episode of DIC a patient can suffer irreparable damage secondary to hypovolemia or intracranial or intraperitoneal bleeding. Ischemia secondary to hemorrhage and/or anemia is also a life-threatening event in any patient with acute fulminating DIC. The milder cases may have no overt signs of clotting disruption (Lavery, 1982; McGillick, 1982).

Laboratory Studies

If approached systematically, laboratory findings associated with DIC provide a logical system for differential diagnosis. Because DIC occurs secondary to a disruption of multiple hemostatic mechanisms, laboratory assessment should reflect an alteration in clotting physiology. If DIC is present, laboratory studies will reflect the disruption of hemostasis in two or more of its essential components. Initial clotting studies should include hemoglobin, hematocrit, phase platelet count, thrombin time, fibrinogen level, prothrombin time (PT), partial thromboplastin time (PTT), clotting time, and clot retraction. The PT tests the extrinsic pathway of coagulation, the PTT assesses the intrinsic pathway of coagulation, and the thrombin time quantitates fibrinogen to fibrin conversion (Bick and Adams, 1974; Lavery, 1982).

In patients with clinically significant DIC, all of these studies will be abnormal, supporting a presumptive diagnosis of DIC. To verify the diagnosis, a test for early soluble fibrin monomers should be performed to differentiate between DIC and a primary hyperfibrinolytic syndrome (Bick and Adams, 1974; Gambino and Altman, 1979). For this purpose, a positive protamine sulfate test is utilized and, if positive, is highly diagnostic of DIC (Table 23–1).

There are other laboratory tests that are

Table 23–1. Laboratory Findings in DIC

Test	Result
Partial thromboplastin time	prolonged
Prothrombin time	prolonged
Platelet count	decreased
Thrombin generation time	prolonged
Fibrinogen	decreased
Fibrin/fibrinogen degradation products	increased
Protamine paracoagulant test	positive
Blood smear	microangiopathic changes

useful for the patient in whom DIC is suspected. Laboratory testing time prohibits or limits the diagnostic usefulness of these tests. They are, however, useful in the long-time management of a patient. Essential information regarding fibrinolysis may be derived from the euglobin lysis time, the fibrin plate assay for plasminogen and plasmin, and assays for demonstrating fibrin degradation products. The tanned red cell hemagglutination inhibition immunoassay is probably most suitable for quantitative evaluation of fibrin degradation resulting from antigen-antibody reaction. These tests do not distinguish between primary fibrinolysis and secondary fibrinolysis secondary to DIC. Hence, they must be considered useful only in reinforcing a presumptive diagnosis. Also useful for the presumptive but not definitive diagnosis of DIC are assays to document decreased factor V or VIII levels. (Bick and Adams, 1974; Gambino and Altman, 1979; Lavery, 1982).

All of these laboratory studies must be used in conjunction with the clinical symptomatology to determine the appropriate management of a patient. Laboratory values should be used primarily to confirm clinical impressions and secondarily to collect data for ongoing and retrospective understanding of the disease process (Bick and Adams, 1974) (Table 23–2).

MANAGEMENT (Tables 23–3 and 23–4)

The management of DIC should be approached in a systematic and timely fashion, prioritizing and addressing problems one at a time. Foremost is the elimination of the underlying disease process that precipitated the DIC. In obstetrics this generally means termination of the pregnancy. Once this goal is achieved, the DIC may be eliminated by

Table 23–2. A Systematic Approach to the Diagnosis of DIC*

Responsible Pathology	Screening Tests	Presumptive Tests	Definitive Tests	Adjunctive Tests	Clinical Hints
Fibrin deposition Thrombocytopenia Platelet function defects	(Combinations of abnormalities are highly significant) Smear for platelets and RBC fragments Platelet count Bleeding time Tourniquet test	Progressive thrombocytopenia		Platelet adhesion Platelet aggregation Complement levels Endotoxin	Bruising Petechiae Purpura Ecchymoses Epistaxis
Hypofibrinogenemia Factor V decreased Factor VIII decreased Circulating anticoagulants (fibrinolytic degradation)	Thrombin time Fibrinogen screen (FI, Fibrindex) Prothrombin time Partial thromboplastin time	Factor V assay Factor VIII assay Quantitative Fibrinogen FDP (IEOP, latex, staph, clumping)	Protamine sulfate test or ethanol gelation test	?	Gastrointestinal, genitourinary, intracranial, or interperitoneal bleeding
Secondary fibrinolysis Circulating plasma	Clot retraction	Fibrin plate for plasminogen depletion and circulating plasmin Clot lysis Long ELT			Associated clinical conditions

*Reprinted with permission from Bick, R. L., and Adams, T.: Disseminated intravascular coagulation. Medical Counterpoint, 1974, p. 41.

facilitating a return to control of the coagulation mechanism by intact hemostatic pathways. On the other hand, if the underlying process cannot be eliminated or if the DIC has progressed beyond the point of a possible spontaneous, compensatory response, additional therapy is essential (Bick and Adams, 1974; Pritchard and Brekken, 1967).

Table 23–3. Management of DIC

Basic Principles
1. Understand pathophysiology
2. Prioritize clinical problems
3. Eliminate underlying cause
4. Utilize perinatal team approach for support of patient and family

Procedures
1. Stabilize vital signs
2. Maintain adequate urinary output
3. Institute and maintain appropriate blood component therapy to replace consumable blood clotting factors and platelets
4. Conduct prudent fluid replacement
5. Perform constant CVP or Swan-Ganz monitoring
6. Use anticoagulant therapy only in critical, individual situations

The perinatal team approach is essential for the diagnosis and optimal treatment of DIC. Outcome for the parturient and her neonate may be greatly improved by early identification and assessment of clinical manifestations of DIC. The most subtle sign of bleeding or vascular occlusion may be observed by the care provider and followed by a laboratory assessment to form the basis for diagnosis. Sophisticated laboratory capability is useful only if skilled personnel recognize the need for its use. Open communication and coordination with the blood bank are essential for a consistent, systematic approach to patient care. The initial goal of management should be to stabilize the patient's vital signs and maintain adequate urinary output while plans are being made to terminate the pregnancy as soon as possible. A urinary catheter system is helpful to assess urinary output.

The secondary goal should be to institute and maintain appropriate blood component therapy to replace consumable blood clotting factors and platelets. AT III is replaced in the form of fresh frozen plasma or cryo-

Table 23–4. Patient Care Summary for DIC

	Out-patient	Antepartum Inpatient	Intrapartum	Postpartum
BP, P, R	—	q 15 min	q 15 min	q 15 min until stable
T	—	q 4 hr	q 4 hr	On admission to RR; then q 4 hr
CVP line/Swan-Ganz	—	Yes	Yes	Yes
FHR	—	Continuous fetal monitoring	Continuous fetal monitoring, internal if possible	—
Contractions	—	Continuous fetal monitoring	Continuous fetal monitoring, internal if possible	Fundal heights q 15 min until stable; then q 30 min × 2; then q 1 hr
Laboratory assessment	—	Clot observation Fibrinogen Platelets Fibrinogen-fibrin degradation products Thrombin time Prothrombin time Partial thromboplastin time	Clot observation Fibrinogen Platelets Fibrinogen-fibrin degradation products Thrombin time Prothrombin time Partial thromboplastin time	Clot observation Fibrinogen Platelets Fibrinogen-fibrin degradation products Thrombin time Prothrombin time Partial thromboplastin time
I & O	—	q 1 hr	q 1 hr	q 1 hr
Observation for signs of shock	—	Continuously	Continuously	Continuously
Observation for level of consciousness	—	Continuously	Continuously	Continuously

Note: Nurse–patient ratio, 1:1.

precipitate. Two or three units of plasma are given initially and then followed by subsequent doses as necessary to replace consumed factors. Cryoprecipitate should be given as needed to attain a fibrinogen level greater than 100 mg/100 ml. This will replace not only fibrinogen but factor VIII as well. Generally, each unit of cryoprecipitate raises the fibrinogen level by 2 to 5 mg/100 ml. Cryoprecipitate is the therapy of choice because fibrinogen, once commercially available, has been removed from the market in the United States owing to the significant risk of hepatitis associated with its use (Talbert and Blatt, 1979) (Table 23–5).

Prudent fluid replacement along with component therapy is necessary with constant CVP or Swan-Ganz monitoring of intravascular volume. Infrequently there is a need for whole blood in the treatment of DIC, since component therapy including fresh frozen plasma, cryoprecipitate, and platelets can usually be used quite effectively. When available, blood component therapy can be used with greater effectiveness and versatility, less cost, and a smaller total volume of fluid than fresh whole blood (Lavery, 1982).

One of the longstanding controversies about the management of DIC in obstetrics is related to the appropriate use of antico-

Table 23–5. Blood Component Replacement Therapy*

Factor	Volume (ml)†	Supplies
Platelet concentrate	40–60	Increased count of viable platelets by 25,000–35,000
Cryoprecipitate	30–50	Fibrinogen Factors VIII, XIII (3 to 10 times the equivalent volume of plasma)
Fresh frozen plasma	200	All factors except platelets; 1 g fibrinogen
Packed RBC	200	Hematocrit 60 to 65%
Fibrinogen‡	300	Increased fibrinogen (1–2 g)

*Reprinted with permission from Lavery, P.: When coagulopathy threatens the pregnant patient. Contemporary OB/GYN 20:198, 1982.
†Depends on local blood bank service.
‡Not available in the United States.

agulant therapy. Heparin generally is not used because, following factor replacement therapy and removal of the cause of DIC, it is not needed. The major risk of heparin therapy is hemorrhage due to the enhanced interaction of the serine proteinases and AT III (Corrigan and Jordan, 1970). There is general agreement that heparin is not needed in the treatment of DIC *unless* total defibrination has occurred or the patient has minimal disruption of the vascular system. The hallmarks of decision making regarding the utilization of heparin are caution and careful evaluation of risk-benefit ratio (Saltzman et al., 1975).

Patients with a retained dead fetus in utero may require heparin. Normalization of fibrinogen levels and control of chronic consumption of clotting factors are attempted until vaginal delivery can be performed (Pritchard, 1973). Heparin is also used in cases of fulminating disease in which almost total defibrination has occurred and patient stabilization is necessary to facilitate delivery. When heparin is administered in the treatment of DIC, fresh frozen plasma should be given as well. Heparin can be administered by constant infusion pump at approximately 500–1000 units/hr with adjustments in dosage based on clinical and laboratory response.

Emotional support for the patient and her family is extremely important, since DIC can be life-threatening to the woman and her fetus. The nurse should stay with the patient for constant physical assessment as well as emotional support. If the partner can remain with the patient this is good for his understanding and support as well as emotional support for his mate. If the woman is bleeding, it may be very frightening, and the patient and her mate should be kept apprised of her condition and the fetus's condition at all times. In an emergency such as this it is sometimes difficult to take the time for these explanations but it will save time in the long run if the patient and her family are informed so they can fully cooperate with treatment modalities.

OBSTETRIC CONDITIONS ASSOCIATED WITH DIC

There are several well-known events in obstetrics that can precipitate DIC. Abruptio placentae, dead fetus syndrome, amniotic fluid embolism, saline-induced abortion, hemorrhagic shock, pregnancy-induced hypertension, and sepsis have been studied specifically in relation to DIC. Each condition poses specific challenges for the perinatal care team. Therefore, it is important to understand and manage the underlying problem as well as the DIC.

Abruptio Placentae

Depending on the criteria used for diagnosis, premature separation of the placenta has been reported to range in incidence from 1 in 55 to 1 in 150 deliveries (Knobs, 1978). Patients with abruptio placentae whose babies do not survive have a 38 percent incidence of severe hypofibrinogenemia; thus, any patient with a placental abruption should be considered at risk for the development of DIC (Pritchard and Brekken, 1967). At the time of placental separation, retroplacental hemorrhage occurs. Thromboplastin is released from the traumatized placenta and decidua, activating the extrinsic clotting pathway. Simultaneously, the fibrinolytic mechanisms are activated by thromboplastin and activated procoagulants entering the maternal circulation from the implantation site (Sutton et al., 1971). Pritchard and Brekken recommend prompt vaginal delivery, if possible, with judicious use of oxytocin and amniotomy. In the event of fetal demise, 20 mg PGE$_2$ suppositories can be used to encourage delivery without cesarean section. Cesarean section should be used to deliver the patient with abruptio placentae if severe DIC is present and in those who do not progress in labor (Pritchard and Brekken, 1967; Pritchard, 1973). Specific management of DIC is carried out as outlined previously with blood component therapy and fluid replacement based on clinical manifestations and laboratory studies.

Retained Dead Fetus

Historically, it has been consistently recognized since the early to mid 20th century that the in utero retention of a dead fetus can precipitate abnormal maternal bleeding (Delee, 1901). Significant clotting defects have been linked particularly to the fetus retained for more than 4 weeks after demise. The triggering mechanism for DIC seems to be the release of thromboplasin from the dead fetus. Hence the ensuing coagulation is slow and chronic in nature with resultant gradual depletion of clotting factors (Pritchard, 1959, 1973). In this situation where depletion of clotting factors is chronic rather than acute, heparin occasionally is useful in normalizing fibrinogen levels so that vaginal delivery can be facilitated (Pritchard, 1973). Prostaglandins as well as oxytocin may be used to induce labor (Bailey et al., 1975; Gordon and Pite, 1975). Component therapy is used to stabilize the patient for delivery or at any time when the chronic DIC process becomes more severe or acute in nature.

Amniotic Fluid Embolism

Amniotic fluid embolism is a rare complication of pregnancy that is often fatal and always extremely serious. Characterized by respiratory distress, circulatory collapse, and shock, this maternal condition is fatal in 25 percent of patients in the first hour after onset. The secondary complication of hemorrhage is often seen if the patient survives the initial pathophysiologic insult (Pritchard, 1973). Consumptive coagulopathy with hypofibrinogenemia has been the most consistent finding in the surviving parturient secondary to the clot-promoting properties of the amniotic fluid and gestational debris that entered the maternal circulation (Phillips and Davidson, 1972). Management of this acute emergency is immediate recognition and support for the intensive cardiorespiratory distress and shock with constant clinical and laboratory surveillance for DIC. Life-sustaining therapy, including fluid and blood replacement, oxygen therapy, ventilatory support, and digitalization, may be necessary (Halmagyi et al., 1962; Peterson and Taylor, 1970). When diagnosed, DIC should be treated as outlined previously with blood component therapy, fluid replacement, and prompt delivery of the infant.

Saline-Induced Abortion

Saline-induced abortion has been shown to frequently produce coagulation and fibrinolytic changes. It is hypothesized that DIC is due to thromboplastin release from the uterus or its contents secondary to hypertonic saline injection (Laros and Penner, 1976; Stander et al., 1971; Weiss et al., 1972). Following the intraamniotic instillation of hypertonic (20 percent) saline to patients desiring second trimester pregnancy termination, Cohen and Ballard found a 0.01 to 0.25 percent incidence of DIC severe enough to require therapeutic intervention (1974). Medical management is based on the severity of clinical manifestations and laboratory findings.

Pregnancy-Induced Hypertension

Pregnancy-induced hypertension (PIH) appears to be a predisposing factor to DIC. The two disease processes are separate entities but occasionally coexist. In the patient with PIH, the triggering mechanism for the development of DIC seems to be vascular endothelial damage secondary to the underlying disease state rather than thromboplastin release from the placenta into the maternal circulation (Roberts and May, 1976). The complexity of both PIH and DIC poses an extraordinary challenge for the perinatal care team. Management should include expeditious delivery and blood component therapy in conjunction with treatment for the underlying PIH disease process.

Sepsis

Sepsis commonly incites some level of DIC. It has been speculated that bacterial toxins cause release of platelet phospholipids, which result in platelet clumping (Yoshiwa et al., 1971). Exposure of collagen in the capillary walls very likely also plays a role in the DIC process by activating factor XIII (Coleman et al., 1972). Management should reflect a primary concern for treatment of the underlying cause by appropriate antibiotic administration or surgical drainage if necessary. Once the sepsis itself has been treated, DIC is managed as previously outlined with blood component therapy and supportive therapy as needed.

Idiopathic (Autoimmune) Thrombocytopenic Purpura

INCIDENCE

Idiopathic or autoimmune thrombocytopenic purpura (aITP) is an acquired immunologic disorder caused by the abnormal development of IgG immunoglobulin, which attaches to platelets and results in their removal by the reticuloendothelial system (McMillan, 1977, 1981; Karpatkin, 1980; Kelton and Gibbons, 1982). It occurs most frequently in young women and is the most common autoimmune disease occurring in the childbearing years. This disease probably affects more pregnant women than had been recognized previously. Both the parturient and the fetus are exposed to significant risks.

PATHOPHYSIOLOGY

1 *Thrombocytopenia is defined as a platelet or thrombocyte count less than 150,000/ mm³.* The normal adult platelet count in pregnancy is 150,000 to 350,000/mm³ (Romero and Duffy, 1980). As indicated in Table 23–6, thrombocytopenia may complicate several obstetric syndromes (Perkins, 1979), and several types of thrombocytopenia may complicate pregnancy. Actually the disease of aITP is often referred to as a syndrome because there is a wide spectrum of possible clinical presentations (Baldini, 1966, 1972). Most parturients with aITP have a primary form of aITP, whereas others develop the condition secondary to a drug reaction or in

Table 23–6. Classification of Thrombocytopenia

I. Nonfunctional Platelet Disorders
  A. Disorders of decreased platelet survival
    1. Immunologic mechanisms
      a. Autoimmune disease–associated
        (1) aITP (acute/chronic)
        (2) Alloantibodies (posttransfusion, neonatal)
        (3) Collagen disorders
        (4) Lymphoproliferative disorders
      b. Drug-induced
      c. Acute infection (viral, bacterial, parasitic)
      d. Localized consumption
    2. Dilution with platelet-poor blood
      a. Massive blood transfusion
      b. Extracorporeal
  B. Disorders of decreased platelet production
    1. Aplasia or hypoplasia of bone marrow
      a. Toxic
      b. Idiopathic
    2. Bone marrow malignancy
    3. Megaloblastic anemias
II. Functional Platelet Disorders
  A. Congenital
    1. Storage pool disease/defective release
    2. Glanzmann's thrombasthenia
  B. Acquired
    Drug-induced platelet dysfunction (see I A1b above)
III. Combined Platelet and Plasma Abnormalities
  von Willebrand's disease

Table 23–7. Clinical Features of aITP

Mild to Moderate Disease
None if platelets > 50,000/mm³
Ecchymoses (scattered purplish patches, especially in areas exposed to trauma)
Petechiae (generalized pinpoint hemorrhagic lesions that do not disappear with applied pressure)
Areas of purpura (hemorrhage into the skin or mucous membranes)
Oozing from puncture wound (venipuncture)

Severe Disease
Epistaxis
Hematemesis
Hematuria
Melena
Generalized purpura
Hemorrhagic vesicles or bullae (blood blisters) in the oral mucosa
CNS symptoms
Prolonged bleeding time (especially if platelets ≤ 20,000)

association with other diseases such as systemic lupus erythematosus (SLE), lymphoma, or lymphocytic leukemia. The acute form of aITP typically is found in very young children. In contrast, most young adults with aITP are afflicted with a chronic variety that may last for many years with multiple episodes of relapse and remission. In milder cases, the chronic disease form may be unsuspected unless a screening maternal platelet count taken at the initial visit or at the time of delivery is found to be low or a thrombocytopenic neonate is delivered.

Thrombocytopenia is not always associated with clinical manifestations. The severity of bleeding in this disorder can range from minimal to life-threatening, beginning with easy bruising or small petechiae, then minor cutaneous and subcutaneous hemorrhages that progress to form purpuric lesions of the skin. More serious mucosal membrane bleeding from the gastrointestinal, genitourinary, or respiratory tract can occur with increasingly severe disease (Table 23–7). In pregnancy the most frequent manifestations of aITP are epistaxis, gingival bleeding, and ecchymosis. Even with severe thrombocytopenia, maternal intracranial hemorrhage and hemarthroses are uncommon in parturients with aITP.

DIAGNOSIS

The diagnosis of aITP is generally one of exclusion (Wintrobe, 1971). Nonimmune causes of thrombocytopenia, such as tox-

Table 23–8. Critically Important Components of Maternal History and Examination

---

Previous operations (especially splenectomy)
History of easy bruising or bleeding
Family history (especially maternal) of bleeding complications
Previous obstetric history
Recent or current infections
Medications taken during or immediately before pregnancy
Collagen vascular diseases
Maternal physical examination (look for splenomegaly)
Laboratory assessment

---

emia, infection, or intravascular coagulation, and immune etiologies secondary to other diseases, such as SLE, usually are evident from their clinical presentation and can be confirmed by appropriate testing. A thorough medical and obstetric history is very important (Table 23–8). Once thrombocytopenia is detected in a parturient, the finding should be verified by a phase manual platelet count because automated counts can be falsely low. If thrombocytopenia is confirmed, further testing should include a complete blood count and a sternal bone marrow aspiration. If the megakaryocytes appear normal and are present in normal or increased numbers, the thrombocytopenia is probably secondary to platelet destruction. Hematocrit, hemoglobin, and white blood cell count are usually within normal limits unless there has been a recent hemorrhage. Abnormal megakaryocytes and platelets may be seen on a peripheral blood smear. Although the bleeding time is prolonged, clotted blood

Table 23–9. aITP Diagnostic Findings

Isolated thrombocytopenia ($< 150,000/mm^3$) in the complete blood count
Normal coagulation screens (PT, PTT, thrombin clotting time)
Increased mean platelet volume
Elevated antiplatelet antibody/platelet-associated IgG
Negative antinuclear antibody
Normal to increased megakaryocyte mass in bone marrow aspirate
Absence of splenomegaly
Other causes excluded such as:
    Recent transfusion
    Identified sources of platelet destruction
    Drug ingestion
    Exposure to noxious substances
    Recent infections
    Family history of bleeding

---

fails to retract and the tourniquet test is positive; in patients with aITP, the usual coagulation tests (coagulation time, prothrombin time, and partial thromboplastin time) are all within normal limits. Unless aITP is secondary to another disease, the spleen usually is not enlarged. A demonstration of free or bound platelet-associated antibodies serves to support the diagnosis of an autoimmune thrombocytopenia. Criteria for the diagnosis of aITP are summarized in Table 23–9.

The maternal antiplatelet factor responsible for aITP is a circulating 7S gamma-globulin blocking ("incomplete") antibody, which attaches to target cell surface antigens on the maternal platelet (Dixon et al., 1975; Harrington et al., 1951; Sprague et al., 1952; Schulman et al., 1965; McMillan et al., 1975). Because the human placenta has receptors for the Fc portion of the IgG molecule and actively transports IgG antibodies of all types from the maternal circulation into the fetal circulation (Kohler and Farr, 1966; Schlamoritz, 1976), these antiplatelet antibodies can cross the placenta to cause fetal and neonatal thrombocytopenia and do so in over half the cases of maternal illness (McMillan et al., 1975; Goodhue and Evans, 1963; Territo et al., 1973; Kernoff et al., 1979; Kelton et al., 1980; Minchinton et al., 1980; Van Leeuwen et al., 1980). Until recently, attempts to detect the presence of platelet antibody have been difficult, inaccurate, and unreliable (McMillan, 1977; Schreiber, 1982).

Severity of the thrombocytopenia depends on the balance between platelet production and destruction (Ahn and Harrington, 1977). This, in turn, varies with the type and quantity of antibody coating the platelet. The usual number of IgG molecules adsorbed upon the normal platelet's surface (6,000 to 12,000) can be increased from 2 to 20 times in patients with aITP (Dixon et al., 1975). Greater amounts of attached (adsorbed) antibody are related to faster rates of clearance by the spleen and liver. Whereas the spleen preferentially seems to clear lightly coated platelets, the liver can remove from circulation more heavily coated platelets as well as those carrying attached complement.

In the absence of the spleen, the liver acts similarly but less efficiently as an alternative site for platelet sequestration and destruction.

RISKS OF ITP

The overall course and severity of primary aITP do not seem to be affected by pregnancy in any significant way (Heys, 1966, Tancer, 1960). In contrast, it has been well demonstrated that aITP may have an adverse effect upon mother and baby (Kitzmiller, 1978). The principal maternal risk is hemorrhage associated with either genital tract injury or abdominoperineal incisions employed for operative delivery. Since 1954, only a single maternal death has been attributed in published literature to aITP (O'Reilly and Taber, 1978; Noriega-Guerra et al., 1979). Corticosteroid administration and platelet transfusion, along with the expertise of specialists in medical centers, are significant factors in the virtual elimination of maternal mortality with this disease process, in contrast to the rates as high as 5 to 10 percent reported as recently as the mid 1950s (Heys, 1966; Robson and Davidson, 1950; Rogers, 1959; Murray and Harris, 1976).

Intrapartum and postpartum hemorrhage occur with greater frequency in this disease since bleeding tends to occur during the expulsive efforts of the second stage. Postpartum hemorrhage from trauma to the genital tract still must be anticipated and carefully managed with meticulous surgical technique. Uterine bleeding is not increased markedly, apparently a reflection of the efficient manner in which the uterus contracts to promote postpartum hemostasis. The principle of gentle delivery encouraged primarily out of neonatal concern is also advantageous for the mother to minimize the possibility of cerebral hemorrhage provoked by expulsive efforts in the second stage of labor (Scott, 1976).

There also are sobering concerns for the fetus in the aITP pregnancy. The risk of spontaneous abortion in parturients with aITP has been reported to range from 5 to 33 percent as compared with 10 to 15 percent in normal women (O'Reilly and Taber, 1978; Schenker and Polishuk, 1968). Adverse effects on the fetus and neonate are more frequent and more serious, overall perinatal mortality rates having been reported in association with aITP pregnancies to range upward as high as 15 to 25 percent (Scott, 1976; Laros and Sweet, 1975). In the last decade, reported perinatal mortality rates in carefully managed series have been at or less than 5 percent (Romero and Duffy, 1980; Jones, 1979; Horger and Keane, 1979). Reasons for perinatal demise most commonly have been linked to fetal prematurity, intracerebral hemorrhage, and fetal death resulting from maternal hemorrhage and shock (Territo et al., 1973; O'Reilly and Taber, 1978; Laros and Sweet, 1975; Flessa, 1974).

Traditionally perinatal deaths have been ascribed to intracerebral hemorrhage occurring in thrombocytopenic infants delivered vaginally. Morbidity and mortality, however, may occur more commonly and much earlier in gestation than during labor and delivery. In O'Reilly and Taber's review (1978) of 133 pregnancies in women with aITP, 24 gestations were unsuccessful for a failure rate of 18 percent. Six were lost by first trimester spontaneous abortion, 13 were stillborn, and 5 infants died in the neonatal period. Six of the stillborn infants had evidence of hemorrhage preceding labor and delivery, and three of the neonatal losses were considered due to hemorrhage. Thus, only 9 deaths altogether in the 133 gestations (7 percent) were directly attributable to thrombocytopenia (O'Reilly and Taber, 1978).

A variant of the aITP syndrome may occur in some parturients within 4 to 6 weeks after delivery, miscarriage, or spontaneous abortion. Ahn and Harrington have managed 17 such episodes in 8 postpartum women, describing a pattern of recurring puerperal thrombocytopenia in these parturients that follows successive pregnancies. No other recognizable instigating factor or relationship to medication was discovered (Ahn and Harrington, 1977; Harrington, 1977a, 1977b).

MANAGEMENT

Antepartum Period

Once a diagnosis of aITP is made, therapy can be instituted (Table 23–10). *The primary goal of management should be to prevent maternal-fetal hemorrhage.* The overall management of aITP in pregnancy is based on the same general principles as those used in the nonpregnant state. Although it is true in nonpregnant patients that the platelet count alone should not be treated since some nonpregnant individuals tolerate marked thrombocytopenia without complications, marked thrombocytopenia during pregnancy

Table 23–10. Antepartum Management Considerations for aITP

Frequent outpatient clinic evaluations
Collaboration between obstetrician and
  hematologist
Periodic platelet counts
Oral iron and folate supplementation
Avoidance of salicylates and related
  prostaglandin synthetase inhibitor
  medications
Avoidance of trauma
Rapid treatment of fever and infections
Careful clinical, ultrasound, and biophysical
  surveillance of the fetus
Possible use of corticosteroids
Possible use of other immunosuppressant drugs
Possible second trimester splenectomy
Possible use of platelet transfusion
Possible plasma exchange procedure
Possible use of intravenous immunoglobulins

---

even without hemorrhage may be harmful to fetal well-being. A "safe" platelet count for pregnant women with aITP has never been determined. Not unlike any other individual with aITP, the pregnant woman should be under the careful medical supervision of a well-trained hematologist as well as a competent perinatal team. Obstetric and neonatal care for optimal perinatal outcome probably are best delivered at medical centers where the expertise and resources to respond appropriately to any eventuality are continuously available. Hospitalization should occur whenever there is a platelet count of 20,000 or less or if there is an episode of hemorrhage.

General measures of aITP pregnancy management include the avoidance of not only agents such as aspirin and aspirin-like drugs that impair platelet function but also factors such as trauma (intramuscular injections), fever, infection, azotemia, and increased metabolic rate. These complications must be avoided or remedied promptly because they can enhance an aITP patient's tendency to bleed by slowing platelet production, increasing platelet consumption, or impairing platelet function (Ahn and Harrington, 1977; Higby et al., 1974). Adequate vitamin and iron intake must be encouraged to maintain accelerated hematopoietic thrombopoiesis (Karpatkin et al., 1974; Smith et al., 1962).

Specific therapeutic modalities include corticosteroids, splenectomy, immunosuppressive drugs, plasma exchange procedures, platelet transfusions, and high-dose immunoglobulin therapy.

Corticosteroids. *Corticosteroids represent the cornerstone of aITP therapy* and are used in the absence of any contraindications. Use of these agents appears to be associated with decreased antiplatelet antibody production and binding, decreased antibody-coated platelet destruction, and improved capillary stability (Ahn and Harrington, 1977; McMillan et al., 1976; Suhrland et al., 1958; Doan et al., 1960; Cines and Schreiber, 1979; McMillan et al., 1974; Handin and Stossel, 1975; Fallon et al., 1952; Robson and Duttie, 1950; Handin and Stossel, 1975; Fallon et al., 1952; Robson and Duttie, 1950; Stefanini and Martino, 1956). Large doses of prednisone (60 to 100 mg or 1.0 to 1.5 mg/kg/day) are employed initially for 2 to 4 weeks or until the platelet count climbs to a range of 250,000/mm^3 or more. Higher starting doses may be appropriate if the initial platelet count is less than 10,000/mm^3. A favorable response to corticosteroid therapy is evidenced by a rise in the platelet count within 7 to 21 days and a lessening in new purpura and hemorrhagic tendencies. Daily therapy by divided dosage has been found to be more effective than single dose or alternate-day therapy (Lacey and Penner, 1977). After remission is achieved, the drug is tapered gradually at 2-week intervals, usually by decreasing the dose 10 to 20 percent. Tapering is continued until the lowest possible dosage compatible with hemostasis is reached (platelet count > 50,000/mm^3) and maintained at this level. Relapse following discontinuation of corticosteroid therapy is quite common. Some patients with aITP will not respond to steroids. *If a significant rise in the platelet count has not been observed after 21 days of corticosteroid treatment, another mode of therapy must be considered.*

The majority of parturients treated initially with corticosteroids for aITP respond to them, but the quantity and quality of individual responses are highly variable and depend on the duration of disease and level of antibody production (Ahn and Harrington, 1977; O'Reilly and Taber, 1978; Heys, 1966; Brennan et al., 1975). Unfortunately, a sustained remission has been reported in only 14 to 38 percent of treated patients (Thompson et al., 1972). If the platelet count has not reached 50,000/mm^3 after 21 days of therapy, splenectomy (Ahn and Harrington, 1977) or immunosuppressive drugs other than corticosteroids should be considered. In the absence of complications secondary to the drug itself or when indications for splenectomy are not met, it has been recommended that corticosteroids be continued throughout pregnancy on at least a daily maintenance level of 5 to 20 mg prednisone, especially in those patients with severe or chronically relapsing disease (O'Reilly and Taber, 1978; Laros and Sweet, 1975; Flessa, 1974). It may be particularly important to administer corticosteroid therapy during the first trimester. Further study is required to accept or refute the alleged beneficial effects on fetal morbidity and mortality during the various stages of gestation.

Following a suggestion of Laros and Sweet (1975) that the near-term maternal administration of corticosteroids might prevent or ameliorate fetal thrombocytopenia and Horger and Keane's (1979) suggestion that the antenatal administration of betamethasone to mothers with aITP might reduce fetal platelet destruction and peripartum hemorrhage, Karpatkin and coworkers (1981) recommended recently that all women with aITP be treated with a short course of corticosteroids prior to delivery. Although Karpatkin's clinical results were suggestive of a positive effect from such a treatment plan, most other investigators have not been as successful (Heys, 1966; Robson and Davidson, 1950; Flessa, 1974). Indeed, *the administration of corticosteroids in such a fashion may be contraindicated.* Corticosteroids are known to alter the interaction between IgG antiplatelet antibodies and platelet surface antigens in patients with aITP (Rosse, 1971). Recently Cines and colleagues (Cines and Schreiber, 1979; Cines et al., 1981, 1982) recorded that high doses of prednisone were noted to be associated with a fall in the level of platelet-associated IgG and a positive clinical response in the treated mothers. However, the level of circulating antiplatelet antibody simultaneously increased in the mothers and was associated with the delivery of severely thrombocytopenic infants.

Corticosteroid administration can be detrimental to the mother and fetus in one of several ways. Although the increased incidence of cleft palate in animal studies has not been substantiated in human investigations and first trimester steroid therapy is not thought to be of great risk in the human, an adverse impact on several human body systems early or later in pregnancy may be possible. Maternal and fetal adrenocortical insufficiency, steroid-induced diabetes mellitus, pregnancy psychosis, and an increased incidence of preeclampsia/eclampsia may occur secondary to prolonged corticosteroid therapy (Flessa, 1974; Gowda et al., 1977; Heys, 1966). Recently a report has appeared of an increased incidence of intrauterine fetal growth retardation in the offspring of parturients taking more than 10 mg of prednisone per day (Machover Remisch, 1978).

Splenectomy. Chronic autoimmune thrombocytopenic purpura is a relapsing disease process requiring lifelong therapy beyond the conclusion of pregnancy. Because corticosteroids usually do not effect a permanent remission and long-term medical therapy can be somewhat hazardous, splenectomy usually becomes necessary at some time in most adults with chronic aITP. Removal of the spleen is associated with a permanent remission in 70 to 80 percent of these patients because it eliminates the primary site of platelet destruction (Ahn and Harrington, 1977; Karpatkin et al., 1972). Ideally, splenectomy should be performed prior to pregnancy in women with aITP who are planning a family. *Indications for performance of splenectomy during pregnancy* include the failure to respond initially to high dose corticosteroids (platelet count < 50,000 after 21 days of therapy), a continuing need for intensive medical therapy to remain in remission, and life-threatening hemorrhage (Ahn and Harrington, 1977; Caplan and Berkman, 1976). After splenectomy, a rise in platelet count may be detected within a few hours. Maximum benefit will be achieved within 1 to 3 weeks (O'Reilly and Taber, 1978). For cases in which the platelet count rises above 500,000/mm^3, anticoagulation has been recommended but not tested rigorously to reduce an alleged increased risk of thromboembolism (Zwaan et al., 1974).

Benefit of the splenectomy to the parturient must be weighed carefully against potential risk to the fetus. In one series, performance of splenectomy was noted to be associated with a 30 percent fetal mortality rate (Peterson and Larson, 1954). In a parturient whose fetus is preterm (ideally midtrimester) and whose aITP is medically unmanageable, splenectomy may be the optimal therapeutic choice. Late in pregnancy prior to fetal maturity, splenectomy can be carried out through a transthoracic approach (Ahn and Harrington, 1977) or the more standard transabdominal approach. Removal of all accessory splenic tissue if present is important. In selected cases where the mother has poorly controlled severe aITP and a fetus that is term and/or has mature lungs, splenectomy can be combined with cesarean section. The mother's disease may thus be controlled and an atraumatic delivery advantageously performed for the potentially thrombocytopenic infant.

Although there is not a consensus regarding therapeutic merit or degree of use, platelet transfusions often are used preoperatively and intraoperatively in association with splenectomy procedures. Use of platelet transfusions, corticosteroids, better anesthesia, and improved surgical techniques for pregnant splenectomies is responsible for today's much lower operative maternal and perinatal mortality rates than those recorded in the older obstetric literature. Formerly, approximately one in ten mothers and one in every four fetuses were lost (Heys, 1966; Tancer, 1960; O'Reilly and Taber, 1978; Laros and Sweet, 1975).

Splenectomy prior to pregnancy usually decreases the frequency and severity of maternal complications during pregnancy (Heys, 1966). However, the impression of maternal well-being may lead to a false sense of security on the part of the patient and her obstetrician that the *fetus is not in danger. Previous splenectomy has not been shown to effect any improvement in either perinatal mortality or neonatal thrombocytopenia* (Territo et al., 1973; Tancer, 1960; O'Reilly and Taber, 1978; Robson and Davidson, 1950). Splenectomy often results in remission of the aITP disease process, but it does not necessarily cure it (Jones, 1979; Cines and Schreiber, 1979; Veenhoven et al., 1980; Karpatkin and Lackner, 1975). After removal of the spleen, platelet-associated antibody can be produced by the liver, bone marrow, and other reticuloendothelial tissue. Absence of the spleen permits longer survival of antibody-coated platelets and more normal maternal platelet counts but would not be expected to decrease the transplacental passage of free antibody targeted for the fetal platelets (McMillan, 1977).

Immunosuppressive Drugs. If severe thrombocytopenia persists despite splenectomy and corticosteroid administration, the ad-

ministration of other immunosuppressive agents must be considered. Although a number of drugs, including azathioprine, cyclophosphamide, and the vinca alkaloids, have been shown to be beneficial in the treatment of a small number of pregnant patients with severe aITP, controlled clinical trials are sorely needed to investigate the benefit versus risk ratio of this therapy as well as its role in treatment (Ahn and Harrington, 1977; Gowda et al., 1977; Caplan and Berkman, 1976). Understandably, immunosuppressive therapy during gestation has been avoided owing to fears of fetal and maternal toxicity, teratogenicity, oncogenicity, fetal growth retardation, and prematurity. Experience recently with immunosuppressant-treated parturients who had undergone organ transplants revealed only an increased frequency of premature growth-retarded infants (Scott, 1977). There is at least one report in which a parturient with aITP was treated successfully during the third trimester with cyclophosphamide, and there were no obvious fetal side effects (Horger and Keane, 1979). Much work needs to be done to clarify the uncertainty surrounding the therapeutic indications and to elucidate recommendations for this type of intervention in the pregnant aITP patient. It is especially here that expert hematologic consultation is most valued.

Plasmapheresis. An alternative approach to therapy for some parturients with severe aITP is the removal of antiplatelet antibodies by automated plasmapheresis with fresh plasma or purified IgG preparations as part of the replacement medium (Marder et al., 1981; Imbach et al., 1981; Taft, 1982). Published results are mixed, with the best outcome in some patients with acute aITP who respond after only one or two exchanges and the worst outcome in patients with longstanding chronic disease (Imbach et al., 1981; Branda et al., 1975, 1978; Novak and Williams, 1978; Weir et al., 1980). Patient selection criteria must be refined and more investigations performed to study how plasma exchange can effect a cure. At present, *plasmapheresis should be considered only as an emergency or secondary adjunct* (Taft et al., 1981) *to the primary therapeutic tools* already discussed (Table 23–11).

Platelet Transfusion. Platelet transfusion in parturients with severe aITP is a temporary measure useful therapeutically for the arrest of life-threatening hemorrhage and useful

Table 23–11. Potential Applications for
Plasmapheresis in aITP

As preoperative treatment for the adult patient
following failed intravenous immunoglobulin
and/or corticosteroid therapy

As emergency treatment for life-threatening
hemorrhage

As alternative treatment when other modes of
therapy are absolutely or relatively
contraindicated

prophylactically as part of the preparation prior to operative procedures such as splenectomy and cesarean section (Baldini, 1972). Although fresh whole blood, platelet-rich plasma, and platelet concentrate are all considered vehicles for platelet administration, in general only platelet concentrates are utilized therapeutically for patients with aITP. In terms of platelet function, platelet-rich plasma and platelet concentrates begin to lose efficacy with time, with exposure to the 4°C temperature of blood refrigerators, with treatment by the anticoagulant solution acid citrate dextrose (ACD), and with placement in plastic storage containers (Murray and Gardner, 1969; Abbott Laboratories, 1971). Optimal practice is to minimize turnaround time from donor to recipient, storing platelets in containers at 4°C for as little as possible of the deadline time of 72 hours. Ideally, platelets should be obtained by single-donor plateletpheresis to reduce the hazards of hepatitis transmission, increases in numbers of transfused platelet antigens, and febrile reactions. Also ideally, platelets should be matched not only for ABO and RH blood groups but also for histocompatibility (HLA) and platelet (PL) antigens (Horger and Keane, 1979).

Depending on how much circulating antiplatelet antibody is present and how well the donor platelets have been matched with the patient and her antibody, transfusion of a single unit of platelet concentrate from a carefully collected unit of ABO-compatible very fresh blood will raise the aITP patient's platelet count significantly less than the

7000 to 11,000/mm³/M² increase observed in normal individuals (Harker and Finch, 1969). There is much variation from one patient to another, and more exact individual needs can be calculated by inserting into the formula depicted in Figure 23–5 the results of blood sampling taken 1 hour after transfusion (Laningham, 1975; American Association of Blood Banks, 1975). For instance, Anguillo and coworkers demonstrated an increment of 3200 platelets/mm³ per unit of platelet concentrate infused into their patient with aITP (1977). Survival of platelets transfused into an individual with aITP is shortened to 48 to 230 minutes (Harker and Finch, 1969).

Because platelets of patients with aITP are younger and larger and function more efficiently as cofactors of coagulation, it may not be necessary to transfuse enough platelet concentrates to achieve the preoperative platelet count of 60,000 to 70,000/mm³ recommended by Anguillo and colleagues. A maternal count of 50,000/mm³ or less may be adequate (Cavanagh, 1982). In our experience, the bleeding time of aITP patients may not be prolonged with only 10,000 to 20,000 platelets. As a reflection of the uncertainty of critical requirements for coagulation, some protocols for aITP management of parturients recommend preset transfusion amounts (Cruickshank, 1982). However, the least amount necessary for hemostasis is recommended because platelet transfusion is expensive and carries with it the risk of transmission of hepatitis and development of platelet isoantibodies and alloantibodies. Aisner recommends that corticosteroids always be administered prior to platelet transfusion to enhance longevity of the transfused platelets (1977).

The most recent innovation for the therapy of aITP is the intravenous infusion of high-dose monomeric polyvalent human immunoglobulin, usually administered in amounts of 400 mg/kg daily for 5 days. Adult as well as pediatric patients with chronic aITP have been shown to experience at least

$$\text{Increment in Platelet Count per Unit of Platelets Transfused} = \frac{\left[\begin{array}{c}\text{Platelet}\\\text{Count One}\\\text{Hour After}\\\text{Transfusion}\end{array}\right] - \left[\begin{array}{c}\text{Platelet}\\\text{Count}\\\text{Before}\\\text{Transfusion}\end{array}\right] \times \left[\begin{array}{c}\text{Body}\\\text{Surface}\\(m^2)\end{array}\right]}{\text{Number of Units of Platelets Given}}$$

Figure 23–5. Calculation of platelet response after transfusion.

a transient increase in the circulating platelet count (Imbach et al., 1981; Schmidt et al., 1981; Fehr et al., 1982; Bierling et al., 1982; Newland et al., 1983; Carroll et al., 1983). Preliminary studies suggest that mechanical and/or immunologic mechanisms are involved. Although a long-term response has been seen in some patients, most often there has not been a sustained response following rapid improvement unless the IgG infusions were followed closely by splenectomy. Investigations are continuing to further evaluate the utility of this therapeutic modality in three special areas: (1) prior to splenectomy in corticosteroid-refractory patients; (2) as a preoperative medication for all patients with aITP; and (3) to control bleeding in acute aITP.

Intrapartum Period

The most critical and controversial aspect of aITP pregnancy management is the optimal planning of labor and delivery. Because of the transplacental passage of antiplatelet antibody, infants of women who have undergone platelet transfusion may be born with thrombocytopenia. The most feared perinatal complication is intracranial hemorrhage. Because birth trauma is a major cause of perinatal morbidity and mortality, efforts have been directed toward identification of the fetus at risk and delivery by atraumatic cesarean section. Optimal outcome might be achieved by early identification of the thrombocytopenic fetus and its abdominal delivery prior to the onset of labor. Any attempts to select for cesarean delivery only the compromised fetus are advantageous also for the aITP mother's welfare so that she is not subjected to any unnecessary operative intervention and risk.

The maternal platelet count has been observed by many to be an unreliable predictor of the fetal or neonatal platelet count (Territo et al., 1973; Tancer, 1960; O'Reilly and Taber, 1978; Noriega-Guerra et al., 1979; Murray and Harris, 1976; Laros and Sweet, 1975; Cines et al., 1982; Carloss et al., 1980; Kornstein et al., 1980; Baele and Thiery, 1978). The discrepancy between maternal and fetal platelet counts may be particularly evident in the splenectomized parturient in whom a normal platelet count can be detected despite the presence of considerable amounts of antiplatelet antibodies (Jones, 1979; Cines and Schreiber, 1979; Veenhoven et al., 1980;

Karpatkin and Lackner, 1975). In large numbers the unbound IgG antibodies can traverse the placenta, attach themselves to fetal platelets, and render the antibody-coated platelets subject to destruction by the intact fetal spleen. Clinically, these fetuses have proven to be at greater risk for purpura and death than their counterparts in aITP mothers who have not yet undergone splenectomy.

The measurement of venous platelet counts in fetal scalp blood by direct sampling during early labor was first reported in 1978 by Ayromlooi (1978). Because this determination should accurately reflect the venous platelet count and reliably predict the risk of fetal hemorrhage, Scott and coworkers used this novel approach in a small series of parturients and found it to be reliable (1980). Sampling was done either during labor or immediately after amniotomy to induce labor at term when the cervix became favorable. If the platelet count was below 50,000/mm^3, these investigators delivered the fetus abdominally, but more usually it was higher and a vaginal delivery was supported unless traditional obstetric concerns interfered. Three of 12 parturients with aITP underwent cesarean section for fetal counts less than 50,000/mm^3, and in all three infants neonatal platelet counts were less than 20,000/mm^3. In fetuses delivered vaginally, the lowest count was 76,000/mm^3. Scott and coworkers recommended sampling for all parturients with aITP, whether they are in remission, are taking steroids, or have had a splenectomy (1980).

Fetal scalp sampling (Table 23–12) is not without some risk, and it cannot be accomplished in all patients. Membranes must be ruptured, the head must be the descending part, and the cervix must be partially dilated and effaced. Intracranial hemorrhage may already have occurred at the point in pelvic descent when sampling can be performed. Significant bleeding may occur secondary to the scalp laceration itself. In the hands of Scott and colleagues, there were no untoward fetal bleeding episodes in those fetuses with platelet counts as low as 3000/mm^3 so long as pressure was kept on the scalp puncture site through two subsequent uterine contractions (1980).

If vaginal delivery is elected, a prolonged and difficult labor should be avoided. Electronic fetal monitoring and vigilant attention to basic obstetric principles are critical. For instance, the supine position and overstim-

Table 23–12. Fetal Scalp Sampling Technique

1. Place the patient comfortably on her side in a "curled up" position with the vaginal introitus near one side of the labor bed; this usually ensures maternal comfort, maximizes uteroplacental blood flow to the fetus, and facilitates a careful performance of the procedure by the obstetrician.
2. Introduce a plastic cone from a fetal scalp pH set into the vagina and place it against the fetal scalp.
3. Cleanse the designated area on the scalp and make a small stab wound in the area chosen for sampling.
4. Hold the plastic pipette (from a set such as the Becton-Dickinson Unopipette Test 5855 system, which is used in hospital labs for manual platelet determinations) against the bleeding point and allow it to fill by capillary action; obtain at least two samples.
5. With the Unopipette System, the pipette is then quickly inserted into a reservoir containing diluent and the blood sample is rapidly evacuated into this solution.
6. The platelets are then counted using a standard hemocytometer method.
7. After sampling is completed, maintain steady pressure against the scalp stab wound with a long-stem cotton swab until oozing has ceased and at least two uterine contractions have occurred.

ulation with oxytocin should be avoided to prevent fetal hypoxia. Platelet counts in term infants are significantly lower in those who have suffered hypoxic episodes (Chadd et al., 1971). Obstetric analgesia will be influenced by the patient's hematologic status as well as the skills and preferences of the

Table 23–13. Intrapartum Management Considerations for aITP

Periodic manual platelet counts
Avoidance of intramuscular injections
Avoidance of fetal hypoxia and neonatal asphyxia
Avoidance of difficult or prolonged labor
Avoidance of difficult forceps deliveries
Preferred midline episiotomy
Continuous external electronic fetal monitoring
Internal scalp electrode can be placed after normal scalp sampling for platelet count
Fetal scalp sampling for platelet count
Readiness for C section immediately after scalp sampling
Appropriate maternal platelet transfusion
Ready availability of blood products for potential maternal/neonatal use
Appropriate corticosteroid use
Potential use of intravenous immunoglobulin therapy
Optimal analgesia/anesthesia
Meticulous operative technique
Selective cesarean delivery
Excellent neonatal care accessibility

obstetric anesthesiologist. General endotracheal anesthesia is used for preplanned cesarean delivery, avoiding potential coagulation problems associated with the placement of an epidural catheter. Achievement of a platelet count of at least $50,000/mm^3$ is necessary to provide normal maternal hemostasis prior to vaginal delivery or a possible emergent abdominal delivery. If the parturient received corticosteroids at any time during gestation, hydrocortisone 200 mg IV as a bolus probably should be given early in labor or preoperatively. A continuous infusion of 100 mg hydrocortisone every 6 hours should be administered through delivery and the immediate puerperium. Difficult forceps manipulations should be avoided. Episiotomies and any lacerations must be repaired meticulously. Likewise, cesarean section technique must be meticulous, the operator making extra efforts to minimize tissue trauma and maximize hemostasis in the surgical field. Intrapartum management considerations for aITP are listed in Table 23–13.

Postpartum Period

Intensive fetal and maternal surveillance during parturition must be maintained, especially in the immediate postpartum period. Neonatal thrombocytopenia occurs in as many as 70 percent of infants born to women with aITP (Noriega-Guerra et al., 1979; Laros and Sweet, 1975; Goldswerg and Chediak, 1977). It may be severe enough to cause hemorrhagic complications prior to, during, or immediately after the birth process. A review of 98 infants born to women with aITP by Scott and coworkers (1980) revealed no serious bleeding recorded in any infant with a platelet count greater than or equal to $50,000/mm^3$. Because the passive acquisition of antibody from the mother ceases after the umbilical cord is severed, neonatal thrombocytopenia usually is mild and a self-limited process that peaks 4 to 6 days after delivery and then disappears over a course of weeks to, at the most, 3 months (Scott, 1976; Pearson and McIntosh, 1978). Regardless of the postdelivery platelet count, each neonate of an aITP mother should be monitored for at least 1 week or longer until improvement is noted.

Most often the neonate requires no special therapy. In unusually severe situations, an exchange transfusion with fresh whole blood should be performed (Nelson et al., 1979). Platelet packs can be given after exchange transfusion. In cases in which only purpura or petechiae develop, some investigators have used corticosteroid therapy for 3 weeks until the platelet antibodies of maternal origin ultimately have disappeared (Laros and Sweet, 1975). This approach to therapy is controversial (Pitkin, 1977).

Early in the puerperium, breast-feeding may induce thrombocytopenia owing to the passage of platelet antibodies in the colostrum (Kelman et al., 1978). In view of this as well as the possible passage of corticosteroids across to the fetus via breast milk, lactation usually is discouraged in these patients (Katz and Duncan, 1975).

For the mother, concerns about future fertility must be addressed prior to hospital discharge (Table 23–14). Because intrauterine devices have an increased failure rate in mothers taking corticosteroids and are associated with increased risks of menorrhagia and uterine perforation in aITP women, low-dose combination birth control pills may be the optimal mode of contraception. If sterilization is desired, we prefer an inpatient procedure via minilaparotomy incision for optimal visualization and handling of tissue for hemostasis.

CONCLUSION AND RECOMMENDATIONS

The utility of platelet antibody measurement as a tool to facilitate clinical management decisions is under intense study and debate at this writing (Kelton et al., 1980, 1981, 1982; Cines et al., 1982). Because this role must be further defined before these platelet antibody assays can enter into our diagnosis and management schemes, we must at present make clinical decisions often without optimal data. Where the equipment and expertise exist, fetal scalp sampling

Table 23–14. Postpartum Management of aITP

Continued intensive fetal and maternal surveillance
Reproductive counseling
Contraception by birth control pills or barrier method; avoidance of IUDs
Consider later splenectomy if future childbearing desired
Inpatient sterilization by minilaparotomy if desired; avoidance of laparoscopy
Avoidance of breast-feeding

---

prior to or early in labor as practiced by Scott and coworkers may facilitate decision making (1980). If determination of the fetal platelet count is not available, a regimen such as that proposed by Carloss and colleagues appears at this time to be a rational management scheme (1980). Thus, *all mothers with platelet counts less than 100,000/mm³ and all mothers with a history of aITP at any time in the past and who have undergone splenectomy, regardless of current platelet count, should undergo cesarean section prior to labor.*

It is apparent that, while great strides have been made recently to improve the maternal and perinatal outcome of pregnancies complicated by aITP, there remain many unknowns. As answers become available, our clinical management plans can evolve responsibly into ever more rational efforts to improve the maternal, fetal, and neonatal care of the aITP pregnancy.

A summary of patient care procedures in the management of aITP is presented in Table 23–15.

Hemoglobinopathies

ETIOLOGY

Maternal anemia is the *most common* maternal complication noted during gestation and occurs in more than 50 percent of all pregnancies (Morrison, 1981). These anemias can be categorized as acquired and inherited disorders. Of the congenital disorders, there are over 1000 possible genetic abnormalities, and most involve the structure of the globin chains of the hemoglobin molecule. Examples of these defects include hemoglobin S (Hb-S) and hemoglobin C (Hb-C), which differ from the normal adult hemoglobin (Hb-A and Hb-A_2) or fetal hemoglobin (Hb-F) only by the substitution of one amino acid in the globin chain (Morrison, 1979). Other types of abnormalities involve the diminished production of either the alpha or beta globin chain of the hemoglobin molecule, such as thalassemia (Hb-Thal). Fortunately, most of these abnormalities are quite rare and are imbedded in an autosomal codominant or recessive manner. Sickle hemoglobin is one of the most common structural variants and is also clinically important because of the increased maternal mortality and morbidity as well as fetal/neonatal wastage encountered during

Table 23–15. Patient Care Summary for aITP

| | Antepartum | | Intrapartum | Postpartum |
	Outpatient*	Inpatient		
BP, P, R, T	With each clinic visit	Minimum q 4 hr, depending on patient's condition	Minimum q 1 hr	On admission to RR; then q 15 min × 4; then q 30 min × 2; then q 1 hr until stable
FHR	With each clinic visit	Weekly NST/CST	After normal scalp sampling, continuously with fetal monitor, preferably internal; if monitor not available, q 15–30 min in first stage, and q 5 min in second stage	—
Scalp sampling	—	—	× 1 in labor room to establish fetal aITP	—
Contractions	—	—	q 1 hr	Fundal checks on admission q 15 min × 4; then q 30 min × 2; then q 1 hr until stable
Lochia	—	—	—	Lochia checks q 15 min until stable; then q 30 min × 2; then q 1 hr until stable; then q 4–8 hr
Sonograms	q 4 wk after 26 wk			
Possible plasma exchange	See discussion of management schemes in text; maintain individualized care			
Possible platelet transfusions				
Laboratory values				
Platelet count				
Observation for signs of shock	—	—	Continuously	Continuously
I & O	—	q 8 hr	q 1 hr	q 1 hr until stable

*Frequent clinic visits (frequency will depend on patient's condition).
Note: Nurse–patient ratio, 1:6 to 8 ante partum; 2:3 intra partum; 1:6 to 8 post partum.

pregnancy in parturients with severe disease.

INCIDENCE

Inherited abnormal hemoglobins may be divided into mild or severe type, depending on their clinical appearance (Table 23–16). The *most common type of hemoglobinopathy* is sickle cell trait (Hb-S) (Foster, 1980), which occurs in 1 in 12 black Americans or those of Mediterranean descent. Fortunately, this is usually a benign syndrome during pregnancy, and sickle cell patients are not usually treated differently than patients with normal hemoglobin with the exception that Hb A-S patients receive intensive antepartum scrutiny for infections, specifically those related to the urinary tract. Other var-

iants, such as hemoglobin S-E, S-D, and S-Memphis, are usually benign during pregnancy and are exceedingly rare (Morrison, 1979). Finally, hemoglobin C disease (Hb C-C and Hb A-C) is the 6th most common

Table 23–16. Classification of Hemoglobinopathies

Mild (Benign Forms)
  Sickle cell trait (Hb A-S)
  Hemoglobin S-E disease (Hb S-E)
  Hemoglobin S-D disease (Hb S-D)
  Hemoglobin S-Memphis (Hb S-Memphis)
  Hemoglobin C disease (Hb C-C)
Sickle Cell Disease
  Sickle cell anemia (Hb S-S)
  Hemoglobin S-C disease (Hb S-C)
  Hemoglobin S-thalassemia (Hb S-Thal)
  Hemoglobin B-thalassemia

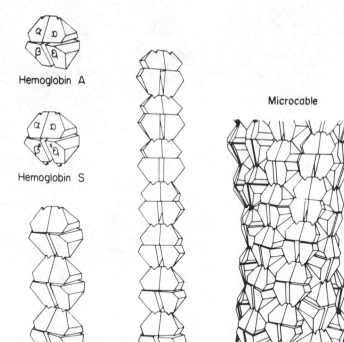

Hemoglobin A

Hemoglobin S

Microcable

Hydrophobic Bonding   Micro Filament

Figure 23–6. Sickle cell microcables. Hemoglobin filaments coalesce into a semisolid gel to form microcables. These microcables further polymerize to form helical structures that distort the cell into its characteristic sickle shape.

hemoglobinopathy and affects 1 in 4400 black Americans. It also does not have a significant adverse effect on either the mother or the fetus.

As shown in Table 23–16, patients with severe hemoglobinopathies include those with clinically significant forms of thalassemia and those with sickle cell disease. Sickle cell disease is composed of sickle cell anemia (Hb S-S), hemoglobin S-C (Hb S-C), and hemoglobin S-thalassemia (Hb S-Thal), which occur in 1 per 600, 1 per 850, and 1 per 1600 patients, respectively (Foster, 1980). In pregnant patients these hemoglobinopathies are usually thought to increase the risk for the mother/fetus/neonate. Those with homozygous beta thalassemia or Cooley's anemia usually do not live to conceive, and those with homozygous alpha thalassemia are rarely born alive (Morrison, 1981). Therefore, the disorders that constitute sickle cell disease are the ones most clinically applicable to the perinatologist.

PATHOPHYSIOLOGY

The molecular alteration that distinguishes Hb-S from normal hemoglobin A (Hb-A) is a minor structural change that involves only 2 of the 574 amino acids in normal hemoglobin. The substitution of the amino acid valine for glutamic acid in the two beta chains of each hemoglobin molecule drastically diminishes the oxygen-carrying capacity and survival time of the red blood cell in those patients who have sickle hemoglobin. As shown in Figure 23–6, this amino acid replacement allows the beta chains of various hemoglobin molecules within the red cells to interlock by hydrophobic bonding with other Hb-S molecules. Long microfilaments form, which then coalesce into large microcables. Once these helical structures polymerize in the deoxygenated state they distort the cell into its characteristic sickled shape. Once the cell loses water the cell membrane may be hardened by calcium deposits and thus the cell becomes irreversibly sickled and is destroyed.

If a sickle cell patient is exposed to acidosis or hypoxia, the sickling of the Hb-S–containing cells occurs more often, which causes sludging of the cells in the microcirculation (Fig. 23–7). With subsequent capillary obstruction there is increased blood viscosity within the capillaries and more sickling occurs, which leads to further deoxygenation. This completes the vicious cycle of increased intravascular sickling, and thus a painful vasoocclusive crisis is clinically

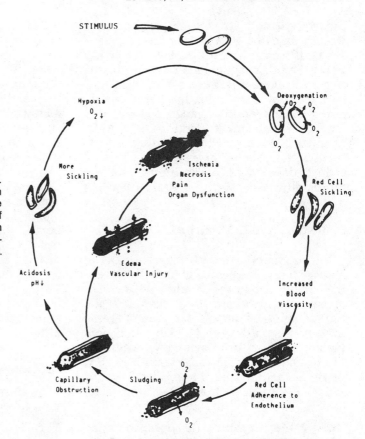

Figure 23–7. The sickle cell crisis cycle. A dangerous sequence is set in motion when HbS-containing red cells become deoxygenated, sickled, and obstructive of blood flow in the microvasculature. (From Martin, J. N., Jr., and Morrison, J. C.: Managing the parturient with sickle cell crisis. Clin. Obstet. Gynecol. 27:39, 1984.)

set in motion (Martin and Morrison, 1982). Clinically, these crises produce sudden pain involving the abdomen, chest, vertebrae, and extremities. The manifestations usually follow a repetitive pattern from one crisis to the next, but during pregnancy such findings may be intensified. Although vasoocclusive crises are more common during pregnancy, hematologic crises can occur and are characterized by reticulocytopenia and a rapid decline in the hematocrit (Hct). These patients are usually more pale but less icteric than patients having a vasoocclusive crisis.

EFFECTS ON PREGNANCY

Older reports regarding pregnant patients with sickle cell disease (Hb-SS, Hb-SC, Hb S-Thal) revealed maternal mortality figures

Table 23–17. Pregnancy Outcome with Severe Sickle Hemoglobinopathies

Reference	Number of Gestations	Maternal Values (%)		Neonatal Values (%)	
		Morbidity	*Mortality*	*Morbidity*	*Mortality*
Statistics prior to 1970					
Adams (1953)	25	65	35	17	22
Curtis (1959)	64	35	8	46	42
Anderson (1960)	28	0	48	—	80
Rimer (1961)	25	0	—	—	42
McCurdy (1964)	34	75	3	17	29
Laros (1967)	67	15	—	—	19
Freeman (1969)	67	—	—	21	42
Statistics after 1970					
Perkins (1971)	109	13	0	12	12
Hendricks (1972)	61	13	0	12	12
Horger (1972)	54	96	8	51	24
Pritchard (1973)	128	—	1.5	29	33
Morrison (1976)	36	4	0	16	3
Charache (1979)	74	45	1.4	33	28
Milner (1980)	181	—	—	—	5.3
Morrison (1980)	75	14	0	9	2.6

between 10 and 20 percent and perinatal wastage rates of 40 and 60 percent (Table 23–17) (Freeman and Ruth, 1969; Fort et al., 1971). Through meticulous care and intensive medical therapy, these percentages have been reduced to the point that it is no longer rare to expect a normal pregnancy outcome for mother and infant (Perkins, 1971; Morrison and Wiser, 1976). Nevertheless, patients with sickle cell disease are considered at high risk and are a continuing problem for the physician (Morrison et al., 1980a).

DIAGNOSIS AND COUNSELING

It is prudent that each black parturient be assessed for sickle hemoglobin. If the screening test is positive she should have a hemoglobin electrophoresis to differentiate the type of abnormal hemoglobin present (Table 23–18). It is unlikely that sickle cell anemia patients without prior symptoms would be discovered, but some subjects with Hb S-C or Hb S-Thal have been found, and even if milder disorders such as HB A-S are diag-

Table 23–18. Diagnosis of Hemoglobinopathies

A. Screening Tests (Sickledex—Ortho, etc.)
  1. Based on solubility and color change
  2. High false positive rate, rare false negative result
  3. Confirm with sodium metabisulfate slide test
  4. Definitive diagnosis—hemoglobin electrophoresis
B. Genetic Diagnosis
  1. Amniotic fluid uncultured cells by restrictive endonuclease
  2. Fetal blood sampling by fetoscopy
  3. Family pedigree
C. Hemoglobin Electrophoresis
  1. HbA-S: 25 to 35%-S, 60%-A_1, normal A_2, F
  2. HbS-S: 90 to 95%-S, normal A_2, normal to increased F, no A_1
  3. HbS-C: normal A_2 and F, 45 to 48% of both S and C, no A_1
  4. HbS-Thal: 35 to 50%-S, 40 to 60% A_1, normal to increased A_2 and F
  5. B-Thal heterozygous: 90%-A_1, increased A_2 and F
  6. A-Thal heterozygous: 95%-A_1, normal A_2 and F
D. Hemoglobin/Hematocrit Values
  1. HbA-S: Hb 11 to 12 g%, Hct 32 to 37%
  2. HbS-S: Hb 5 to 8 g%, Hct 15 to 22%
  3. HbS-C: Hb 8 to 10 g%, Hct 25 to 30%
  4. HbS-Thal: Hb 9 to 10 g%, Hct 28 to 32%
  5. B or A-Thal: Hb 9 to 12 g%, Hct 28 to 36%
E. Other Indices
  1. Blood films of sickling (Hb-S), target cells—thalassemia
  2. Indices—normochromic, normocytic unless associated iron deficiency
  3. Reticulocyte count increased 3 to 20%
  4. Serum iron—variable
  5. Bilirubin elevated in HbS-S and SC even when not in crisis

nosed, proper education and counseling can be offered. The detection of subjects with hemoglobinopathies allows proper patient education. For those with mild disorders, the avoidance of stress, high altitudes, infection, and hypoxia should be mentioned, but reassurance of their normalcy is underscored. Avoidance and early recognition of infection and crises are very important in those with major hemoglobinopathies. Educating the public as to the extent of the disease and its cause is also important. Therefore, antepartum screening is recommended for black Americans to detect sickle hemoglobinopathies. It is also essential to test the cord blood to determine the presence of Hb-S in the newborn so that the family can be counseled if necessary (Kramer et al., 1979). Infants rarely have crises before 3 to 6 months of age, because there is ample fetal hemoglobin to protect the cells from sickling.

Laboratory Findings

As shown in Table 23–18, the most common laboratory finding in patients with hemoglobinopathies is anemia (Morrison, 1981). In general, those with Hct less than 20 or Hb less than 6 g/dl usually have Hb S-S or Cooley's beta thalassemia. Patients with Hb S-C or Hb S-Thal may have a hematocrit value of 20 to 25 percent and even 30 percent on some occasions. Patients with heterozygous beta or alpha thalassemia as well as the mild sickle hemoglobinopathies including sickle cell trait have hematocrit values of 30 to 35 percent. The reticulocyte count is usually elevated in the range of 10 to 20 percent, and thrombocytosis is common in patients with sickle hemoglobinopathies. The serum bilirubin is normally elevated (1 to 7 mg/dl) and can reach 15 to 20 mg/dl during crisis. The prothrombin, partial thromboplastin, and clotting times are normal in patients with hemoglobinopathies, but platelet counts, fibrinogen, and fibrin split products may be abnormal, particularly during crisis (Martin and Morrison, 1982).

MANAGEMENT

Antepartum Period

Conservative versus Transfusion Therapy. *All authorities recommend careful and frequent antepartum visits* beginning early during gestation. The severity of anemia, retic-

Table 23–19. Antepartum Assessment of Pregnant Patients with Hemoglobinopathies

A. Hemoglobin Testing
   1. Sickle screen to black patients with unknown hemoglobin
   2. Hemoglobin electrophoresis with unexplained or unresponsive anemia
   3. Husband, family members of known hemoglobinopathy patients
   4. Consider genetic amniocentesis if both parents have hemoglobinopathy
B. Education and Counseling After Identification
C. Prenatal Visits
   1. Encourage early entry into prenatal clinic
   2. If asymptomatic, visits every 2 weeks until 20 weeks, then weekly
   3. Close scrutiny for signs of infection, crisis, or labor
D. Laboratory Tests
   1. Routine prenatal assessment
   2. Baseline fibrinogen, platelet count, and SMAC
   3. Reticulocyte count, bilirubin, hematocrit, hemoglobin, urinalysis twice monthly
   4. Hemoglobin electrophoresis twice monthly if patient has received transfusions
E. Fetal Assessments
   1. NST/OCT weekly beginning 34 weeks
   2. USG 16 to 18 weeks, repeat at 28 to 30 weeks
   3. Fetal movement—30 minutes, three times daily beginning 32 weeks

ulocyte counts, bilirubin levels, degree of sickling, and presence of infection and/or crisis should be intensively assessed at each visit (Table 23–19). Many authors recommend continued observation during gestation if the patient with a severe sickle hemoglobinopathy has a benign prior history, elevated Hb-F, or no hint of infection or crisis (Perkins, 1971; Desforges and Warth, 1974; Charache et al., 1980). On the other hand, others who have noted deterioration in such patients during pregnancy recommend prophylactic treatment with partial exchange or simple transfusions to remove Hb-S–containing cells, replacing them with normal donor cells containing Hb-A (Morrison et al., 1980b; Cunningham et al., 1979). Therefore, one group advocates conservative management of pregnant patients with severe sickle hemoglobinopathies, whereas another recommends intensive therapy with prophylactic transfusions. Each group has good statistics to warrant the use of its approach (see Table 23–18). During infection or crisis most authors recommend the use of blood products as a major therapeutic modality.

For those recommending prophylactic transfusions, several techniques are available. Prior to 1978 most persons used the manual method, but this type of therapy is expensive and cumbersome (Morrison and

Wiser, 1976; Cunningham et al., 1979). More recently, continuous automated erythrocytopheresis has been recommended by several authors as a method that can lead to a more accurate estimation of the amount of blood infused and withdrawn as well as allow the clinician to perform these transfusions on an ambulatory basis (Key et al., 1980; Keeling et al., 1980; Morrison et al., 1982). The IBM 2997 Cell Separator and the Haemonetics Model 30 have both been useful in this maneuver. If the newer methods are not available the manual method can be used (Table 23–20). The method of manual transfusion as well as critical levels for follow-up are listed in Table 23–20. The benefits and risks of this technique are listed in Table 23–21.

Crisis Management. If a vasoocclusive crisis does occur during pregnancy, one must consider medical and surgical or obstetric disorders in the differential diagnosis, since pain does not always mean crisis in a sickle cell patient. Up to one third of crises during adulthood are associated with apparent or occult infections and most commonly include the lung and urinary and intestinal tracts. To differentiate bacterial infection from simple vasoocclusive crisis without infection, the total number of segmented leu-

Table 23–20. Protocol for Manual Partial Exchange Transfusion

1. Obtain hematocrit (HCT) and Hb-A %; match, type, and cross-match.
2. Infuse 200 to 500 ml of normal saline (60 min).
3. Phlebotomize 500 ml (30 min).
4. Give 2 units (150 to 200 ml per unit) buffy coat–poor, washed RBC (90 min).
5. Repeat entire procedure.
6. Allow 12 hours for equilibration.
7. Obtain Hct and Hb-A %.
8. If Hct > 30% and Hb-A > 40%, discharge patient; if not, repeat procedure.
9. Assess Hct and Hb-A every 2 weeks
10. Repeat entire procedure:
    a. At 36 to 38 weeks.
    b. When Hct < 25% and Hb-A < 20%.
    c. If crisis occurs.
    d. If labor ensues.
Comments:
    a. Infuse buffy coat–poor, washed RBC warmed and under pressure.
    b. If HCT falls rapidly (1 to 2 weeks) posttransfusion, check hemolysis:
       (1) reticulocyte count
       (2) bilirubin
       (3) antibody screen
       (4) plasma hemoglobin
    c. In HbS-C patients it may be difficult to raise Hb-A > 35%.
    d. Interval between exchanges usually 4 to 8 weeks.

Table 23–21. Benefits and Risks of Transfusion Therapy

Benefits	Risks
Decreases number of Hb-S cells	Hepatitis
Increases number of Hb-A cells	Transfusion reaction
Decreases erythropoiesis of Hb-S cells	Isosensitization
Can abort a crisis	Febrile reactions
Increased sense of well-being	Premature labor
Can be used in congestive heart failure or renal disease	Temporary measure only

kocytes (rarely above 1000 bands/mcl in crisis), leukocyte alkaline phosphatase activity (normal in vasoocclusive crisis alone), and isoenzymes (1 and 2) of serum lactate dehydrogenase (higher during crisis) are helpful assessments (Martin and Morrison, 1982).

The treatment of the crisis itself should be directed toward relieving the pain, preventing dehydration, and treating intercurrent infections as well as other complications. Acetaminophen is the antipyretic/mild analgesic of choice, although during crisis meperidine is usually required for alleviating severe pain. Morphine is avoided because of its potential smooth muscle constrictive properties. It is important to use these drugs only for severe pain because of the possibility of drug abuse or addiction. If infection is thought to be a problem, then antibiotics should be begun as soon as appropriate cultures are taken. Fluid and electrolyte replacement are essential because of the increased insensible fluid loss and hyposthenuria that occur during sickle cell crisis. Many compounds to alkalize the maternal serum (and prevent further sickling) have been assessed as therapeutic agents but have not been effective. The efficacy of oxygen administration is also questionable unless the patient has evidence of a respiratory infection or other problems that would cause the PaO_2 level to be less than 70 mm.

The administration of blood components with Hb-A–containing cells is the cornerstone of crisis therapy. Routine crisis or labor is a contraindication to the use of blood components. We prefer the exchange transfusion method using the IBM 2997 for erythrocytopheresis. Only if the Hct is less than 15 is it necessary to give packed red cells prior to initiating an exchange transfusion. Buffy coat–poor washed erythrocytes are returned to the patient with her own plasma and leukocytes by erythrocytopheresis. Usually this method aborts the crisis within 30 minutes after beginning the infusion. It is critically important to make certain that properly matched and administered red blood cells are used. Impeccable blood banking technique is important in assuring the patient the maximal benefits and minimal risks of transfusion therapy. Table 23–22 outlines a step-wise fashion for antepartum management of these patients with suggested nursing actions.

Intrapartum Period

General Principles. During the intrapartum period spontaneous labor is managed with intensive maternal and fetal surveillance. Blood smears for potential crisis (assessment of the percentage of sickle cells), coagulation studies, serial maternal blood gases, and determination of Hct, Hb, and percentage of

Table 23–22. Antepartum Management of Hemoglobinopathy Crisis

A. General
   1. Environment—quiet, comfortable, supportive
   2. Prevent dehydration—Ringer's lactate, NS, fresh frozen plasma
   3. Monitor I & O
   4. Monitor vital signs during labor
B. Analgesia
   1. Acetaminophen
   2. Meperidine
   3. Sedatives
C. Blood Component Replacement (most important)
   1. Method—simple, manual partial exchange transfusion, antenatal erythrocytopheresis
   2. Meticulous blood banking, volunteer donor, fresh as possible
   3. Buffy coat–poor washed donor RBCs, S, VDRL, and hepatitis B
D. Antibiotics
   1. 25 percent of crises associated with infection
   2. Use broad spectrum coverage until culture return
E. Others
   1. Oxygen—may or may not be of benefit (3 l/min nasal/biprong)
   2. Alratinization—not useful
   3. Catheters (bladder, uterine, central venous)—avoid if possible
   4. Laboratory test—SMAC, blood film, hemoglobin studies
F. Special Cases
   1. Labor—continuous FHR monitoring and scalp sampling, maternal ABG
   2. Hemolytic crisis—plasma hemoglobin, but no increased bilirubin
   3. Infection—urinary tract, pulmonary, bone, gallbladder—unusual organisms

hemoglobin A are all useful during the intrapartum period. Frequent vital signs assessments in the mother as well as adequate fluid administration to avoid dehydration are recommended. Central venous lines and Foley and uterine catheters should be avoided, unless necessary, to reduce infectious morbidity. Although oxygen is not generally recommended, it may be used in labor, particularly if there are signs of fetal compromise. Intensive electronic monitoring of the fetal heart rate (FHRM) and maternal contractions is helpful to assess the fetal response to the contractions. Likewise, fetal scalp sampling can be helpful when alarming patterns are seen on the FHRM.

Blood Component Therapy. It is best if the hemoglobin Hb-A level is greater than 20 percent and the Hct is greater than 25 percent. If transfusions are needed because the patient is in crisis during labor or there is a low Hct/Hb-A, labor is not a contraindication to the infusion or exchange transfusion of blood. Adequate pain relief with meperidine can be used during early labor, and this can be combined with pudendal, local, or nitrous oxide anesthesia at delivery. If an obstetric anesthesiologist is present, conduction anesthesia with a light segmental epidural block may be used, but spinal, caudal, and paracervical blocks are best avoided. For cesarean birth, balanced endotracheal general anesthesia has provided best results.

Postpartum Period

During the postpartum period the patient should be assessed for signs of crisis due to the stress of labor. These patients are also prone to infection, and early recognition of signs of fever or foul-smelling lochia with prompt treatment is essential.

Sterilization is often recommended to these patients because of the risk not only to the fetus but to the patient. If the patient desires future pregnancies, an effective means of birth control is imperative so that future pregnancies can be planned. Estrogen-progestin combination oral contraceptives are probably contraindicated in women with sickle cell anemias, because erythrocyte sequestration and vascular occlusion may be intensified. Contraception is a difficult issue but is probably best handled by barrier techniques. It is possible that the use of the progestin-only pill ("mini-pill") as well as the extremely low-dose estrogen pill (< 35 mg) may prove safe in the future. Nevertheless, the association of coagulation changes with sickle cell anemia and estrogens makes the use of the oral contraceptives undesirable at this time. Similarly, use of the intrauterine device, because it is associated (in Hb-S patients) with infectious problems, cannot be recommended.

Counseling for these patients is important. If the patient is newly diagnosed, emotional support as well as education regarding her disease is needed. Information on the effects of chronic illness on the mother and her family is necessary to help these families cope. If the patient has had the disease for some time, the effect of pregnancy on her disease should be discussed, including the maternal and fetal morbidity and mortality. Emotional support is important if the patient chooses permanent sterilization. If the couple had desired more children, they may have a grief reaction to their loss of fertility.

Genetic counseling is important in helping the couple decide on sterilization. If both parents have the trait form of the disease, there is a 25 percent chance with each pregnancy that the child will be affected. If one parent has the trait and the other has the hemoglobinopathy, there is a 50 percent chance with each pregnancy that the child will develop the hemoglobinopathy; in such cases, a child born without the hemoglobinopathy will have the trait form. If both parents have a hemoglobinopathy, then all of their children will be affected.

Hemoglobinopathy in the Newborn

Since most of the hemoglobin in the red blood cells is fetal hemoglobin, hemolytic anemia characteristics of these hemoglobinopathies are not operational in utero or at birth. As more red blood cells that contain more abnormal hemoglobin are synthesized, the disease will become clinically apparent.

NEW DEVELOPMENTS

Therapeutics

The prospects for new and successful therapy for sickle cell hemoglobinopathies have never looked brighter. Most of these new therapeutic regimens are aimed at the atomic interaction that actually triggers a sickle cell crisis (Klotz et al., 1981). The new agents are divided into three major categories: (1) those that inhibit the actual polymerization of sickle hemoglobin by disrupting the hydrophobic bonding (see Fig. 23–6); (2) those that inhibit the polymerization by decreasing the concentration of deoxygenated Hb-S; and (3) those that interact with the erythrocyte membrane. Of the agents that effect molecular bonding, several drugs, such as urea, organic solvents, and detergents, have been used but have proven too toxic for use in humans. New agents in this category that are most promising are the small peptides that can bind to the surface of the Hb-S molecule and prevent the intramolecular contacts necessary for polymerization. The major advantage of the use of these peptides is that they contain only amino acids, which (because they are naturally occurring compounds) have very low toxicities.

The second approach to this problem (decrease in the concentration of deoxy Hb-S) simply involves an increase in the oxygen affinity so that Hb-S binds to oxygen more tightly. The drug cyanate has been used in humans but produced toxic effects such as peripheral damage and has been withdrawn. One possible solution would be to use this

Table 23–23. Patient Care Summary for Hemoglobinopathies

| | Antepartum | | Intrapartum | Postpartum |
	Outpatient	*Inpatient*		
BP, P, R	q visit	Minimum q 4 hr	q 1 hr	On admission q 15 min × 4; then q 30 min × 2; then q 1 hr until stable
T	q visit	Minimum q 4 hr	q 4 hr	On admission; then q 4 hr
FHR	Weekly NST/CST	Weekly NST/CST	Continuous electronic fetal monitoring, preferably internal; if no monitor available, q 15 to 30 min in first stage, and q 5 min in second stage	—
Contractions	—	—	Continuous electronic monitoring; if no monitor available, q 1 hr	Fundal checks on admission; then q 15 min × 4; then q 30 min × 2; then q 10 min until stable; then q 4 hr Lochia checks as above
Laboratory values				
Hemoglobin/ hematocrit	q visit	Weekly	At onset of labor	On admission to RR; qod until discharge
Screening	First visit of all black and Mediterranean patients	—	—	—

Observation for signs of:
  Pulmonary complications
  Infection
  Congestive heart failure
  Sickle cell crisis
	q visit	q shift	q 1 hr	q 1 hr until stable; then q 4 hr

Sonogram	As appropriate to rule out IUGR			

Note: Nurse–patient ratio, 1:6 to 8 antepartum, 2:3 intrapartum, 1:6 to 8 postpartum.

drug in an extracorporeal method; a clinical trial is in progress (Maugh, 1981). Another way of attacking the deoxyhemoglobin is to increase the volume in the erythrocyte itself, as in creating hyponatremia. In one clinical trial, chronic hyponatremia has reduced (in nonpregnant patients) the frequency of painful crises. Unfortunately, this is an extreme form of therapy with the potential for water intoxication and probably would not be applicable except for the most severely affected patients. The most exciting modality in this group, however, is the induction of fetal Hb-F or hemoglobin A in patients with hemoglobinopathies by inserting DNA into their marrow. Studies in animals have been carried out, and this method is being seriously considered as one of the better methods on the horizon (Maugh, 1981).

In the category of agents that would act on the erythrocyte membrane, there are several drugs that inhibit the cell membrane from stiffening so that the cell becomes permanently sickled. Among these, cetiedil, a local anesthetic, zinc acetate, and thioridazine, a tranquilizer, have all been used with good results. Human studies are beginning in this area. Therefore, it is apparent that the near future may hold exciting potential treatment agents for those with sickle hemoglobinopathies. Genetic engineering to induce normal hemoglobin in persons with structurally deficient hemoglobin such as S and C could also be applied to those who produce less hemoglobin A than they should, such as patients with major thalassemia. Inherited disorders that were previously thought to be incurable may at last be eliminated.

Diagnosis

An exciting development in counseling enables restrictive endonucleases, adapted by Kan and coworkers using uncultured amniotic fluid cells during the midtrimester, to detect those infants who would have severe sickle or other major hemoglobinopathies (1978). The advantage of this technique would be obvious for a couple who had the propensity to produce a severely affected offspring. Clearly, then, the choice of continuation of the pregnancy or abortion would be open to the parents. Here again, education and diagnostic testing of the mother and father play very important roles.

SUMMARY

The hemoglobinopathies can drastically affect the mother/fetus/neonate during gestation. Through aggressive prenatal care and current as well as future therapeutic interventions, the risk of sickle cell and other major hemoglobinopathies has been reduced to a much lower level than in the past. Continued progress in this area is expected in the future.

A summary of patient care procedures in the management of hemoglobinopathies is presented in Table 23–23.

REFERENCES

Disseminated Intravascular Coagulation

Abildgaard, C. F.: Recognition and treatment of intravascular coagulation. J. Pediatr. 74:163, 1968.

Bailey, C. D. H., Newman, C., Elinas, S. P., et al.: Use of prostaglandin E$_2$ vaginal suppositories in intrauterine fetal death and missed abortion. Obstet. Gynecol. 45:110, 1975.

Bennett, B., and Ratnoff, O. D.: The normal coagulation mechanism. Med. Clin. North Am., 56:95, 1972.

Bick, R. L., et al.: Disseminated Intravascular Coagulation: Etiology, Pathophysiology, Diagnosis, and Treatment. Medical Counterpoint, October, 1974, p. 38–43.

Cohen, E., and Ballard, C. A.: Consumptive coagulopathy associated with intra-amniotic saline instillation and the effect of intravenous oxytocin. Obstet. Gynecol. 43:300, 1974.

Colman, R. W., Robboy, S. J., and Minna, J. D.: Disseminated intravascular coagulation: an approach. Am. J. Med. 52:679, 1972.

Colman, R. W., Minna, J. D., and Robboy, S. J.: Disseminated intravascular coagulation: a problem in critical-care medicine. Heart Lung 3:789, 1974.

Corrigan, J. J., and Jordan, C. M.: Heparin therapy in septicemia with disseminated intravascular coagulation. N. Engl. J. Med. 283:778, 1970.

Davie, E. W., and Ratnoff, O. D.: Waterfall sequence for intrinsic blood clotting. Science 145:1310, 1964.

Delee, J. B.: A case of fatal hemorrhagic diathesis with premature detachment of the placenta. Am. J. Obstet. 44:45, 1901

Deykin, D.: The clinical challenge of disseminated intravascular coagulation. N. Engl. J. Med. 283:636, 1970.

Gambino, S. R., and Altman, P.: The FDP test. Lab. 79, Jan/Feb, 1979, pp. 34–36.

Gordon, H., and Pipe, N. G. H.: Induction of labor after intrauterine fetal death. A comparison between prostaglandin E$_2$ and oxytocin. Obstet. Gynecol. 45:44, 1975.

Guyton, A. C.: Disseminated intravascular clotting. In Textbook of Med Physiology, 5th ed. Philadelphia, W. B. Saunders Co., 1976, p. 109.

Halmagyi, D. F. J., Starzecki, B., and Shearman, R. P.: Experimental amniotic fluid embolism: mechanism and treatment. Am. J. Obstet. Gynecol., 84:251, 1962.

Kaplan, A. P., Castellino, F. J., Collen, D., et al.: Molecular mechanisms of fibrinolysis in man. Thromb. Hemostasis 39:263, 1978.

Knob, D. R.: Abruptio placentae: an assessment of the time and method of delivery. Obstet. Gynecol. 52:625, 1978.

Laros, R. K., and Penner, J. A.: Pathophysiology of disseminated intravascular coagulation in saline-induced abortion. Obstet. Gynecol. 48:353, 1976.

Lavery, J. P.: When coagulopathy threatens the pregnant patient. Contemp. Obstet. Gynecol. 20:191, 1982.

McGillick, K.: DIC: The deadly paradox. RN 42:41, 1982.

McNichol, G. P., and Davis, J. A.: Fibrinolytic enzymes system. Clin. Haematol. 2:23, 1973.

Moore, M. L.: Realities in Childbearing, 2nd ed. Philadelphia, W. B. Saunders Co., 1983.

O'Brian, B. S., and Woods, S.: The paradox of DIC. Am. J. Nurs. 78:1878, 1978.

Ogston, D.: The protease inhibitors of blood coagulation, fibrinolysis and the complement system. Rec. Adv. Hematol. 2:375, 1977.

Perez, R. H.: Protocols for Perinatal Nursing Practice. St. Louis, C. V. Mosby Co., 1981.

Peterson, E. P., and Taylor, H. B.: Amniotic fluid embolism. An analysis of 40 cases. Obstet. Gynecol., 35:787, 1970.

Phillips, L. L., and Davidson, E. C.: Procoagulant properties of amniotic fluid. Am. J. Obstet. Gynecol. 113:911, 1972.

Pritchard, J. A.: Fetal death in utero. Obstet. Gynecol. 14:573, 1959.

Pritchard, J. A., and Brekken, A. L.: Clinical and laboratory studies on severe abruptio placentae. Am. J. Obstet. Gynecol. 97:681, 1967.

Pritchard, J. A.: Hematologic problems associated with delivery, placental abruption, retained dead fetus and amniotic fluid embolism. Clin. Haematol. 2:563, 1973.

Pritchard, J. A., and MacDonald, P. C.: Williams Obstetrics, 16th ed. New York, Appleton-Century-Crofts, 1980.

Roberts, J. M., and May, J. W.: Consumptive coagulopathy in severe pre-eclampsia. Obstet. Gynecol. 48:163, 1976.

Salzman, F. W., Deykin, D., Shapiro, R. M., et al.: Management of heparin therapy. N. Engl. J. Med. 292:1046, 1975.

Stander, R. W., Flessa, H. C., Gleuck, H. I., et al.: Changes in maternal coagulation factors after intra-amniotic injection of hypertonic saline. Obstet. Gynecol. 27:660, 1971.

Stefanini, M.: Disseminated intravascular coagulation: how to recognize an insidious culprit. Mod. Med. Feb. 1974, pp. 31–39.

Sutton, D. M. C., Houser, R., Kulapongs, P., et al.: Intravascular coagulation in abruptio placentae. Am. J. Obstet. Gynecol. 109:604, 1971.

Talbert, L. M., and Blatt, P. M.: Disseminated intravascular coagulation in obstetrics. Clin. Obstet. Gynecol. 22:889, 1979.

Weiss, A. E., Esterling, W. E., Odom, M. H., et al.: Defibrination syndrome after intra-amniotic infusion of hypertonic saline. Am. J. Obstet. Gynecol. 113:868, 1972.

Wiman, B., and Collen, D.: Molecular mechanism of physiological fibrinolysis. Nature 272:549, 1978.

Yoshikawa, T., Tanaka, K. R., and Guze, L. B.: Infection and disseminated intravascular coagulation. Medicine 50:237, 1971.

Ziegel, E. E.: Disseminated intravascular coagulation. In Ziegel, E. E., and Van Blarcom, C.: Obstetric Nursing, 7th ed. New York, Macmillan, 1979, p. 638.

Idiopathic Thrombocytopenic Purpura

Ahn, Y. S., and Harrington, W. J.: Treatment of idiopathic thrombocytopenic purpura. Ann. Rev. Med. 28:299, 1977.

Abbott Laboratories: The Use of Blood. Chicago, 1971.

Aisner, J.: Platelet transfusion therapy. Med. Clin. North Am. 61:1133, 1977.

American Association of Blood Banks: Blood Component Therapy, 2nd ed. 1975.

Angiulo, J., Temple, J. T., Corrigan, J. J., et al.: Management of cesarean section in a patient with idiopathic thrombocytopenic purpura. Anesthesiology 46:145, 1977.

Ayromlooi, J.: A new approach to the management of idiopathic thrombocytopenic purpura in pregnancy. Am. J. Obstet. Gynecol. 130:235, 1978.

Baele, G., and Thiery, M.: Management of gravidas with idiopathic thrombocytopenic purpura. Am. J. Obstet. Gynecol. 130:248, 1978.

Baldini, M. G.: Idiopathic thrombocytopenic purpura. N. Engl. J. Med. 274:1245, 1302, and 1360, 1966.

Baldini, M. G.: Idiopathic thrombocytopenic purpura and the ITP syndrome. Med. Clin. North Am. 56:47, 1972.

Bierling, P., Farcet, J. P., Duedari, N., et al.: Increased platelet IgG in patient on high dose gammaglobulin for autoimmune thrombocytopenic purpura. Lancet 2:388, 1982.

Branda, R. F., McCullough, J. J., Tate, D. Y., et al.: Plasma exchange in the treatment of fulminant idiopathic (autoimmune) thrombocytopenic purpura. Lancet 1:688, 1978.

Branda, R. F., Moldow, C. F., McCullough, J. J., et al.: Plasma exchange in the treatment of immune disease. Transfusion 15:570, 1975.

Brennan, M. F., Rappeport, J. M., Maloney, W. C., et al.: Correlation between response to corticosteroids and splenectomy for adult idiopathic thrombocytopenic purpura. Am. J. Surg. 129:490, 1975.

Caplan, S. N., and Berkman, E. M.: Immunosuppressive therapy of idiopathic thrombocytopenic purpura. Med. Clin. North Am. 60:971, 1976.

Carloss, H. W., McMillan, R., and Crosby, W. H.: Management of women with immune thrombocytopenic purpura. JAMA 244:2756, 1980.

Carroll, R. R., Noyes, W. D., and Kitchens, C. S.: High-dose intravenous immunoglobulin therapy in patients with immune thrombocytopenic purpura. JAMA 249:1748, 1983.

Cavanagh, D.: Clotting disorders in pregnancy. In Cavanagh, D., and Woods, R. F. (eds.): Obstetric Emergencies, 3rd ed. Philadelphia, J. B. Lippincott, 1982, p. 7.

Chadd, N. A., Elwood, P. P., and Gray, O. P.: Coagulation defects in hypoxic full term newborn infants. Br. Med. J. 4:516, 1971.

Cines, D. B., and Schreiber, A. D.: Immune thrombocytopenia use of Coombs' anti-globulin to detect platelet IgG and C_3. N. Engl. J. Med. 300:106, 1979.

Cines, D. B., Dusak, B., Tomaski, A., et al.: Immune thrombocytopenia in pregnancy. Clin. Res. 29:516A, 1981.

Cines, D. B., Dusak, B., Tomaski, A., et al.: Immune thrombocytopenic purpura and pregnancy. N. Engl. J. Med. 306:826, 1982.

Cruickshank, D. P.: Idiopathic thrombocytopenic purpura. In Quennan, J. T., and Hobbins, J. C. (eds.): Protocols for High Risk Pregnancies. A contemporary Ob/Gyn book. Oradell, NJ, Medical Economics Co. 1982, p. 89.

Dixon, R., Rosse, W., and Ebbert, L.: Quantitative determination of antibody in idiopathic thrombocytopenic purpura. N. Engl. J. Med. 292:230, 1975.

Doan, C. A., Bouroucle, B. A., and Wiseman, B. K.: Idiopathic and secondary thrombocytopenic purpura. Clinical study and evaluation of 381 cases over a period of 28 years. Ann. Intern. Med. 53:861, 1960.

Fainstat, T.: Cortisone-induced congenital cleft palate in rabbits. Endocrinol. 55:502, 1954.

Fallon, W. W., Greene, R. W., and Losner, E. L.: the hemostatic defect in thrombocytopenia as studied by the use of ACTH and cortisone. Am. J. Med. 13:12, 1952.

Fehr, J., Hofmann, V., and Kappeler, V.: Transient reversal of thrombocytopenia in idiopathic thrombocytopenic purpura by high-dose intravenous gammaglobulin. N. Engl. J. Med. 306:1254, 1982.

Flessa, H. C.: Hemorrhagic disorders and pregnancy. Clin. Obstet. Gynecol. 17:236, 1974.

Goldswerg, H., and Chediak, J.: Quantitative and qualitative platelet disorders that complicate pregnancy. J. Reprod. Med. 19:205, 1977.

Goodhue, P. A., and Evans, T.: Idiopathic thrombocytopenic purpura in pregnancy. Obstet. Gynecol. Surv. 18:671, 1963.

Gowda, V. J., Appuzio, J., Langer, A., et al.: Pregnancy complicated by refractory idiopathic thrombocytopenic purpura and diabetes mellitus. J. Reprod. Med. 19:147, 1977.

Handin, R. I., and Stossel, T. P.: Effect of corticosteroid therapy on the phagocytosis of antibody-coated platelets. Blood 46:1016, 1975.

Harker, L. A., and Finch, C. A.: Thrombokinetics in man. J. Clin. Lab. Invest. 48:963, 1969.

Harrington, W. J.: Chronic idiopathic thrombocytopenic purpura. In The Blood Platelets, 1971, p. 264.

Harrington, W. J.: Differential diagnosis and management of thrombocytopenia. Med. Times 99:53, 1971b.

Harrington, W. J., Sprague, C. C., Minnich, V., et al.: Demonstration of a thrombocytopenic factor in the blood of patients with thrombocytopenic purpura. J. Lab. Clin. Med. 38:1, 1951.

Heys, R. F.: Childbearing and idiopathic thrombocytopenic purpura. J. Obstet. Gynecol. Br. Commonw. 73:205, 1966.

Heys, R. F.: Steroid therapy for idiopathic thrombocytopenic purpura during pregnancy. Obstet. Gynecol. 23:532, 1966.

Higby, D. J., Cohen, E., Holland, J. F., et al.: The prophylactic treatment of thrombocytopenic leukemic patients with platelets: a double blind study. Transfusion 14:440, 1974.

Horger, E. O., and Keane, M. W. D.: Platelet disorders in pregnancy. Clin. Obstet. Gynecol. 22:843, 1979.

Imbach, P., Barandum, S., and d'Apuzzo, V.: High dose intravenous gamma globulin for idiopathic thrombocytopenic purpura in childhood. Lancet 1:1228, 1981.

Imbach, P., d'Appuzzo, V., Hirt, A., et al.: High dose intravenous gamma globulin for idiopathic thrombocytopenic purpura in childhood. Lancet 1:1228, 1981.

Jones, W. R.: Tissue-specific autoimmune diseases in pregnancy. Clin. Obstet. Gynecol. 6:473, 1979.

Karpatkin, M., Porges, R. F., and Karpatkin, S.: Platelet counts in infants of women with autoimmune thrombocytopenia: effect of steroid administration to the mother. N. Engl. J. Med. 305:936, 1981.

Karpatkin, S.: Autoimmune thrombocytopenic purpura. Blood 56:329, 1980.

Karpatkin, S., Gang, S. K., and Freedman, M. L.: Role of iron as a regulator of thrombopoiesis. Am. J. Med. 57:521, 1974.

Karpatkin, S., and Lackner, H. L.: Association of anti-platelet antibody with functional platelet disorders: autoimmune thrombocytopenic purpura, systemic lupus erythematosus and thrombopathia. Am. J. Med. 59:599, 1975.

Karpatkin, S., Strick, N., and Suskind, G. W.: Detection of splenic anti-platelet antibody synthesis in idiopathic autoimmune thrombocytopenic purpura. Br. J. Med. 23:167, 1972.

Katz, F. H., and Duncan, B. R.: Entry of prednisone into human breast milk. N. Engl. J. Med. 293:1154, 1975.

Kelemen, E., Szalay, F., and Petefy, M.: Autoimmune (idiopathic) thrombocytopenic purpura in pregnancy and the newborn. Br. J. Obstet. Gynaecol. 85:239, 1978.

Kelton, J. G., Blanchette, V. S., Wilson, W. E., et al.: Neonatal thrombocytopenia due to passive immunization: prenatal diagnosis and distinction between maternal platelet alloantibodies and autoantibodies. N. Engl. J. Med. 302:1401, 1980.

Kelton, J. G., and Gibbons, S.: Autoimmune platelet destruction: idiopathic thrombocytopenic purpura. Semin. Thromb. Hemostas. 8:83, 1982.

Kelton, J. G., Inwood, M. J., Barr, R. M., et al.: The prenatal prediction of thrombocytopenia in infants of mothers with clinically diagnosed immune thrombocytopenia. Am. J. Obstet. Gynecol. 144:449, 1982.

Kelton, J. G., Moore, J., Gaudie, J., et al.: The development and evaluation of a serum assay for platelet bindable IgG (S-PBI IgG). J. Lab. Clin. Med. 98:272, 1981.

Kernoff, L. M., Malan, E., and Gunston, R.: Neonatal thrombocytopenia complicating autoimmune thrombocytopenia in pregnancy: evidence for transplacental passage of anti-platelet antibody. Ann. Intern. Med. 90:55, 1979.

Kitzmiller, J. L.: Autoimmune disorders: maternal, fetal and neonatal risks. Clin. Obstet. Gynecol. 21:385, 1978.

Kohler, P. F., and Farr, R. S.: Elevation of cord over maternal IgG immunoglobulin: evidence for an active placental IgG transport. Nature 210:1070, 1966.

Kornstein, M., Smith, J. R., and Stockman, J. A., III: Idiopathic thrombocytopenic purpura: mother and neonate. Ann. Intern. Med. 92:128, 1980.

Lacey, J. V., and Penner, J. A.: Management of idiopathic thrombocytopenic purpura in the adult. Semin. Thromb. Hemostas. 3:160, 1977.

Laningham, J. E. T.: Platelet transfusion. Bull. Lab. Med. Univ. N. Carolina, 1975, p. 3.

Laros, R. K., and Sweet, R. L.: Management of idiopathic thrombocytopenic purpura during pregnancy. Am. J. Obstet. Gynecol. 122:182, 1975.

Machover-Reinisch, J., Simon, N. G., Karow, W. G., et al.: Prenatal exposure to prednisone in human and animal retards intrauterine growth. Science 202:436, 1978.

Marder, V. J., Nusbacher, J., and Andersen, F. W.: One-year follow-up of plasma exchange therapy in 14 patients with idiopathic thrombocytopenic purpura. Transfusion 21:291, 1981.

McMillan, R.: Chronic idiopathic thrombocytopenic purpura. N. Engl. J. Med. 304:1134, 1981.

McMillan, R.: The pathogenesis of immune thrombocytopenic purpura. CRC Crit. Rev. Clin. Lab. Sci. 8:303, 1977.

McMillan, R.: Platelet-associated IgG: an assay of anti-platelet antibodies in immune thrombocytopenic purpura. Blood 46:1039, 1975.

McMillan, R., Longmire, R. L., Tavassoli, M., et al.: In vitro platelet phagocytosis by splenic leukocytes in idiopathic thrombocytopenic purpura. N. Engl. J. Med. 290:249, 1974.

McMillan, R., Longmire, R., and Yelenosky, R.: The effect of corticosteroids on human IgG synthesis. J. Immunol. 116:1592, 1976.

Minchinton, R. M., Dodd, N. J., O'Brien, H., et al.: Autoimmune thrombocytopenia in pregnancy. Br. J. Haematol. 44:451, 1980.

Morgan, A. D.: An update on the clinical application of blood components. JSC Med. Assoc. 74:532, 1978.

Murray, J. M., and Harris, R. E.: The management of the pregnant patient with idiopathic thrombocytopenic purpura. Am. J. Obstet. Gynecol. 126:449, 1976.

Murray, S., and Gardner, F. H.: Effect of storage temperature on maintenance of platelet viability—deleterious effect of refrigerated storage. N. Engl. J. Med. 280:1094, 1969.

Nelson, W., Vaughan, V., and McKay, R. (eds.): Textbook of Pediatrics, 11th ed. Philadelphia, W. B. Saunders Co., 1979, p. 1416.

Newland, A. C., Treleaven, J. G., Minchinton, R. M., et al.: High-dose intravenous IgG in adults with autoimmune thrombocytopenia. Lancet 1:84, 1983.

Noriega-Guerra, L., Aviles-Miranda, A., de la Cadena, O. A., et al.: Pregnancy in patients with autoimmune thrombocytopenic purpura. Am. J. Obstet. Gynecol. 133:439, 1979.

Novak, R., and Williams, J.: Plasmapheresis in catastrophic complication of idiopathic thrombocytopenic purpura. J. Pediatr. 92:434, 1978.

O'Reilly, R., and Taber, B.: Immunologic thrombocytopenic purpura and pregnancy. Obstet. Gynecol. 51:590, 1978.

Pearson, H. A., and McIntosh, S.: Neonatal thrombocytopenia. Clin. Haematol. 7:111, 1978.

Perkins, R. P.: Thrombocytopenia in obstetric syndromes: a review. Obstet. Gynecol. Surv. 34:101, 1979.

Peterson, O., and Larson, P.: Thrombocytopenic purpura in pregnancy. Obstet. Gynecol. 4:454, 1954.

Pitkin, R. M.: Autoimmune diseases in pregnancy. Semin. Perinatol. 1:161, 1977.

Robson, H. N., and Davidson, L. S. P.: Purpura in pregnancy, with special reference to idiopathic thrombocytopenic purpura. Lancet 2:164, 1950.

Robson, H. N., and Duttie, J. J. R.: Capillary resistance and adrenocortical activity. Br. J. Med. 2:971, 1950.

Rogers, T. E.: Thrombocytopenia in pregnancy following splenectomy. Am. J. Obstet. Gynecol. 78:806, 1959.

Romero, R., and Duffy, T. P.: Platelet disorder in pregnancy. Clin. Perinatol. 7:327, 1980.

Rosse, W. F.: Quantitative immunology of immune hemolytic anemia. II. The relationship of cell-bound antibody to hemolysis and the effect of treatment. J. Clin. Invest. 50:734, 1971.

Schatz, M., Patterson, R., Zeitz, S., et al.: Corticosteroid therapy for the pregnant asthmatic patient. JAMA 233:804, 1975.

Schenker, J. G., and Polishuk, W. Z.: Idiopathic thrombocytopenia in pregnancy. Gynecologia 165:271, 1968.

Schlamoritz, M.: Membrane receptors in the specific transfer of immunoglobulins from mother to young. Immunol. Communications 5:481, 1976.

Schmidt, R. E., Bodde, V., Schafer, G., et al.: High-dose intravenous gammaglobulin for idiopathic thrombocytopenic purpura. Lancet 2:475, 1981.

Schreiber, A. D.: Immunohematology. JAMA 248:1380, 1982.

Schulman, N. R., Marder, V. J., and Weinrack, R. S.: Similarities between known antiplatelet antibodies and the factors responsible for thrombocytopenia in idiopathic purpura: physiologic, serologic and isotopic studies. Ann. NY Acad. Sci. 124:499, 1965.

Scott, J. R.: Fetal growth retardation associated with maternal administration of immunosuppressive drugs. Am. J. Obstet. Gynecol. 128:668, 1977.

Scott, J. R., Cruikshank, D. P., Kochenour, N. K., et al.: Fetal platelet counts in the obstetric management of immunologic thrombocytopenic purpura. Am. J. Obstet. Gynecol. 136:495, 1980.

Scott, J. S.: Immunological diseases in pregnancy. In Scott, J. S., and Jones, W. J. (eds.): Immunology of Human Reproduction. London, Academic Press, 1976, p. 229.

Sitarz, A. L., Driscoll, J. M., Jr., and Wolff, S. A.: Management of isoimmune neonatal thrombocytopenia. Am. J. Obstet. Gynecol. 124:39, 1976.

Smith, M. D., Smith, D. A., and Fletcher, M.: Hemorrhage associated with thrombocytopenia in megaloblastic anemia. Br. Med. J. 1:982, 1962.

Sprague, C. C., Harrington, W. J., Lange, R. D., et al.: Platelet transfusions and the pathogenesis of ITP. JAMA 150:1193, 1952.

Stefanini, M., and Martino, N. B.: Use of prednisone in the management of some hemorrhagic states. N. Engl. J. Med. 254:313, 1956.

Suhrland, L. G., Anguilla, E. R., and Weisberger, A. S.: The effect of prednisone on circulating antibody formulation in animals immunized with human platelet antigen. J. Lab. Clin. Med. 51:724, 1958.

Taft, E. G.: Apheresis in platelet disorders. Plasma Ther. 2:181, 1982.

Taft, E., et al.: Apheresis in platelet disease states. In Kasprisin, D. O., and Vaithianathan, T.: Proceedings of the Second Annual Apheresis symposium. Chicago, 1981, p. 138.

Tancer, M. L.: Idiopathic thrombocytopenic purpura and pregnancy. Am. J. Obstet. Gynecol. 79:148, 1960.

Territo, M., Finklestein, J., Oh, W., et al.: Management of autoimmune thrombocytopenia in pregnancy and in the neonate. Obstet. Gynecol. 41:579, 1973.

Thompson, R. L., Moore, R. A., Hess, C. E., et al.: Idiopathic thrombocytopenic purpura: long-term results of treatment and the prognostic significance of response to corticosteroids. Arch. Intern. Med. 13:730, 1972.

Van Leeuwen, E. F., Kr von dem Borne, A. E. G., Oudesluijs-Murphy, A. M., et al.: Neonatal alloimmune thrombocytopenia complicated by maternal autoimmune thrombocytopenia. Br. Med. J. 281:27, 1980.

Veenhoven, W. A., van der Schans, G. S., and Nieweg, H. O.: Platelet antibodies in idiopathic thrombocytopenic purpura. Clin. Exp. Immunol. 39:645, 1980.

Weir, A. B., III, Poon, M., and McGowan, E. I.: Plasma exchange in idiopathic thrombocytopenic purpura. Arch. Intern. Med. 140:1101, 1980.

Wintrobe, M. M.: Clinical Hematology, 7th ed. Philadelphia, Lea & Febiger, 1974, p. 1071.

Zwaan, F. E., deKoning, J., and Eernisse, J. G.: Idiopathic thrombocytopenic purpura. Neth. J. Med. 17:140, 1974.

Hemoglobinopathies

Charache, S., Scott, J., Niebyl, J., et al.: Management of sickle cell disease in pregnant patients. Am. J. Obstet. Gynecol. 55:407, 1980.

Cunningham, F. G., Pritchard, J. A., Mason, R., et al.: Prophylactic transfusion of normal red blood cells during pregnancy complicated by sickle cell hemoglobinopathy. Am. J. Obstet. Gynecol., 135:994, 1979.

Desforges, J. E., and Warth, J.: The management of sickle cell disease in pregnancy. Clin. Perinatol. 1:385, 1974.

Fort, A. T., Morrison, J. C., Berreras, L., et al.: Counseling the patient with sickle cell disease about reproduction: pregnancy outcome does not justify the maternal risk. Am. J. Obstet. Gynecol. 11:324, 1971.

Foster, H. W.: Managing sickle cell anemia in pregnant patients. Contemp. Obstet. Gynecol. 16:21, 1980.

Freeman, M. G., and Ruth, G. J.: SS disease and CC disease: obstetric considerations and treatment. Clin. Obstet. Gynecol. 12:134, 1969.

Kan, Y. W., and Dozy, A. M.: Antenatal diagnosis of sickle cell anemia by DNA analysis of amniotic fluid cells. Lancet 2:910, 1978.

Keeling, M. M., Lavery, J. P., Clemons, A. U., et al.: Red cell exchange in the pregnancy complicated by a major hemoglobinopathy. Am. J. Obstet. Gynecol. 138:185, 1980.

Key, T. C., Horger, E. O., Walker, E. M., et al.: Automated erythrocytopheresis for sickle cell anemia during pregnancy. Am. J. Obstet. Gynecol. 138:731, 1980.

Klotz, I. M., Haney, D. N., and King, L. C.: Rational approaches to chemotherapy: antisickling agents. Science, 213:724, 1981.

Kramer, M. S, Rooks, Y., Johnston, D., et al.: Accuracy of cord blood screening for sickle hemoglobinopathies. JAMA 241:139, 1979.

Martin, J. N., Jr., and Morrison, J. C.: Sickle cell crisis: recognizing it and treating it. Contemp. Obstet. Gynecol. 20:171, 1982.

Maugh, T. H.: Sickle cell (II): many agents near trials. Science 211:468, 1981.

Moore, M. L.: Realities in Childbearing, 2nd ed. Philadelphia, W. B. Saunders Co., 1983.

Morrison, J. C.: Anemia associated with pregnancy. In Sciarra, J. J. (ed.): Gynecology and Obstetrics, Vol. 3. New York, Harper & Row, 1981, pp. 1–38.

Morrison, J. C.: Hemoglobinopathies and pregnancy. Clin. Obstet. Gynecol. 22:819, 1979.

Morrison, J. C., Douvas, S. G., Martin, J. N., et al.: Methods of exchange transfusion in pregnant patients with sickle hemoglobinopathies. Obstet. Gynecol. In press.

Morrison, J. C., Propst, M. G., and Blake, P. G.: Sickle hemoglobin and the gravid patient: a management controversy. Clin. Perinatol. 7:273, 1980a.

Morrison, J. C., Schneider, J. M., Whybrew, W. D., et al.: Prophylactic transfusions in pregnant patients with sickle hemoglobinopathies: Benefit versus risk. Obstet. Gynecol. 56:274, 1980b.

Morrison, J. C., and Wiser, W. L.: The use of prophylactic partial exchange transfusion in pregnancies associated with sickle cell hemoglobinopathies. Obstet. Gynecol. 48:516, 1976.

Perkins, R. P.: Inherited disorders of hemoglobin synthesis and pregnancy. Am. J. Obstet. Gynecol. 111:120, 1971.

24

ADDITIONAL MEDICAL COMPLICATIONS IN PREGNANCY

CHARLES J. INGARDIA

Pregnancy causes or aggravates many medical conditions in addition to those presented in the preceding chapters. Some of its effects can be minor; others may cause major difficulties for the parturient. Some of the more frequently observed medical complications are presented in this chapter.

Rh Isoimmunization

Rh ANTIGEN AND SENSITIZATION

Although the actual structure of the Rh antigen is still unclear, unlike the A and B antigens, its presence is confined to the surface of red blood cells (RBCs). The genetic locus for the Rh antigen is on the short arm of chromosome number 1, but the actual number of genes controlling Rh expressivity as well as the number of Rh antigens is unclear. There have been several systems proposed for their nomenclature, the Fischer-Race concept being the most popular. In this model there are three closely linked genes and their alleles controlling antigenic variation (Dd, Cc, Ee) (Race, 1948).

In this concept, all alleles (except for "d") have a corresponding distinct cell surface antigen. The frequency of distribution of these antigens varies, with geographic and racial differences noted. CeDe, CDe, and cde are the most common antigenic arrangements and are present in 35, 20, and 16 percent of the population, respectively. The presence of D determines Rh positivity, whether in a homozygous or heterozygous

individual. Each of the other Rh antigens is capable of engendering a specific antibody reaction (i.e., anti-e), but multiple antibody reactions can be seen, particularly if anti-D is present.

An Rh-negative individual is at risk when exposed to Rh-positive RBCs. Two major determinants affect the risk of sensitization: the volume of Rh-positive cells transfused (i.e., transplacental hemorrhage) and the ABO compatibility status of mother and infant. As little as 0.1 to 0.25 ml of Rh-positive blood can engender an immune response.

Following exposure to Rh-positive antigen, an initial response of primarily IgM (saline reacting) is followed by an IgG antibody (albumin reacting) response. The IgG antibody produced is of the IgG_1 and IgG_3 subclasses. Immune suppression appears to be effective until the appearance of the IgG response. A secondary immune response can be elicited with a very small transplacental hemorrhage (0.1 ml) (Bowman, 1978).

By 6 months up to 8 percent of exposed Rh-negative individuals will have a detectable antibody response. In another 8 to 10 percent, however, the antibody response may only be detectable in subsequent pregnancy when the fetus is Rh-positive. The overall risk then of an ABO compatible pregnancy of Rh immunization following delivery is approximately 16 to 17 percent.

Tests to Detect Transplacental Hemorrhage

Acid Elution (Kleihauer-Betke) Test. Fetal red cells are detected by adding an acid

472

buffer, which causes adult hemoglobin (HbA) to leave the RBC membrane, leaving "ghost" cells. Fetal hemoglobin (HgF), however, is resistant to this acid elution and remains intact. Fetal red cells then can be distinguished from maternal RBCs on smear (Fig. 24–1).

Although fetal hemoglobin can almost always be assumed to be from RBCs, persistent *hemoglobin F* exists in about 2 percent of the population and has been associated with a false-positive acid elution test in a patient transfused with blood from such an individual.

The fetomaternal bleed can be calculated using the following formula:

$$\frac{\dfrac{\text{number of fetal RBCs}}{\text{number of maternal RBCs}} \times (\text{ml FMH})}{\text{estimated maternal blood volume (ml)}} =$$

Other Tests. Other tests that can be utilized to detect fetal/maternal hemorrhage (FMH) are Fetaldex test, alpha fetoprotein test, microscopic Du test, Rho-gam cross match test, and enzyme-linked antiglobulin test (ELAT).

ABO Incompatibility

The presence of ABO-incompatible blood decreases the risks of sensitization probably owing to removal of fetal RBCs from maternal circulation at a faster rate or to sequestration of fetal RBCs at a site in the maternal reticuloendothelial system (e.g., liver) where recognition lymphocytes are scarce. Both anti-A and anti-B are complement fixing;

therefore, intravascular hemolysis of fetal red cells occurs with destruction of the Rh antigen.

It has been demonstrated by Bowman (1978) that the risk of Rh sensitization with ABO incompatibility between mother and infant is about 2 percent. In ABO-compatible pregnancies the risk is 16 to 17 percent. Other influences of sensitization are paternal genotype (homozygous or heterozygous) and fetal genotype (Rh antigenic position affects antigenicity).

ERYTHROBLASTOSIS FETALIS

Pathogenesis

The basic pathogenetic process in erythroblastosis fetalis (EBF) is the destruction of fetal Rh-positive erythrocytes by maternal anti-D (IgG) antibody. The mechanism of hemolysis is not completely understood. It is known that anti-D (mostly IgG_1 and IgG_3) can activate the complement cascade but cannot fix complement; therefore, direct erythrolytic activity is unlikely. Most IgG-tagged red cells are hemolyzed through the extravascular phagocytic system in the spleen.

The resultant fetal anemia leads to an increased production of erythropoietin and eventual extramedullary erythropoiesis in the liver and spleen, resulting in enlargement of these organs. Immature red cell erythroblasts are released into circulation. Further progression leads to extensive erythropoiesis with enlargement and distortion of liver parenchyma. Although it was once be-

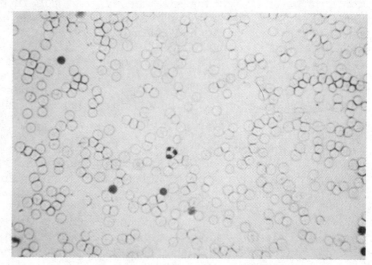

Figure 24–1. Acid elution smear depicting fetal RBCs and maternal "ghost" RBCs. (From Scott, J. R., and Warenski, J. C.: Tests to detect and quantitate fetomaternal bleeding. Clin. Obstet. Gynecol. 25:279, 1982.)

lieved that myocardial failure was primarily related to the anasarca and ascites associated with EBF, it is more likely the result of increased portal hypertension due to hepatosplenomegaly. Fetal edema is further complicated by fetal hypoproteinemia due to decreased hepatic protein synthetic function. This increased portal hypertension is probably also related to the increase in placental edema and hypertrophy (placentomegaly) characteristic of the disease. The placental enlargement probably alters the flow of oxygen and nutrients across the placental bed and, along with the significant anemia, places the fetus at risk for hypoxia and fetal demise.

Ultrasound Detection

Sonographic analysis of sensitized pregnancies, although not as sensitive as spectrophotometric analysis of amniotic fluid bilirubin, is a helpful adjunct to detect signs of erythroblastosis. Ultrasonographic changes consistent with hydrops fetalis include polyhydramnios, placental enlargement, fetal hepatosplenomegaly, umbilical vein dilation, fetal ascites, fetal scalp edema, and fetal cardiomegaly.

Antibody Detection

Antibodies can be detected in several ways.

Saline Agglutination. If Rh-positive RBCs are suspended in isotonic saline they will not agglutinate if anti-D is added to the solution. The RBC membranes lie relatively too far to be bridged by the IgG antibody (160,000 mw). IgM, however, can bridge this gap owing to its larger molecular size (900,000 mw). The absence of agglutination in saline, then, cannot rule out significant anti-D (IgG) production.

Albumin Agglutination. With the addition of a 22 percent bovine albumin solution, the RBC membranes are aligned closer and subsequently agglutinate and/or hemolyze when anti-D (IgG) or anti-D (IgM) is added. The presence of a negative saline agglutination and a positive albumin agglutination indicates an anti-D (IgG) response.

Antiglobulin Testing (Indirect Coombs'). The introduction of anti-human globulin (produced by rabbits, goats, and so on) to a suspension of known washed Rh-positive RBCs mixed with the patient's serum, which has anti-D antibody, will agglutinate those RBCs (positive indirect Coombs'). This indirect method for testing for RBC antibody is very sensitive. Other techniques include enzyme-treated RBCs and autoanalyzer analysis.

Evaluation and Management

Use of Titers. The Rh-negative patient who is identified by initial prenatal laboratory analysis should have an associated antibody screen test performed to rule out the presence of anti-D antibody. Even if the antibody screen is initially negative, it must be repeated at 24, 28, 32, and 36 weeks, because in one half of sensitized women the antibody cannot be detected until subsequent pregnancy. Negative titers at these weeks warrant no further investigation.

Queenan (1977) and Bowman (1981), in reviewing the relationship between antibody titers and perinatal outcome, found a relationship between titers and outcome only if pregnancy represented the "first immunized pregnancy," i.e., one characterized by a negative antibody titer at the initial visit with subsequent detection of anti-D antibody. Previous history should be negative for stillbirths or previous infants that required exchange transfusion. In Bowman's experience with titers of less than 1:8 (Queenan <1.32), no intrauterine death has occurred. These patients are not followed by serial amniocentesis but rather have serial antibody titers done every 3 to 4 weeks. If a rise over this critical titer occurs, spectrophotometric analysis of amniotic fluid bilirubin is performed.

If the patient has anti-D antibody on initial screen or has a previously affected infant, titers alone are not predictive of outcome. An important point to remember is that each laboratory must determine its own "critical titer." With the general decline in Rh immunization, some authors conclude it is impossible for most laboratories to develop their own "critical titer." Even in the first Rh-isoimmunized pregnancy the presence of an Rh-positive fetus can be associated with severe involvement in up to 20 percent of cases.

At the present time, then, it is clear that spectrophotometric analysis of amniotic fluid for bilirubin pigment remains the most important index of severity of fetal hemolytic involvement.

Spectrophotometric Analysis. This technique was pioneered by Liley and is based on the measurement of the deviation, or "peak," produced by bilirubin pigment in amniotic fluid at 450 mu on the spectra absorption curve. The values are plotted on semilogarithmic paper with wave length as the linear horizontal coordinate and optical density as the vertical coordinate (see Fig. 24–2).

Timing of the initial analysis can be based on both previous pregnancy history and serial antibody titers. With previous severely affected neonates or stillbirths, the initial analysis may be performed as early as 22 to 24 weeks. A sudden increase in titer level over previous values may also indicate an earlier analysis. With the typical presentation of a patient with no previously affected children but with a significant, but stable, anti-D titer, the initial amniocentesis is performed at 28 weeks. Subsequent analyses are gauged by the result of spectrophotometric examination and usually range from 1 to 3 weeks but may be repeated as early as 5 days following the previous amniocentesis. Declining trends allow for spacing every 3 weeks. This spacing allows for the bilirubin trend to be clearly revealed and removes the likelihood that spectrophotometric distortion has occurred because of an amniotic fluid blood contamination from the previous tap. Sources of error in interpretation include:

- Blood (peak 415 mu)
- Meconium (peak at 410 to 415 mu)
- Polyhydramnios (fall in Δ OD 450 values)
- Light (reduction in Δ OD 450 values)
- Congenital anomalies (elevation of values)

Liley's "zone" method. In 1961, Liley (1961) reported on a method of amniotic fluid spectrophotometric analysis that offered ongoing evaluation of fetal hemolysis utilizing bilirubin absorption curves plotted against gestational age. Liley demonstrated in over 100 cases that the trend in normal pregnancy is declining levels toward term. He subdivided these trends into three prediction zones (Fig. 24–2). Declining levels into zone 1 heralded no in utero mortality and generally little fetal involvement. Increasing trends into zone III indicated an ominous prognosis with severe hydrops fetalis or fetal death in 7 to 10 days. Zone II values needed to be followed closely to determine whether they would move into zones I or III. The zone boundaries decline with advancing gestation. The significance of a normal trend is that values that are initially in high zone II but plateau on serial examination will move into zone III with advancing gestational age. With regard to singular values, extremely high (> 0.28 to 0.30) or extremely low (< 0.02) values may be helpful in predicting outcome, but only after sequential sampling do trends emerge that more adequately anticipate fetal/neonatal status.

Three basic trends emerge in serial evaluation. Rising values into zone III or the upper 20 percent of zone II indicate significant fetal involvement and the need for intervention. With significant prematurity (< 30 weeks), this intervention should be intrauterine transfusion. Once evidence of pulmonary lung maturity is obtained, delivery

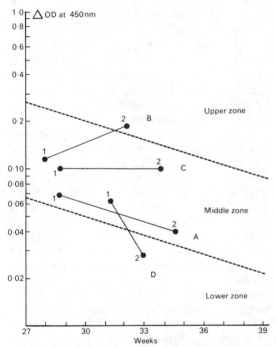

Figure 24–2. Liley's prediction zones. *A,* Usual reduction in Δ OD 450 results with advancing gestational age. *B,* Upward trend indicating severe hemolytic involvement. *C,* Plateauing of Δ OD 450 results, indicating need to intervene because the normal fall with gestational age is not seen—indicates moderate to severe involvement. *D,* Steeply falling values indicate unaffected or mildly affected neonate. (From Whitfield, C. R.: Amniotic fluid analysis. *In* Beard, R. W., and Nathanielsz, P. W. [eds.]: Fetal Physiology and Medicine. London, W. B. Saunders Co. Ltd., 1976. p.333.)

should be accomplished. Plateauing values can be watched without intervention with serial analysis unless they enter zone III or upper zone II; treatment is similar to that used for rising values. Declining values can be watched until term with serial analysis. A recent review suggests that all patients with evidence of anti-D production be delivered by 38 weeks, since some morbidity can occur even with very low Δ OD 450 values.

Whitfield's "action line" method. Whitfield and coworkers (1968), in their analysis of 641 spectrophotometric values during a 3-year period, proposed a curve "action line," which delineated at any one point in gestation when intervention is mandatory (Fig. 24–3). In general, the action line follows Liley's zone III and zone II border until about 34 weeks, when it drops into zone II range. If the Δ OD 450 remains less than 0.035 the pregnancy is allowed to continue until term.

In Whitfield's original series, intrauterine transfusion was performed if the action line was crossed (or extrapolated to be crossed) at less than 33 weeks gestational age. Beyond 33 weeks, delivery was accomplished when the action line was crossed.

Intrauterine Transfusion. Since Liley introduced the technique of intrauterine transfu-

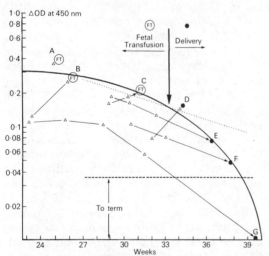

Figure 24–3. Whitfield's "action line." When Δ OD 450 results cross or are extrapolated to be crossed, intervention is mandatory. If this crossing occurs at less than 33 weeks, fetal intrauterine transfusion (FIT) is performed. If over 34 weeks, delivery is indicated. The horizontal broken line indicates initial Δ OD 450 value of 0.035 mu (no serial amniocentesis is performed). (From Whitfield, C. R.: Amniotic fluid analysis. *In* Beard, R. W., and Nathanielsz, P. W. [eds.]: Fetal Physiology and Medicine. London, W. B. Saunders Co. Ltd., 1976, p. 334.)

sion (IUT) in 1963, many refinements have been proposed to reduce the risks involved. The goal of IUT is the deposition of unsensitized (Rh-negative) packed RBCs into the fetal peritoneal cavity. There, they are taken up by the subdiaphragmatic lymphatics and eventually deposited into the intravascular compartment. These unsensitized RBCs help correct severe fetal anemia and help to postpone the onset of hydropic changes associated with poor prognosis.

Blood to be utilized for the transfusion should be fresh (< 24 hours old) buffy coat–poor, packed O-negative RBCs. The use of O blood (with no A or B antigen) eliminates the possibility of intravascular hemolysis from the presence of fetal antibody (anti-A or anti-B) against these antigens. Absorption of RBCs, in the absence of significant ascites, is about 12 percent of transfused RBCs/day.

Several variations in IUT technique have appeared over the years. Fetal radiographic exposure has for the most part been discontinued in favor of B mode or real time scanning. IUTs should be performed by experienced clinicians in a tertiary care center. Important points in technique follow.

1. Preliminary ultrasound should be performed to assess fetal position and presentation, placental localization and size, and umbilical cord location. The fetus can also be evaluated for evidence of fetal ascites or other hydropic changes.

2. After skin prep, a 16-gauge Touhy needle is entered into the fetal abdominal cavity at an angle under real time ultrasound, and a small amount of radiographic contrast medium is injected into a threaded catheter. If the medium does not seem to disperse freely around the bowel gas pattern or the "stream" or bubbles from the catheter and cannot be visualized with ultrasound, an x-ray may be taken to help determine dispersion.

3. The amount of blood to be transfused can be calculated by the following formula: number of weeks gestational age − 20 × 10 = ml packed RBCs to be transfused.

4. The transfusion begins at a rate of 5 to 10 cc/min. A sudden increase in intraperitoneal pressure could lead to a cessation of umbilical blood flow and fetal death. The fetal heart rate is monitored continuously via real time ultrasound or Doppler.

5. Repeat transfusion is planned on an average of 10 days in the fetus less than 30 weeks, with subsequent intervals of 4 weeks.

Maternal risks, theoretical and real, associated with the procedure are rare but include local abdominal infection and inadvertent placental injury that leads to consumptive coagulopathy or premature ruptured membranes with resultant chorioamnionitis.

Fetal risks are not uncommon and may range from minor fetal function to fetal demise. Risks to the fetus may be characterized as early and late. Early complications include extraperitoneal placement of the catheter (i.e., spine, thoracic cavity, and so on), fetal/placental vessel laceration, and fetal puncture injury. The risks are greatly increased with an anterior placenta. In earlier reports, mortality rates from the procedure ranged from 6 to 24 percent (Queenan, 1969), but more recent data suggest a mortality rate of 3 to 9 percent (Bowman and Manning, 1983). Later fetal complications include a possible graft versus host reaction because of the lymphocytes in transfused blood.

Subsequent survival rates of the fetus that has undergone IUT depend on the gestational age and hydropic condition of the fetus at transfusion. With early gestations (< 26 weeks) and/or hydropic changes, the survival rate drops. It appears that the affected fetus that survives IUT is not at added risk for delayed mental or physical development compared with a controlled population (White et al., 1978).

SUPPLEMENTAL ANTEPARTUM TESTING IN Rh ISOIMMUNIZATION

NST/OCT

Routine antepartum fetal heart rate monitoring should be performed from 32 weeks until delivery in the Rh-sensitized pregnant patient. The frequency of testing should be based in part on the degree of fetal involvement suspected by Δ OD 450 analysis. A nonstress test (NST) should be performed twice a week when values place the fetus in upper zone II or zone III or if there is a rising trend in values. With declining levels the NST may be performed weekly. All nonreactive NSTs should be followed by an oxytocin challenge test (OCT).

The presence of a sawtooth or sinusoidal fetal heart rate pattern (Fig. 24–4) has been described in the fetus with erythroblastosis (Baskett and Koh, 1974). It has also been reported with fetal acidosis, alphaprodine administration, and acute fetal anemias (Modanlou et al., 1977; Grey et al., 1978). The presence of a persistent sinusoidal fetal heart rate pattern in an Rh-sensitized pregnancy

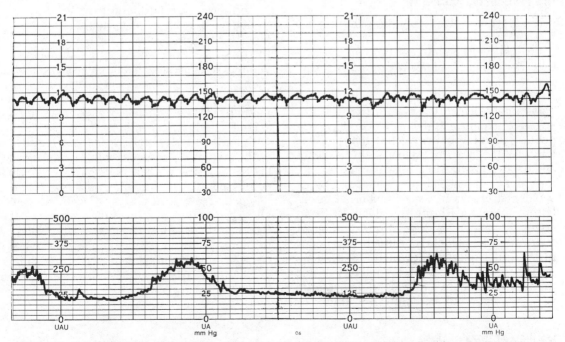

Figure 24–4. Sinusoidal heart rate pattern. (From Veren, D., Boehm, F. H., and Killam, A. P.: The clinical significance of sinusoidal fetal heart rate pattern associated with alphaprodine administration. J. Reprod. Med. 27:412, 1982.)

indicates significant anemia and mandatory intervention.

Estriol Determination

The determination of plasma or urinary estriol levels in the Rh-immunized patient is of little value. The placental hypertrophy associated with this condition and its associated elevated estriol production lead to a false sense of reassurance, even in the face of impending fetal demise.

Ultrasound—Dynamic Testing (Biophysical Assessment)

The recently introduced modality of dynamic fetal evaluation can help in the assessment of fetal status. By assessing fetal breathing movements, body tones and flexion, amniotic fluid production, and fetal movements, a composite "picture" of fetal status can be obtained. Although these parameters have not been extensively studied in regard to the isoimmunized pregnancy, they will probably prove invaluable in the ongoing evaluation in these patients.

Rh-IMMUNE GLOBULIN (RhIg) IN TREATMENT OF Rh ISOIMMUNIZATION

The Remaining Problems

It has become clear that although RhIg has reduced sensitization, certain problems remain that have prevented its total elimination. The major problems of underutilization and inadequate dosage still need to be corrected. Another still unproven theory, the "grandmother theory," asserts that the Rh-negative female infant is sensitized by Rh-positive blood from her mother at birth (Taylor, 1967). More important is the issue of antenatal sensitization that occurs during the course of normal pregnancy owing to accidental breaks in the fetomaternal circulation, allowing Rh-positive fetal RBCs to enter the maternal circulation. The great majority (> 95 percent) of these breaks occur in the last trimester (Bowman, 1978). This transplacental leak prior to delivery is for the most part silent and goes undetected by the usual means of acid elution testing.

Routine Antenatal Use

If accidental breaks in placental circulation occur regularly, with the antenatal transfusion of fetal RBCs accounting for up to 2 percent of cases of Rh sensitization, then routine antenatal administration of RhIg prior to the third trimester can eliminate this problem. A clinical trial of antenatal RhIg prophylaxis in Canada (300 mcg at 28 and 34 weeks' gestation) (Bowman, 1978) was followed by a trial of only one dose (300 mcg at 28 weeks), with equal efficacy (Bowman, 1978). If at delivery the infant is found to be Rh-positive, another injection is given. It is apparent that RhIg reduces the incidence of antenatal sensitization by 93 percent.

Du Variant

About 3 to 5 percent of Rh-negative mothers are Du-positive (variant). Because the Du factor represents an incomplete D antigen, its antigenicity and ability to produce anti-D are also variable. Hemolytic disease of the newborn has been reported in a Du variant infant born to an Rh-sensitized Rh-negative mother (Lacey, 1978). Conversely, an Rh-negative, Du-positive, Coombs-negative mother who delivers an Rh-positive fetus does run the risk, albeit small, for full anti-D sensitization and antibody production (Hill et al., 1974).

Another problem that may arise is the detection of the Du factor. In the postpartum period, enough fetal blood from an Rh-positive fetus may enter maternal circulation to modify the interpretation of her Rh status. In these circumstances, the Rh-negative woman with a large fetal/maternal hemorrhage from an Rh-positive fetus will be inaccurately classified as Du-positive. If these mothers are then mistakenly assumed to be "genetically" Du-positive, RhIg is often withheld. Unfortunately, it is these mothers with the large transplacental hemorrhage (TPH) who are at even higher risk of being sensitized. These problems could be eliminated by routine administration of RhIg to all Rh-negative, Du-positive mothers or those mothers found to be only Du-positive in the postpartum period. In mothers found to be Du-positive after delivery, the volume of fetal-maternal bleeding should be determined.

Atypical Antibodies

With the development of prophylactic immune globulin, the incidence of hemolytic disease of the newborn (HDN) has declined

Table 24–1. Atypical Antibodies Associated With Moderate To Severe HDN

Kelly (k)	Public Antigens
Duffy (Fyᵃ)	Ytᵃ
Kidd (Jkᵃ, Jkᵇ)	ENᵃ
MNSₛ	Coᵃ
Diego (Diᵃ, Diᵇ)	Private Antigens
P	Biles
	Good
	Heibel
	Radin
	Wrightᵃ
	Zd

dramatically. Although 98 percent of all HDN is related to the Rh antigen, approximately 2 percent is due to antibody produced by other blood group antigens, the so-called irregular or atypical antibodies. Sources of sensitization are similar to those of the Rh antigen (i.e., fetal blood and/or transfused blood). It is clear that not all atypical antibodies are capable of producing HDN, either because of the nature of the immunoglobulins (IgM versus IgG) that may prevent transplacental transfer or because the antibodies have no effect on RBC integrity, sequestration, or clearance. Other antibodies can produce HDN⁻ similar in appearance to Rh hemolytic disease, and amniotic fluid studies need to be performed (Weinstein, 1976).

The finding of an atypical antibody indicates the need for analysis of paternal blood. If the father is antigen-negative, no further analysis is performed. If he is positive for the antigen in question, the management scheme proposed by Weinstein should be followed (1976). A partial list of common atypical antibodies that can lead to HDN is seen in Table 24–1.

Table 24–2. General RhIg Dosage Guidelines for Obstetric Conditions

Condition	Dosage (mcg)
Spontaneous vaginal delivery	300
Cesarean section	300
Cesarean section with hemorrhage*	
Abortion	
< 12 weeks	50
> 12 weeks	300
Ectopic pregnancy	50
Transfusion mix	20 (per ml packed RBCs)
match†	10 (per ml whole blood)
Amniocentesis†	300

*Need Kleihauer-Betke test to determine dosage.
†Need Kleihauer-Betke test if blood amniocentesis of anterior placenta.

Clinical Use

To be effective in preventing Rh isoimmunization, RhIg must be given in sufficient amounts to compensate for the extent of antigen (Rh-positive fetal RBCs) exposure. Presently, RhIg is available in 300- (Rhogam) and 50-mcg doses (Mic-Rhogam). Greater than expected fetal-maternal hemorrhage can be associated with abruption, cesarean section, manual exploration, and so on, and these situations warrant an acid elution (Kleihauer-Betke) or ELAT test to determine the amount of fetal-maternal hemorrhage. No delay in the administration of RhIg should be tolerated after delivery of an Rh-positive infant to an Rh-negative Coombs' mother. General dosage guidelines for the usual obstetric conditions are listed in Table 24–2.

OTHER MODALITIES OF TREATMENT

Other methods in the treatment of Rh isoimmunization include plasmapheresis, oral desensitization, and the use of immunosuppressive drugs such as steroids and promethazine hydrochloride.

DELIVERY CONSIDERATIONS

Once the decision is made to deliver the isoimmunized patient, the choice of delivery method and labor conduction should be based on the usual obstetric indications with very few modifications. Vaginal delivery should be conducted with direct fetal heart rate monitoring and utilization of fetal scalp sampling when worrisome fetal heart rate patterns exist. The association of polyhydramnios with isoimmunization can lead to uterine overdistention, abruption, and occasional desultory labor patterns. With an unfavorable cervix, where internal monitoring is not possible from the onset, or with significant fetal distress and/or fetal malpresentation, primary cesarean section is indicated. Care of the isoimmunized patient is summarized in Table 24–3.

Cardiopulmonary Complications

ASTHMA

Bronchial asthma complicates approximately 0.5 to 1 percent of all pregnancies.

Table 24-3. Patient Care Summary for Rh Isoimmunization*

	Antepartum		Intrapartum	Postpartum
	Outpatient	*Inpatient*		
BP, P, R	Each visit	q 8 hr (if normal, BP may be deleted during the night)	q 1 hr	On admission to RR: q 15 min × 4; then q 30 min × 2; then q 1 hr until stable On postpartum floor: q 4 hr
T	Same as above	Same as above	q 4 hr	Same as above
FHR	Weekly NST/CST starting at 32 wks	Weekly NST/CST starting at 32 wks	Continuous electronic fetal monitoring, preferably internal; if no monitor available, q 15 min in 1st stage and q 5 min in 2nd stage	—
Contractions	Each visit	q shift	Continuous electronic fetal monitoring, preferably internal; if no monitor available, q 1 hr by palpation	Same as BP, P, R Lochia same as above
Laboratory studies				
RH titers	24, 28, 32, and 36 weeks	24, 28, 32, and 36 weeks	—	—
Amniocentesis	Performed at any maternal titer or "critical titer" as established by your lab		—	—
Sonograms	At 24 weeks (dating ultrasound plus R/O hydropic changes); then q 3–4 wks to detect early hydropic changes			
Rho-gam administration	—	—	—	Given within 72 hr after delivery to Rh-neg mothers with Rh-pos babies

*Nurse–patient ratio: *Antepartum,* 1:6 to 8; *intrapartum with fetal distress,* 1:1; *intrapartum without fetal distress,* 2:3; *postpartum,* 1:6 to 8.

The disease may present as episodic attacks of various degrees of severity or may be more chronic in nature with persistent dyspnea. Bronchoconstriction is the basic pathophysiologic mechanism, although this "hyperactivity" may be triggered by a number of antigenic stimuli that lead to release of chemical mediators (histamine, kinins, slow reactivity substance (SRS), and 5-hydroxy tryptamine). Prostaglandins and beta adrenergic receptors also play a role in mediating bronchospasm.

Arterial hypoxemia, occasionally severe, results from ventilation perfusion inequity. This is due to varying degrees of airway obstruction produced by bronchoconstriction, bronchial edema, and/or bronchial mucus plugging. Decreased CO_2 is a major deflection of the disease severity and an important management guideline. Although decreased arterial pCO_2 is most commonly observed pCO_2 may be elevated because of hypoventilation. Carbon dioxide retention (increased pCO_2) occurs in approximately 15 to 20 percent of patients with severe disease, and when renal bicarbonate concentration is not adequate, respiratory acidosis ensues. Death due to asthma is a result of "asphyxiation." Pathologically, widespread mucous impactions and distentions of bronchioles, which are approximately 5 ml wide, are found throughout the lungs. The importance of mucous stagnation must be remembered, particularly in the context of management.

Effect of Pregnancy on the Course of Asthma

One might expect that, owing to the increase in plasma cortisol, prednisone, and histaminase in normal pregnancy, some predictable clinical improvement in most asthmatic patients should occur, particularly during the first trimester. However, clinical observations of pregnant asthmatic patients have not demonstrated any consistent ameliorative effect. Asthma in pregnant patients may remain stable, may worsen, or may improve. In a study by Gluck and Gluck (1976), the authors followed 47 pregnant asthmatics through delivery. Compared with their prepregnant asthmatic state, 20 patients became worse (43 percent), 20 patients were the same (43 percent), and 7 patients improved (14 percent). These changes were examined in relation to severity of their preconceptual asthma. In the mild group 12 percent improved, 72 percent were unchanged, and 16 percent became worse. In the moderate group, 40 percent improved, 60 percent became worse, and there were three admissions for asthma conditions. Finally, in the severe group, no patients improved, 17 percent were unchanged, and 83 percent became worse, with nine hospitalizations for asthma. The authors felt that the severity of asthma before pregnancy definitely correlated with the response of asthma in pregnancy; patients with mild asthma were generally unchanged, whereas those with severe asthma were usually worse (Gluck and Gluck, 1976).

A common problem in evaluating the response of asthma in pregnancy is the fact that in normal nonasthmatic pregnancies there can be breathing difficulties and orthopnea. Hence the appearance of these symptoms during pregnancy, particularly in the last trimester, does not necessarily indicate the presence of asthma or its worsening.

It has been shown by most authorities that worsening of the asthmatic condition during pregnancy never occurs before the 4th month of gestation and that the majority occur in the 6th or 7th month. It was also noted by Gluck and Gluck (1976) that rising or stable IgE levels (normally decreased in pregnancy) in pregnant asthmatic patients prognosticated worsening of the disease during the pregnancy. The severe asthmatic is at the highest degree of deterioration during the second half of her pregnancy, and one can anticipate improvement after delivery. Likewise, patients who had improvement of their asthma during pregnancy noted it primarily during the 1st trimester. In a large study by Schaffer and Silverman (1961), there was no improvement in asthmatic patients after the 16th week of pregnancy.

Effect of Asthma on the Pregnant Woman, the Fetus, and the Neonate

Severe asthma may severely affect pregnancy. A study by Gordon and colleagues (1970) reviewed 277 patients under active treatment for asthma in which 16 were classified as severe asthmatics. Those 16 women with severe asthma had the highest perinatal mortality and morbidity, with an incidence of 35 percent low birth weight infants and 12.5 percent neurologically abnormal infants at 1 year of age. There were also four deaths among the women with severe asthma. However, with mild to moderate disease, asthma had little effect on pregnancy outcome. In a review of 293 pregnant patients with asthma by Schaffer and Silverman (1961), the spontaneous abortion rate and prematurity rate did not exceed those of their normal controls.

The issue of desensitization during pregnancy has been raised. In a review by Schaffer and Silverman (1961), desensitization was performed in 44 of their patients; they noted no deleterious effects from desensitization. In a survey of the literature of 212 pregnant patients who were desensitized during gestation, 11 percent showed constitutional reactions, including mild cramping and/or bleeding, but none had abortions.

Management (Table 24–4)

History and Physical Examination. Inquiries into the duration of the attack, precipitating events, present medications, and presence of associated cough, fever, upper respiratory infection (URI), and so on should be made. Physical examination should be conducted with vital signs (rectal temperature) recorded. Findings specifically concerned with pulmonary status, i.e., associated rales, wheezing, bronchi, decreased breath sounds, and so on, should alert the physician to bronchospasm as well as a contributing factor (e.g., pneumonia, bronchitis).

Laboratory Studies. Management of the pregnant woman with asthma should include the following laboratory studies:
• Blood gases
• CBC with differential

Table 24–4. Patient Care Summary in Asthma*

	Antepartum		Intrapartum	Postpartum
	Outpatient	Inpatient		
BP	Each visit	q 8 hr	q 1 hr	On admission; then q 15 min × 4; then q 30 min × 2; then q 1 hr until stable; then q 4–8 hr
P, R	Same as above	q 4 hr	q 30 min	Same as above
T	Same as above	Same as above	q 1 hr	On admission; then q 4 hr
FHR		With acute attack	Continuous electronic fetal monitoring, preferably internal	
Laboratory values Blood gases CBC with differential Electrolytes Sputum with gram stain and culture Chest x-ray with abdominal shielding		On admission and repeated as needed		

*Nurse–patient ratio: *Antepartum,* 1:6 to 8; *intrapartum,* 2:3; *postpartum,* 1:6 to 8.

- Electrolytes
- Sputum with Gram stain and culture
- Chest x-ray with abdominal shielding if there is no immediate improvement or if fever, rales, and so on are present

Medications

Aqueous epinephrine
Dose—0.3 to 0.5 ml (1/1000 solution) every 15 to 20 minutes SC (in the absence of severe hypertension or cardiac arrhythmias).

Theophylline
Loading dose—250 mg in anhydrous theophylline (6 mg/kg) in 50 to 100 ml D$_5$W over 20 minutes.
Maintenance dose—0.9 mg/kg/hr IV (50 to 70 mg/hr in D$_5$W solution).
Long-term maintenance—Theodur 100 to 300 mg bid; Staphylline 125 to 250 mg q-8 hr; Quibron t/SR 200 to 300 mg bid. Theophylline level should be 10 to 20 mcg/ml.

SIDE EFFECTS. If persistent nausea and vomiting, tachycardia, hypotension, cardiac arrhythmias, or convulsions occur, the dosage should be reduced or discontinued.

USE IN PREGNANCY. At the present time, theophylline is considered safe in pregnancy without evidence of teratogenic effect. Theophylline toxicity (jitteriness, tachycardia, and so on) has been reported, however, in neonates who received the drug transplacentally near delivery as well as those who were breast-fed. Theophylline concentration in breast milk peaks 1 to 3 hours after oral dosage.

Beta Agonist

Terbutaline (Brethine)

Loading Dose—0.25 mg SC every 30 min.
Maintenance Dose—0.25 mg q 5 hr.
Long-Term Maintenance—5 mg tid.

SIDE EFFECTS. The use of beta agonists has been associated with a number of metabolic and clinical side effects. The most common side effects include tachycardia, widening of pulse pressure, anxiety and restlessness, and increased water retention. Hyperglycemia, hyperlipemia, and increased renin production also occur.

USE IN PREGNANCY. Betamimetics should be used with caution because of the frequency of at least minor side effects. Pulmonary edema has been reported, particularly with intravenous administration for preterm labor. Experience with patients in preterm labor demonstrates few neonatal problems, but if they occur, they center on cardiac stimulation effects (i.e., tachycardias) as well as hypoglycemia due to hyperinsulinism. No serious neonatal adverse reactions have been reported in medicated mothers breast-feeding their infants.

INHALANT THERAPY. Intermittent positive pressure breathing (IPPB) can be given with isoproterenol via nebulizer, 20 to 30 breaths every 45 minutes. Aerosols, 2 to 3 breaths every 2 to 3 hours, can also be used with bronchodilators such as terbutaline (Brethine), 2.5 to 5 mg, and metaproterenol (Alupent), 10 to 20 mg.

Glucocorticoids

Loading Dose—hydrocortisone (Solucortef) 100 to 200 mg IV, then 100 mg q 8 hr in D_5W.
Maintenance Dose—Prednisone 60 to 100 mg/day with gradual tapering to lowest effective dose.

SIDE EFFECTS. Glucocorticoid's side effects include hypertension, hypokalemia, hypernatremia with water retention, hyperglycemia, susceptibility to infections, peptic ulcers, and cushingoid features. Osteoporosis and ecchymosis have been associated with long-term use.

USE IN PREGNANCY. Glucocorticoids should be utilized with caution in pregnancy. Their use as a therapy to enhance fetal pulmonary lung maturity is still controversial. Long-term studies are incomplete; however, animal data indicating a potential problem with neurologic development suggest they be utilized only in cases of asthma that are resistant to other therapy (theophylline, betamimetics). Patients should seek advice from their pediatrician as to whether they may breast-feed while taking these drugs.

Antibiotics (Ampicillin)

Initial Dose—1 gm IV, then 500 mg q 6 hr.
Maintenance Dose—500 mg p.o. qid × 10 to 14 days.

Utilize with evidence of bronchitis, pneumonia, and so on.

PULMONARY EDEMA

Acute pulmonary edema is a medical emergency that demands prompt diagnosis and early therapy. The most common causes of pulmonary edema in the pregnant and nonpregnant state are cardiac disease (atherosclerosis, hypertension, cardiomyopathy) and excessive positive fluid balance. The latter is especially true in pregnant patients treated for preterm labor with beta sympathomimetics with or without associated glucocorticoid use for acceleration of fetal pulmonary lung maturity.

Acute myocardial failure occurs in all instances when left ventricular function can no longer effectively eject normal (or increased) stroke volume. This failure of complete left ventricular ejection during systole causes a rise in left ventricular diastolic pressure, which leads to a rise in left atrial and pulmonary venous pressures. Under normal circumstances, the plasma oncotic pressure prevents a substantial diffusion of intravascular fluid into interstitial tissues. However, with the increased hydrostatic pressure of the elevated pulmonary venous system, movement of the fluid into the lung, interstitium, and alveoli occurs. This movement of fluid into interstitium and alveoli interferes with alveolar/capillary bed oxygen exchange, which results in hypoxia. The various etiologies of pulmonary edema are listed in Table 24–5.

Diagnosis

Diagnosis of acute pulmonary edema should be considered when any patient complains of acute shortness of breath, whether at night (paroxysmal nocturnal dypsnea) or any other time the patient assumes a sitting or upright position (orthopnea). The condition may be accompanied by cough and occasional hemoptysis. Chest pain (substernal) can accompany other symptoms.

Confirmatory signs include presence of rales at lung bases, engorged hepatojugular veins, and a protodiastolic gallop (S3) on cardiac auscultation. With progressive disease, patients may become cyanotic and semicomatose or may display confusion.

Management (Table 24–6)

Initial management should involve seeking the mechanism of left ventricular failure. Adjuvant testing that should proceed while therapy is initiated includes:
• ECG
• Chest x-ray
• Serial blood gas analysis
• Electrolytes
• Hemodynamic monitoring—CVP or pulmonary arterial balloon catheter

Once the initial management is under way, secondary management steps can be taken. Betamimetic therapy and steroids should be discontinued if they are being used. Steps to improve ventilation and oxygenation should be initiated. The goals are P_{CO_2}, 35 to 45 mm Hg; P_{O_2}, 80 mm Hg; and normal pH. The patient can be placed in a sitting position. Or oxygen can be administered via nasal prongs. If the P_{CO_2} is greater than 50 mm Hg or the P_{O_2} is less than 60

Table 24–5. Etiologies of Acute Pulmonary Edema in Pregnancy

Cardiac Etiology	Noncardiac Etiology

A. Left ventricular failure
  1. Acute decompensation of chronic left ventricular disease (i.e., hypertensive heart disease)
  2. Myocardial infarction
  3. Cardiomyopathy
B. Mitral valve disease
  1. Congenital (i.e., mitral stenosis)
  2. Acquired (i.e., rheumatic valvular disease)
C. Volume overload—particularly with risk factors
  1. Pre-eclampsia/eclampsia with or without renal impairment
  2. Beta mimetic use with or without associated glucocorticoid use
  3. Transfusion therapy
  4. Underlying cardiac disease
	A. Altered capillary membrane permeability
	  1. Bacteremia
	  2. DIC
	  3. Uremia
	  4. Toxic agent inhalation
	B. Decreased plasma oncotic pressure—hypoalbuminemia
	C. Pulmonary embolism

mm Hg despite therapy, intubation and mechanical ventilation are indicated. *Caution:* High Fio$_2$ (greater than 50 to 60 percent) seen with assisted ventilation can lead to oxygen toxicity and adult respiratory distress syndrome.

Diuretic Therapy

Dose—Furosemide 40 mg IV.

Diuretic therapy causes a prompt diuresis, which reduces the hydrostatic pressure as well as directly affects the venous vasculature, causing vasodilatation. These two effects cause a reduction in the pulmonary wedge pressure and improved cardiac output. Ethacrynic acid has been associated with fetal and maternal ototoxicity and therefore should not be used if possible.

Side effects. Commonly reported complications include hypovolemia, nausea, vomiting, abdominal pain, and diarrhea. Furosemide decreases uric acid excretion and hyperuricemia may develop. Tinnitus has

Table 24–6. Patient Care Summary for Pulmonary Edema*

	Antepartum	Intrapartum	Postpartum
BP, P, R	q 15 min until stable	q 15 min	q 15 min until stable; then q 30 min × 2; then q 1 hr
T	q 4 hr	q 4 hr	q 4 hr
FHR	NST/CST	Continuous electronic monitoring, preferably internal; if no monitor available, then q 15 min in 1st stage and q 5 min in 2nd stage	—
Contractions	q 1 hr	Continuous electronic monitoring, preferably internal; if no monitor available, then q 1 hr	Fundal checks on admission to RR; then q 15 min × 4; then q 30 min × 2; then q 1 hr until stable; then q 4 hr Lochia: Same as above
ECG Chest x-ray Blood gases Electrolytes	On admission and as needed	As needed	As needed
CVP/Pulmonary arterial balloon catheter	If necessary	If necessary	If necessary
I & O	q 1 hr	q 1 hr	q 1 hr until stable; then q 8 hr

*Nurse–patient ratio: *Antepartum,* 1:6 to 8; *intrapartum,* 1:1; *postpartum,* 1:6 to 8.

been also reported. Significant other complications from diuretic therapy include hypokalemia, hyponatremia, and occasionally metabolic alkalosis. Severe hypokalemia is a contraindication to diuretic therapy, although potassium supplementation may help correct depletion so that it may subsequently be utilized.

USE IN PREGNANCY. The use of furosemide during pregnancy has been associated with increased maternal and fetal uric acid. Fetal urinary output does increase following maternal administration. Severe volume depletion, which can occur following its use, can lead to decreased uterine blood flow. No serious neonatal reactions have been reported in breast-fed infants of medicated mothers.

Morphine

Dose—Morphine sulfate 3 to 4 mg IV repeated as needed.

Morphine helps to improve the status of acute pulmonary edema via a reduction in the work of breathing by reducing hyperventilation (central effect). It can also act directly as an agent to cause vasodilatation, which leads to reduced volume return to the decompensated ventricles. Small intravenous doses of morphine are the method of choice, since intramuscular or subcutaneous depositions are erratically absorbed.

SIDE EFFECTS. Morphine's side effects include nausea and vomiting and occasionally profound hypotension and decreased respirations. Therefore, it should be utilized with great caution in patients with preexisting hypotension (systolic < than 100 mm Hg), chronic obstruction pulmonary disease, or AV block. Respiratory acidosis is a contraindication to its use.

USE IN PREGNANCY. Morphine can depress the fetal CNS if given close to delivery. Breast milk excretion has been shown. Morphine has also been associated with vasoconstriction of placental vessels (impairing O_2 and CO_2 transfer); however, human documentation of deleterious effects is lacking. Narcotic antagonists should be available at the time of delivery.

Digitalis

Dose—(Complete digitalization)
  Digoxin 0.50 mg; then 0.25 mg q 6 hr × 3 doses. Follow with digoxin levels (< 3 ng/ml).

Although probably not necessary in many patients, digitalis should be utilized in patients who exhibit cardiac disease, particularly those with cardiomegaly. Digitalis, however, should not be used when there has been a recent myocardial infarction (increased cardiac oxygen requirement). When used for pulmonary edema it should be given as an intravenous dose. Ionotropic effect can be seen prior to full digitalization.

SIDE EFFECTS. Common side effects with digitalis include nausea, vomiting, skin rashes, eosinophilia, and occasionally AV block and arrhythmias due to digitalis intoxication. As previously mentioned, digitalis increases myocardial contractility while increasing cardiac oxygen requirement, and recent myocardial infarction militates against its use. It must not be used in patients with preexisting heart block (second or third degree), bradycardia, obstructive cardiomyopathies, and digitalis toxicity (toxic effects may be seen in patients with digoxin levels > 3 ng/ml). Hypokalemia potentiates the cardiotoxic effects and should be corrected prior to its use.

USE IN PREGNANCY. Digoxin crosses the placenta and can concentrate in the fetal heart. It may even be utilized to treat fetal tachyarrhythmias with congestive changes. Fetal toxic effects have not been reported.

Vasodilatory Therapy (Afterload Reduction)

Dose—Nitroprusside 20 mcg/min (hemodynamic monitoring is essential).

Newer agents have been proposed that reduce peripheral vascular resistance and/or dilate venous capillary bed in the patient with acute pulmonary edema. This reduced resistance causes a lowering of the impedence to left ventricular ejection, thereby allowing improved ventricular emptying. These drugs, although helpful in refractory cases, should not be used in initial therapy. Nitroprusside is the drug of choice since the ganglionic blockers phentolamine, trimeth-aphan, and hexamethonium primarily lead to arterial vasodilatation, whereas nitroprus-side affects both arterial and venous vascular tone. Nitroprusside should be given intra-venously as a continuous drip.

SIDE EFFECTS. Nitroprusside's side effects center on its hypotensive effects, and there-fore patients in shock should not receive the drug. Cyanide toxicity has been reported since this is a byproduct of its metabolism.

USE IN PREGNANCY. Although increased fetal serum cyanide levels are reported with ma-ternal administration, the risk to the fetus is unclear.

Phlebotomy and Rotating Tourniquets. Once considered a mainstay of therapy, phlebotomy and rotating tourniquets should only be used to temporize prior to initiating other therapy. Removal of 500 cc initially helps to reduce plasma volume and thereby decreases an end-diastolic ventricular vol-ume. Patients may, if necessary, be reinfused with their own blood (packed cells) after plasmapheresis. Rotating tourniquets can be utilized to help reduce venous return, but care must be taken not to impede arterial flow to the extremities in the process.

Thromboembolic Complications

DEEP VEIN THROMBOSIS (THROMBOPHLEBITIS)

The true incidence of superficial and deep thrombophlebitis in pregnancy is unknown, but in a review by Aaro and Juergens (1971) it has been estimated to complicate approx-imately 1 in 70 pregnancies. Friend and Kakkar (1970) estimated that deep vein thrombosis is less common than superficial veins and that thrombosis occurs in 1.6 to 4.7 per 1000 deliveries. The onset of throm-bophlebitis is three times more likely to occur in the postpartum period than ante-natally. Factors associated with increased pregnancy risk include: maternal age greater than 35 years, obesity, immobilization, car-diopulmonary disease, diabetes mellitus, and previous history of thromboembolism. Mode of delivery also seems to be a risk

factor, with cesarean section three times more likely to engender thromboembolic problems than vaginal delivery. Thrombi are often bilateral, although only one calf ap-pears affected. The most common sites in-clude the venous sinuses within the soleus muscle, the pocket of valve cups, and the left ileofemoral venous segment.

Pathophysiology

In 1846, Virchow described a classic triad of venous stasis, hypercoagulable blood, and venous intimal injury as the prerequisite for thromboembolism.

Pregnancy is characterized by an increase in venous stasis in the lower extremities and groin area due to the enlarging gravid uterus. Compression of the inferior vena cava caus-ing this stasis is most pronounced when the pregnant patient is in the supine or sitting position. Pregnancy is also characterized by some marked changes in the coagulation and fibrinolytic systems. There is a moderate rise in all coagulation factors except factors XI and XIII. A dramatic rise in fibrinogen and factors III, X, and VIII can be seen. In addi-tion to this rise in coagulation factors, there is also a suppression of the fibrinolytic sys-tem, specifically a depression of plasmino-gen activator and anti-thrombin III, both of which play crucial roles in clot lysis. Intimal vessel injury probably plays no role in ini-tiation of thrombosis in pregnancy except for the possibility of injury during cesarean section, which could conceivably trigger a pelvic vein thrombophlebitis.

Diagnosis

The clinical signs of calf tenderness, swelling, erythema, and pain elicited with dorsal flexion of the foot (Homans' sign) are the most common manifestations. The pain may be particularly noticeable with ambu-lation. The swelling may not be discernible to the naked eye, and calf measurements should be taken. A difference of 2 cm in circumference (measured equidistant from the patella) is significant. An area of warmth or distinct erythema may be noted over the involved area.

Confirmatory testing of the presence of thrombosis can be accomplished by the non-invasive techniques of Doppler ultrasound or plethysmography or the invasive techniques of venography or ^{125}I-fibrinogen scanning.

Noninvasive Testing

Doppler ultrasound. Doppler testing is based on ultrasonic velocity detection. The flow pattern after Valsalva's manuever, respirations, or alternating compression is noted. Distortions in the flow pattern indicate thrombosis. Small nonocclusive thrombi can be missed, but major emboli can be detected. It is less effective in detecting emboli above the groin area.

Plethysmography. This testing is based on electrical impedence of the calf and its alteration when thrombosis is present. The plethysmographic tracing is a measurement of the rate of emptying after venous occlusion induced by inflating and rapidly releasing a thigh cuff. Respirations also cause a fluctuation in the impedence tracings. Deviation from normal patterns is diagnostic of thrombosis.

Both the Doppler ultrasound and plethysmographic techniques have interpretation problems in the gravid patient. Approximately 10 to 15 percent of normal pregnant patients will have abnormal tests if they are supine. It is imperative, then, that all abnormal tests be confirmed while the patient is in the lateral recumbent position.

Invasive Testing

Venography. The injection of radioopaque dye into a vein in the foot with follow-up x-rays has remained a mainstay of diagnosis for many years. Because it is difficult to adequately shield the fetus from radiation, particularly while examining the inguinal area, this technique has become less popular during pregnancy. If utilized, a pronounced collateral venous system can be visualized in the affected calf due to thrombosis. Subiliac lesions can be missed occasionally. The contrast medium can also induce phlebitis in and of itself.

[125]I-fibrinogen scan. The incorporation of radioactive tracer compound into the thrombus leads to a "hot spot" that can be detected. The use of radioactive iodine, however, is contraindicated in pregnancy because of fetal thyroid concentration, although the radiation risk is probably small.

Management (Table 24–7)

Initial Management. The initial management of thrombophlebitis consists of the following elements:
1. Bedrest with elevation of affected leg for 5 to 7 days or until symptoms clear.
2. Analgesia.
3. Support hose—thigh-high lightweight elastic.
4. Laboratory studies:
   a. PT, PTT
   b. Fibrinogen
   c. CBC with platelets
5. Anticoagulation—heparin 40,000 U/day as continuous drip infusion (1500 to 1700 U/hr) until PTT is 2.5 to 3 times control and/or plasma heparin is 0.3 U/ml.

Initial therapy continues for 10 to 14 days.

Subsequent Anticoagulation

Maintenance dose. Heparin, 20,000 U/day (or 10,000 units bid) SC, may be given throughout pregnancy. Warfarin, 5 mg tid (15 mg/day) until PT is 1.5 to 2 times controlled values, may be given to postpartum patients *only*.

Intrapartum management. Heparin can be stopped when labor commences without risk of excessive intrapartum or postpartum bleeding. Rarely is there a need to reverse heparin, but if excessive bleeding exists protamine sulfate (1 mg IV push inactivates approximately 100 U heparin) can be utilized. Heparin is again initiated post partum, and a switch to warfarin can be made over the next few days. Anticoagulation should be continued for 4 to 6 weeks.

Anticoagulation in pregnancy is discussed more fully elsewhere in this chapter.

PULMONARY EMBOLISM

Pulmonary embolism occurs once in every 2500 to 3000 pregnancies. Untreated, the condition can result in a mortality rate of 50 percent. It is believed that the underlying pathophysiology is similar to that of deep vein thrombosis. Approximately 35 percent of patients who develop pulmonary embolism give an antecedent history of deep vein thrombosis. The remaining pulmonary embolism patients may develop silent deep vein thrombosis with migration to the pul-

Table 24–7. Patient Care Summary for Deep Vein Thrombosis*

| | Antepartum | | Intrapartum | Postpartum |
	Outpatient	Inpatient		
BP, P, R	Each visit	q 4 hr	q 1 hr	On admission to RR; then q 15 min × 4; then q 30 min × 2; then q 1 hr until stable; then q 4 hr PP
T	Each visit	q 4 hr	q 4 hr	On admission to RR; then q 4 hr
FHR	Each visit	q shift	Continuous electronic monitoring, preferably internal; if no monitor available, q 15 min in 1st stage and q 5 min in 2nd stage	—
Contractions	Each visit	q shift	Continuous electronic monitoring; if no monitor available, q 1 hr by palpation	Fundal checks on admission to RR; then q 15 min × 4; then q 30 min × 2; then q 1 hr until stable; then q 4 hr Lochia: Same as above
Bedrest	Yes	Yes	Yes	Yes
Support hose	Yes	Yes	Yes	Yes
Laboratory studies PT PTT Fibrinogen CBC with platelets	At initial visit; then q month	Yes	Yes	q month until therapy discontinued
Assessment of thrombosis site	Each visit	q 4 hr	q 1 hr	q 1 hr in RR q 4 hr on PP floor

*Nurse–patient ratio: *Antepartum,* 1:6 to 8; *intrapartum,* 2:3; *postpartum,* 1:6–8.

monary arterial branches or thrombi that arise de novo as cardiopulmonary emboli without deep vein origin.

Diagnosis

Dypsnea remains the most common symptom of pulmonary embolism and is present in over 80 percent of cases. Pleuritic chest pain (72 percent) and apprehension (60 percent) are also commonly present. Other signs and symptoms may include hemoptysis (34 percent), rales, tachypnea (90 percent), a loud pulmonic closure, and/or pleuritic friction rub. Confirmatory findings include a P_{O_2} less than 80 mm Hg and an abnormal ventilation-perfusion lung scan or angiography. A chest x-ray may reveal an infiltrate indicating an elevated hemidiaphragm or pleural fluid. ECG often reveals a right axis shift or right bundle branch block. Lactic dehydrogenase and bilirubin levels are often elevated.

The mainstays of diagnosis are arterial blood gas analysis and lung scanning. If the P_{O_2} is greater than 90 mm Hg, one can rule out pulmonary embolism. Values less than 90 mm Hg can represent smaller emboli. Ventilation perfusion lung scans utilizing ^{99}Tc and xenon gas can be most useful, particularly when a "mismatch" pattern is seen. This "mismatch" pattern indicates normal ventilation with decreased perfusion. Fetal irradiation risks from these agents are probably minimal, and the importance of establishing the diagnosis is so great that the physician should not hesitate to use this technique. The specificity of lung scan can be reduced if the patient has congestive heart failure or chronic obstructive lung disease.

Table 24–8. Patient Care Summary for Pulmonary Embolism*

	Antepartum	Intrapartum	Postpartum
BP, P, R	q 15 min	q 15 min	q 15 min until stable; then q 30 min × 2; then q 1 hr; then q 4 hr on PP floor
T	q 4 hr	q 4 hr	On admission; then q 4 hr
FHR	Weekly NST/CST	Continuous electronic monitoring, preferably internal; if no monitor available, q 15 min in first stage and q 5 min in second stage	—
Contractions	q 8 hr	Continuous electronic monitoring, preferably internal; if no monitor available, q 1 hr by palpation	Fundal checks on admission; then q 15 min × 4; then q 30 min × 2; then q 1 hr until stable; then q 4 hr on PP floor
			Lochia: Same as above
I & O	q 1 hr until stable; then q 8 hr	q 1 hr	q 1 hr until stable; then q 8 hr
CVP	Yes	Yes	Yes
ECG	Yes	Yes	Yes

Laboratory studies
  Serial blood gases
  PT
  PTT
  CBC with differential
	At initial evaluation; then as needed during anticoagulation therapy	—	—

Chest x-ray	At initial evaluation; then as needed	—	—
O₂ therapy	1 to 2 L/min nasal prong	1 to 2 L/min face mask	1 to 2 L/min nasal prong

*Nurse–patient ratio = 1:1.

In equivocal cases, pulmonary angiography with abdominal shielding can be helpful, although smaller emboli can be missed.

Management (Table 24–8)

The management of pulmonary embolism consists of the following elements:
1. Laboratory studies
   a. Serial blood gas analysis
   b. PT
   c. PTT
   d. CBC with differential
2. ECG
3. Chest x-ray
4. O_2 therapy—1 to 2 L/min via nasal prongs
5. Sedation—10 mg morphine sulfate SC or 4 mg IV
6. Aqueous theophylline—250 mg in 50 ml D_5W over 15 to 20 minutes
7. Digitalization (with massive pulmonary embolus) 0.50 mg IV, then 0.25 mg q 8 hr × 3
8. Anticoagulation therapy, fibrinolytic therapy, or surgical intervention

Anticoagulation Therapy

Heparin

Initial Dose—10,000 U IV bolus, then 1000 to 2000 U/hr as continuous IV infusion until PTT is 2.5 to 3 times controlled (plasma heparin 0.3 U/ml).
Maintenance Dose—1000 U/hr continuous IV for 10 days, then 10,000 U bid as SC injection. This lower dose rarely affects PTT.

SIDE EFFECTS. Hemorrhage is the most frequent side effect associated with heparin. Other side effects include anaphylactoid reactions, alopecia, thrombocytopenia, and, with long-term use, osteoporosis. The use of salicylates, phenylbutazone, indomethacin, clofibrate, and dipyridamole may increase the risk of excessive bleeding. Quinine drugs and d-tubocurarine may decrease the anticoagulant effect.

USE IN PREGNANCY. The use of heparin appears to be safe during the course of pregnancy without added risks to mother or fetus. Since heparin does not cross the placenta, it does not lead to fetal anticoagulation and perinatal hemorrhage. It remains the drug of choice for anticoagulation during pregnancy.

Warfarin

Maintenance Dose (in postpartum patients *only*)– 5 mg tid (15 mg/day) until PT is 1.5 to 2 times controlled.

SIDE EFFECTS. The major side effect of warfarin is hemorrhage. This hemorrhage may be so brisk that administration of fresh frozen plasma and blood may be required. Less frequently encountered side effects include nausea, vomiting, diarrhea, alopecia, and dermatitis. Overdosage may be managed by intravenous or subcutaneous vitamin K administration. Certain drugs, including phenylbutazone, anabolic steroids, broad spectrum antibiotics, salicylates, and chloramphenicol, enhance the anticoagulant response to warfarin. Barbiturates, griseofulvin, and glutethimide may diminish anticoagulant response.

USE IN PREGNANCY. The fetus and neonate appear to be extremely sensitive to warfarin and warfarin drugs because of their lower concentration of vitamin K–dependent coagulation factors. Risk of perinatal hemorrhage in up to 5 to 10 percent of cases has been reported. Warfarin drugs may also induce fetal malformation (warfarin embryopathy), which is reported to occur in approximately 15 to 25 percent of prenatal exposures (Hall et al., 1980). This syndrome includes nasal hypoplasia, stippling of bones, ophthalmologic abnormalities, intrauterine growth retardation, and mental delay. Because of these concerns, warfarin should be considered contraindicated in pregnancy.

Warfarin is excreted in breast milk, but whether neonatal effects can be seen is controversial.

Intrapartum management. Heparin dosage can be lowered to 20,000 units the day of delivery and increased to previous levels after delivery. Warfarin can be added post partum. Anticoagulation therapy at maintenance levels should be continued for 6 to 8 months following pulmonary embolism.

Fibrinolytic Therapy. The thrombolytic agents streptokinase and urokinase are available for clot dissolution. Both act to increase active plasmin, which then hydrolyzes the fibrin in clots. Lytic therapy has been demonstrated to result in quicker lysis of clots than heparin therapy; however, whether this translates into reduced recurrence risks or overall improvement in long-term status is unclear. These agents need to be used with great caution, since frank hemorrhage may occur with biopsies, arterial punctures, and so on. Patients need to be at strict bedrest, and blood products (packed RBCs, fresh frozen plasma) should be available. Allergic and pyrogenic side effects have also been reported. The experience with these agents in pregnancy is limited, and they should be used only in very selective cases.

Surgical Intervention. Emergency surgical removal of a pulmonary embolus has limited applicability, since most patients respond to anticoagulation therapy and over 90 percent of the fatalities associated with pulmonary embolism occur within 1 hour, usually before surgical intervention could be initiated. At the present time, embolectomies are reserved for those few patients who do not respond to anticoagulation therapy yet demonstrate persistent hypotension and/or hypoxemia. When performed in a timely manner the survival rate approaches 50 percent (Sasahara and Barsamian, 1973).

Vena cava interruption is another surgical technique used in patients with pulmonary embolism in whom deep vein origin is demonstrated and in whom anticoagulation is contraindicated or deep vein thrombosis failed to resolve after anticoagulation. Other candidates include patients with septic pulmonary emboli from pelvic vein thrombophlebitis.

A variety of procedures (clip, ligation, filters) of vena cava interruption have been proposed. Recurrence risks, however, are approximately 10 percent owing to emboli arising from areas above the ligation or from ovarian vein thromboembolism or even emboli arising from the ligation site itself (Bernstein, 1973).

Side effects include vena stasis of the legs and perineum. Clearly, this is a procedure to be utilized selectively.

REFERENCES

Aaro, L. A., and Juergens, J. L.: Thrombophlebitis associated with pregnancy. Am. J. Obstet. Gynecol. 109:1128, 1971.

Baskett, T. F., and Koh, K. S.: Sinusoidal fetal heart rate pattern—a sign of fetal hypoxia. Obstet. Gynecol. 44:379, 1974.

Bernstein, E. F.: The place of venous interruption in the management of pulmonary embolism. *In* Moser, K. M., and Stein, M. (eds.): Pulmonary Thromboembolism. Chicago, Year Book Medical Publishers, 1973.

Bowman, J. M.: Blood-group incompatibilities. *In* Iffy L., and Kaminetzky, H. A. (eds.): Principles and Practice of Obstetrics and Perinatology. New York, John Wiley & Sons, 1981, p. 1193.

Bowman, J. M.: The management of Rh-isoimmunization. Obstet. Gynecol. 52:1, 1978.

Bowman, J. M., Chown, B., Lewis, M., et al.: Rh-isoimmunization during pregnancy: antenatal prophylaxis. Can. Med. Assoc. J. 118:623, 1978.

Bowman, J. M., and Pollack, J. M.: Antenatal Rh prophylaxis: 28 weeks gestation service program. Can. Med. Assoc. J. 118:627, 1978.

Bowman, J. M., and Manning, F. A.: Intrauterine fetal transfusions: Winnepeg, 1982. Obstet. Gynecol. 61:203, 1983.

Friend, J. R., and Kakkar, V. V.: The diagnosis of deep vein thrombosis in the puerperium. J. Obstet. Gynaecol. Br. Commonw. 77:820, 1970.

Gluck, J. C., and Gluck, P. A.: The effects of pregnancy on asthma: a prospective study. Ann. Allergy 37:164, 1976.

Gordon, M., Niswander, K. R., Barendes, H., et al.: Fetal morbidity following potentially anoxigenic obstetric conditions. VII. Bronchial asthma. Am. J. Obstet. Gynecol. 106:421, 1970.

Gray, J. H., Cudmore, D. W., Luther, E. R., et al.: Sinusoidal fetal heart rate pattern associated with alphaprodine administration. Obstet. Gynecol. 52:678, 1978.

Hall, J. G., Pauli, R. M., and Wilson, K.: Maternal and fetal sequelae of anticoagulation during pregnancy. Am. J. Med. 68:122, 1980.

Hill, Z., Vacl-Kalasova, E., Clabkova, M., et al.: Hemolytic disease of the newborn due to anti-D antibodies in Du positive mothers. Vox Sang. 27:92, 1974.

Lacey, P.: An unexpected case of severe hemolytic disease of the newborn due to anti-D (Abstract). Transfusion 18:642, 1978.

Liley, A. W.: Liquor amnii analysis in management of pregnancy complicated by rhesus sensitization. Am. J. Obstet. Gynecol. 82:1359, 1961.

Liley, A. W.: Intrauterine transfusion in the foetus in haemolytic disease. Br. Med. J. 2:1107, 1963.

Modanlou, H. T., Freeman, R. K., Ortiz, O., et al.: Sinusoidal fetal heart rate pattern and severe fetal anemia. Am. J. Obstet. Gynecol. 49:537, 1977.

Queenan, J. T.: Intrauterine transfusion—a cooperative study. Am. J. Obstet. Gynecol. 104:397, 1969.

Queenan, J. T.: Modern Management of the Rh Problem, 2nd ed. Hagerstown, MD, Harper & Row, 1977.

Race, R. R.: The Rh genotype and fisher's theory. Blood 3:27, 1948.

Sasahara, A. A., and Barsamian, E. M.: Another look at pulmonary embolectomy. Ann. Thorac. Surg. 16:317, 1973.

Schaffer, G., and Silverman, F.: Pregnancy complicated by asthma. Am. J. Obstet. Gynecol. 82:182, 1961.

Taylor, J. F.: Sensitization of Rh negative daughters by their Rh positive mothers. N. Engl. J. Med. 276:547, 1967.

Weinstein, L.: Irregular antibodies causing hemolytic disease of the newborn. Obstet. Gynecol. Surv. 31:581, 1976.

White, C. A., Goplerud, C. P., Kissker, C. T., et al.: Intrauterine fetal transfusion, 1965–1976, with an assessment of surviving children. Am. J. Obstet. Gynecol. 130:933, 1978.

Whitfield, C. R., Neely, R. A., and Telford, M. E.: Amniotic fluid analysis in rhesus iso-immunization. J. Obstet. Gynecol. Br. Commonw. 75:121, 1968.

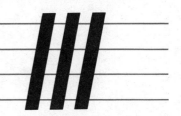

FOLLOW-UP

NEWBORN CARE IN THE DELIVERY ROOM

M. DOUGLAS CUNNINGHAM
KATHRYN E. TePAS

The birth of all infants is a moment of uncertainty. Modern obstetrics and neonatology seek to maximize the options for effective therapy of complications befalling the fetus or infant of a woman with a high-risk pregnancy. It is essential for newborn care in the delivery room of high-risk pregnancies to declare the presence of fetal-neonatal compromise, document severity, and immediately treat the adverse physiologic states. Delivery room care for sick newborn infants begins with a high state of preparedness for the rapid implementation of resuscitation measures.

Perinatal asphyxia presents the neonatologist-pediatrician with the pathophysiologic effects of impaired respiration. Hypoxia and acidosis are the overriding events to be relieved by ventilation of the newborn lungs. The transformation from dependence on maternal respiration to independent respiration requires a great deal of energy and vitality on the part of normal newborn infants but may be an impossible task for compromised neonates. Prior to delivery, the lungs are filled with fluid and largely bypassed from the standpoint of cardiac output. At the moment of birth they must be rapidly relieved of the fluid and instantly inflated and perfused. Impediments to this transformation preclude the infant's only immediate means for reversing the metabolic acidosis of perinatal asphyxia and the deterioration of vital signs. Successful newborn resuscitation depends on effective restoration of respiratory function.

Antepartum Considerations

PREGNANCY RISK FACTORS

Numerous maternal conditions can be related to an increased risk for fetal well-being and birth asphyxia. Table 25–1 lists most conditions that allow time to prepare for a high risk delivery and prompt resuscitation of the sick newborn.

Pregnancy risk scoring systems have been advocated for nearly 15 years, but their acceptance has been variable and generally limited to larger medical centers. Indexing high-risk pregnancies affords the opportunity to weigh various risk factors and distinguish the more ominous situations. Numerous scoring systems have been proposed. A simple $1+$, $2+$, $3+$ system initiated at the University of Colorado and adapted for the University of California, San Diego, (Resnick, 1976) weighs breech delivery as $1+$, drug abuse $2+$, and premature rupture of membranes $3+$. Another scoring system, the Maternal-Child Health Care Index, offered by Nesbitt and Aubry (1969), relies on maternal history and physical examination and subtracts positive risk data from a perfect score of 100. Irrespective of form, some manner of high-risk assignment sets the stage for anticipatory measures to be taken should an asphyxiated infant be delivered.

A retrospective analysis of 96 cases of cerebral palsy revealed that many high-risk pregnancies did not receive special care and

Table 25–1. Pregnancy Risk Factors

Antepartum Conditions Suggesting Advanced
Preparations for Delivery and Resuscitation
  Rh isoimmunization
  Toxemia
  Diabetes mellitus
  Prolonged rupture of fetal membranes
  Premature delivery
  Prolonged labor (especially prolonged second
    stage)
  Postterm delivery
  Breech presentation
  Chorioamnionitis
  Thyroid disease
  Acute pyelonephritis or other urinary tract infection
  Severe anemia (such as sickle cell or thalassemia)
  Severe maternal respiratory distress
  Myasthenia gravis
  Multiple gestation
  Oligo- and polyhydramnios
  Maternal drug therapy or usage:
    Propylthiouracil
    Propranolol
    Reserpine
    Lithium
    Magnesium
    Alcohol
    Heroin
    Methadone
    Ritodrine
  Intrauterine growth disturbance
    Very low birth weight
    Intrauterine growth retardation
    Small- or large-for-gestational-age fetuses
  Meconium staining of amniotic fluid
  Apparent anomalies
    Myelomeningocele
    Omphalocele
    Gastroschisis

Intrapartum Events that Occur with Little Notice and
Require a Constant State of Preparedness
  Abruptio placentae
  Placenta previa
  Precipitous labor
  Mid-forceps rotation
  Prolapsed umbilical cord
  Maternal hypotension
  Cord tightly around neck (nuchal cord)
  Shoulder dystocia
  Ruptured uterus

that potentially avoidable problems, of either obstetric or neonatal care, could have been identified ante partum (McManus et al., 1977). Of 94 severely asphyxiated infants studied by Brown and colleagues (1974), 56 percent involved specific antepartum and intrapartum disorders. Birth injury and subsequent neurologic and behavioral disorders developed in 13 percent. Whether or not the stress is prolonged or acute, identifiable high-risk factors (as in Table 25–1) may have similar neurologic sequelae.

ASSESSMENT OF FETAL WELL-BEING

Fetal assessment for growth and development seeks to establish normal growth and allows for the assumption that the fetus can withstand the stresses of labor, birth, and the adaptation to an extrauterine existence. Various methods are now available for assessing fetal condition and intrauterine environment.

Ultrasonography affords detection and monitoring of intrauterine growth and the presence of anomalies. Decreased biparietal diameters for fetal head growth suggest intrauterine growth retardation. Anomalies such as hydrocephalus, omphalocele, and myelomeningocele can be documented as well as estimates of uterine size and amniotic fluid volume. Ultrasound examinations revealing disproportionate twin growth and the presence of hydramnios have led to the diagnosis of twin-to-twin transfusion.

Amniotic fluid studies obtained by amniocentesis have aided fetal assessment. Resuscitation preparations are mandatory for those Rh-sensitized pregnancies with rising amniotic fluid Δ OD 450 levels. Phospholipid analysis of amniotic fluid for lung maturation has led to improved awareness and preparation for prematurity. Low L/S ratios and absence of PG are associated with increased risk for birth asphyxia (Gluck, 1978). Falling L/S ratios have been associated with maternal renal disease (nonhypertensive glomerulonephritis), anomalies of the lung (diaphragmatic hernia and hypoplastic lung), Pierre Robin syndrome, and multiple congenital anomalies.

Antepartum contraction stress tests and nonstress testing using electronic fetal heart rate monitoring establish fetal heart rate response and beat-to-beat variability prior to the onset of labor. During labor, awareness by the resuscitation team of loss of beat-to-beat variability with variable or late decelerations of fetal heart rate alerts them to possible fetal compromise.

Fetal heart rate monitoring should be complemented by sampling of scalp capillary blood to determine intrapartum fetal acid base status if a problem is noted on the fetal monitor. Scalp blood pH values of 7.25 or less signal a diminishing capability of the fetoplacental unit to maintain acid base balance. Fetal blood pH values of 7.15 or less are associated with at least a 90 percent incidence of birth asphyxia.

COMMUNICATION

Introduction of the parents to the neonatal physician and nurses by the obstetric team before delivery confirms continuity of care and prepares them for future interaction. A myriad of strangers under difficult circumstances is an unnecessary burden for the parents. If a patient has been identified as high risk before the intrapartum period, a tour of the neonatal intensive care nursery may also help to alleviate stress. If labor has already begun, pictures of the unit may be useful, if the timing is appropriate.

Interdisciplinary communication between anesthesiology, obstetrics, and neonatology personnel eliminates confusion and enhances sharing of information and coordination of efforts. The use and effects of analgesic and anesthetic agents must be made known to the resuscitation team. Airway placement and ventilatory management of the asphyxiated infant require smooth and proficient performance: neonatologists and anesthesiologists cannot jostle one another in attempts to intubate the infant. Early designation of resuscitation responsibilities by the obstetrician-in-charge sets in motion lines of responsibility.

Once a high-risk delivery has been defined and plans for infant resuscitation established, notification of the neonatal intensive care unit should be made. Advance notice allows for preparation of an acute care bed and the placement of additional nursing personnel on standby status. Sick infant transport to the nearest neonatal intensive care facility may also be required. Advance notice to the transporting agency allows time to assemble equipment and alert personnel.

Anticipation of Resuscitation

As delivery of the high-risk infant becomes imminent, communication and preparations for the event continue. Ideally, the neonatal intensive care nurses and physicians are made aware early on of the presence of a woman with risk factors including the maternal history, course of management for the mother, anesthesia and analgesia, condition of the fetus, and planned route of delivery. During final preparations for delivery, the obstetric staff need only update the neonatal resuscitation team. The physical environment, equipment, and medications required for resuscitation of an infant must be organized in the delivery area at all times. Last-minute scrambling by the neonatal team in preparation for the arrival of a sick infant is inexcusable. Daily inventories and rechecking before and after each delivery are necessary to ensure smooth and orderly resuscitations.

DESIGNATION AND PREPARATION OF PERSONNEL

If the infant is known beforehand to be at risk for asphyxia, then a neonatal resuscitation team is requested. All deliveries should be attended by a nurse qualified to perform initial newborn assessments and capable of initiating resuscitation measures. The nurse should be free to deal with the infant and devoid of responsibilities for the mother.

The neonatal resuscitation team should consist of at least one neonatal physician and two nurses or two neonatal nurse clinicians and one special care nurse. One clinician must be experienced in endotracheal intubation of infants, especially low birth weight premature newborns. One member must assume the role of team leader to determine and delegate specific tasks and responsibilities before the actual delivery. One attendant should control the airway, perform laryngoscopy, suction and/or intubate, and maintain ventilation. Another attendant must concern himself with cardiovascular function by assessing heart rate and perfusion and providing external cardiac massage when needed. A third team member is recommended for preparation and administration of medications and for recording the sequence of events in the resuscitation.

Korones (1981) emphasizes the need for a well-coordinated effort for infant resuscitation:

Obviously the continuous presence of someone adept and knowledgeable is essential for the care of all infants, especially the sick ones—wasted minutes are crucial to survival and the preservation of intact central nervous system function.

The objective of the team is to function together smoothly, quickly reverse the effects of asphyxia, and stabilize the infant. To achieve these goals, physicians and nurses committed to maintaining their expertise in resuscitation techniques and who frequently work comfortably as a unit are required.

THE PHYSICAL ENVIRONMENT

In many cases delivery room management of the sick newborn is just the beginning of many days of intensive care. In others it will constitute an intensive period of care for the infant, albeit for an hour or less. Bearing in mind the nature of care, the physical space allocated for newborn resuscitation should meet the recommendations of the American Academy of Pediatrics (1978) for a neonatal intensive care station. One hundred square feet of floor space meets minimal requirements for a resuscitation bed, two to three team members, and usable space for monitoring equipment and supplies. It also must provide space for the set-up of sterile trays for umbilical catheterization or thoracostomy trays when needed.

The resuscitation area can be either within the delivery room or in an immediately adjacent room. The latter is often preferred by neonatologists. A large delivery room may adequately accommodate the 100 square foot space requirement of the station and have the advantage of avoiding a three-step transfer of the infant to a resuscitation bed. Properly equipped, a resuscitation area in the delivery room should suffice for all low-risk and most high-risk deliveries.

The advantages of a resuscitation room include having an isolated environment dedicated entirely to the needs of a neonate requiring vigorous resuscitation. It provides space for mounted equipment and storage of supplies (Fig. 25–1). If emergency x-rays are required, portable equipment can be brought in without disturbing the obstetric team. If mechanical ventilation is required, respiratory therapy technicians can enter without violating sterile field set-ups. Lastly, a resuscitation room buffers parents and professionals from the sights, sounds, and dialogue of full scale resuscitation, and the resuscitation team can work without being distracted by frightened and distraught parents.

Temperature and air flow in the delivery room are traditionally regulated for the comfort of the mother and obstetric staff. A complicating feature of birth asphyxia is hypothermia (Sheldon, 1977), and the advent of effective radiant heat warmers in the delivery room is often accompanied by a

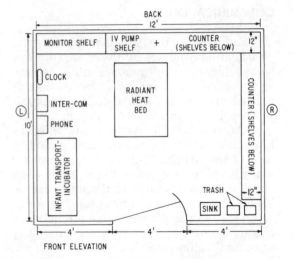

Figure 25–1. Overhead schematic for distribution and arrangement of resuscitation room facilities. Note counter space and shelving for monitoring and support equipment. (Courtesy of K. TePas and University of Kentucky Medical Illustrations Department.)

false sense of security that thermal stability is no longer a problem. The high-risk infant quickly loses heat following delivery by evaporation, conduction, radiation, and convection. The design of the resuscitation area must take into account all four routes of heat loss. Evaporative, conductive, and radiant heat loss can be minimized by placing the infant in warm blankets or towels under a radiant warming bed and rapidly drying the skin. As soon as the skin is dry, towels and blankets should be removed and a servo control probe attached to allow for temperature stabilization. However, convective heat loss (dependent upon ambient temperature and the velocity of air flow over the infant) must be considered separately. Air conditioning ducts are a major source of convective losses in many delivery rooms. It is important to assure that the resuscitation area is not within the cross draft of ducts. Keeping the delivery room temperature at or above 76°F (usual nursery or neonatal intensive care room temperature) helps minimize convective losses.

The resuscitation station must include adequate utilities to supply today's technical support systems. Good ceiling lighting is essential for accurate assessment of the neonate. A surgical spotlight is most helpful for umbilical vessel catheterizations. If attached to the bed, the spotlight is available without taking up additional floor space.

Sufficient numbers of electrical outlets for

the operation of support equipment is critical to any intensive care (resuscitation) setting. Ten outlets with emergency generator back-up are usually adequate to power the radiant warmer, infusion pumps, spotlight, cardiac monitor, and blood pressure monitor. The electrical outlets should be immediately adjacent to the neonatal station (Fig. 25–2) and should not in any way be required by the obstetric staff for care of the mother.

Two vacuum outlets are required; one for airway suction, and the other for use with thoracostomy drainage systems. The station should have two oxygen outlets and one air outlet. One oxygen outlet attaches to the respirator flow meter and supports hand bag ventilation. An air outlet and the second oxygen outlet are made available for a ventilator, should one be needed. Air, oxygen, and vacuum outlets should also be separate from the maternal supply.

Although seldom considered, waste materials are a fact of resuscitative efforts. A large amount of trash accumulates (syringe packages, sterile wrappings, empty vials and ampules, expended syringes, and used linens). A waste receptacle within arm's reach is convenient and decreases the clutter associated with rapid intervention. A wastebasket behind the bed or a large plastic trash bag taped to the back of the bed in an open position minimizes this problem.

EQUIPMENT

It is imperative that equipment be organized and immediately accessible to the infant resuscitation team: this means within an arm's reach of the infant's bed. Supplies should be checked periodically throughout the day and kept restocked at all times. Responsibility for this should be delegated to each nursing shift.

The items required for delivery room management of the high-risk infant are listed in Table 25–2. The radiant warmer should be turned on prior to delivery to avoid warm-up time. Stethoscope, facemasks, anesthesia bag, and laryngoscope blade should be on the bed to be kept warm and in plain view. The infant servo control temperature probe for the radiant warmer should be ready for attachment to the infant.

Mounting the cardiac monitor on a wall

Table 25–2. Equipment for Resuscitation

Large surface radiant warmer with:
  Servo mechanism and probe
  Observation lights
  Spotlight
  Thermometer
Anesthesia bag with:
  Pressure manometer
  Positive end expiratory pressure valve
  Masks; premature and newborn
Flowmeters for oxygen and air with tubing
Simple suction with extension tubing
Stethoscope with infant dome and diaphragm
Laryngoscope: Miller "0" blade (8 cm) and extra
  batteries and light bulbs
Endotracheal tubes—2.5 mm to 4.5 mm inner diameter
Soft wire stylet
DeLee suction trap #10 Fr
Hand suction bulb
Cord clamps
Suction catheters, sizes 6.5, 8, and 10 Fr
Umbilical catheterization trays with umbilical catheters,
  sizes 3.5, 5, and 8 Fr
Betadine solution
Cardiac monitor with leads and electrodes
Blood pressure device with infant cuffs, sizes 2.5, 3.5,
  and 4.0 cm
Needles, 27 to 18 gauge
Scalp vein needles, 21 to 25 gauge
Syringes, size 1 to 60 cc
Sterile gloves
Benzoin solution
Tape, ½" and 1"
Three-way stopcocks
Scissors
Thoracostomy tray
Thoracostomy catheters, sizes 10, 12 and 16 Fr
Chest drainage system with underwater seal
Intravenous fluids: dextrose 5% in water and dextrose
  10% in water in 250-ml or 500-ml containers

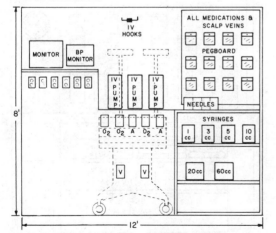

BACK WALL DETAIL

Figure 25–2. View of wall behind resuscitation bed. Easy access to supplies and visibility of monitors is stressed. Note number of oxygen (O$_2$), air (A), and vacuum (V) outlets behind the bed. (Courtesy of K. TePas and University of Kentucky Medical Illustrations Department.)

Table 25–3. Medications for Use in Resuscitation

Principal Medications			
Drug	*Indications*	*Route*	*Dose*
Atropine	Sinus bradycardia	IV	0.02–0.04 mg/kg
Sodium bicarbonate	Metabolic acidosis	IV	1–2 mEq/kg
Calcium chloride (10% solution)	Low cardiac output	IV	0.3 ml/kg
Glucose (10% solution)	Hypoglycemia	IV	4–8 mg/kg/min
Epinephrine (1:10,000 dilution)	Bradycardia	IV	0.1–0.3 ml/kg
Naloxone	Opiate narcosis	IV	0.01 mg/kg
Alternative and Ancillary Medications			
Albumin (5% solution)	Hypovolemia	IV	10–20 ml/kg
Calcium gluconate (10% solution)	Low cardiac output	IV	1 ml/kg
Glucose (25% solution)	Hypoglycemia	IV	2 ml/kg
THAM (0.3 molar solution)	1–2 doses only Metabolic acidosis	IV	1 cc/kg dose

Heparin for anticoagulation of syringes and intravascular catheters

Normal saline without preservatives for mixing medications

Sterile water without preservatives for mixing medications

shelf conserves floor space. Blood pressure monitoring is made easier by the use of pneumatic monitors or Doppler pulse sensors. Several small arm cuff sizes are necessary. Blood pressure monitoring is essential for evaluating the recovery of an infant from asphyxia.

PHARMACEUTICALS

The most essential drugs for use in resuscitation efforts are listed in Table 25–3. These drugs have been divided into two groups—principal and ancillary. Drugs listed are either basic to resuscitation of the newborn or reserved for alternative use or special circumstances. Drugs are listed alphabetically by their common name to minimize errors of identification during resuscitation. Crisis medications are generally *requested* by common name ("bicarb" rather than sodium bicarbonate and Valium rather than diazepam). Displaying both medications and supplies on a pegboard seems to be the most practical storage system (Fig. 25–3). It provides immediate visualization of the presence or absence of items, takes up no counter space, and allows for the individual labelling of items. Color-coded and easy-to-read labels will facilitate quick retrieval of appropriate items. Obvious labelling discourages errors when two preparations of a drug are present, such as calcium gluconate and calcium chloride or 10 and 25 percent solutions of glucose.

Figures 25–1, 25–2, and 25–3 are examples of a resuscitation station with equipment and supplies that meet American Academy of Pediatrics (1977) criteria for space, organization, and use for resuscitation.

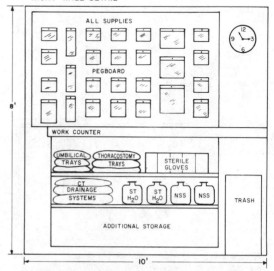

Figure 25–3. Schematic for supply storage and pegboard storage of frequently used supplies requiring easy and quick retrieval. (Courtesy of K. TePas and University of Kentucky Medical Illustrations Department.)

Need for Resuscitation

PATHOPHYSIOLOGY OF ASPHYXIA

Asphyxia is the failure to exchange carbon dioxide and oxygen and maintain body acid base balance. Survival of the fetus is dependent upon the continued respiratory function of the placenta. Intermittent intrauterine asphyxia may occur for periods lasting several days if marginal respiratory compensation can be achieved by the feto-placental circulation. Progressive fetal asphyxia and intrauterine death may result, or the fetus may survive until the onset of labor only to suffer increasing asphyxia with the stress of advancing labor. Fetal asphyxia may also occur acutely as in maternal shock following abruptio placentae, uterine rupture, or compromise of the umbilical vessels by prolapse of the cord. In the fetus, asphyxia usually causes a loss of heart rate beat-to-beat variability. Late and prolonged fetal heart rate decelerations are signs of limited myocardial ability to withstand the stress of uterine contractions because of acute or chronic intrauterine asphyxia.

In contrast to the fetus, asphyxia in the newborn is always acute and related to intrapartum events or failure of the newborn airway to become established with sustained spontaneous ventilation. Most commonly the newborn lungs fail to become adequately aerated or perfused owing to central nervous system depression and absence of respiratory drive or airway obstruction by secretions. Failure to establish spontaneous ventilation immediately leads to asphyxia or greatly aggravates the existing consequences of intrauterine asphyxia.

Oxygen deprivation leads to the deteriorating pathophysiologic events listed in Table 25–4. Hypoxia, especially of the larger muscle masses and organs, causes tissue metabolism to revert to an anaerobic state with an accumulation of blood lactic acid. Failure of respiration leads to carbon dioxide accumulation, increasing production of carbonic acid, and respiratory acidosis. The end result is uncompensated metabolic and respiratory acidosis. The increased hydrogen ion concentration leads to a failure of bicarbonate buffering of the blood. Other blood buffering mechanisms, principally phosphates and hemoglobin, are overwhelmed and whole blood buffering capability fails, a base deficit rapidly accrues, and blood pH falls rapidly.

Worsening hypoxia and hypercarbia at first cause a maximal ventilatory effort in either the fetus or the newborn, but with advancing asphyxia ventilatory efforts fail and apnea ensues (see Table 25–4). A second effort at ventilation occurs at approximately 5 minutes in the form of gasping movements. Dawes (1968) described the second effort to breathe and noted that it gives way to a final period of apnea after 10 minutes of asphyxia. Secondary, or terminal, apnea may last up to 20 minutes with occasional agonal gasping movements, usually associated with fixed blood pH values of 6.8 or less.

Concomitant to these metabolic derangements of respiratory failure are changes in cardiac rhythm. Heart rate increases initially, causing increased cerebral vascular flow, myocardial perfusion, and slightly increased cardiac output.

Table 25–4. Pathophysiologic Events and Consequences of Birth Asphyxia

Physiologic Factor	Time from Birth			
	1 min	*3 min*	*5 min*	*10 min*
Respiratory Effort	Increased	Fails, becomes apneic	Returns briefly	Fails again, becomes agonal
Approximate Blood pH	7.25	7.15	7.00	6.75
Heart Rate	Increased	Falls	Plateau about 50 bpm	<50 bpm, becomes idioventricular
Cardiac Output	Slightly increased	Decreasing	Falling	Minimal
Pulmonary Blood Flow	Decreases rapidly	Decreasing	Minimal	Negligible
Cerebral Blood Flow	Slightly increased	Decreasing	Rapidly falling	Ischemia resulting in brain damage
Renal Perfusion	Unchanged	Decreasing	Rapidly declining	Ischemia, cortical necrosis

Like the fetal heart rate, the asphyxiated newborn heart will be tachycardic initially, followed by progressive bradycardia (see Table 25–4). After 5 minutes of asphyxia, a plateau of bradycardia at 50 beats per minute is usually noted. If resuscitation is not effective the heart rate declines further to a slow dysfunctional rhythm with increasing electrocardiographic R-R intervals, idioventricular contractions, and finally asystole.

Following the initial increased cardiac output, progressive asphyxia and bradycardia result in an ever diminishing cerebral blood flow. Cerebral ischemia and brain damage are most likely between 5 and 10 minutes of severe asphyxia in both the fetus and newborn. Similar perfusion losses occur in the gut and kidneys.

In the fetus pulmonary vascular flow is unchanged, but the newborn experiences a rapid decrease in pulmonary blood flow. In addition to the severe acid base derangements brought on by asphyxia, glucose and calcium metabolism are also disturbed. Because of poor cardiac output and decreased peripheral perfusion, large muscle groups and abdominal organs are deprived of oxygen and revert to anaerobic metabolism. Glucose utilization becomes inefficient, and energy demands of the brain and myocardium are met by an increased glucose consumption and rapid depletion of glycogen stores. Intravenous 10 percent glucose in water is required, but excessive glucose administration is to be avoided (Phibbs, 1981). Hyperglycemia may lead to increased lactic acid levels until adequate ventilation reestablishes normal oxidative metabolic processes.

Hypocalcemia has long been recognized as a frequently occurring clinical condition accompanying birth asphyxia (Tsang et al.,

1974). Total and ionized calcium values may be decreased. Increased hydrogen ion concentration may drive ionized calcium into bone or free it to complex with lactate in the face of the ever increasing lactic acidemia of asphyxia. Normal values for ionized calcium below 1.4 mEq/L are indicative of hypocalcemia. Total calcium to ionized calcium ratios of 2:1 should be maintained.

Intracellular red cell potassium depletion resulting from shifting of hydrogen ions into the red cells for hemoglobin binding and buffering action can lead to hyperkalemia. Depending on resuscitation success, the hyperkalemia may persist because of renal ischemia and anuria, or renal excretion of potassium may lead to hypokalemia once the acidosis is relieved and potassium ions begin to return to the intracellular space. Repeated serum determinations are required to assure potassium balance.

IMMEDIATE ASSESSMENT OF THE NEONATE

The need for resuscitation is dictated by the pathophysiologic events of asphyxia, but clinical indicators for initiating vigorous resuscitative procedures must be recognized immediately at birth from the infant's appearance. Dr. Virginia Apgar (1953) proposed a scheme for rapid clinical assessment that has become known as the Apgar Scoring System (Table 25–5). The severely compromised infant with a heart rate of 50 or less is hardly overlooked (Apgar score = 1), but varying degrees of birth asphyxia between scores of 1 and 7 require immediate attention and extended periods of close observation.

Any distressed infant (asphyxiated or suf-

Table 25–5. Apgar Scoring System

Criteria	Scores		
	2	1	0
Heart Rate	>100	<100	Asystole
Respiratory Effort	Crying with regular breath wounds easily heard	No crying, irregular efforts, gasping, weak breath sounds	Apnea
Reflex Irritability	Crying, grimacing, and withdrawal from painful stimuli	No crying, grimacing only, apathetic, minimal to no withdrawal from painful stimuli	Areflexia
Muscle Tone	Limb flexion, fetal positioning, voluntary activity	Minimal movement, weak response to stimulation	Amyotonia
Color	Completely pink	Central pinkness with blue hands and feet	Ashen

fering from other forms of shock) will give evidence for the Apgar scoring parameters. Gluck (1978) described variations of the basic Apgar observations for initial asphyxia for which prompt corrective measures will assure a return to normal. Like the fetus, the newborn will signal early distress (shock and/or asphyxia) with tachycardia (heart rate 140 to 160) with periods up to 200. With deepening but still reversible distress, heart rate begins to decline to rates of 120 to 100. Other signs of early but reversible neonatal asphyxia and distress noted by Gluck include heightened respirations, overreaction to stimuli, excessive body movements, and exaggerated reflexes.

Skin color and the general appearance of a distressed infant are difficult to consistently describe. In practice, a duskiness of forehead, lips, hands, and feet overlaying a deeper pinkish color has been referred to as "pink-on-blue" or "blue-on-pink" to connote the unusualness of color and to call attention to an early sign of neonatal distress. It is distinct from poor peripheral perfusion or vasoconstriction with mottling and an underlying gray cyanosis.

Steps for Resuscitation

AIRWAY AND VENTILATION

Recognition of respiratory failure requires immediate attention and the establishment of a patent airway in any resuscitation attempt. In the neonate, clearing of the airways

should have taken place with delivery of the head on the perineum and prior to the infant taking the first breath. As the head and neck of the fetus present, bulb suctioning of the nares and oropharynx should be routine. If excessive secretions appear in the pharynx, a DeLee suction catheter with trap can be passed to clear the upper airway and then advanced to empty the stomach (Fig. 25–4). If delivery is by cesarean section, a similar approach to clearing the airways can be taken. A 10 or 12 French suction catheter is more effective if thick or tenacious secretions are encountered. Immediately upon delivery of the infant, the head should be held slightly downward in a Trendelenburg position to avoid aspiration of any retained secretions.

As soon as the cord has been clamped and cut, the high-risk infant should be transferred to an overhead radiant warmer in either the delivery room or an adjacent resuscitation room. From the moment of the appearance of the head, visual examination gives some idea as to the infant's respiratory capabilities. Monitoring of heart rate should begin with the first minute by stethoscope and later electronically when time permits lead attachment. Heart rate greater than 100 by 1 minute of age allows for continued attempts to give tactile stimulation and observe for spontaneous respirations. This sequence of events is known as primary apnea and may continue as long as the heart remains above 100 in the first 1 to 3 minutes of life. During this period, suctioning of the upper airway should be avoided. Care must

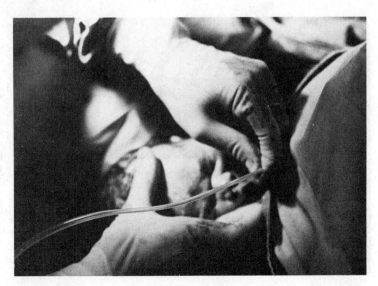

Figure 25–4. Fetus's head presenting on the perineum and obstetrician using DeLee trap suctioning of nasopharynx. This procedure is of special importance before the first breath in the presence of meconium-stained amniotic fluid. (Courtesy of K. TePas and University of Kentucky Medical Illustrations Department.)

be taken not to overly stimulate the posterior pharynx and produce vagal stimulation with reflex bradycardia. Tactile stimulation during primary apnea can take the form of brisk rubbing with a warm towel to dry the infant. Drying the infant reduces heat loss by evaporation while providing safe stimulation. Stimulating the birth-depressed infant by slapping the buttocks and soles of the feet or rasping the infant's back with the physician's knuckles can only be condemned.

If apnea persists and heart rate falls below 100 (within 1 to 3 minutes of life) asphyxia is worsening. Suctioning to provide a clear upper airway permits the next step: bag-and-mask ventilation using a properly fitting (newborn versus premature) soft rubber facemask with good seal about the nasal bridge, cheeks, and chin (Fig. 25–5). A collapsible rubber anesthesia bag, fitted with a connector, adapter, and elbow, is preferred. The bag is inflated from wall oxygen outlet and flowmeter. The volume of the bag should not exceed 750 ml. Other resuscitation bags and masks are available and include self-inflating bags and triggered mechanisms with preset oxygen and pressure limits. Self-inflating bags have valves that limit flow to 5 L/min, but this also limits oxygen concentration to less than 60 percent (usually about 40 percent). Pressure pop-off valves are built in and preset to inflating pressures of usually 30 to 35 cm H_2O. Airway pressure monitoring is not practical while ventilating with a self-inflating type of bag as opposed to the anesthesia flow-dependent bag. Triggered positive pressure ventilatory mechanisms as applied to some infant beds have excessively high pressure limits (50 cm H_2O), which may be inadvertently set too high, and excessively prolonged inspiratory times.

A major requirement and advantage of this system is the in-line aneroid manometer for breath-to-breath pressure monitoring. One is cautioned to closely watch the manometer to avoid overfilling of the bag and pressure buildup and transfer to lungs. For infant resuscitation, 100 percent oxygen is preferred for the short time required. Flows of 10 to 15 L/min are usually sufficient to inflate the bag and refill it after each breath at a ventilatory rate of 20 to 30 breaths/min. Adequate flow is also required to maintain flow through the bag to avoid carbon dioxide rebreathing. An inflation pressure of approximately 20 cm H_2O is usually adequate. Adequate lung inflation can be judged by the rise of the chest with each mechanical breath and by equality of breath sounds heard by stethoscope. Adequate ventilation is noted by a surge in heart rate from below 100 to a rate of 120 or higher. Mucous membrane color change to pinkness, increased skin perfusion, and spontaneous breathing movements are additional signs of the infant's improving condition and the abatement of asphyxia.

The majority of term infants with prolonged apnea and early bradycardia in the first 2 minutes of life will respond satisfactorily to airway management and recover from mild to moderate asphyxia at birth, but low birth weight infants, premature infants,

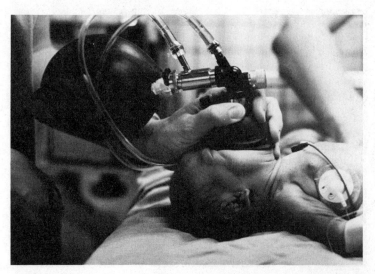

Figure 25–5. Bag and mask ventilation with adequate seal about face. Seal is supported by fourth and fifth fingers of attendant below the infant's chin and with the base of the attendant's palm against the infant's forehead. The seal should not be achieved by pressing the mask against the face and forcing the occiput against the mattress. (Courtesy of K. TePas and University of Kentucky Medical Illustrations Department.)

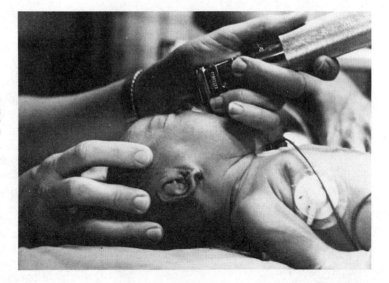

Figure 25–6. Left-handed laryngoscopy, leaving right hand free to pass endotracheal tube. Note only slight neck extension with insertion of blade. (Courtesy of K. TePas and University of Kentucky Medical Illustrations Department.)

and infants who have prolonged and chronic intrauterine hypoxia are less likely to do so.

With persistence of heart rate less than 100 with no return of respiratory effort, the infant is declared to have secondary apnea. At this point endotracheal intubation becomes mandatory to begin mechanical ventilation and reverse the effects of lost respiration and worsening hypoxia.

Establishment of an adequate airway and initiation of effective ventilation and respiration are the keys to successful infant resuscitation. All other measures are secondary to placing an adequate airway.

The apneic and bradycardiac newborn is severely hypoxic and acidotic by 3 minutes of life, and death is imminent unless effective ventilation and respiration can be established. The following steps must be taken:

1. Resuscitate the infant beneath a radiant warmer to maintain body heat.

2. Place the infant in a supine position with the neck slightly extended (Fig. 25–6).

3. Perform direct laryngoscopy using straight blades (either 10 cm for full term infant or 7 cm for premature infant).

4. Suction the hypopharynx under direct vision if secretions preclude visualization of epiglottis and vocal cords.

5. Pass a straight endotracheal tube (with or without a plastic-coated soft wire stylet) through the vocal cords (see Table 25–6 for size of tube to use).

6. Pass the tip of the tube through the cords:

    0.5 to 1.0 cm for infants 1000 g or less

    1.0 to 1.5 cm for 1000 to 2000 g infants

    1.5 to 2.0 cm for infants 2000 g or more

7. Immediately connect the endotracheal tube to a 500- to 750-ml anesthesia bag.

8. Begin ventilation at 20 to 30 breaths/min. Ventilate with 20 cm H_2O pressure per attached manometer. Inspiratory time to expiratory time should be in a ratio of approximately 1:2.

9. Listen for equality of breath sounds on the left and right sides of the chest. Look for a symmetric rise and fall of the chest with each mechanical breath.

10. Listen for a quickening heart rate and look for an improving color of mucous membranes.

11. If the heart rate improves to 120, fix an endotracheal tube by adequately taping it in place on the upper lip and anchoring it to the cheeks side-to-side (Fig. 25–7).

Table 25–6. Endotracheal Tube Size

Birth Weight (g)	Endotracheal Tube Internal Diameter (mm)	Comments
>3000	4.0	Needed for passage of 10 Fr suction catheter to clear larger volume of secretions; expect good fit
1250–3000	3.5	Usually passes easily into trachea; easy to pass 8 Fr suction catheter
850–1250	3.0	Most likely size to pass
<850	2.5	Larger endotracheal tube not likely to fit

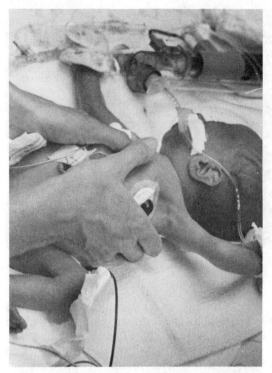

Figure 25–7. Simulated two-handed chest-encircling midsternal method of external cardiac massage. Note that in this very small infant the thumbs override, but in a larger infant, the thumbs would be side-by-side. (Courtesy of K. TePas and University of Kentucky Medical Illustrations Department.)

12. Continue ventilation manually with bag until the infant respirator can be attached or until the infant is able to regularly and effectively breathe with assistance and support his heart rate and color.

As soon as possible after resuscitation, a chest roentgenogram should be taken for lung appearance and endotracheal tube placement. Blood gas determinations should also be made as soon as possible to verify effectiveness of ventilation (i.e., restoration of oxygenation and compensation of acidosis).

After endotracheal intubation, arterial and/or venous umbilical catheters should be considered. Umbilical artery catheters afford blood gas sampling and central arterial blood pressure monitoring. An umbilical vein catheter allows for venous blood gas monitoring and central venous pressure monitoring if it can be documented by roentgenography to be above the diaphragm. Umbilical vein catheters can be quickly placed and secured and can serve as routes for drug, intravenous fluid, or colloid solution administration.

CIRCULATION

Support of circulation of the asphyxiated infant begins with effective ventilation and restoration of respiration. However, if heart rate should fail to rise above 100, external cardiac massage must be considered. If heart rate is documented at 80 bpm or less, external cardiac massage is mandatory (Chameides et al., 1980). During the first minute of life only estimates of heart rate can be made. The stethoscope is usually used to count heart rate, but palpation of cord pulse may also be useful. Attachment of electronic monitor leads may be difficult to impossible, and time should not be lost attempting technological finesse. Continuous stethoscope monitoring in the first 1 to 2 minutes by an assistant with estimates of heart rate made quickly will inform the resuscitation team of cardiac status and responses to airway placement and management.

Cardiac compression for the newborn infant, and especially the low birth weight infant, is specifically different from that described in most basic life support courses and guidebooks. First noted by Todres and Rogers (1975) and later included in Standards for Advanced Cardiac Life Support for Neonates (Chameides et al., 1980), it calls for open-handed encirclement of the newborn chest with thumb over sternum for cardiac compression (see Fig. 25–7). The fingers of both hands interlace to form posterior support of the spine and ribs. The palms stabilize the lateral walls of the chest, localizing the mediastinum medially. The thumbs (side-by-side in larger infants, or overlapped on smaller infants) are pressed downward (posteriorly) 1 to 2 cm. The chest should be compressed approximately 100 times per minute with maximum thumb pressure over the lower third of the sternum. Adequate cardiac compression can be documented if an umbilical artery line is in place and a pulse wave form can be observed. Occasionally palpation of the femoral artery by an assistant can be used to confirm adequate external cardiac compression. If continued mechanical ventilation and cardiac compression do not bring about improved heart rate (> 100 bpm) and improved color of the infant, drug therapy must then be considered.

PHARMACOLOGIC ADJUNCTS

Severe birth asphyxia may not respond to the previously mentioned measures, and drug support may be needed. It must be emphasized that only severe asphyxiating circumstances should be expected to include drugs for support of continued resuscitative efforts.

Certain medications have become recognized as the principal choices for infant resuscitation. Extensive lists of drugs for inclusion in resuscitation preparations lead to confusion. Table 25–3 lists those drugs most frequently noted for use in standardized resuscitation of neonates (Chameides et al., 1980).

Atropine is used for bradycardia with heart rate persisting below 100 but usually above 50. This suggests vagal overplay or vasovagal reflex that may follow pharyngeal suctioning or endotracheal intubation, and a single intravenous dose should increase heart rate. Complications of atropine may be excessive tachycardia and diminished cardiac output (Gregory, 1975). If heart rate continues at 50 or less, repeated doses of atropine will probably be to no avail.

Persistent bradycardia with severe metabolic acidosis may not be readily relieved by ventilation within the first 3 to 5 minutes. Alkali use may have to be considered. Sodium bicarbonate given intravenously should improve the pH and support improved cardiac responsiveness to ventilation. It is important to continue ventilation during the administration of sodium bicarbonate. Moreover, the use of alkalizing agents can improve cardiac response to both endogenous and exogenous catecholamines with a concomitant chronotropic effect. Trishydroxymethyl aminomethane (THAM) has proven to be an effective alkalinizer (Avery et al., 1981). Although not commonly used, it has been used clinically for more than two decades. Disadvantages of THAM include respiratory suppression in high concentrations (0.6 molar or greater), hyponatremia, hypokalemia, and hypoglycemia. Disadvantages of sodium bicarbonate include increased carbon dioxide content with rebound acidosis and hypernatremia. Central

nervous system hemorrhage following sodium bicarbonate use in low birth weight infants has been associated with resuscitation and the need to give large volumes of hypertonic solutions. Studies to date raise concerns about rapid expansion of blood volume in the absence of autoregulation of cerebral blood flow. Infusions of alkali and colloid substances in volumes of 5 to 10 cc must be given slowly in asphyxiated newborns, especially those of low birth weight with a propensity to central nervous system hemorrhage.

Epinephrine administered intravenously is indicated for refractory bradycardia (heart rate less than 50) following continued ventilation, external cardiac compression, and attempts at alkalization. Schematically, this would follow in time beyond 5 minutes, provided the umbilical vessel has been quickly catheterized. Intraarterial administration is absolutely contraindicated because of possible irreversible lower limb or organ ischemia. Intracardiac epinephrine may lead to myocardial ischemia, necrosis, and irreversible dysrhythmias. Additionally, the blind introduction of a needle into the chest carries the risk of pneumothorax, hemopericardium, and coronary artery laceration. Endotracheal administration of epinephrine via the endotracheal tube has been observed with chronotropic effects in resuscitation comparable to those observed when using nebulized racemic epinephrine in the treatment of bronchospastic disorders. Gregory (1975) also advocated using epinephrine in an attempt to convert a "flat-line" electrocardiogram in agonal birth asphyxia. Complications of excessive epinephrine use include tachycardia, hypertension, and ventricular fibrillation.

Hypoglycemia complicates birth asphyxia, and initiating a continuous infusion to keep intravenous and intra-arterial lines open also allows supplementation of body glucose. Monitoring capillary glucose by test strips through the first hour of life is essential.

In severe and protracted asphyxia and acidosis, calcium metabolism may be deranged and may result in low circulating ionized calcium. Subsequently the failing myocardium may continue to have low cardiac output because of altered contractility secondary to hypocalcemia. Calcium infusions are indicated when heart rate has increased but output remains low as evidenced by low blood pressure, poor peripheral perfusion, and weak pulses. Calcium is prepared in several forms, but the readily dissociable form of $CaCl_2$ is preferred (Chameides et al., 1980). Intravenous calcium infusions must be given slowly and with constant cardiac monitoring to avoid bradycardia. Intracardiac and intraarterial infusions of calcium solutions should not be undertaken because of the risk of vessel and tissue injury.

Occasionally, antepartum analgesia with morphine or other opiates will result in respiratory depression of the newborn. Usually respiratory depression is seen as primary apnea with heart rate remaining stable and tactile stimulation transiently improving heart rate and respirations. If the immediate antepartum history is positive for opiate analgesia, naloxone (Narcan) is a rapidly acting antagonist. Special packaging for neonatal unit dosage is available and should be used rather than ampules for adult dosage.

Administration of drugs during resuscitation carries considerable risk because of the uncertainty of route of administration. Umbilical vessels are used because of availability and the need for expediency. Hypertonic and sclerosing solutions are dangerous to hepatic portal vessels, and if administered through umbilical arteries renal, intestinal, and lower limb arteries are threatened. Intravenous routes are recommended. Umbilical vessels must be cautiously used.

Throughout the process of resuscitation following a high risk pregnancy, attention must be paid to the environment. Thermoregulation to avoid hypothermia in the infant is paramount. Hypothermia alone causes hypoglycemia, acidosis, dysrhythmia, and shock. If allowed to occur, no amount of resuscitative effort can successfully reverse both asphyxia and profound hypothermia. No data exist to support the notion that hypothermia is protective or helpful to the asphyxiated infant. Availability and use of servo control mechanisms for conserving infant body heat are mandatory for all resuscitation settings.

Accidents can occur if care in handling electrical outlets and high pressure lines is not exercised. Unnoticed suction lines have found their way to the skin of infants and produced suction-induced blisters.

After Resuscitation

At some point in the management of a sick infant, it is necessary to reassess the infant's condition with regard to moving him from the resuscitation area to either the neonatal intensive care unit or a tertiary care facility. This depends largely on the infant's response to intervention. The resuscitation team leader decides when and where the infant should be moved. Following a brief physical examination, the infant's destination is confirmed and the receiving facility notified of the mode of transport, expected time of arrival, and current condition of the infant. The parents should be apprised as soon as possible of the plans for transfer, their infant's condition, and the immediate expectations for the infant.

PHYSICAL EXAMINATION

A brief physical examination of the infant should be completed before the infant leaves the delivery/resuscitation area, with special consideration being given to cardiovascular and respiratory function (Table 25–7). Inspection for bruising, lacerations, paralysis, and fractures is necessary. An attempt to establish gestational age should be made, especially looking for age:size discrepancies. An evaluation of pulmonary and cardiovascular adjustment to extrauterine life includes:

1. Color (in and out of oxygen).
2. Ease of respirations.
3. Presence of excessive secretions.
4. Quality of breath sounds.
5. Peripheral perfusion.
6. Blood pressure.
7. Presence of murmurs.

A general assessment of the infant's overall condition should note tone, activity, and alertness with a final determination of body temperature, heart rate, respiratory rate, and blood pressure.

DISPOSITION AND OBSERVATION

All infants in high-risk delivery situations should be observed closely for at least 4 to 6 hours whether mother and child are bond-

Table 25–7. Guide for General Assessment in the Delivery Room

Feature	General Condition	Trauma	Maturity ≥ 36 weeks
General	Color and peripheral perfusion		Pink skin Flexion all limbs Diminishing vernix

Head	Appropriate size
	Dysmorphologic features
		Large cephalohematoma
		  or caput
		Bruising
		Petechiae
		Lacerations
		Depressed skull fracture
			Quick ear pinnae recoil
			Incurving ⅔ pinnae
			Head circumference
			  > 31 cm

Face	Alertness Obvious defects of palate and lip Copious secretions	Bruising Lacerations Paralysis (7th cranial nerve)	Absent facial lanugo
Thorax	Ease of respirations Quality of breath sounds Peripheral perfusion Blood pressure Murmur	Pneumothorax Diaphragmatic paralysis	1–2 mm breast tissue
Abdomen	Distended or scaphoid Number of cord vessels Masses Liver size Patent anus		Few visible vessels
Back	Deformities	Bruising Petechiae Lacerations	Patchiness or absence of lanugo

Limbs	Color
	Deformities
	Range of motion
	Muscle tone
		Bruising
		Lacerations
		Fractures
			Sole creases, anterior ⅔:
			  100° popliteal angle
			  20° ankle angle
			  45° wrist angle

Genitals	Sex distinction		Testes in scrotum
			Anterior scrotal rugae
			  and rubor
			Labia majora cover labia
			  minora
			Mons pubis present

Neuromuscular Condition	Alertness Spontaneous activity Muscle tone	Upper extremity paralysis (Erb's or Klumpke's)	Recoil arms and legs Strong grasp reflex Strong rooting reflex Complete Moro reflex

ing in a recovery room or if the infant has been removed to an observation nursery. Constant observation by skilled personnel includes 15-minute reassessment of temperature, respirations, heart rate, color, tone, and behavior. Generally, this should continue until all vital signs have been continuously normal for 1 hour.

Thermal control is a major concern, even for seemingly normal infants, but should not be a problem if the naked infant is placed against the mother's skin with warm blankets covering both. Overhead radiant warmers may provide supplemental heat if needed, but Freeman (1979) found that infant temperatures were warmer with skin-to-skin contact and blankets than with the use of a radiant warmer. If, for reasons of maternal health, a bonding period is not feasible with this attention to thermal control, then admission of the infant to the observation nursery is strongly recommended rather than a protracted period of observation in the delivery suite.

Special care facilities are required for any infant who has not made a smooth transition to extrauterine life. A preterm infant requiring oxygen and ventilation should be admitted to an intensive or special care nursery. Infants who require immediate special care include those with suspected pneumothorax, asphyxia, poor peripheral perfusion, poor muscle tone, hypertonia, or seizure-like activity. Any infant for whom vigorous resuscitation was required should be monitored in intensive care for the sequelae of birth asphyxia. If the delivering institution does not have facilities for intermediate or critical intensive care, consultation with a neonatal referral center may be considered.

PARENT CONTACT

The only circumstance under which an infant should leave the delivery area without parental contact is if the father is not present and the mother is under general anesthesia. If appropriately transported, a few moments can be made available for the parents to have face-to-face contact with the infant and time to touch a hand or foot. Usually it is unlikely that this will jeopardize the infant's condition. Failure to have even this brief contact may interfere with the parental attachment process later. Marut (1978) describes the earliest phase of the postpartum attachment process as the time in the delivery room when the mother identifies the child as her own. A few seconds of contact establish reality and assist the woman in assuming her new role as a mother.

During this brief contact, the parents should be informed of the general condition of the infant and the immediate plans for his care. Although it is important to be honest with the parents when they ask the inevitable, "Will the baby be all right?" it is also important to be as supportive as possible. Parents may have difficulty dealing with the reality of having an infant in crisis. Benfield and coworkers (1976) describe grief reaction in parents as often being out of proportion to the level of illness in the infant. The resuscitation team members should accept the parents' behavior and allow them to use their coping mechanisms to deal with their grief. The many technical details of the infant's condition or predicted hospital course can be relayed to them as their awareness of reality develops. The prime objectives of the resuscitation team at the time of transport are to allow parent-infant contact, establish the beginnings of reality, and build rapport with the parents.

TRANSPORT

During transport of the infant from the resuscitation area to an observation nursery or special care unit, three things should be provided for: thermal control, maintenance of required ventilatory support, and visibility of the infant. Much ground is lost if, after extensive resuscitation efforts, a sick infant becomes cold or disconnected from life support equipment while en route to a special care nursery. Radiant heat warming with skin temperature control allows personnel attending the infant and the parents to touch the infant without interruption of thermal control. New disposable thermal pads can be placed under the infant and can maintain temperature for 4 hours. A transport incubator equipped with a ventilator and cardio-pulmonary monitors is recommended for referral to special care centers. Good visibility of the infant is of special importance to prevent life support mechanisms from becoming dislodged.

Special Considerations

Some high-risk infants will require special attention in addition to resuscitation because of certain problems.

MECONIUM STAINING

The passage of meconium in utero is a presumed fetal response to asphyxia, but it is uncommon before 34 weeks gestation despite other signs of fetal distress. Amniotic fluid that is stained dark green and appears thickened poses a greater risk to the newborn (Phibbs, 1981) than yellowish fluid. The mere presence of meconium-stained fluid increases the risk of perinatal morbidity and mortality. Preventing the neonate from aspirating meconium present in the hypopharynx before delivery of the chest is the most effective means of minimizing pulmonary complications (Perez, 1981). As soon as the head and neck are delivered upon the perineum or through an abdominal incision, the obstetrician should suction the nasopharynx (see Fig. 25–4). Immediately after delivery, the infant should be examined with a laryngoscope to visualize the vocal cords. If meconium is seen on or below the vocal cords, the infant should have endotracheal intubation and mouth-to-tube suction. If significant meconium is found in the endotracheal tube, the procedure should be quickly repeated. Positive pressure ventilation should not be administered until after direct laryngoscopy and suction. The infant should receive free oxygen during the procedure via a catheter held close to the nose or mouth. Many of these infants will be depressed at birth, but some may be vigorous and crying. Nevertheless, it is recommended that after suctioning on the perineum by the obstetrician these infants be considered for laryngoscopy to clear any aspirated meconium in the upper airway. The morbidity and mortality of infants with meconium aspiration may be significantly decreased if they are thoroughly suctioned on the perineum and undergo direct tracheal suction immediately following birth (Bascik, 1977).

IMMATURITY

Birth asphyxia is a major hazard for the premature infant. Primarily owing to the immature respiratory system, it is often complicated by such perinatal conditions as antepartum hemorrhage, intrauterine infection, breech presentation, or protracted labor.

During aggressive delivery room management to reverse asphyxia, it is especially difficult to keep premature infants warm. Their absence of subcutaneous fat (as an insulator) and large surface-to-volume ratio leads to exaggerated heat losses. Quick, gentle drying, removing wet linen, and servo-operated radiant warmers will help to maintain normal body heat.

Bruising as a result of delivery trauma and excessive stimulation after delivery are common, as these infants have poor capillary integrity. Bruising may lead to excessive red blood cell breakdown and neonatal hyperbilirubinemia later. Gentle handling is a must.

Intraventricular hemorrhage, a common complication of asphyxia associated with prematurity, may be precipitated or exacerbated by a sudden rise in arterial pressure and a concomitant rise in cerebral blood flow. Rapid administration of "bolus" medications is to be avoided during resuscitation efforts because of the potential loss of cerebral blood flow autoregulation. Arterial pressure can also be elevated following infusion of hyperosmolar solutions and colloids. In-

fusion of all solutions and volume expanders should be done *slowly* to minimize the risk of intracranial hemorrhage (Volpe and Koenigsberger, 1981).

Although representing less than 1 percent of all live births, the extremely immature infant of less than 30 weeks gestation accounts for most neonatal deaths and neurologically handicapped infants born without congenital malformations. Today, many infants of 27 to 30 weeks' gestation (800 to 1500 grams) respond well to intensive care. If at all possible, these infants should be delivered in a setting with tertiary obstetric and neonatal services.

Birth asphyxia is the leading cause of death for very low birth weight infants. Delivery room resuscitation must be swift and effective. Gentle handling is a must. The skin of these infants is translucent with a friable capillary base that bruises with otherwise normal handling. Tactile stimulation of any kind is to be avoided. Heat loss is exaggerated in the infant less than 1500 grams. Blot the skin dry, remove all wet linens, and allow maximum exposure to radiant heat. Care must be taken not to obstruct the radiant heat by leaning over the infant or by covering the infant with drapes if umbilical catheterization is required.

MULTIPLE BIRTHS

Twin births require provisions for two resuscitation teams. Advance preparations for extra supplies and equipment should be made to assure readiness at the time of delivery. Although the second twin is more at risk for intrapartum asphyxia, the teams should be prepared for asphyxia in either infant. Premature onset of labor, premature rupture of membranes, and the need for cesarean section due to malpresentation are common complications of preterm deliveries. Birth weight discrepancies between the twins can be a sign of fetus-to-fetus transfusion and the resulting polycythemia of one infant and anemia of the other.

If intrauterine screening determines the presence of more than two fetuses, the incidence of both preterm delivery and neonatal complications increases markedly, and it is strongly recommended that these pregnancies be transported in utero to a tertiary center for obstetric and neonatal care.

Table 25–8. Some Birth Anomalies Whose Presence Alters Delivery Room Management

Anomaly	Recognition	Problems	Intervention
Encephalocele Myelomeningocele		Contamination leading to infection Respiratory impairment Increased heat loss through defect	Sterile gloves Moist-to-dry sterile saline dressings May require continued assisted ventilation
Choanal Atresia	Cyanotic and distressed at rest Pink when cries	Hypoxia Acidosis	Tape oral airway in place Position on back or abdomen
Diaphragmatic Hernia	Scaphoid abdomen Absent breath sounds Cyanosis	Severe respiratory distress secondary to abdominal contents in chest Hypoplastic lung Pneumothorax	Nasogastric tube to suction If ventilation required, intubate trachea
Esophageal Atresia with Tracheo-esophageal Fistula	Hoarse cry Excess oral secretions Respiratory distress	Aspiration of saliva Aspiration of stomach contents	Elevate head Prevent aspiration Continuous upper airway suction
Gastroschisis Omphalocele	External abdominal contents with or without protective membrane	Increased heat loss through exposed viscera Risk of infection Risk of bleeding if traumatized	Maintain thermal control Sterile gloves Sterile saline wet-to-dry dressings
Ambiguous Genitalia			Make parents aware of problem early Do not assign sex role
Epidermolysis Bullosa	Large fluid-filled bullae Excoriated skin	Increased risk of infection Increased fluid loss Increased heat loss Exfoliated skin obstructing airway or GI tract	Sterile linen, gloves Mask Minimal handling No tape Do not apply identification bands

BIRTH ANOMALIES

Although 4 per cent of children are born with some major birth defect, few require alteration in delivery room management of the infant. However, some conditions can be identified as requiring special attention in the delivery room (Table 25–8).

Myelomeningocele and encephalocele are examples of neural tube defects that are obvious in the delivery room. Care must be taken to prevent infection due to contamination of the exposed meninges. Use sterile technique, wet-to-dry sterile dressings. Position the infant on his abdomen to avoid pressure on the lesion.

Infants are obligate nasal breathers. Choanal atresia must be suspected if the newborn is distressed and cyanotic at rest yet pink when crying (mouth breathes). The diagnosis is strongly suggested if a soft rubber catheter cannot be easily passed through each nostril. Position the infant on his side or abdomen and tape an oral airway in place to provide adequate intake of air.

Diaphragmatic hernia occurs once in every 3000 live births and should be suspected in the infant who has a scaphoid abdomen and is greatly distressed at birth. These infants should be intubated but ventilated with caution, as hypoplastic lungs and pneumothoraces are common complications. A nasogastric tube is required to keep the stomach decompressed and reduce thoracic pressure caused by the displacement of dilated bowel. These infants require rapid transport for emergency surgery.

Infants who have esophageal atresia with tracheoesophageal fistula may present in the delivery room with excess oral secretions, a hoarse cry, and respiratory distress. Aspiration pneumonia is the immediate danger. These infants should be positioned with the head elevated to reduce gastric acid aspiration through the fistula; with a nasogastric tube placed in the pouch, intermittent suction will help to avoid aspiration of saliva.

Gastroschisis and omphalocele present with bowel external to the abdominal wall. Omphaloceles are covered with a translucent membrane that may or may not survive delivery. In either instance, risk of trauma to the bowel and infection are of prime concern. Delivery room management should include gentle handling with sterile gloves and wrapping the sac and/or bowel with wet-to-dry saline dressings. The infant will have increased heat loss via the exposed bowel, and added thermal control is needed.

Ambiguous genitalia are mentioned because all parents are anxious to know whether their infant is a boy or a girl. Hurried sex assignment without understanding the infant's anatomy, endocrine physiology, and chromosome constitution can have serious social and emotional consequences for the family in later years. If the genitalia appear indeterminate, the problem of sex assignment should be discussed with the parents in the delivery room.

DRUGS

There are many medications that affect the growth and development of the fetus if taken by the mother during pregnancy. Certain drugs, regardless of their long-term effect on the fetus, alter or compromise the fetus/newborn's ability to adapt to extrauterine life. Drugs that may affect the newborn in the delivery room are listed in Table 25–9 (narcotic agents have been mentioned with birth depression).

INFANTS OF DIABETIC MOTHERS

Despite careful obstetric and anesthetic management, infants of diabetic mothers (IDM) remain at greater risk for birth asphyxia. The incidence of hyaline membrane

Table 25–9. Drugs That May Affect the Newborn in the Delivery Room

Antepartum Drugs	Immediate Effects on Neonate
Propylthiouracil	Fetal goiter with airway obstruction
Propranolol	Hypoglycemia Respiratory depression Bradycardia
Reserpine	Respiratory depression Lethargy Nasal obstruction
Lithium	Hypotonia Respiratory distress
Magnesium	Respiratory depression Hypotonia Hypotension Hypocalcemia
Alcohol	Hypoglycemia Hypotonia
Heroin	Respiratory depression (reversed with Naloxone)
Ritodrine	Hypoglycemia Hypotension (may be unresponsive to volume expansion) Hypocalcemia

disease is 5 to 6 times greater for premature and near-term IDM. Maternal hyperglycemia predisposes the infant to hypoglycemia, and continuous serum glucose monitoring is mandatory until values remain within normal limits and regular feedings are established.

Rh ISOIMMUNIZATION AND HYDROPS FETALIS

Erythroblastosis fetalis following Rh isoimmunization of the mother may be mild and may require only minimal attention at delivery. However, hydrops fetalis is a severe manifestation of Rh disease, and delivery room preparations for resuscitation must be maximal. In addition to airway management, circulatory assessment is especially important. Most Rh affected hydropic infants have low hematocrit and hemoglobin values. The resuscitation team must plan for an early packed red blood cell exchange transfusion. O-negative, low-titer, anti-A and anti-B blood should be immediately available. A packed red blood cell isovolumetric exchange transfusion to increase the hematocrit to 32 to 40 percent within the first hour of life may be life-saving in the face of severe hydrops fetalis or cardiopulmonary failure.

Routine Care

When the newly delivered infant requires vigorous resuscitation for survival, some of the routine newborn procedures may be forgotten. Identification procedures, gonococcal eye prophylaxis, and vitamin K administration remain important aspects of the newborn infant's delivery room care.

The infant should be identified before leaving the delivery room even if he is in crisis at the time. Identification bands (prepared before delivery and including mother's name, hospital number, infant's sex, and date and time of delivery) can be attached to the infant's arm and leg without interrupting resuscitation efforts. Footprinting can be omitted. Individual institutional protocols differ, but arm and leg banding is the *minimal* recommendation for identification before the infant leaves the delivery room. If properly banded, the infant's footprint impressions may be done after he is admitted to a nursery.

Documentation of gonococcal eye prophylaxis will assure that, if the procedure has not been completed in the delivery room (commonly owing to the poor condition of the infant), the nursery staff will be aware of the need to complete it.

The neonate is deficient in vitamin K–dependent coagulation factors and may develop significant bleeding. The administration of 0.5 to 1.0 mg of intramuscular vitamin K corrects prolonged prothrombin time. Stressed and premature infants are at a great risk for developing these bleeding problems and should receive vitamin K in the delivery room or upon admission to the nursery.

Long-Term Outcome

Low Apgar scores and ultimate infant outcome are difficult to correlate. Information originating from the Collaborative Project on Cerebral Palsy, Mental Retardation, and Other Neurological and Sensory Disorders of Infancy and Childhood (Drage and Berendes, 1966) reported poor neurologic outcome with low 1- and 5-minute Apgar scores. More recent studies, however, especially of very low birth weight infants, reveal more encouraging results. Nelson and Ellenberg (1981) found that for children who had Apgar scores of 0 to 3 at 10 minutes or later and had survived with intensive resuscitation, 80 percent were free of major handicap at early school age. Similarly, Westgren and colleagues (1982) have reported that intensive obstetric and neonatal management of 72 infants weighing less than 1500 grams resulted in 88 percent of all surviving infants being neurologically normal at 2 years of age. One third of these infants had prolonged asphyxia with Apgar scores of less than 7 at 10 minutes. On a case by case basis, the chances for recovery in normal development following severe birth asphyxia can be documented. In a series of 31 children surviving severe birth asphyxia, Thompson and coworkers (1977) reported 93 percent of the infants to have no serious neurologic or mental handicap at 5 to 10 years of age at follow-up. They defined severe birth asphyxia as a condition in which infants have a 1-minute Apgar of 0 or a 5-minute Apgar of less than 4. They concluded that the quality of life enjoyed by the majority of survivors was a clear justification for a positive approach for intensive resuscitation of all severely asphyxiated neonates.

Apgar scoring should not be looked upon as a predictor of outcome but as a scheme to call forth appropriate resuscitative measures. Attempts to correlate scores with fetal and newborn scalp serum pH values have shown wide discrepancies (Sykes et al., 1982). Apgar scores of 0 at 1 to 5 minutes should not preclude a maximal first response by the resuscitation team.

Seizure activity during the first week of life is currently being evaluated by Dennis and Chalmers (1982) as an indicator of the efficacy of perinatal care and the effectiveness of resuscitation measures. They suggest that a seemingly successful resuscitation followed by serious seizure disorder may be an index of either chronic intrauterine asphyxia with ineffective intervention or inadequate postdelivery resuscitation measures for birth asphyxia. A study of severely asphyxiated infants followed to 5 years of age by Mulligan and coworkers (1980) revealed that the most common neurologic abnormalities were spastic diplegia and choreoathetosis. They reported that most of the neurologically impaired children also had serious intellectual deficits. Postasphyctic seizures were closely associated with both the severe neurologic and intellectual deficits.

Parent Information and Education

All too often parents are given only a brief view of their high-risk infant before he is transferred to the intensive care area. To understand the impact this may have on the parent-infant unit, it is necessary to briefly look at the development of parent-infant attachment and how the imperfect child may interfere with that process.

Although a common worry for all pregnant couples is that their infant will not be normal, they may become anxious with the onset of labor. Prospective mothers and fathers carry set expectations with them to the delivery suite, and if all has gone well up to the time of admission, they expect a healthy infant. Delivery of the healthy infant tends to reinforce their previous expectations of their baby. Contact with the infant facilitates the bonding process. Indeed, bonding at this stage (in the first hours after delivery) is primarily unidirectional (parent-to-infant), rapid, and facilitated by physical contact (Taylor, 1980).

High-risk parents have different perceptions of their pregnancies. Johnson (1979) has identified several feelings that are associated with parents during high-risk pregnancies, including denial, guilt, feelings of failure, and anticipatory grief. Denial may be used as a defense against prenatal attachment to an infant who may die. Pregnancy is thought of as a normal physiologic process, and parents (especially the mother) may feel guilty, blaming themselves for being unable to have a normal pregnancy. If the parents associate success as a man or woman with successful childbearing, they may have feelings of failure. Anticipatory grief is used by these parents to prepare themselves for loss of the child they envision. These feelings develop with their increasing knowledge of the high-risk pregnancy and accompany the parents to the delivery room.

During the activity of preparation in the delivery room, it is important for the parents to receive ongoing support from the staff. Honesty is crucial. Johnson (1979) reports that although information regarding the status of the fetus may be stressful, lack of information is more stressful. Relating positive as well as negative information is important. A positive statement about fetal heart tones sounding good, when spoken in an encouraging manner, will help parents to cope with their fears.

If the high-risk mother has required prolonged hospitalization in the labor area, it is helpful if the obstetrician introduces the parents to members of the neonatology team. Parents are reassured to see familiar persons whose only concern is the welfare of their baby. Since most people have a great fear of the unknown, it is helpful if the neonatology team has briefly described to the parents what immediate steps will be taken for their infant.

After delivery, both parents focus immediately on the infant. During the resuscitation it is vital that someone provide them with information about the baby. Unfortunately, the parents' need for information comes at a time when the resuscitation team is most preoccupied. The leader of the neonatal team should decide what is to be said and how, so that the parents do not receive conflicting reports.

If the infant is immature or ill, the parents must be told the reality of the situation. The mother's condition may not permit her to visit the nursery for hours or days, and the initial delivery room contact will help her to begin to know her real infant. Pictures may be provided to help her identify with her infant until she is able to visit. Unless healthy, the infant will differ from the infant the parents have anticipated during the pregnancy. Delivery room personnel must be prepared for the anxiety and grief displayed by parents when faced with the appearance of their infant (Affonso, 1976). Generally the specifics of long-term outcome are not dealt with in the delivery room for the simple reason that they are usually not known at the time.

Before leaving the delivery room, the neonatal team should assure the parents that they will return with specific information regarding the child's status as soon as possible. At this time, the neonatology team can begin to explain how the infant is doing and what interventions are to be undertaken once the infant reaches the special care nursery.

For the parents, delivery of an immature, sick, or deformed infant is just the beginning of a period of attachment and adjustment to the fact that the infant is not healthy. The maternal/infant dyad is most fragile when the infant is imperfect. Although the delivery room time is brief, supportive behavior by the obstetric and neonatal staff can have a positive influence by reducing stress for the parents by providing honest information, understanding their grief, supporting their coping mechanisms, and promoting contact with their infant.

REFERENCES

Affonso, D.: The newborn's potential for interaction. J. Obstet. Gynecol. Nurs. 5:9, 1976.

Apgar, V.: A proposal for a new method of evaluation of the newborn infant. Anesth. Analg. 32:260, 1953.

Avery, M. E., Fletcher, B. D., and Williams, R. G.: The lung and its disorders. In The Newborn Infant. Philadelphia, W. B. Saunders Co., 1981, p. 338.

Bascik, R. T.: Meconium aspiration syndrome. Pediatr. Clin. North Am. 24:463, 1977.

Benfield, D., Leib, S., and Reuter, J.: Grief response of parents after referral of the critically ill newborn to a regional center. N. Engl. J. Med. 294:975, 1976.

Brown, J. K., Purvis, R. J., Forfar, J. O., et al.: Neurological aspects of perinatal asphyxia. Develop. Med. Child Neurol. 16:567, 1974.

Chameides, L., Melker, R. J., Raye, J. R., et al.: Advanced cardiac life support for neonates. In Standards and Guidelines for Cardiopulmonary Resuscitation and Emergency Cardiac Care. JAMA 244:495, 1980.

Dawes, G.: Foetal and Neonatal Physiology. Chicago, Year Book Publishers, 1968, p. 149.

Dennis, J., and Chalmers, I.: Very early neonatal seizure rate: A possible epidemiological indicator of the quality of perinatal care. Br. J. Obstet. Gynecol. 89:418, 1982.

Drage, J. S., and Berendes, H.: Apgar scores and outcome of the newborn. Pediatr. Clin. North Am. 13:635, 1966.

Freeman, M.: Giving family life a good start in the delivery room. Am. J. Maternal Child Nurs. 4:51, 1979.

Gluck, L.: Special problems of the newborn. Hosp. Pract. 13:75, 1978.

Gluck, L.: Fetal lung maturity. In Proceedings of the Seventy-Eighth Ross Conference on Pediatric Research. Columbus, 1979, p. 256.

Gregory, G. A.: Resuscitation of the newborn. Anesthesiology 43:225, 1975.

Johnson, S. H.: High Risk Parenting. Philadelphia, J. B. Lippincott Co., 1979, p. 10.

Korones, S. B.: High Risk Newborn Infants: The Basis for Intensive Nursing Care. St. Louis, C. V. Mosby Co., 1981, p. 68.

Marut, J. S.: Special needs of cesarian mothers. Am. J. Maternal Child Nurs. 3:202, 1978.

McManus, F., Rang, M., Chance, G., et al.: Is cerebral palsy a preventable disease? Obstet. Gynecol. 50:71, 1977.

Mulligan, J. C., Painter, M. J., O'Donooyhue, P. A., et al.: Neonatal asphyxia. II. Neonatal mortality and long-term sequelae. J. Pediatr. 96:903, 1980.

Nelson, K. B., and Ellenberg, J. H.: Apgar scores as predictors of chronic neurologic disability. Pediatrics 68:36, 1981.

Nesbitt, R. E. L., and Aubry, R. H.: High-risk obstetrics. II. Value of semi-objective grading system in identifying the vulnerable group. Am. J. Obstet. Gynecol. 103:972, 1969.

Perez, R.: Protocols for Perinatal Nursing Practice. St. Louis, C. V. Mosby Co., 1981, p. 224.

Phibbs, R. H.: Delivery room management of the newborn. In Avery, G. B. (ed.): Neonatology: Pathophysiology and Management of the Newborn. Philadelphia, J. B. Lippincott Co., 1981, p. 199.

Resnick, R.: Principles of organization of an obstetrical unit from scratch. Clin. Perinatol. 3:323, 1976.

Sheldon, R.: Management of perinatal asphyxia and shock. Pediatr. Ann. 6:15, 1977.

Standards and Recommendations for Hospital Care of Newborn Infants. Evanston, IL, American Academy of Pediatrics, 1977, p. 25.

Sykes, G. S., Johnson, P., Ashworth, F., et al.: Do Apgar scores indicate asphyxia? Lancet i:494, 1982.

Taylor, P. M.: Parent-Infant Relationships. New York, Grune & Stratton, 1980, p. 81.

Thompson, A. J., Searle, M., and Russel, G.: Quality of survival after severe birth asphyxia. Arch. Dis. Child. 52:620, 1977.

Todres, I. D., and Rogers, M. C.: Methods of external cardiac massage in the newborn infant. J. Pediatr. 86:781, 1975.

Tsang, R. C., Chen, I., Hayes, W., et al.: Neonatal hypocalcemia in infants with birth asphyxia. J. Pediatr. 84:428, 1974.

Volpe, J. J., and Koenigsberger, R.: Neurologic disorders. In Avery, G. B. (ed.): Neonatology: Pathophysiology and Management of the Newborn. Philadelphia, J. B. Lippincott Co., 1981, p. 943.

Westgren, M., Ingemarsson, I., Ahlström, H., et al.: Delivery and long-term outcome of very low birth weight infants. Acta Obstet. Gynecol. Scand. 61:25, 1982.

26

GENETIC COUNSELING

ANNE L. MATTHEWS
ANN C. M. SMITH

Genetic counseling is "a communication process which deals with the human problems associated with the occurrence or the risk of occurrence of a genetic disorder in a family" (Ad Hoc Committee on Genetic Counseling, 1975). The multifaceted process of genetic counseling involves a team approach to assist families or individuals in dealing with genetic disorders and their implications for the family now and in the future. In general, the process includes five major areas of concentration:

1. Providing information concerning the disorder or problem and all its ramifications, i.e., diagnosis, prognosis, future risk, etc.
2. Helping the family comprehend the information provided.
3. Discussing client management options and referring to appropriate health care resources.
4. Presenting alternatives with respect to future family planning.
5. Supporting the family in their decisions and assisting them in making the best possible adjustment to the problem.

By its very nature, genetic counseling demands the expertise, effort, and time of many health professionals in order to be an effective avenue of health care maintenance and prevention. The following chapter will discuss the overall impact of genetic disease, basic patterns of inheritance, environmental influences, appropriate indications for genetic counseling, and the genetic counseling process. Emphasis has been placed on the family's most common questions and concerns regarding pregnancy and reproduction.

Incidence of Genetic Disease

Health professionals have become increasingly aware of a need for genetic services in virtually every aspect of health care. Since the time of Gregor Mendel in the 1800's, the knowledge base in the arena of human genetics has dramatically increased, with huge strides having been made since the 1950's. McKusick's catalog presently lists over 2500 disorders with known inheritance patterns (McKusick, 1979). Additionally, many common disorders such as cancer, mental illness, diabetes, coronary heart disease, and gout are now known to have a genetic component. For the woman who is pregnant or considering pregnancy, a normal healthy infant is the hoped-for outcome. And yet, 0.5 to 1 percent of all liveborn infants are documented to have a chromosome abnormality; 4 to 7 percent of perinatal deaths are said to be due to chromosome aberrations; and it is estimated that at least half of all first trimester miscarriages have abnormal chromosome complements (Pawlowitski, 1972). Among the newborn population, 3 to 5 percent will have a major congenital malformation, most of which are found to have a genetic component. In the United States alone, this accounts for more than a quarter of a million affected children each year. If one then examines the impact (social, financial, emotional, and so on) of these children on their families, birth defects affect more than 15 million Americans in one way or another.

Another area of importance is mental retardation. It is stated that approximately 3 percent of the general population is mentally retarded (Opitz, 1980). In the severe form of mental retardation, the risk of illness and death early in life is high. Further, it is estimated that 70 percent of mental retardation in the general population can be attributed to genetic causes (Opitz, 1980). Clearly, then, the effect of genetic disorders is not isolated to a few affected individuals but extends to thousands of individuals or at risk individuals and their families. Certainly, pregnancy initiates a heightened awareness of particular risks and concerns. The future of genetic counseling services in the detection, treatment, and prevention of genetic disorders is very promising. Through increased awareness by health care providers and collaborative efforts, genetic counseling services offer a reasonable and important avenue of preventive health care.

Development of Cytogenetic Techniques

In 1956, Tjio and Levan opened a new era in the field of human cytogenetics by developing an effective technique for analyzing human chromosomes. Based on their technique, it was documented that humans have 46 chromosomes in each somatic cell, instead of 48 as previously reported (Tjio and Levan, 1956). In 1959, Lejeune and colleagues described the chromosomal basis of Down's syndrome, thereby opening the way for rapid advances in clinical genetics (Lejeune et al., 1959). Since that time, cytogenetic techniques have become more precise, and many syndromes have now been documented to have a chromosomal etiology.

THE HUMAN GENOME

In each human somatic cell, there are 46 chromosomes (*diploid* number). The germ cells, i.e., sperm and egg, contain the *haploid* number of chromosomes, 23. Chromosomes are the structural elements in the cell nucleus composed of DNA (deoxyribonucleic acid) and proteins that contain genes, the smallest inherited unit of the genome. For each somatic cell there are 23 pairs of

homologous chromosomes, with one member of each pair being inherited from each parent. Of the 23 homologous pairs, 22 are known as autosomes (non sex chromosomes), and one pair is known as the sex chromosomes, X and Y. In the normal female, the sex chromosomes are represented by two X chromosomes, and in the normal male, they are represented by an X and Y chromosome (Figs. 26–1 and 26–2).

During the metaphase stage of cell division, human chromosomes can be seen under the microscope as distinct entities with identifiable landmarks. Chromosomes are described as having two arms joined at a central region, the *centromere* (Fig. 26–3). Chromosomes are then arranged according to a standardized format based on size known as a *karyotype*. This pictorial display of chromosomes can be obtained by doing a chromosome analysis. Although any tissue in the body can be used (e.g., skin, bone marrow, amniotic fluid), the analysis is usually performed on peripheral blood lymphocytes. The obtained cells are first stimulated to undergo mitosis and are then arrested during metaphase by the use of colchicine. The preparation is then placed in a hypotonic solution so that the cell membrane swells and bursts, allowing the chromosomes to spread. The preparation is stained and placed under a microscope. The chromosomes are then photographed, enlarged during the printing process, and cut out to be arranged so that a complete karyotype is provided.

With the advent of new banding techniques (G, R, C, and high resolution banding), it is now possible to identify not only abnormalities of chromosome number but small additions or deletions of chromosome material as well as rearrangements of chromosome material (Caspersson et al., 1968). The new banding techniques have identified many individuals who were said to have normal chromosomes as actually having abnormal chromosome constitutions. This becomes an important finding, since even small aberrations in chromosomes can cause clinical abnormalities such as slow growth and development of mental retardation. What is important for the clinician to note is that a child need not have gross major malformations to be affected by a chromosome abnormality. Thus, chromosome analysis may be appropriate even when clinical

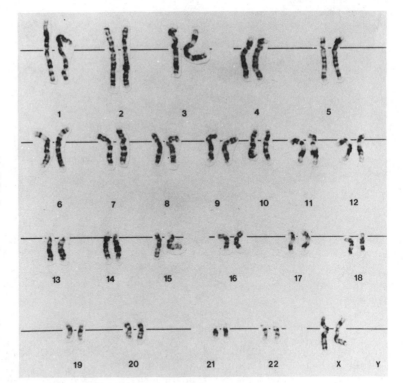

Figure 26–1. Normal female karyotype: 46,XX. (Courtesy of The Children's Hospital, Denver, CO.)

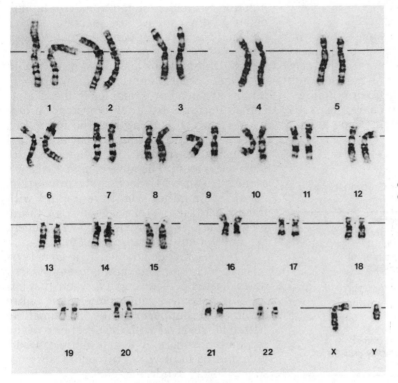

Figure 26–2. Normal male karyotype: 46,XY. (Courtesy of The Children's Hospital, Denver, CO.)

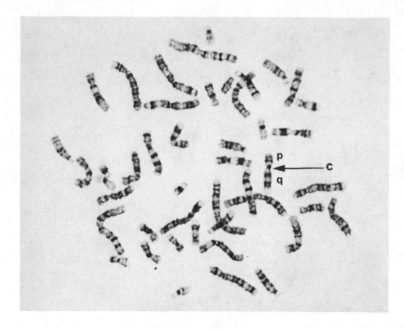

Figure 26–3. Metaphase spread. Note: p = short arm of chromosome; q = long arm of chromosome; c = centromere. (Courtesy of The Children's Hospital, Denver, CO.)

manifestations are mild (Table 26–1). In either case, it would appear that too much or too little chromosome material produces adverse effects on normal physical and/or mental development.

CLASSIFICATION OF CHROMOSOME ABNORMALITIES

Abnormalities of chromosomes occur in both the autosomes and sex chromosomes. Two major categories of abnormalities can occur: (1) those of chromosome number, and (2) those of chromosome structure. Following the discussion of these categories, specific clinical aspects of chromosome abnormalities will be presented.

Table 26–1. Indications for Chromosome Analysis

Suspected chromosome syndrome
Multiple malformations with or without associated mental retardation
Positive family history of X-linked mental retardation (fragile X syndrome)
Ambiguous genitalia
Abnormal sexual development (primary amenorrhea, lack of secondary sexual characteristics)
Multiple miscarriages
Possible balanced translocation carrier
Acquired chromosomal abnormality (leukemias, environmental hazards)

Numerical Abnormalities (Aneuploidy)

Cells with abnormalities of chromosome number (aneuploidy) have an unbalanced set of chromosomes due to either an excess or deficiency of an entire chromosome. Aneuploidy can arise by a variety of mechanisms. The most common cause is *nondisjunction*, which is the failure of two homologous chromosomes to separate during meiosis. The resulting gamete may then contain one too many or one too few chromosomes. Union of this aneuploid gamete with a normal gamete then leads to aneuploidy in the zygote. For example, if the gamete containing the extra chromosome unites with a normal gamete, then the individual will have 47 chromosomes. That individual is considered *trisomic* for whatever chromosome is extra. The most common trisomy seen is trisomy 21, Down's syndrome (Fig. 26–4). For families who have a child with trisomy 21, the risk of recurrence for future pregnancies is approximately 1 percent (Thompson and Thompson, 1980).

A *monosomy* occurs when a gamete is missing a chromosome and is united with a normal gamete, resulting in a zygote that has 45 chromosomes. Monosomy of an entire chromosome appears to be incompatible with fetal survival with the exception of the sex chromosomes. A female fetus can survive and be born with only one X chromosome, Turner syndrome, 45,X.

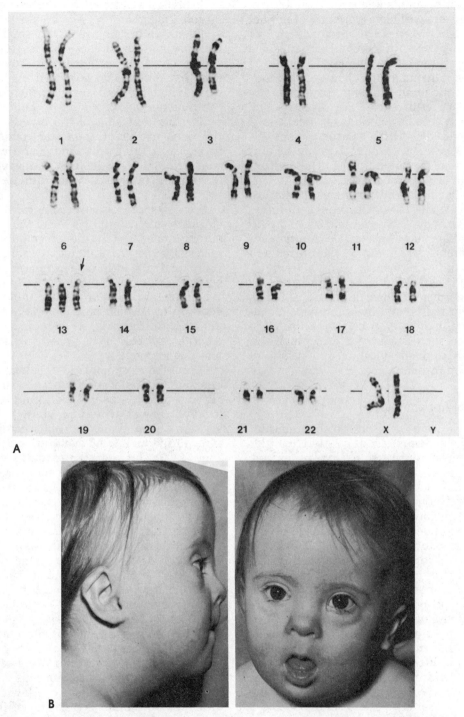

Figure 26–4. *A,* Karyotype of a patient with trisomy 21, Down's syndrome: 47,XY, + 21. Arrow denotes extra chromosome 21. *B,* Infant with Down's syndrome. (*A* courtesy of The Children's Hospital, Denver, CO. *B* from Smith, D. W.: Recognizable Patterns of Human Malformation, 3rd ed. Philadelphia, W. B. Saunders Co., 1982, p. 13.)

If nondisjunction occurs after fertilization (i.e., mitotic nondisjunction), then the resulting zygote will have a mixture of normal and aneuploid cells. This produces two or more cell lines with different chromosome numbers within the individual. This specific type of nondisjunction is known as *mosaicism*. Mitotic nondisjunction may occur any time after fertilization. For example, in Down's syndrome mosaicism, one tissue may contain cells with 47 chromosomes (trisomy 21), whereas another contains the normal number of chromosomes. The concept of mosaicism becomes particularly important in diagnosis and prognosis for the individual. Again, in the situation of an infant with Down's syndrome mosaicism, the clinical findings may be classic, minimal, or nonapparent, depending on the degree and location of the mosaicism. Thus, an individual with Down's syndrome who has normal or near normal intelligence should be investigated for the possibility of mosaicism. Additionally, it may be necessary to examine more than one tissue system (e.g., blood and skin) to define the location and degree of mosaicism present.

Structural Abnormalities

Thus far, we have discussed abnormalities of chromosome number only. Abnormalities of chromosome structure involve a loss, gain, or repositioning of the chromosome material. Structural abnormalities are deletions, additions, duplications, inversions, and translocations. Presently, over 100 structural abnormalities have been described (deGrouchy and Turleau, 1977). A deletion is a loss of chromosome material. In humans, the most common deletion seen involves a loss of chromosome material at the end of the chromosome (terminal deletion). Occasionally, loss of an intervening segment (interstitial deletion) occurs. Deletions may be lethal or they may be associated with severe phenotypic effects. One of the more common deletion syndromes is the cri du chat syndrome (cat cry syndrome) caused by the deletion of the short arm of chromosome 5 (5p-).

Structural abnormalities involving the presence of additional chromosome material are classified as duplications or additions. Duplications arise through errors in chromosome replication or errors in crossing over during cell division. The term *partial* trisomy is used to describe the presence of segments of additional or duplicated chromosome material.

When two breaks occur in a single chromosome and the intervening segment becomes inverted (turned upside down), the resulting abnormality is known as an *inversion*. If the inverted segment includes the centromere, the inversion is known as a *pericentric inversion*. If the inverted material does not involve the centromere, the inversion is known as a *paracentric inversion*. Prior to the availability of new banding techniques, inversions were difficult to detect.

A translocation involves the exchange of chromosome material between two or more chromosomes. If all the essential genetic material is present, although rearranged, the individual is said to be a *balanced translocation carrier* and is phenotypically normal. When the translocation results in the loss or addition of chromosome material, the individual is said to have an *unbalanced translocation* and may have an associated abnormal phenotype.

One of the most common unbalanced Robertsonian translocations occurs between chromosomes 21 and 14, resulting in translocation Down's syndrome. These individuals are phenotypically indistinguishable from individuals who have the classic trisomy 21. In this case, the karyotype reveals 46 individual chromosomes with a structurally abnormal number 14 chromosome. On further analysis, there is an extra number 21 chromosome fused to the number 14 chromosome (Fig. 26–5). Unlike the karyotypically normal parents of children with trisomy 21 Down's syndrome, some cases of translocation Down's syndrome have been inherited from one of the parents. The parental karyotype reveals 45 chromosomes with one of the number 21 chromosomes fused to a number 14 chromosome (Fig. 26–6). Figure 26–7 illustrates the possible zygotes resulting from the mating of a balanced translocation carrier and his spouse.

The risk of occurrence of Down's syndrome if the mother is a carrier of the balanced translocation is stated to be approximately 10 percent. If the father carries the translocation, then the risk is lower, approximately 2 to 5 percent (Thompson and Thompson, 1980). Although the 14/21 translocation appears to be one of the most common, any chromosome may be involved, and

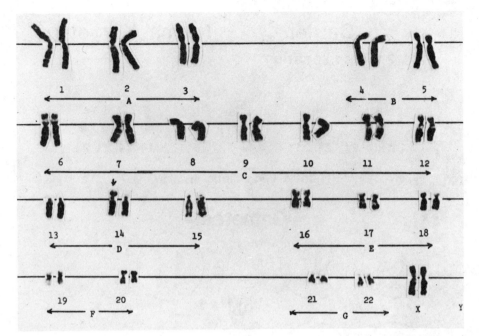

Figure 26–5. Karyotype of a patient with Down's syndrome as a result of an unbalanced 14/21 translocation. Arrow denotes an extra 21 chromosome fused to a 14 chromosome. (Courtesy of Dr. Arthur Robinson, Denver, CO.)

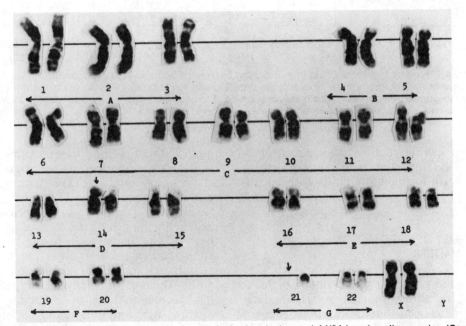

Figure 26–6. Karyotype of a clinically normal parent who is a balanced 14/21 translocation carrier. (Courtesy of Dr. Arthur Robinson, Denver, CO.)

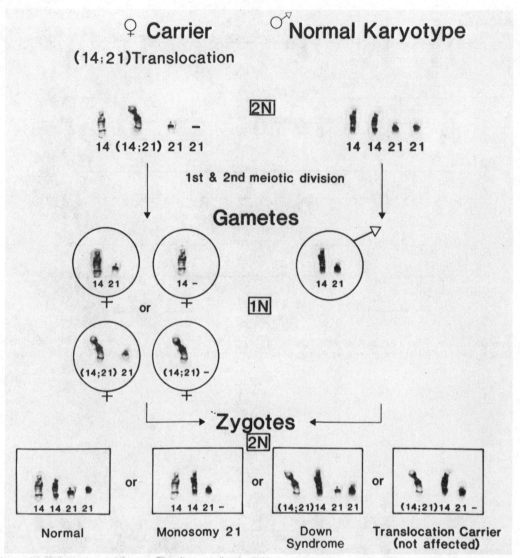

Figure 26–7. Possible zygotes resulting from a mating between a balanced (14/21) translocation carrier female and a karyotypically normal spouse. Note that the zygote giving rise to a fetus with Down's syndrome results from the maternal gamete, which contains both the translocated chromosome and a normal chromosome 21. Monosomy 21 is lethal, and this pregnancy would result in early spontaneous abortion. (Courtesy of The Children's Hospital, Denver, CO.)

a parent having such a balanced chromosomal rearrangement is potentially at increased risk for having a child with an unbalanced chromosomal rearrangement.

ETIOLOGIES OF CHROMOSOME ABNORMALITIES

With the continuing refinement of techniques for chromosome analysis, medical genetics has been able to illuminate some of the possible etiologies of chromosome abnormalities. Three major areas have been

identified that are important for the primary health care provideer to be aware of: (1) advanced parental age; (2) radiation; and (3) gene regulation.

Advanced parental age historically has dealt with the age of the mother at conception. It has been well documented that women 35 years and older are at an increased risk for a fetal chromosome abnormality (Goad et al., 1976). It is hypothesized that the maternal age of the ovum in combination with environmental factors interferes with normal spindle function during meiosis and results in nondisjunction. Paternal age has traditionally been associated with an increase of mutations at the gene level and has only recently been investigated as a possible cause for chromosome abnormalities (Stene et al., 1977). Recent studies of data from live births and amniocentesis registries have indicated no evidence for a consistent paternal age effect independent of maternal age (Cross and Hook, 1982).

X-ray and other sources of radiation have been documented to cause chromosomal breakage and possible rearrangements, thereby increasing the risk for a chromosome abnormality (Uchida, 1977). Routine preventive measures to minimize the amount of radiation exposure should be taken whenever possible (i.e., shielding and not scheduling elective x-rays within 10 days of the onset of the last menstrual period).

Genes regulating nondisjunction have been documented in other species and thus similar hypotheses have been raised in human beings (Thompson and Thompson, 1980). Empiric data have demonstrated that in some families who have a family member with a trisomy there is an increased risk for future offspring to also have a trisomy. This genetic predisposition does not include families where there is a familial translocation.

CLINICAL ASPECTS OF AUTOSOMAL ABNORMALITIES

A few common chromosome disorders are discussed in this section. The following is intended as an outline or guide and is not an exhaustive discussion of any of the disorders.

Down's Syndrome

Down's syndrome is the most common chromosome abnormality, with an incidence of approximately 1 in 600 live births. In the absence of major complications such as severe cardiac abnormalities, individuals with Down's syndrome live fairly long lives and are usually moderately to severely mentally retarded (Penrose and Smith, 1966; Gayton and Walker, 1974). Since the disorder has significant sequelae, it is important to diagnose it as soon after birth as possible. When the diagnosis is suspected, a chromosome analysis should be performed to delineate the specific etiology of the disorder (trisomy versus translocation). This information be-

comes paramount in providing the family with accurate genetic counseling.

The phenotypic features of individuals with Down's syndrome are often obvious at birth. The major clinical features are (see Fig. 26–4, B):

CNS: Mental retardation
Hypotonia at birth; improving with age
Head: Depressed nasal bridge
Mongoloid slant of eyes
Epicanthic folds
Brushfield spots (white speckling of the iris)
Protruding tongue
High arched palate
Low set ears
Flattened occiput
Broad short neck
Extremities: Shortened metacarpals
Abnormal dermatoglyphics:
Transverse palmar crease (simian line)
Increased number of ulnar loops
Arch tibial on hallucal area

Congenital heart disease is present in approximately one half of individuals affected with Down's syndrome; gastrointestinal and urinary tract abnormalities are also seen. There are no reported cases in the literature of affected males reproducing (unless mosaicism was present), but affected females have been known to reproduce (Riccardi, 1977).

Trisomy 18

Trisomy 18 (Edwards' syndrome) is a severe chromosome abnormality seen in approximately 1 in 6000 live births. Major features include (Fig. 26–8):

CNS: Mental retardation
Severe hypertonia
Microcephaly
Head: Prominent occiput
Low set and/or malformed ears
Corneal opacity
Ptosis (drooping of the eyelids)
Micrognathia
Extremities: Overriding clenched fingers
Abnormal dermatoglyphics
Rocker bottom feet
Other: Congenital heart disease
Single umbilical artery

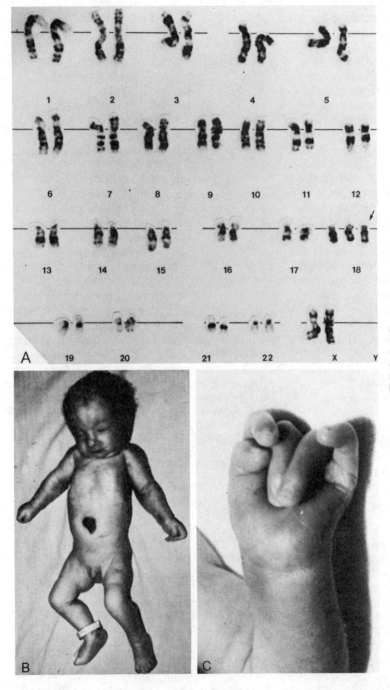

Figure 26–8. *A,* Karyotype of a patient with trisomy 18: 47,XX,+18. Arrow denotes extra chromosome 18. *B,* Newborn with trisomy 18. *C,* Characteristic posturing of the fingers of a newborn with trisomy 18. (Courtesy of The Children's Hospital, Denver, CO.)

Renal abnormalities
Cryptorchidism
Gastrointestinal tract abnormalities

The diagnosis of trisomy 18 should be confirmed since the prognosis is grim; 30 percent of affected infants die within the first month of life, 90 percent by 1 year, and 99 percent by age 10. Those infants who have survived the first year of life have been found to be profoundly retarded (Taylor, 1968).

Trisomy 13

Trisomy 13 (Patau's syndrome) is seen in about 1 in 5000 live births. The major clinical findings include (Fig. 26–9):

CNS: Mental retardation
Brain abnormalities
Head: Microcephaly
Microphthalmia
Malformed ears
Micrognathia
Cleft lip and palate

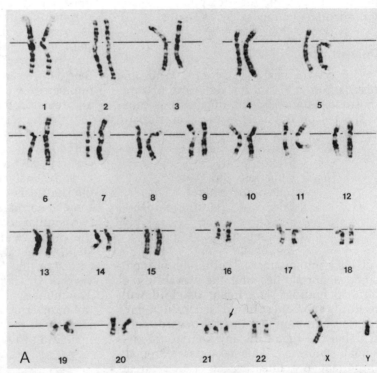

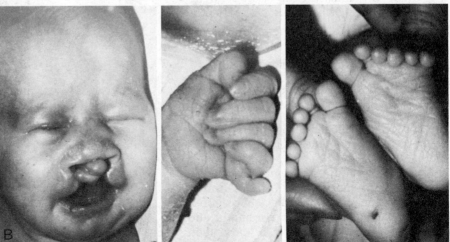

Figure 26–9. *A,* Karyotype of a patient with trisomy 13: 47,XX,+13. Arrow denotes extra chromosome 13. *B,* Newborn with trisomy 13. Note bilateral cleft lip and palate and polydactyly of hands and feet. (Courtesy of The Children's Hospital, Denver, CO.)

Extremities: Polydactyly
              Abnormal posturing of fingers
              Abnormal dermatoglyphics
    Other: Congenital heart defects
              Gastrointestinal tract defects
              Reproductive system defects
              Hemangiomas
              Scalp defects

As in trisomy 18, the prognosis for infants born with trisomy 13 is extremely poor. Over one half of the affected individuals die within the first month of life, and 95 percent succumb by age 3 years. All affected individuals have been profoundly retarded, and no individuals are known to have survived to adulthood with the exception of those with documented mosaicism (Taylor, 1968).

Deletion 5p-

The cri du chat, or cat cry, syndrome results from a loss of the short arm of chromosome number 5. The diagnosis is often suspected on the basis of the characteristic cat-like cry. Other features include:

    CNS: Mental retardation
            Microcephaly
    Head: Hypertelorism
            Epicanthic folds
            Downward slanting palpebral
              fissures
            Low set ears
            Micrognathia

Given the number of different chromosome abnormalities and the variability of clinical findings, any infant or child with multiple anomalies should be considered for banded chromosome analysis regardless of whether the infant fits any known chromosomal syndrome. This becomes extremely important in delineating the etiology, treatment, and prognosis of such an affected child.

Sex Chromosome Abnormalities

Abnormalities of the sex chromosomes are relatively common, occurring in approximately 1 in 500 live births (Gerald, 1976). In addition, they account for approximately 25 percent of spontaneous abortions (Riccardi, 1977).

A discussion of the abnormalities involving the sex chromosomes requires an understanding of the Lyon hypothesis. In response to questions concerning sex chromatin and gene dosage compensation, Dr. Mary Lyon

(1961) published her *inactive X hypothesis*, which proposes the following:

1. Females at an early embryonic stage inactivate one of the two normal X chromosomes present.

2. All descendants of that cell have the same inactivated X.

3. Inactivation is a random and independent process in each individual cell.

The inactive X forms a dark staining mass in the nucleus known as the *Barr body*, or X chromatin body (Fig. 26–10, A). Cells containing one or more X chromatic bodies are said to be chromatin-positive; those lacking these bodies are chromatin-negative. The most common procedure used to observe X chromatin is the buccal smear. Cells, which are scraped from the inside of the cheek, are stained and microscopically examined for the presence of Barr bodies. The number of Barr bodies seen is always one less than the number of X chromosomes present. In normal females, there is one Barr body, representing the inactive X chromosome. A normal male is Barr body–negative since he has only one X chromosome. Since a buccal smear is only a screening technique, a chromosome analysis should be done to confirm the diagnosis of the suspected sex chromosome abnormality.

A similar technique is used to screen for the presence of the Y chromosome. After staining buccal mucosal cells with a fluorescent dye, the Y chromosome appears as a very bright body within the cell nucleus. The number of Y bodies in a cell is equal to the number of Y chromosomes present. Normal males have one Y body and normal females have no Y bodies (Fig. 26–10, B).

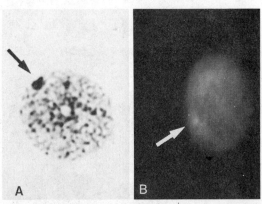

Figure 26–10. *A*, Positive buccal smear. Arrow denotes Barr body within the cell nucleus. *B*, Nucleus of lymphocyte noting fluorescent Y body. (Courtesy of The Children's Hospital, Denver, CO.)

Two of the most common sex chromosome abnormalities are Turner's syndrome (45,X) and Klinefelter's syndrome (47,XXY).

Turner's Syndrome

Turner's syndrome has a frequency of approximately 1 in 10,000 female live births. However, the 45,X karyotype represents the most common chromosome abnormality found in spontaneous abortions (Carr and Gedeon, 1977). Major clinical findings in females with Turner's syndrome include:

Short stature
Webbed neck
Low posterior hairline
Shield-like chest
Widely spaced nipples
Cubitus valgus
Primary amenorrhea
Streak ovaries
Underdeveloped secondary sex characteristics
Congenital heart disease (50 percent with coarctation of the aorta)
Renal abnormalities

Intellectually, females with Turner's syndrome are usually within the normal range, although some learning disabilities, particularly perceptual difficulties, have been noted (Robinson et al., 1979).

The diagnosis of Turner's syndrome is often not made until puberty, when the absence of menses and short stature become concerns. Occasionally the diagnosis can be suspected in female infants at birth by the presence of redundant skin on the back of the neck and marked lymphedema of the dorsum of the hands and feet (Fig. 26–11).

Klinefelter's Syndrome

The incidence of 47,XXY karyotype in newborn males is approximately 1 per 1,000 (Hook and Hamerton, 1977). In general, the term Klinefelter's syndrome refers to those males with a 47,XXY chromosome constitution and the following phenotype:

Tall stature
Eunuchoid body shape
Underdeveloped secondary sex characteristics
Gynecomastia
Small testes
Azoospermia

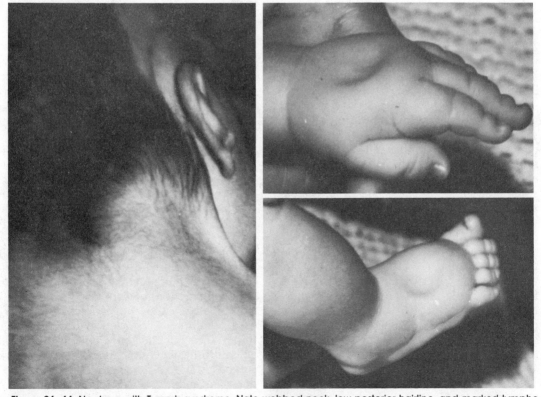

Figure 26–11. Newborn with Turner's syndrome. Note webbed neck, low posterior hairline, and marked lymphedema of hand and foot. (Courtesy of The Children's Hospital, Denver, CO.)

Intellectual development ranging from normal intelligence to mild mental retardation has been reported in males with Klinefelter's syndrome (Robinson et al., 1979).

A number of other sex chromosome abnormalities have been described. It would appear that in most cases an increasing number of X and/or Y chromosomes leads to an increasing number of physical and mental abnormalities.

Fragile X Syndrome

In his description of a family with X-linked mental retardation, Lubs (1969) identified a fragile site on the X chromosome (Xq28). With the identification of other affected individuals, the fragile X syndrome (marker X) is now recognized as one of the most common causes of mental retardation in the male population (Herbest and Miller, 1980). The major physical characteristics are large ears, prominent maxilla, large hands, and macroorchidism. Mental retardation varies from mild to severe, with the greatest delays noted in language development.

MENDELIAN INHERITANCE

Single gene disorders that follow the classic Mendelian patterns of inheritance are classified as autosomal dominant, autosomal recessive, X-linked dominant, or X-linked recessive. In these disorders the abnormality occurs at the gene level and is the result of either a single gene or pair of abnormal genes. For any given trait an individual possesses, there is a pair of genes working in concert with one another. The paired genes are located on homologous chromosomes and occupy a specific place on the chromosome, known as the *locus*. An individual is said to be *homozygous* for a particular trait when two genes at a given locus are identical. The individual is said to be *heterozygous* for a particular trait when two different genes are present at a given locus. Alternate forms of genes occurring at a given locus are known as *alleles*. For many traits, there may be only one form of a particular gene; for others, multiple alleles may exist. For example, an individual may be homozygous for blood type A (AA), in which both genes at the ABO locus are identical. Or, the individual may be heterozygous for blood type, such as AB. In this case, one gene is the A allele and the other gene is the B allele. Any change in a gene's form is known as a *mutation*. Although the majority of mutations are inconsequential to normal growth and development, on occasion a gene mutation results in a disease process or malformation. We will now discuss the major types of Mendelian inheritance patterns.

Autosomal Dominant Inheritance

A condition is inherited in an autosomal dominant fashion when the disorder manifests itself in the heterozygous state. That is, the abnormal or mutant gene overshadows the normal gene. Autosomal dominant disorders are characterized by the following (Fig. 26–12):

1. Multiple generations of affected individuals. An affected individual usually has one affected parent.

2. Both males and females are affected and both sexes can transmit the gene.

3. There is male-to-male transmission. This concept is important, as it rules out X-linked inheritance.

4. Offspring of affected individuals have a 50 percent risk (one half) of inheriting the gene.

5. Individuals who do not have the abnormal gene cannot transmit the disorder to their offspring.

6. New mutations may occur. Given a negative family history and normal parents, a child with an autosomal dominant disorder is presumed to represent a new mutation. Parents in this case would not be at increased risk in future pregnancies.

7. Variable expressivity may exist with respect to phenotype. That is, clinical findings may differ among affected individuals. This becomes important to the clinician when making a diagnosis, as there may only be mild symptomatology in affected individuals.

McKusick's catalog currently lists over 1200 autosomal dominantly inherited disorders. Some of the more common are Huntington's chorea, neurofibromatosis (von Recklinghausen's disease), and polycystic kidney disease. Dominant disorders with particular importance for the pregnant woman are achondroplasia; connective tissue disorders such as Marfan's syndrome; bleeding disorders, particularly von Willebrand's disease; and acute intermittent porphyria.

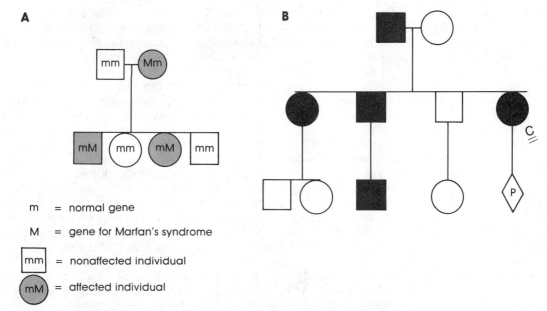

m = normal gene

M = gene for Marfan's syndrome

mm = nonaffected individual

mM = affected individual

Figure 26–12. *A,* Potential genotypes of a mating between an affected female and an unaffected spouse. *B,* Autosomal dominant pedigree.

Autosomal Recessive Inheritance

A condition is inherited in an autosomal recessive fashion when the disorder manifests itself in the homozygous state. To be affected, the individual must have two abnormal genes. The individual is considered to be a carrier in the heterozygote state with the normal gene overshadowing the abnormal gene. Carriers are usually phenotypically normal. Autosomal recessive disorders are characterized by the following (Fig. 26–13):

1. Most affected individuals have phenotypically normal parents. Pedigrees show affected individuals within sibships.

2. Both males and females are affected and both sexes can transmit the gene.

3. Parents who are carriers of the same abnormal gene have a 25 percent risk (one fourth) with each pregnancy of having an affected child.

4. Unaffected offspring of two carrier parents have a two thirds chance of being a carrier.

5. The incidence of consanguineous mat-

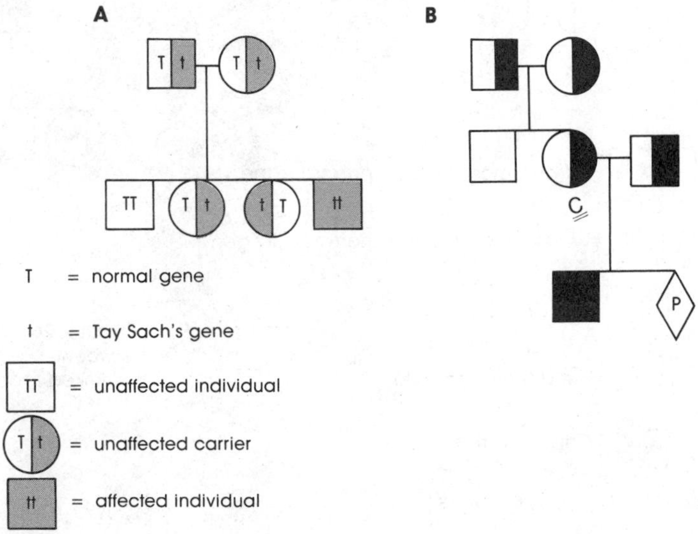

Figure 26–13. *A,* Potential genotypes of a mating between two carrier parents. *B,* Autosomal recessive pedigree.

T = normal gene

t = Tay Sach's gene

TT = unaffected individual

T t = unaffected carrier

tt = affected individual

ing is often increased. There is a higher probability that two related individuals will have the same gene in common than that two unrelated individuals will.

6. The clinical picture is often relatively severe.

7. In instances where affected individuals reproduce, all of the offspring must be carriers for the disorder.

The vast majority of biochemical disorders are inherited in an autosomal recessive manner. For a number of these disorders, biochemical assays are available to detect the heterozygote carrier state. For example, carriers of Tay-Sachs disease have approximately half the normal enzyme activity for hexosaminidase A. Thus, the phenotypically normal carrier is biochemically abnormal.

Common autosomal recessive disorders seen are cystic fibrosis, galactosemia, and phenylketonuria (PKU). Recessive disorders that should have special consideration during pregnancy are PKU and the hemoglobinopathies, e.g., sickle cell anemia and SC disease.

X-Linked Recessive Inheritance

X-linked (or sex-linked) disorders are those for which the abnormal gene is located on the X chromosome. Females who have two X chromosomes are considered to be heterozygote carriers; i.e., the normal gene on the chromosome overshadows the abnormal gene on the other X chromosome. In general, carrier females are clinically normal. Males who have a gene for an X-linked recessive disorder are affected since they have only one X chromosome. Genes located on the Y chromosome have not been shown to be paired with those on the X chromosome. The most distinguishing characteristic delineating X-linked disorders from autosomal disorders is the absence of male-to-male transmission. As males pass on their Y chromosomes to sons, a son cannot receive an X-linked disorder from his father. Only females are able to pass on an X-linked disorder to male offspring. Other major characteristics of X-linked recessive disorders are (Fig. 26–14):

1. Usually only males are affected. On rare occasions, carrier females may manifest some clinical signs and symptoms of the disorder.

2. Affected males are related through carrier females.

3. There is a 50 percent risk (one half) that a female carrier will have an affected son.

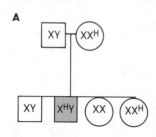

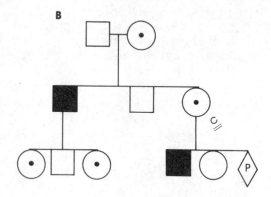

X = X chromosome with normal gene

X^H = X chromosome with hemophilia gene

XY = unaffected male

XX = unaffected female

$X^H Y$ = affected male

XX^H = carrier female

Figure 26–14. *A,* Potential genotypes of a mating between a carrier female and an unaffected spouse. *B,* X-linked recessive pedigree.

4. There is a 50 percent risk (one half) that a female carrier will have a carrier daughter.

5. Males affected with an X-linked disorder cannot pass the disorder on to their sons; conversely, all of their daughters are *obligate* carriers.

6. If only one affected male is seen in a pedigree, the possibility of a new mutation should be considered. Approximately one third of lethal disorders affecting males are caused by new mutations (Thompson and Thompson, 1980).

There are approximately 200 X-linked disorders now described (McKusick, 1979). Common X-linked disorders include glucose-6-phosphate dehydrogenase deficiency (G-6-PD), Duchenne's muscular dystrophy, color blindness, hemophilia, and Lesch-Nyhan syndrome. X-linked disorders that need to be followed closely during pregnancy are hemophilia A and B.

X-Linked Dominant Inheritance

Relatively few genetic disorders exhibit X-linked dominant inheritance. The most common is the Xg blood group system. In this particular pattern, the abnormal gene located on the X chromosome overshadows the normal gene; therefore, heterozygous females as well as males are affected. The major characteristics include the following:

1. No male-to-male transmission.

2. All daughters of an affected male will be affected.

3. Affected females have a 50 percent risk (one half) of having affected offspring regardless of sex.

MULTIFACTORIAL INHERITANCE

In contrast to Mendelian disorders where a single gene pair is involved, multifactorial disorders are thought to result from an additive effect of *many genes* interacting with environmental factors. In the majority of cases, the environmental factors cannot be identified. Usually, this pattern of inheritance is more complex and less straightforward than Mendelian inheritance and is associated with smaller risk figures. The frequency of multifactorial disorders may vary with respect to ethnic background. For example, neural tube defects have an increased incidence among English and Irish populations. Some of the most common and familiar isolated malformations are inherited in a multifactorial fashion, such as cleft lip and palate, neural tube defects (anencephaly and meningomyelocele), clubfoot, dislocated hips, hypospadias, and pyloric stenosis. Additionally, there are many other common disorders considered to have a multifactorial etiology: diabetes, allergies, cancers, cardiac disorders, affective disorders, and some forms of mental retardation. Major characteristics of multifactorial inheritance include:

1. Risk figures are based on empiric data. In general, there is a 2 to 5 percent risk of recurrence among first degree relatives of an affected individual.

2. There is often a sex bias; e.g., pyloric stenosis is more common in males; congenital dislocated hips are more common in females.

3. The risk of recurrence is greater if the affected individual is of the less commonly affected sex.

4. The risk of recurrence increases with the severity of the disorder. For example, parents of a newborn with congenital aganglionic megacolon (Hirschsprung's disease) involving a long segment of bowel have a greater risk of recurrence in future offspring than if only a small segment of bowel was affected.

5. The more family members affected, the greater the risk of recurrence. This is in contrast to Mendelian disorders, where the risk remains constant.

THE ENVIRONMENTAL ETIOLOGY OF MALFORMATIONS

In the newborn population, 2 to 4 percent of infants will have a recognizable malformation. If the period of ascertainment is extended beyond the first year of life, this figure increases to 4 to 6 percent as those previously unrecognized malformations present themselves. A portion of the previous section of this chapter has dealt with congenital malformation of a known genetic etiology. This section will concentrate on the environmental causes of malformations.

Congenital malformations are structural defects present at birth resulting from abnormal tissue differentiation and/or abnormal tissue/organ interaction during fetal development (Warkany, 1971). Approximately

10 percent of congenital anomalies are known to have an environmental etiology (Wilson, 1973). Since Gregg (1941) first demonstrated a relationship between maternal rubella during pregnancy and fetal malformations, it has become increasingly evident that a variety of environmental agents can have a deleterious effect on the developing fetus. Those agents capable of causing malformation are classified as teratogens and include drugs and chemicals, radiation, congenital infection, and maternal environment.

Prerequisites for a Teratogenic Effect

When considering the teratogenic effect of agents on the developing embryo, four major factors must be considered: (1) genetic susceptibility of the fetus; (2) time of exposure to the agent; (3) pharmacologic properties of the agent; and (4) dosage.

The *genetic susceptibility (or predisposition) of the fetus* is an important factor in determining whether a specific agent will be teratogenic. Although the majority of research regarding the teratogenicity of agents has been generalized from animal models, caution must be taken when extrapolating these data to humans. Agents shown to be teratogenic in certain animals may have no association with birth defects in humans, and vice versa. For example, evidence implicating the drug thalidomide as a teratogen in the human embryo was overwhelming, whereas early animal data demonstrated little or no evidence of a teratogenic effect. Additionally, susceptibility within species may vary according to individual genetic make-up. Thus, the risk to the fetus may vary even in the presence of a documented teratogenic agent.

The *time of exposure* to a teratogenic agent is an important determinant of the effect on the developing fetus. The period of embryogenesis from 2 to 8 weeks postconception appears to be the most vulnerable time for the fetus. Exposure to a teratogenic agent during this time may result in multiple malformations. Exposure prior to this time (conception through implantation) results in either early fetal wastage or no apparent effect. During the second and third trimesters, exposure to these agents does not result in gross malformations but may produce functional pathology.

The *nature and pharmacologic properties of an agent* determine its interaction with developing fetal tissues. Prior to the early 1960's, it was a common belief that the placental barrier offered effective protection to the fetus. However, current data have shown that a number of agents and/or their breakdown products readily cross the placental barrier in both animals and humans. Thus, a single agent may not prove to be teratogenic, but its breakdown products will represent a significant risk to the developing embryo.

The *dose of an agent* represents another important determinant in producing a teratogenic effect. In many animal models, a dose response relationship has been demonstrated (McClearn, 1977). This hypothesis has now been extrapolated to humans and appears to be appropriate, at least in some instances. For example, a dose response curve has been demonstrated in fetal alcohol syndrome, with a higher blood alcohol level being associated with a more severe clinical picture (Smith, 1980).

Teratogenic Agents

Radiation. Ionizing radiation was the first environmental agent shown to be teratogenic in humans (Warkany, 1971). During the 1920's, pregnant women who were treated with therapeutic doses of radiation for pelvic malignancy gave birth to children with severe birth defects including microcephaly, skeletal defects, and mental retardation (Heinonen et al., 1977). An increased incidence of congenital malformations was also noted in children born to women who were pregnant at the time of the Hiroshima and Nagasaki atomic bomb explosions (Wood, 1969; Satow and West, 1955).

From a genetic standpoint, radiation exposure is cumulative and may result in a variety of outcomes. Radiation may produce a change at the gene level (multigenic), at the chromosome level (clastogenic), at the cell level (oncogenic), or at the tissue/organ level (teratogenic). The effects of radiation depend on the dosage and time of exposure. Fetal tissues are most susceptible to radiation damage during the first trimester when the cells are rapidly dividing and differentiating. Exposure to high doses of radiation (>10 rads) during the first 3 weeks following conception is more likely to result in spontaneous abortion, whereas weeks 4 through 12 place the fetus at increased risk for major malformations (Swartz and Reichling, 1978). Radiation exposure after the first trimester is not likely to cause either miscarriage or anomalies; however, it has been associated with an increased incidence of childhood leukemias (Stewart and Kneale, 1970).

For couples who wish to minimize their risks, the following precautions are appropriate: shielding of the pelvis and abdomen whenever possible; for females, scheduling of elective x-rays during menses or within 10 days of onset; and, for males, delaying conception for 6 to 8 weeks following exposure.

Drugs and chemicals. It is important to understand the effects of drugs during pregnancy, since they represent an area over which we have some control. In general, the time during gestation when the drug is taken determines whether and what type of embryotoxicity will result. A variety of mechanisms by which drugs produce abnormalities have been hypothesized. Drugs may (1) disturb a critical phase in embryologic development by causing cell death and/or altering cell migration; (2) alter the hormonal environment; or (3) interfere with physiologic functions. Relatively few drugs have been positively implicated as being teratogenic in humans. A variety of drugs are suspected of having a teratogenic potential although they have yet to be clearly established as known teratogens. On the other hand, certain drugs have been used widely enough in control situations to warrant exclusion from the list of potential teratogens.

Table 26–2 lists some of the drugs that have been documented to represent a definite and/or suspected hazard to the fetus. A few of these drugs, as well as alcohol, will now be discussed briefly.

Thalidomide demonstrates the classic example of a teratogen. Introduced as a remedy against influenza in the mid 1950's, thalidomide was also recommended as a sedative and tranquilizer. Five years later after the birth of over 8000 infants with similar limb malformations, the drug was withdrawn. Thalidomide proved to be extremely teratogenic when taken 6 to 8 weeks after the last menstrual period (Goldman, 1980).

Alcohol. In 1973, Jones and colleagues described a group of children with a characteristic phenotype born to mothers who had been chronic alcoholics during their pregnancies. This phenotype, known as the fetal alcohol syndrome, includes the following clinical findings (Fig. 26–15):

Prenatal and/or postnatal growth retardation

Mental retardation

Microcephaly

Microphthalmia and/or short palpebral fissures

Underdeveloped philtrum

Carp-shaped mouth

Thin upper lip and/or flattened maxillary area

Although fetal alcohol syndrome can be di-

Table 26–2. Definite, Suspected, and Nonteratogenic Drugs

Drug	Clinical Findings
Definite Hazards	
Alcohol	Fetal alcohol syndrome
Accutane (isotretinoin)	
Hormones	
Androgens	Labial fusion and clitoral hypertrophy
Folic acid antagonists (aminopterin, methotrexate)	Cranial and skeletal abnormalities; microcephaly
Anticoagulants (Coumadin)	Nasal hypoplasia; fetal hemorrhage; stippled epiphyses; psychomotor delay
Anticonvulsants	
Dilantin	Fetal hydantoin syndrome
Tridione	Craniofacial abnormalities
Thalidomide	Craniofacial skeletal (limbs) and cardiac abnormalities
Suspected Hazards	
Estrogens/progestins	VACTERL syndrome
Amphetamines	Cardiac malformations
Lithium	Cardiac malformations
No Evidence of Teratogenic Effect	
Salicylates	
Antihistamines	
Heparin	
Antibiotics (penicillins, sulfonamides)	
Narcotics	

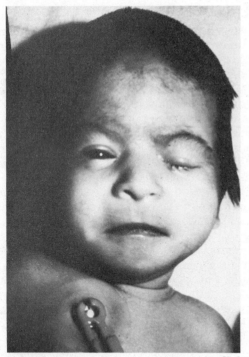

Figure 26–15. Infant with the fetal alcohol syndrome. (Courtesy of The Children's Hospital, Denver, CO.)

agnosed in the neonate, the syndrome may not be recognized until postnatal growth retardation and developmental delay become more apparent at 1 to 2 years of age. Although no one clinical finding is pathognomonic for the syndrome, the diagnosis should be considered in light of the previously mentioned phenotype and a positive history of maternal alcohol use.

In general, infants diagnosed as having the fetal alcohol syndrome have been born to mothers who were chronic alcoholics and drank heavily during pregnancy. It is known that alcohol freely crosses the placenta, reaching the same concentration in the fetus as that in the mother's blood. The critical factor appears to be the blood alcohol level; there is a direct relationship between the amount of alcohol consumed and the severity of the syndrome (Hanson et al., 1978). The fetal alcohol syndrome is felt to be a consequence of disharmonic growth, i.e., a diminished cell number, which is more profound in some tissues than in others (Smith, 1980).

Fetal alcohol syndrome represents the extreme end of the spectrum of problems related to the effects of alcohol during pregnancy. A second term, the fetal alcoholic effect, is now being used to describe those infants who exhibit only mild or partial manifestations of the syndrome (Rosett et al., 1981). There continues to be controversy regarding the minimum amount of alcohol intake necessary to produce an effect. Partial features of the fetal alcohol syndrome were seen in 11 percent of offspring whose mothers consumed two to four drinks ("hard" liquor) per day as opposed to 19 percent of offspring whose mothers consumed four or more drinks per day (Hanson et al., 1978). Additionally, it has been reported that the consumption of two drinks per day is associated with infants whose only clinical findings is decreased birth weight (Little, 1977). Although it is still unclear "how much alcohol is too much alcohol," it has been documented that a reduction of alcohol consumption as late as 24 to 26 weeks gestation is associated with an improved neonatal outcome (Rosett et al., 1981).

Dilantin. Women with documented seizure disorders taking anticonvulsants (Dilantin) during pregnancy have been found to have an increased incidence of offspring with characteristic abnormalities now termed the fetal hydantoin syndrome. The syndrome is characterized by the following:

Prenatal and/or postnatal growth deficiency

Motor and/or mental retardation

Microcephaly

Short upturned nose

Broad and/or depressed nasal bridge

Epicanthic folds

Nail and/or distal phalangeal hypoplasia

Other associated malformations are cleft lip and/or palate (6 percent) and cardiac defects (9 percent) (Hanson et al., 1976).

It is generally felt that there is approximately a 10 percent risk for women on Dilantin to have offspring with serious sequelae of the fetal hydantoin syndrome and a 30 percent risk for offspring with some minor features of the syndrome (Smith, 1977). There continues to be considerable discussion regarding the teratogenicity of Dilantin versus the maternal disease state. Whether it is the seizures or the in utero exposure to Dilantin that acts as a teratogen remains unclear. In any case, pregnant women on Dilantin should be counseled that they are at an increased risk for offspring with anomalies.

Progestins/oral contraceptives. Infants born to mothers taking oral contraceptives or progestins during early pregnancy have been found to have an increased incidence of a cluster of anomalies termed the VACTERL syndrome. VACTERL is an acronym for the types of anomalies seen, including vertebral anomalies, anal anomalies, cardiac anomalies, tracheoesophageal (TE) fistula, renal anomalies, and limb anomalies. The incidence of the VACTERL syndrome has been reported to occur with a two- to fourfold increase over the general population in women on progestational agents during early pregnancy (Nora and Nora, 1975). Given this information, the use of provocative pregnancy tests for pregnancy confirmation is contraindicated.

Since most drugs have not been thoroughly investigated regarding their teratogenic potential, it is best to avoid all unnecessary drugs during pregnancy. If a drug is indicated, the potential benefits for that drug must be weighed against the potential hazards to the fetus.

Congenital Infections. As previously stated, Gregg (1941) was one of the first to recognize an association between maternal rubella infection and abnormal fetal development.

Other infectious diseases that have been documented to produce deleterious effects in the fetus are cytomegalovirus (CMV), toxoplasmosis, herpes simplex, and syphilis.

Congenital infections may result in a wide spectrum of clinical pathology, ranging from major malformations to fetal and/or newborn infection. Figure 26–16 illustrates the major consequences of an intrauterine infection. After the mother is exposed and infected, she develops an acute viremia. The infection itself may or may not produce any maternal symptomatology. The virus then reaches the fetus via the placenta, where it may persist for the remainder of the pregnancy and early neonatal life. The type and severity of pathology seen will be dependent on the nature of the virus and the time of fetal infection. Table 26–3 lists the major types of problems seen with several of the more well-defined congenital infectious agents.

The diagnosis of a congenital infection is important for genetic counseling to help establish the correct recurrence risk in future pregnancies. Thus, when a congenital infection is suspected, appropriate diagnostic tests should be obtained such as viral cultures, antibody titers on both mother and

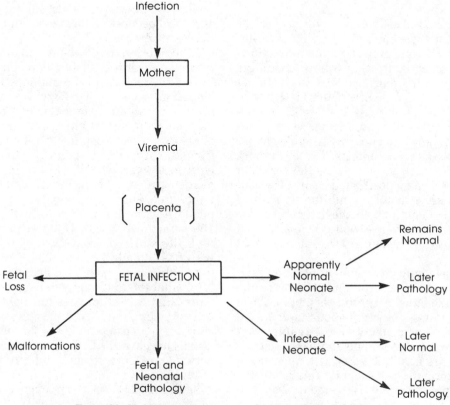

Figure 26–16. Major consequences of an intrauterine infection.

Table 26–3. Intrauterine Infections

Disease	Time of Susceptibility	Infant Findings*
Rubella (Virus)	1st trimester	Microcephaly; cataracts; deafness, congenital heart disease, MR
	2nd and 3rd trimesters	Hearing loss, congenital or progressive
Cytomegalic Inclusion Disease (Virus)	All trimesters	Severe form: Micro- or hydrocephaly; MR; cerebral calcifications; seizures; chorioretinitis; deafness. Some infants excrete virus but are asymptomatic.
Toxoplasmosis (Parasite)	All trimesters	Severe form: Micro- or hydrocephaly; seizures; chorioretinitis
Herpes (Virus)	1st trimester	One half end in miscarriage
	3rd trimester	Encephalitis; chorioretinitis; pneumonitis
Syphilis (Bacteria)	All trimesters (100 percent care if treated by 16 weeks of age)	None at birth 2 to 4 weeks: Lacrimation; snuffles, osteochondritis Later sequelae: Saddle nose; Hutchinson teeth; deafness

*Systemic findings may be seen in all the above infections except syphilis. These include hepatosplenomegaly, jaundice, apnea, tachypnea, cyanosis, hypothermia, fever, lethargy, and poor feeding.

infant, and radiologic examination for intercranial calcifications.

Maternal Environment. The previous discussion centered on fetal exposure to external agents such as drugs, radiation, and congenital infections. We will now briefly discuss the effects of the maternal environment from from both physical and metabolic standpoints.

Constraints placed on the fetus because of the mother's uterine cavity may on occasion result in certain types of malformations known as *deformations*. Uterine constraints may affect different parts of the forming embryo, mimicking other malformation syndromes. For example, the Pierre-Robin sequence can result from a single gene disorder, can be associated with other major anomalies and be indicative of a chromosome abnormality, or may be the result of the infant's being positioned against the wall of the uterus, thereby inhibiting growth of the lower mandible. In the latter case, the Pierre-Robin sequence would be considered a deformation secondary to uterine constraint.

The metabolic environment of the mother may also have a profound effect on the developing fetus. An entire chapter has been devoted to treating the diabetic mother, but from the genetic standpoint it is important to be aware that infants born to diabetic mothers are at an increased risk for congenital malformations. Generally this risk is felt to be approximately 10 percent (Day and

Insley, 1976). The incidence of congenital anomalies has been correlated with the severity of the disease and the degree of maternal control (Karlsson and Kjellmer, 1972). In general, diabetic mothers with vascular complications have approximately a twofold increased risk over controls to have an infant with congenital anomalies as well as a significantly higher risk for fetal wastage. The types of malformations most commonly seen are sacral agenesis, facial clefts, and congenital heart disease.

Phenylketonuria (PKU) is an autosomal recessive disorder involving an abnormality in the metabolism of the amino acid phenylalanine. Lacking the enzyme phenylalanine hydroxylase, women with PKU have high levels of serum phenylalanine. During pregnancy, these high levels represent a serious threat to the developing fetus. Infants born to women with PKU have been documented to have a high incidence of mental retardation and microcephaly. The risk for mental retardation may be as high as 90 to 100 percent (Richards, 1975). Although current literature suggests placing a woman with PKU on a low phenylalanine diet prior to and during pregnancy to decrease the risk for mental retardation, there is no documentation that this eliminates the risk. Clearly, this problem represents a significant risk, since an increasing number of women diagnosed to have PKU during the newborn period have been treated and are currently of reproductive age.

Smoking has been associated with increased perinatal mortality and small for gestational age infants. After adjusting for multiple variables, Mayer and Tonascia (1977) documented an increased risk of approximately 20 percent to infants whose mother smoked one pack a day as opposed to a 35 percent risk of perinatal mortality in women who smoked more than one pack a day. In addition, an increased incidence of placenta previa as well as spontaneous abortions has been reported (Fielding, 1978). Although smoking has not been documented to cause malformations, it certainly must be recognized as a potential hazard to the developing infant.

In terms of genetic counseling, the documentation of a teratogenic etiology is important, since the risk of recurrence in the absence of a teratogen is low for the majority of families and they can be reassured during future pregnancies. The importance of a detailed pregnancy history including exposure to any possible teratogenic agents cannot be overemphasized. With continued careful documentation of exposure to environmental agents during pregnancy, we will gain a better understanding of the potential relationship between these agents and fetal malformations.

Preconception Counseling

In the past, genetic counseling has been primarily provided retrospectively, i.e., after the birth of a child with birth defects or a genetic disorder. With technologic advances and an increasing public awareness, it has become imperative that health care practitioners provide information on a prospective basis. There are three major areas of focus to be considered when counseling a couple who are planning a pregnancy: (1) reproductive history; (2) family history and screening pedigree; and (3) consanguinity.

MATERNAL REPRODUCTIVE HISTORY

From the genetic standpoint, the reproductive history should include any type of pregnancy loss, spontaneous abortion, stillbirth, and perinatal death. For those couples with three or more miscarriages where no maternal anatomic or physiologic explanation can be found, cytogenetic analysis should be considered. In studies of couples

with a history of repeated reproductive failure, 5 to 10 percent have been documented to have a chromosome rearrangement or sex chromosome mosaicism (Ward et al., 1980; Watson, et al., 1981).

Stillbirths and perinatal deaths should be investigated whether or not obvious malformations are present. As previously mentioned, a very small chromosomal deletion or unbalanced rearrangement can produce increased morbidity and mortality without the identification of major structural malformations. Additionally, congenital infections and genetic disorders can go undetected and result in the family not knowing the specific cause of death. Other areas to be included are infertility, duration and types of contraception, how pregnancy was confirmed, environmental exposures, and potential health histories of the couple.

FAMILY HISTORY

The family history and screening pedigree can be extremely helpful in determining the high-risk family. The screening pedigree can identify conditions "running" in a family that may or may not have immediate implications for obstetric management. However, the family should be advised that other conditions may occur that were not predictable from this pedigree.

The pedigree itself is a fairly simple but often productive method for ascertaining high-risk families. The health professional can obtain the necessary information and draw a screening pedigree in approximately 15 to 20 minutes. Information that should be obtained from the family when drawing the pedigree includes the following: full names and maiden names if appropriate; birth dates of the immediate family members; names and ages of the rest of the family with a description of their health status; causes of death and age at death; and any other information that the family feels is pertinent. The screening pedigree usually includes the affected indivdual or the individual for whom the family is concerned and his siblings, parents, aunts, uncles, and grandparents (Fig. 26–17).

Ethnicity is another important aspect of the screening pedigree. A couple's ethnic background may be useful in determining the applicability of screening tests. For example, couples of Ashkenazi Jewish descent

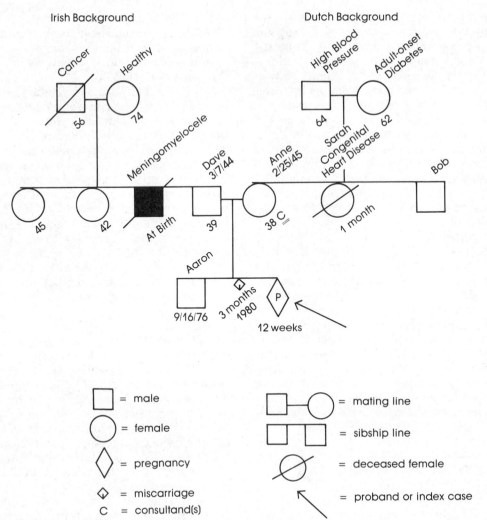

Figure 26-17. Screening pedigree obtained from a couple seeking prenatal diagnosis. Note positive family history for a neural tube defect (■ = affected).

are at an increased risk for being carriers of the gene for Tay-Sachs disease. The carrier rate is approximately 1 in 30 (Greenberg and Kaback, 1982). Blacks are at an increased risk for sickle cell anemia, and the Mediterranean populations have been shown to be at risk for the thalassemias.

CONSANGUINITY

The screening pedigree may also identify those families where consanguinity is an issue; that is, the partners are related to one another. For example, first cousins have one sixteenth of their genes in common. As all individuals are carriers of five to seven lethal recessive genes, related couples may be at an increased risk for having a child with an autosomal recessive condition. For consanguineous couples with a known inherited disorder in the family, more specific risk figures can be provided.

Postconception Counseling

Although preconception counseling is extremely helpful in identifying at risk couples, by far the vast majority of couples seen for genetic counseling are at the postconception stage. These families generally can be grouped into two major categories: (1) those couples who are currently pregnant and have an appropriate indication for prenatal diagnosis, and (2) those couples who have given birth to a child with birth defects or a genetic disorder.

PRENATAL DIAGNOSIS

Prenatal diagnosis, the in utero determination of fetal disease, is an important part of genetic counseling. Rapid advances in natal diagnostic techniques represent a major significant breakthrough in clinical genetics. These techniques have made it increasingly possible for a couple to make more informed reproductive decisions.

A number of different prenatal diagnostic techniques are now available (Table 26–4). The two most widely known and utilized are genetic amniocentesis and ultrasonography. Other techniques are chorionic villus sampling, fetoscopy (amnioscopy), amniography, and x-ray.

Genetic amniocentesis presently allows for the detection of chromosome abnormalities as well as over 100 biochemical disorders. The procedure involves the transabdominal withdrawal of fluid from the amniotic sac at approximately 15 to 16 weeks of pregnancy. Prior to the procedure, couples should receive adequate counseling to discuss the indications for the amniocentesis, the procedure itself, and any risks that may be involved. Ultrasound is performed to localize the placenta and fetus, determine approximate fetal gestation, and rule out the presence of twins. Under sterile conditions, approximately 30 cc of amniotic fluid is removed via a 22-gauge needle. Amniotic cells that originate from fetal skin, amnion, and fetal mucous membranes are then grown in culture and may be analyzed for fetal chromosomes, fetal DNA fragments, or fetal enzyme activity (Huisjes, 1978).

Prenatal diagnosis should be considered for couples presenting with the following indications:

1. Maternal age (35 years or older).
2. Previous child with a chromosome abnormality or positive family history.
3. Parental balanced translocation carrier.
4. Mother a known or at risk carrier for an X-linked disorder.
5. Parents carriers of an autosomal recessive disorder diagnosable in utero.
6. Positive family history for neural tube defects.

Advanced maternal age has been documented to be associated with an increased risk for fetal chromosome abnormalities (Epstein and Golbus, 1977). The actual risk figures given to couples depend on whether figures are quoted from the newborn population or amniocentesis data (Fig. 21–18). Nationwide, genetic amniocentesis is usually offered at maternal age 35, as the risk tends to rise at this time. In general, the risk increases from approximately 1 percent at age 37 to 10 to 12 percent at age 45 or older.

Couples who have had a previous child with trisomy 21 have a 1 to 2 percent recurrence risk in future pregnancies (Epstein and Golbus, 1977). Additionally, there is some evidence that families with children affected with other chromosome aberrations may also be at increased risk in future pregnancies (Hecht, 1979). Prenatal diagnosis should be made available to any couple who have had a child with a chromosome abnormality. Further, if a positive family history for a chromosome abnormality is ascertained, prenatal diagnosis should be considered. As stated previously, a parent who is a carrier of a balanced translocation is at an increased risk for having offspring with an unbalanced rearrangement. Genetic amniocentesis is appropriate for these couples and can delineate the specific chromosome constitution of the fetus.

Mothers who are documented carriers or at risk for being a carrier of an X-linked disorder may find genetic amniocentesis an appropriate option. Even if the disorder itself cannot be diagnosed, the sex of the fetus

Table 26–4. Techniques for Prenatal Diagnosis

Technique	Abnormalities Detectable
Genetic amniocentesis	Chromosomal abnormalities; inborn errors of metabolism; hemoglobinopathies and other biochemical disorders; alpha-fetoprotein detection for neural tube defects
Chorionic villus sampling (CVS)	As above for genetic amniocentesis except does *not* include alpha-fetoprotein analysis
Ultrasonography	Skeletal malformations; major organ malformations; polyhydramnios; oligohydramnios; hydrops
Fetoscopy	Hemoglobinopathies and other disorders detectable via fetal blood; external malformations
X-ray	Skeletal malformations
Amniography	External malformations; GI/GU malformations

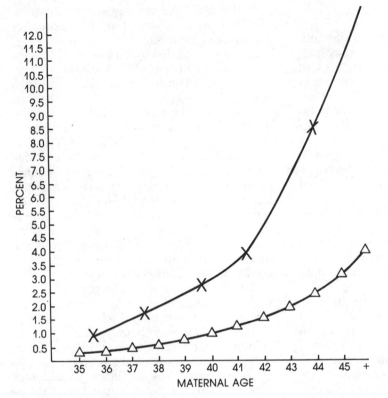

Figure 26–18. Incidence of chromosome abnormalities at midtrimester amniocentesis (X) and Down's syndrome at term (△) as a function of maternal age. (Redrawn from Antenatal Diagnosis. U.S. Department of Health, Education, and Welfare, NIH Publication #79-173, April 1979, p. I-51).

can be determined and the pregnancy electively terminated in the presence of a male fetus. The decision to terminate a pregnancy in light of this knowledge must be discussed at length and the family's decision supported.

Recently, the diagnosis of hemophilia and Duchenne's muscular dystrophy has been attempted in utero via fetoscopy to obtain fetal blood samples. Classic hemophilia A has been diagnosed by measuring ratios of factor VIII coagulant and factor VIII–related antigen (Firschein et al., 1979). The diagnosis of Duchenne's muscular dystrophy by analysis of creatine phosphokinase (CPK) activity in fetal blood has been attempted but, to date, remains an unreliable assay (Golbus et al., 1979). Application of genetic engineering techniques to directly visualize fetal DNA (restriction fragment length polymorphisms) may offer a promising new diagnostic tool for this and many other genetic diseases. With continued research, the family at risk for an X-linked disorder may no longer be faced with having to terminate a male fetus without a definitive diagnosis.

Prenatal diagnosis has been accomplished for a variety of biochemical disorders, some of which are listed in Table 26–5. A diagnosis of specific inborn errors of metabolism is made by analysis of amniotic fluid or cultured fibroblasts. The vast majority of these disorders are inherited in an autosomal recessive fashion, putting couples at a 25 percent risk with each pregnancy.

The diagnosis of neural tube defects is one of the more recent advances made in prenatal diagnosis. The spectrum of neural tube defects ranges from anencephaly and myelomeningocele to spina bifida occulta. Neural tube defects are seen in approximately 1 in 1000 live births and are inherited as multifactorial disorders. Regardless of the numerical risk given, families with a positive history of neural tube defect should be offered prenatal diagnosis. The specific risk can be reduced by as much as 90 percent through alpha-fetoprotein (AFP) determination.

AFP is a glycoprotein and a major component of fetal blood. Small amounts of AFP are found in the amniotic fluid of normal fetuses as well as in maternal serum. In the presence of an open neural tube defect, concentrations of AFP in amniotic fluid are greatly increased (Brock, 1977). Elevated levels may also be associated with a number of other malformations (Seppala and Unnerus,

Table 26–5. Some Inherited Biochemical Disorders that
Can Be Diagnosed Prenatally in Cultured Fetal Cells

Error in the Metabolism of	Disorder	Metabolic Defect	Brief Description of Phenotype
Amino Acids	Maple sugar urine disease (AR)*	Deficiency of enzymes needed in breakdown of some amino acids (leading to large excesses of leucine, isoleucine, and valine)	Poor development, convulsions, and early death. Urine has maple sugar odor. Diet therapy seems promising.
	Cystinosis (AR)	Primary defect unknown (but leading to accumulation of cystine in cells)	Several forms. In severe form, kidney function is impaired, leading to poor development, rickets, and childhood death.
Sugars	Galactosemia (AR)	Deficiency of enzyme needed in the metabolism of galactose (derived primarily from milk)	Liver and eye defects, mental retardation, and early death if untreated. Restrictive diet can control adverse symptoms.
Lipids	Tay-Sachs disease (AR)	Deficiency of enzyme needed in the breakdown of a complex lipid (allowing its accumulation in nervous tissue)	Progressive physical and mental degeneration, paralysis, blindness, and death in infancy.
	Adrenogenital syndromes (AR)	Deficiency of enzymes needed in the synthesis of sex hormones and of steroids controlling salt and water balance.	Mild and severe forms. In the most common form, dehydration and early death. In females, virilization is often seen.
Purines	Lesch-Nyhan syndrome (XR)	Deficiency of enzyme involved in the metabolism of purines (resulting in excessive production of uric acid)	Mental retardation, muscular spasms, compulsive self-mutilation. Patients may survive into adulthood.
Complex Polysaccharides	Hurler syndrome (AR) Hunter syndrome (XR)	Defects of connective tissue (allowing accumulation of mucopolysaccharides in cells)	Dwarfism, grotesque facial features, mental retardation. Hunter syndrome less severe.
Heme	Porphyria (AD)	Deficiency of enzyme needed in the synthesis of heme	Attacks of abdominal pain accompanied sometimes by impairment of mental functions.

*AR = autosomal recessive, AD = autosomal dominant, XR = X-linked recessive. Altogether, about 40 diseases can be detected prenatally.
From Mange, A., and Mange, E.: Genetics: Human Aspects. Copyright © 1980 by Saunders College/Holt, Rinehart and Winston. Reprinted by permission of Holt, Rinehart and Winston, CBS College Publishing.

1974; Seppala, 1975; Campbell et al., 1978). More recently, AFP determination on maternal serum has become a valuable screening method for neural tube defects. Routine AFP screening via maternal serum during pregnancy may prove an effective and economical method of ascertaining at risk families.

The most recent technique under investigation for the prenatal diagnosis of genetic disorders is chorionic villus sampling (CVS) (Fraccaro et al., 1985). The chorionic villus sampling procedure consists of introducing a sterile catheter into the cervix under the guidance of ultrasound to remove a small sample of chorionic villi (placenta). The villi are then selected out from the obtained sample and cultured for chromosomal and biochemical analysis. The advantages of this method of prenatal diagnosis are that it can be done between the 9th and 12th weeks of pregnancy, it requires no local anesthetic, and results are available within a few days. Since the technique is still under investigation (it is covered by most insurances), the disadvantages lie primarily in the establishment of specific risk figures for the procedure. Currently, there is an overall risk of 3 to 4 percent for problems following the procedure (miscarriage or maternal infection). The percentage of miscarriage specifically due to the procedure may approximate 1 percent. A controlled study is currently being conducted to establish more accurate risk figures. The other major disadvantage is that amniotic fluid is not obtainable using this method. Thus, families at risk for neural tube defects would need to employ other techniques, i.e., amniocentesis and ultrasound, for that specific diagnosis.

As ultrasonography techniques and equipment have become more refined, fetal visualization has become more detailed. Gestational age, twinning, placental localization, and the presence of poly- or oligohydramnios are often screened for routinely in many centers by this technique. The number of structural abnormalities being detected has continued to grow. Craniospinal defects (hydrocephalus, anencephaly, and microcephaly); renal malformations (obstruction or dysplasias); gastrointestinal malformation (obstructions, gastroschisis, omphalocele); and skeletal dysplasias are only a few of the disorders that have been diagnosed in utero by ultrasound (Sabbagha et al., 1981). To date, there is no evidence of problems to either the fetus or the mother from exposure to ultrasound.

Fetal visualization can also be achieved by x-ray. The fetal skeleton is sufficiently ossified by approximately 16 weeks of gestation to allow visualization of bony abnormalities and gross limb malformations. An x-ray of the fetus taken on an oblique axis at 20 weeks of pregnancy has been used to rule out such disorders as hypophosphatasia and metatrophic dwarfism. The need for x-ray has steadily declined as other techniques for the prenatal diagnosis of skeletal malformations have been perfected. However, in a few instances, such as when hypophosphatasia is suspected, x-ray is the most appropriate method of evaluation, and should be considered.

Fetoscopy (amnioscopy) via a fiberoptic endoscope allows direct visualization of the fetus. To date, the technique continues to be considered experimental, as the risk for major complications from the procedure has not been fully delineated. Further, it has been found that the field of vision is quite limited. Fetoscopy has been predominantly used for fetal blood sampling. Alter and Nathan (1976) and Jensen and colleagues (1979) have successfully diagnosed beta-thalassemia and sickle cell anemia using this method.

Recent advances in molecular biology have provided additional techniques for the possible prenatal diagnosis of sickle cell anemia and alpha-thalassemia from amniotic fluid cells. DNA obtained from the amniotic fluid cells is subjected to the action of *restriction endonucleases*, which cleave the DNA at specific locations. Separated by electrophoresis, the DNA fragments are hybridized with complementary DNA (Abelson, 1977). A diagnosis of sickle cell anemia or alpha-thalassemia is based on the absence of normal hybridized patterns (Panny et al., 1979; Phillips et al., 1979).

As one can note, prenatal diagnosis does not guarantee the birth of a normal infant but can only provide information regarding those malformations or disorders that are specifically looked for. Unfortunately, many disorders are not amenable to prenatal diagnosis, such as PKU and cleft lip and palate. The family must be apprised of what prenatal diagnosis can and cannot provide. Thus, it becomes imperative that adequate genetic counseling precede any diagnostic procedure.

For some couples, the detection of an abnormal fetus and termination of pregnancy offer an alternative to having affected offspring. For other couples, the abnormalities detected prenatally may be amenable to surgical correction (e.g., omphalocele) or medical management at birth. For those couples who elect to continue the pregnancy after the prenatal detection of a fetal abnormality, counseling and ongoing support should be made available. Resources such as mental health counseling, social services, and spiritual guidance should be sought to help families to begin the grief process as they mourn the loss of the expected "perfect baby" and begin to deal with the anticipated problems or possible death of the malformed infant (Matthews, 1984). In any case, it is appropriate to discuss all the available options with the family. By far, the vast majority of those couples undergoing prenatal diagnosis are given reassuring results and thus find "peace of mind" throughout the remainder of the pregnancy.

POSTNATAL DIAGNOSIS

Infants with birth defects and genetic disorders can usually be grouped into three major categories: (1) those presenting with obvious malformations at birth, (2) those who have a "stormy" neonatal period, and (3) those who appear normal at birth but subsequently develop an abnormal clinical course. As previously stated, the majority of these infants are detected during the early neonatal period.

It is the general expectation of couples and their primary health care team that pregnancy outcome will result in the birth of a normal healthy infant. Consequently, when an infant with an obvious malformation is born, both the parents and the health professionals involved are faced with an emotional crisis and often a medical emergency. The first major step in determining the course of action for the infant is to make an accurate diagnosis. Often a genetic evaluation is warranted to assist in this process. In making an accurate diagnosis, data from a number of sources need to be obtained and evaluated. These sources include but are not limited to:

1. Pregnancy history
2. Family history and pedigree
3. Detailed physical examination
4. Growth and developmental history
5. Laboratory procedures
6. Photographs

Each of these areas will be discussed in the section dealing with the principles and practices of genetic counseling.

When evaluating the infant with a malformation, the clinical geneticist will try to identify specific patterns of abnormalities. Two major questions are considered: (1) Is the malformation restricted to one organ system or does it involve multiple systems, and (2) does the malformation have a genetic or nongenetic etiology? If multiple major and/or minor malformations are present, the geneticist must consider chromosomal, single gene, and nongenetic etiologies. These etiologies frequently have a recognizable pattern of malformations, thus making it imperative that the clinician have expertise in syndrome recognition (Riccardi, 1977). It is the specific combination and frequency of a constellation of clinical findings that are significant for syndrome identification. For example, in Down's syndrome any one of the specific clinical findings can be found in normal infants, i.e., a single flexion crease (simian line), clinodactyly, or mongoloid slant. However, when these findings are found in combination, the diagnosis of Down's syndrome is considered. In the presence of a single malformation or malformations affecting only one organ system, multifactorial, single gene, or developmental etiologies are considered. For example, isolated congenital heart disease is inherited in a multifactorial fashion. Skeletal dysplasias (including achondroplasia and other dwarfisms) usually affect only the skeletal system but may be inherited as autosomal dominant or recessive disorders. These conditions often can only be distinguished on the basis of skeletal x-ray. Some malformations are considered to be developmental in nature and represent an abnormality of embryonic development that is not explained by known or possible genetic mechanisms or by known teratogens (Riccardi, 1977). For example, the presence of an isolated limb anomaly in the absence of a positive family history would make one consider a developmental etiology.

In the case of a stillborn infant, a careful examination (including an autopsy) for any major or minor abnormalities is indicated. Photographs can be of assistance to the geneticist in establishing the correct diagnosis. As previously mentioned, tissue for cytogenetic analysis should be obtained in the presence of minor malformations with or without major malformations.

Many genetic disorders do not present with congenital malformations but may be identified during the neonatal period by a stormy clinical course. Such findings as nausea and vomiting, organomegaly, abnormal CNS function (seizures, hypo- or hypertonia), and metabolic electrolyte imbalances may warrant investigation for a possible genetic cause. Since many inborn errors of metabolism present with these findings, laboratory screening such as that for amino and organic acids is indicated. Documentation of a metabolic condition as early as possible is imperative given the availability of treatment protocols for some of these disorders (e.g., PKU, galactosemia, thyroid abnormalities). If the etiology of the problem is of an infectious nature, a TORCH screen should be requested.

In some instances, infants with inborn errors of metabolism or other genetic disorders have a normal neonatal course and do not present with clinical findings until several months of age. Unfortunately, many of these disorders are not diagnosed until clinical symptoms become more severe. The classic example of a metabolic disorder presenting in this manner is Tay-Sach's disease. The affected infant appears normal with normal developmental milestones until approximately 4 to 6 months of age. At this time, further development ceases and signs of neurologic degeneration are noted.

Since the early 1960's, most states have mandated programs to screen the entire newborn population for phenylketonuria (PKU).

Table 26–6. Newborn Screening*

Phenylketonuria
Hypothyroidism
Sickle cell anemia
Galactosemia
Maple syrup urine disease
Homocystinuria

*Some centers may screen for other disorders.

Newborns in many centers are now screened for additional genetic disorders (Table 26–6). The major purpose of these programs is the early identification and initiation of appropriate treatment modalities for affected newborns. With this approach, devastating irreversible damage is usually avoided, and the affected infant can be expected to have a normal developmental course.

The Practice of Genetic Counseling

Genetic counseling is appropriate for any family that asks the question "Will it happen again?" Referrals to the genetic counseling team may be made by the family itself or any health care professional. Major indications for referral are summarized in Table 26–7.

INFORMATION GATHERING

The multifaceted process of genetic counseling begins at the time of referral. As previously outlined, information is gathered

Table 26–7. Major Indications for Referral for Genetic Counseling

Genetic counseling is appropriate for any family concerned about the diagnosis, etiology, recurrence risk, prognosis, and/or treatment of a specific disorder.
A. Positive family history with:
  1. Congenital malformations
  2. Mental retardation with or without malformations
  3. Chromosome abnormality
  4. Single gene disorders
  5. Family disorders (multifactorial)
  6. Sensory defects
  7. Neurologic and/or neuromuscular disorders
B. Consanguinity
C. High-risk ethnic group
D. Recurrent miscarriages
E. Potential teratogenic effect
F. Prenatal diagnosis

from a variety of sources. The principles involved include establishing an accurate diagnosis, discussing prognosis and treatment when appropriate, providing risks of recurrence, and presenting reproductive alternatives. Two clinical cases are presented to illustrate the genetic counseling process and to outline what families can expect.

Case #1: A gravida III, para 0, AB II 26-year-old mother delivered a male infant with bilateral cleft lip and palate, congenital heart disease, hypotonia, and multiple minor anomalies including abnormal dermatoglyphics.

Case #2: A 38-year-old woman, who is currently pregnant, was referred for prenatal diagnosis for maternal age. The family history indicated that her husband's sibling died at birth with a large meningomyelocele.

PHYSICAL EXAMINATION

The primary purpose of the initial counseling session is to establish an accurate diagnosis. In Case #1, the physical examination is paramount in helping to establish the diagnosis. Beyond the obvious major malformations, special attention should be given to the presence or absence of minor anomalies, which are frequently overlooked. Facial features should be well described, such as positioning of eyes (hypertelorism, hypotelorism, mongoloid slant); configuration of the nose and mouth (depressed nasal bridge, anteverted nostrils, downturned mouth); development of the jaw (micrognathia); positioning and shape of the ears; overall skull shape; sutures; and hair patterns. Neck and trunk features should include such descriptions as webbed neck, low posterior hairline, and chest configuration. Hyperpigmented or depigmented areas of the skin should be well described with attention to size, shape, location, and number.

Dermatoglyphic analysis can be helpful in delineating the etiology of some genetic disorders. Dermatoglyphics is the study of the dermal ridge configurations on the digits, palms, and soles (Preus and Fraser, 1972). The ridges begin development at approximately the 13th week of gestation and are complete by the 19th week. Thus, many genetic disorders that affect multiple sys-

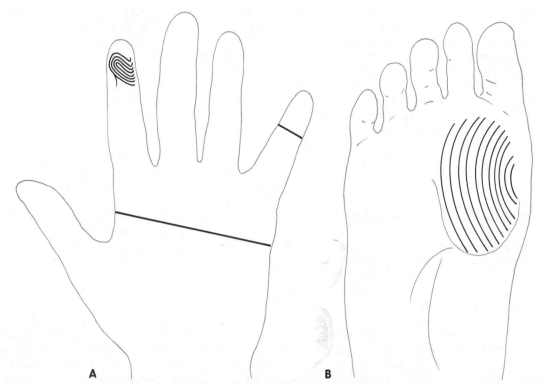

Figure 26–19. Dermatoglyphic findings common in Down's syndrome. Note single palmar crease (simian line), single flexion crease on 5th digit, ulnar loop pattern on index finger, and open field pattern (arch tibial) on hallucal area of foot.

tems will also affect the dermatoglyphics. Some of the more well known aberrations of dermatoglyphics are found in Down's syndrome. A single flexion crease (simian line) on the palms is a common finding as well as an increased number of ulnar loops on the fingertips (Fig. 26–19,A). In addition to changes of the hand print patterns, a very characteristic pattern known as an arch tibial may be found on the hallucal region of the feet (Fig. 26–19,B).

LABORATORY ANALYSES

The next step in evaluating an infant is to collect data from laboratory analyses. Beyond the routine laboratory analyses performed (electrolytes, blood count, x-ray), there are a number of specific studies that may be appropriate in evaluating Case #1. In light of multiple malformations, blood for chromosome analysis should be obtained. If the infant's status is critical and management plans are in question, then cytogenetic analysis of a direct bone marrow preparation may be warranted. Results from bone marrow preparations usually can be obtained

within a day. As a precautionary measure, a blood specimen should also be obtained simultaneously to ensure satisfactory results.

If one suspects an infectious etiology, viral cultures and a TORCH screen are appropriate. In the presence of hypotonia and failure to thrive, a detailed neurologic examination and possibly a CAT scan should be obtained. An ophthalmologic exam is often beneficial since many disorders, including congenital infections, metabolic abnormalities, and chromosome aberrations, are associated with specific eye findings.

FAMILY HISTORY AND PEDIGREE

An extensive family history and pedigree are essential elements of establishing any diagnosis. The family pedigree serves three additional purposes: (1) establishes the mode of inheritance; (2) identifies other areas of concern; and (3) identifies additional family members at risk.

The detailed history should include information concerning conception, pregnancy, labor and delivery as well as neonatal and developmental data. The history may be extremely helpful in determining whether the problem is prenatal (congenital) or postnatal in onset and whether the disorder is familial or nongenetic.

As illustrated by Case #2, the family history identified an additional risk for the couple, i.e., an increased risk for neural tube defects. Had this been overlooked, appropriate testing may not have been offered. When done correctly, the family history and pedigree becomes a powerful tool in the process of genetic counseling.

TIMING OF GENETIC COUNSELING

Another issue of importance is the timing of genetic counseling. Although ideally counseling should be prospective, i.e., before the birth of an affected child, it usually occurs retrospectively. In retrospective counseling, timing is a crucial factor. One needs to appreciate the parameters of the grief process that confronts couples who have just given birth to an abnormal infant and be cognizant of family differences. It may be appropriate for the genetic counselor to approach the family in the newborn nursery, obtain some preliminary information to assist with the immediate evaluation, and suggest counseling at a future date. This allows the family time to recover from the initial stages of shock and be more receptive to "hearing" any information given.

The period of time between the initial referral for genetic evaluation and the final genetic counseling session may include a single consultation or many sessions over a period of months. The final counseling is based on all the available information, published literature, and collaborative expertise of the genetics team. The session includes a discussion of the diagnosis and medical facts, prognosis and management, risk of recurrence, and reproductive alternatives.

DISCUSSION OF REPRODUCTIVE ALTERNATIVES

An important aspect of genetic counseling is a discussion of reproductive alternatives. Options that may be discussed include continuing previous reproductive plans (having another child), sterilization, adoption, artificial insemination, delayed childbearing, prenatal diagnosis, and/or early detection

and treatment. For many families, the risk of recurrence and/or burden of the disorder in question is low or is perceived as low, and the couple elects to have more children. For those couples who view their risk as being too high or the burden too great and for whom prenatal diagnosis is not available, sterilization may represent the only acceptable alternative.

Alternative insemination by donor (AID) may be an appropriate option in specific situations: (1) when the husband has an autosomal dominant disorder AID decreases the recurrence risk to that of the general population; (2) when the husband has an X-linked disorder, AID prevents the continuation of the disorder through obligate carrier daughters; (3) when both parents are carriers for an autosomal recessive disorder, AID decreases the risk of recurrence to considerably less than 25 percent, and if donor carrier testing is available, to 0 percent; and (4) for those couples with a high risk of recurrence for a multifactorial disorder. It is imperative when AID is used for genetic reasons that a careful family history and appropriate carrier tests be obtained on the sperm donor.

Since technology in medical genetics and health care continues to make rapid advances, many couples may decide to delay childbearing until methods of early detection and/or treatment are available. For example, hydrocephalus has been successfully treated surgically via in utero shunting (Clewell et al., 1982).

THE PRINCIPLES OF GENETIC COUNSELING

Geneticists and health professionals must adhere to certain principles of practice in order for genetic counseling to be an effective avenue of health care. These principles include *establishing an accurate diagnosis, offering nondirective counseling, maintaining confidentiality, providing referral and follow-up,* and *utilizing a team approach.* As discussed previously, the importance of an accurate diagnosis cannot be stressed enough. With the establishment of the diagnosis, genetic counseling should proceed in a nondirective manner. A major component of nondirective counseling is the ability to present information in a truthful yet sensitive manner. The counselor must strive to create a nonthreatening and noncoercive atmosphere and refrain from interjecting his own personal biases and opinions. In addition to providing information, the counselor provides assistance and support. The counselor may find that some families need assistance in defining personal properties and making decisions appropriate to their particular situation. Once a family has decided upon a particular course of action, their decision should be supported, regardless of what that course of action is.

As with any patient-professional relationship, confidentiality and trust are paramount features. Occasionally, confidentiality becomes an issue. For example, what is the moral obligation of the counselor if an autosomal dominant disorder is diagnosed and the patient refuses to share this information with at risk relatives? Although this situation is rare, the counselor should encourage the family to share this information with relatives, stressing the reason for doing so.

Families seen for genetic counseling should be provided with a written summary of the discussion. Additionally, the counselor should be in contact with the primary health care provider so that continued follow-up may be coordinated. For some families, referrals to other health services may be appropriate, such as infant stimulation programs, social services, physical therapy, family counseling, special clinics, and parent groups. As an outgrowth of the counseling process, other family members identified to be at increased risk may also benefit from genetic counseling and should be referred.

Genetic counseling is a complex and multifaceted process and therefore *cannot* be done efficiently or effectively in isolation. The genetics team consists of health professionals and scientists representing a variety of backgrounds and expertise. The genetics team is usually composed of a medical geneticist, genetic counselor (genetic associate and/or nurse geneticist), social worker, and laboratory specialists (cytogeneticist, biochemical geneticist, immunogeneticist). The expertise of many other health professionals is drawn upon, including other medical and nursing specialists, population geneticists, and the clergy.

The genetics team continually strives to inform and assist the primary physician or nurse clinician before, during, and after counseling. It is hoped that these primary health care providers utilize the genetics team as a resource group for consultation and assistance in the care of their patients.

REFERENCES

Abelson, J.: Recombinant DNA: Examples of present-day research. Science 196:159, 1977.

Ad Hoc Committee of Genetic Counseling: Genetic counseling. Am. J. Hum. Genet. 27:240, 1975.

Alter, B. P., and Nathan, D. G.: Antenatal diagnosis of haematological disorders—"1978." Clin. Haematol. 7:195, 1976.

Brock, D. J.: Biochemical and cytological methods in the diagnosis of neural tube defects. Prog. Med. Genet. New Series 2:1, 1977.

Campbell, S., Rodeck, C., Thomas, A., et al.: Early diagnosis of exomphalos. Lancet 1:1098, 1978.

Carr, D. H., and Gedeon, M.: Population cytogenetics of human abortuses. In Hook, E. B., and Porter, I. H. (eds.): Population Cytogenetics: Studies in Humans. New York, Academic Press, 1977.

Caspersson, T., Farber, S., Foley, G. E., et al.: Chemical differentiation among metaphase chromosomes. Exper. Call Res. 49:219, 1968.

Clewell, W. H., Johnson, M. L., Neier, R. P., et al.: A surgical approach to the treatment of fetal hydrocephalus. N. Engl. J. Med. 306:1320, 1982.

Cross, P. K., and Hook, E. B.: Paternal age and Down syndrome—a continuing dilemma: Data from prenatal cytogenetic sudies from the New York State chromosome registry and implications for genetic counseling. Am. J. Hum. Genet. 34:121A, 1982.

Day, R. E., and Insley, J.: Maternal diabetes mellitus and congenital malformation. Arch. Dis. Children 51:935, 1976.

deGrouchy, J., and Turleau, C.: Clinical Atlas of Human Chromosomes. New York, John Wiley & Sons, 1977.

Epstein, C. J., and Golbus, M. S.: Prenatal diagnosis of genetic diseases. Am. Sci. 65:703, 1977.

Fielding, J. E.: Smoking and pregnancy. N. Engl. J. Med. 298:337, 1978.

Firshein, S. I., Joyer, L. W., Lazarchick, J., et al.: Prenatal diagnosis of classic hemophilia. N. Engl. J. Med. 300:937, 1979.

Gayton, W. F., and Walker, L.: Down syndrome: Informing the parents. Am. J. Dis. Child. 127:510, 1974.

Gerald, P. S.: Current concepts in genetics: Sex chromosome disorders. N. Engl. J. Med. 294:706, 1976.

Goad, W. B., Robinson, A., and Puck, T.: Incidence of aneuploidy in a human population. Am. J. Hum. Genet. 28:62, 1976.

Golbus, M. S., Stephens, J. D., Mahoney, M. J., et al.: Failure of fetal creatine phosphokinase as a diagnostic indicator of Duchenne muscular dystrophy. N. Engl. J. Med. 300:860, 1979.

Goldman, A. S.: Critical periods of prenatal toxic insults. In Schwartz, R. H., and Yaffe, S. J. (eds.): Drug and Chemical Risks to the Fetus and Newborn. New York, Ian R. Liss, 1980.

Greenberg, D. A., and Kaback, M. M.: Estimation of the frequency of hexosaminidase A variant alleles in the American Jewish population. Am. J. Hum. Genet. 34:444, 1982.

Gregg, N. M.: Congenital cataract following German measles in the mother. Trans. Ophthal. Soc. Aust. 3:35, 1941.

Hanson, J. W., Myrianthopoulos, N. C., Sedgwick, H.,

et al.: Risks to the offspring of women treated with hydantoin anticonvulsants, with emphasis on the fetal hydantoin syndrome. J. Ped. 89:662, 1976.

Hanson, J. W., Streissguth, A. P., and Smith, D. W.: The effects of moderate alcohol consumption during pregnancy on fetal growth and morphogenesis. J. Ped. 92:457, 1978.

Hecht, T.: Chromosome 18 Trisomy syndrome: *In* Bergsma, D. (ed.): Birth Defects Compendium. New York, Alan R. Liss, 1979.

Heinonen, O. P., Slone, D., and Shapiro, S.: Birth Defects and Drugs in Pregnancy. Littleton, MA, PSG Publishing, 1977.

Herbest, D., and Miller, J.: Nonspecific X-linked mental retardation: The frequency in British Columbia. Am. J. Med. Genet. 7:461, 1980.

Hook, E. B., and Hamerton, J. L.: The frequency of chromosome abnormalities detected in consecutive newborn studies—differences between studies—results by sex and severity of phenotypic involvement. *In* Hook, E. B., and Porter, I. H. (eds.): Population Cytogenetics, Studies in Humans. New York, Academic Press, 1977.

Huisjes, H. S.: Cytology of the amniotic fluid and its clinical applications. *In* Fairweather, D., and Eskes, J. (eds.): Amniotic Fluid: Research and Clinical Application, 2nd ed. Amsterdam, Excerpta Medica, 1978.

Jensen, M., Zahn, V., Rauch, A., et al.: Prenatal diagnosis of beta thalassemia. Klin. Wochenschr. 57:37, 1979.

Jones, K. L., Smith, D. W., and Ulleland, N.: Pattern of malformation in offspring of chronic alcoholic mothers. Lancet 1:1267, 1973.

Karlsson, K., and Kjellmer, I.: The outcome of diabetic pregnancies in relation to the mother's blood sugar level. Am. J. Obstet. Gynecol. 112:213, 1972.

Lejeune, J., Gautier, M., and Turpin, R.: Etude des chromosomes somatiques de neuf infants mongoliens. C.R. Acad. Sci. 248:1721, 1959.

Little, R.: Alcohol consumption during pregnancy and decreased birth weight. Am. J. Pub. Health 67:1154, 1977.

Lubs, H. A.: A marker X chromosome. Am. J. Hum. Genet. 21:231, 1969.

Lyon, M. F.: Gene action in the X-chromosome of the mouse (mus musenlus L.). Nature 190:372, 1961.

McClearn, G. E.: Genetics and drug-related behaviors (invited theme symposium). Am. J. Hum. Genet. 31:4A, 1979.

McKusick, V. M.: Mendelian Inheritance in Man, 5th ed. Baltimore, The Johns Hopkins University Press, 1979.

Meyer, M. B., and Tonascia, J. A.: Maternal smoking, pregnancy complications, and perinatal mortality. Am. J. Obstet. Gynecol. 128:494, 1977.

Nora, A. H., and Nora, J. J.: A syndrome of multiple congenital anomalies associated with teratogenic exposure. Arch. Environ. Health 30:17, 1975.

Opitz, J.: Mental retardation: Biologic aspects of concern to pediatricians. Ped. Rev. 2:41, 1980.

Panny, S. R., Scott, A. F., and Phillips, J. A.: Prenatal diagnosis of sickle cell disease by restriction endonuclease analysis. Limitations and advantages. Am. J. Hum. Genet. 31:58A, 1979.

Pawlowitski, I.: Frequency of chromosome abnormalities in abortions. Human Genetik 16:131, 1972.

Penrose, L. S., and Smith, G. F.: Down's Anomaly. Boston, Little, Brown & Co., 1966.

Phillips, J. A., Scott, A. F., Kazazian, H. H., et al.: Prenatal diagnosis of hemoglobinopathies by restric-

tion endonuclease analysis: Pregnancies at risk for sickle cell anemia and S-OArab. Johns Hopkins Med. J. 145:57, 1979.

Preus, M., and Fraser, F.: Dermatoglyphics and syndromes. Am. J. Dis. Child. 124:933, 1972.

Riccardi, V.: The Genetic Approach to Human Disease. New York, Oxford University Press, 1977.

Richards, B. W.: Observations on the familial appearance of diseases associated with metabolic disorders of the mother. Ann. Hum. Genet. 39:189, 1975.

Robinson, A., Puck, M., Pennington, B., et al.: Abnormalities of the sex chromosomes: A prospective study on randomly identified newborns. *In* Robinson, A., Lubs, H. A., and Bergsma, D. (eds.): Sex Chromosome Aneuploidy: Prospective Studies in Children. The National Foundation–March of Dimes, Birth Defects Original Article Series, Vol XV:203, 1979.

Rossett, H. L., Weiner, L., and Edelin, K. C.: Strategies for prevention of fetal alcohol effects. Obstet. Gynecol. 57:1, 1981.

Sabbagha, R. (NMI), Tamura, R. K., and DalCompo, S. (NMI): Antenatal ultrasonic diagnosis of genetic defects: Present status. Clin. Obstet. Gynecol. 24:1103, 1981.

Satow, W. U., and West, E.: Studies on Nagasaki (Japan) children exposed in utero to atomic bomb. Roentgenographic survey of skeletal system. Am. J. Roentgenol. 74:493, 1955.

Seppala, M., and Unnerus, H.: Elevated amniotic fluid alpha fetoprotein in fetal hydrocephalus. Am. J. Obstet. Gynecol. 119:270, 1974.

Seppala, M.: Fetal pathophysiology of human alpha fetoprotein. Ann. N.Y. Acad. Sci. 259:59, 1975.

Smith, D. W.: Teratogenicity of anticonvulsive medications. Am. J. Dis. Child. 131:1337, 1977.

Smith, D. W.: Alcohol effects on the fetus. *In* Schwarz, R. H., and Yaffe, S. J. (eds.): Drug and Chemical Risks to the Fetus and Newborn. New York, Alan R. Liss, 1980, p. 73.

Stene, J., Fischer, G., Stene, E., et al.: Paternal Age effect in Down's syndrome. Ann. Hum. Genet. 40:299, 1977.

Stewart, A., and Kneale, G. W.: Radiation dose effects in relation to obstetric X-rays and childhood cancers. Lancet 1:1185, 1970.

Swartz, H. M., and Reichling, B. A.: Hazards of radiation exposure for pregnant women. JAMA 239:1907, 1978.

Taylor, G. I.: Autosomal trisomy syndrome: A detailed study of 27 cases of Edwards' syndrome and 27 cases of Patau's syndrome. J. Med. Genet. 5:227, 1968.

Thompson, J. S., and Thompson, M. W.: Genetics in Medicine, 3rd ed. Philadelphia, W. B. Saunders Co., 1980.

Tjio, J., and Levan, A.: The chromosome number in man. Hereditas 42:1, 1956.

Uchida, J. A.: Maternal radiation and trisomy 21. *In* Hook, E. B., and Porter, I. A. (eds.): Population Genetics: Studies in Humans. New York, Academic Press, 1977.

Ward, B. E., Henry, G. P., and Robinson, A.: Cytogenetic studies in 100 couples with recurrent spontaneous abortions. Am. J. Hum. Genet. 32:549, 1980.

Warkany, J.: Congenital Malformations. Chicago, Year Book Medical Publishers, Inc., 1971.

Watson, J. D., Ward, B. E., Mosher, G., et al.: Evaluation of 175 couples with reproductive failure. Am. J. Hum. Genet. 33:39A, 1981.

Wilson, J. G.: Environment and Birth Defects. New York, Academy Press, 1973.

Wood, R. W.: Delayed radiation effects in atomic bomb survivors. Science 166:569, 1969.

27

PARENT COUNSELING

JOHN H. KENNELL
MARSHALL H. KLAUS

Study of the mother-infant bond began as recently as 10 to 15 years ago, when nurses and physicians in intensive care nurseries observed that sometimes, after extraordinary efforts had been taken to save small premature infants, they would return to emergency rooms injured by their parents even though they had been sent home intact and thriving. This chapter reviews the recent human attachment studies and applies their findings to the care of the parents of a premature infant, a malformed infant, a stillborn child, or a neonate who has died.

A mother's and father's actions and responses toward their infant are derived from a complex combination of their own genetic endowment, the way the baby responds to them, a long history of interpersonal relations with their own families and each other, past experiences with this or previous pregnancies, the absorption of the practices and values of their cultures, and, probably most important, how each was raised by his or her own mother and father. The mothering or fathering behavior of each woman and man, their ability to tolerate stresses, and their need for special attention differ greatly and depend upon a mixture of these factors.

The actual process of parent-to-infant at-

Table 27–1. Steps in Attachment

Planning the pregnancy
Confirming the pregnancy
Accepting the pregnancy
Fetal movement
(Visualization by ultrasound)
Accepting the fetus as an individual
Birth
Hearing and seeing the baby
Touching and holding the baby
Caretaking

tachment, or bond formation, is not yet completely understood, but a wide diversity of observations are beginning to make it possible to piece together some of the various phases. The time periods that are apparently crucial for this process are shown in Table 27–1.

Many mothers are initially disturbed by feelings of grief and anger when they become pregnant because of factors ranging from economic and housing hardships to intrapersonal difficulties. However, by the end of the first trimester, the majority of women who initially rejected pregnancy have accepted it. This initial stage, as outlined by Bibring, is the mother's identification of the growing fetus as an "integral part of herself."

The second stage is a growing perception of the fetus as a separate individual, usually occurring with the awareness of fetal movement. After quickening, a woman will generally begin to have some fantasies about what the baby may be like, will attribute to the baby some human personality characteristics, and will develop a sense of attachment and value toward him. At this time, further acceptance of the pregnancy and marked changes in attitude toward the fetus may be observed. Unplanned, unwanted infants may now seem more acceptable. (With the frequent use of ultrasound for high-risk patients it is apparent that visualization of a moving fetus has an accelerating effect on the attachment process for both father and mother.) Objectively, the health worker will usually find some outward evidence of the mother's preparation by such actions as the purchase of clothes or a crib, the selection of a name, and the arrangement of space for the baby.

Parenting Considerations in High-Risk Antepartum Care

ASSESSMENT AND COUNSELING

We have found it useful to pick out in advance the mother who is most likely to have special difficulties in relating to her infant. Blau and colleagues noted that mothers who deliver premature infants have more negative attitudes toward their pregnancies, greater emotional immaturity, and more body narcissism (Blau et al., 1963). Cohen emphasizes that after the first trimester behaviors that suggest rejection of pregnancy include (1) a preoccupation with physical appearance, (2) excessive emotional withdrawal or mood swings, (3) excessive physical complaints, (4) absence of any response to quickening, and (5) lack of any preparation for the baby during the last trimester (Cohen, 1966). In our own experience, mothers who have a high incidence of severe mothering difficulties often have one of the following characteristics:

1. The previous loss of a newborn infant, including miscarriage and induced abortion,

2. A fertility problem, with no living children,

3. A previous seriously ill newborn infant,

4. Primiparity if younger than 17 or older than 38 years,

5. A medical problem with which the infant may be affected, such as Rh disease, toxemia, or diabetes, and

6. The unmarried mother and the mother without social support.

Certain management principles for obstetric and pediatric health care professionals apply to all these situations.

1. In almost all high-risk situations, the odds are heavily in favor of the birth of a live baby who will ultimately be healthy and normal, so it is reasonable to stress the positive and be optimistic. This is essential for the mother's later relationship with her baby, which is in turn extremely important for its development. After a physician reads the literature or a physician's report about a woman's new or rare condition, it is tempting to tell her about the problems and pitfalls that may develop. But this may only make the course of the pregnancy more turbulent for the mother and the obstetrician. Mentioning the possibility of a symptom or complication is comparable to telling the young boy just starting to ride a two-wheeler that there is one big tree in the middle of the playground.

2. The obstetric team should include the pediatric team early and continue to involve them in decisions and plans for the management of the mother and baby.

3. Prepare the mother for the anticipated aspects of care for her newborn.

4. Cohen (1966) suggests that the following questions be asked to learn the special needs of each mother:

   a. How long have you lived in this immediate area and where does most of your family live?

   b. How often do you see your mother or other close relatives?

   c. Has anything happened to you in the past (or do you currently have any condition) that causes you to worry about the pregnancy or the baby?

   d. What was your husband's (partner's) reaction to your pregnancy?

   e. What other responsibilities do you have outside the family?

It is wise to inquire about how the pregnant woman was mothered. Did she have a neglected and deprived infancy and childhood or did she grow up with a warm and intact family life? There is evidence that the loss of a parent in the first 11 years of life is a major psychological risk factor for new fathers and mothers, so information about the health of the parents' parents can be valuable (Brown and Harris, 1978).

PRENATAL HOSPITALIZATION

With the advances in high-risk perinatal care, the benefits of prenatal hospitalization for selected patients are well established. The fetus can gain significant medical advantages from this sophisticated hospital care. The nurses and physicians working in high-risk prenatal units are aware of the upsetting emotional effects on pregnant women when they are hospitalized for periods of a month or more for the management of medical problems such as hypertension, diabetes, premature labor, or a slow growing fetus. Investigations by Merkatz (1978) disclosed that mothers who had prolonged antenatal hospitalization were principally concerned about the baby they were carrying and only secondarily about their own medical condition. She reported the great loneliness of these women, their fears about the baby, and their reactions to separation from home and family. Merkatz stressed the need for unlimited visits for the hospitalized woman by her husband or boyfriend, children, and parents. She noted that families need privacy and unrestricted time together so that family members can assist each other to cope with fear, uncertainty, and anxiety. To encourage strong family support will require changes in visiting policies for young siblings-to-be, extra beds for fathers-to-be so that they can stay overnight with their wives, special dining rooms for the family to eat together, and other alterations to make the hospital more like a home. On a number of occasions women who had prolonged prenatal hospitalization mentioned how everybody seemed interested in the high-risk pregnancy but not in them as a person or the baby as an individual. Individualized care plans worked out with the women are necessary because of their highly individualized response to the high-risk pregnancy and hospitalization.

CONTINUITY OF PERINATAL CARE

It is only during this century that the change was made from a system in which there was one continuous caretaker, the family doctor and/or midwife, who was available to the mother during her pregnancy, labor, and birth and who provided the care for both the mother and baby during the postpartum period. Observations by Larson (1980) reveal a significant change in the mother's ability to parent if a home health caretaker, such as a visiting nurse, made contact with the mother before birth and 48 hours after the birth rather than starting 6 weeks post partum. This suggests that interventions in the perinatal period should begin during the pregnancy rather than after the mother has taken her baby home. The study gives added impetus for family physicians, pediatric, obstetric, and public health nurses, and pediatricians to arrange visits to meet and talk with the mother during the pregnancy.

FAMILY-CENTERED CESAREAN CHILDBIRTH

The National Institutes of Health Consensus Development Conference on Cesarean Childbirth (1980) emphasized the importance of the father's presence at a cesarean birth. There has been no evidence of harm to mother, neonate, or father when family-centered maternity care has been extended to the cesarean birth family. The presence of fathers in the operating room and closer contact between mother and neonate appeared to improve all postcesarean behavioral responses of the families. Greater involvement of fathers with their infants has been consistently reported in studies of postcesarean birth families.

The mother who has had a cesarean birth may be somewhat passive and dependent in her early postpartum period. Most of her focus is on her needs. Therefore, the nurse should be respectful and understanding of this and bring the baby to the mother when the mother is the most comfortable. If the baby cannot come out of the nursery to visit with the mother, pictures should be provided to the mother. As the mother becomes more comfortable, she should be assisted to the nursery (sometimes this may necessitate a wheelchair). Some mothers have even been taken on a stretcher if space permits and the condition of the fetus is critical. As the mother is more able to care for herself and her baby, rooming-in can then be made available to her.

During this time of separation, the father may become fatigued and frustrated as he tries to divide his time between the mother and the infant. He too will need support from the nursing staff during this difficult time.

Parenting Considerations in Normal and High-Risk Intrapartum Care

1. The less anxiety the mother experiences during labor and delivery, the better will be her immediate relationship with her baby. Therefore, she and her husband should visit the maternity unit to see where labor and delivery will take place. She should also learn about the anesthetic (if she is to receive one), delivery routines, and all the proce-

dures and medication she will receive before, during, and after delivery. By reducing the possibility of surprise, such advance preparation will increase confidence during labor and delivery. Just as for a child entering the hospital for surgery, the more meticulously every step and event are detailed in advance for an adult, the less the subsequent anxiety.

2. The mother must have continuous support during her labor and delivery, whether from her husband, a midwife, a nurse, or a supportive companion (doula). Doulas are present during an increasing number of labors, to support the mother and family members. This intervention has been shown to reduce the length of labor, perinatal morbidity, and the rate of cesarean sections. The mother also must be satisfied with the arrangements that have been made to maintain her home during her hospitalization. This gives her the freedom to concentrate on the needs of the baby and to enjoy her family in the process, and it relieves the pressure on the father so that he can reserve his energies for the family.

3. In an effort to reduce the amount of tension on the mother, she should labor and deliver in the same room, preventing the need to rush to a delivery room in the last minutes of labor. In some hospitals this option is available not only to low-risk mothers but also to high-risk mothers. Once the delivery is completed and the mother has had a quick glance at the infant, it is important for her to have a few seconds to regain her composure before she proceeds to the next task—taking on the infant. It has been our experience that it is best not to give a mother her baby until she indicates that she is ready to take it on. It should be her decision.

4. In many hospitals it is customary to put the baby on the mother's chest for 1 or 2 minutes shortly after delivery. This is helpful, but the lack of privacy, the narrow table, and the short time period do not allow sufficient opportunity for the mother to touch and explore her baby. Although it is a reasonable procedure, it is not sufficient to optimize maternal attachment.

5. After delivery, it is extremely helpful for the father, mother, and baby to have a period alone in either the delivery room or an adjacent room (labor or recovery room). Obviously, this is possible only if the infant is normal and the mother is well. The mother should have the infant with her on the bed so she can hold him—he should not be off in a bassinet where she can only see his face (Fig. 27–1). She should be given the baby nude and allowed to examine him completely. We have found it valuable to encourage the mother to move over in her regular hospital bed so that she only takes up about half of it, leaving the other half for her partially dressed or nude infant. A heat panel easily maintains or, if need be, increases the body temperature of the infant. Several mothers have told us of the unforgettable experience of holding their nude baby against their own bare chest. The father may also participate in this skin-to-skin contact with his infant. This allows both parents to become acquainted with their new baby. Because the eyes are so important for both the parents and baby, we withhold the ocular application of silver nitrate ($AgNO_3$) or other ophthalmic prophylaxis until after this rendezvous. (Many hospitals now apply an antibiotic ointment, which is not as irritating to the infant's eyes.)

6. We have found it valuable for the mother, father, and infant to be together for at least 1 hour. After 30 to 45 minutes, the mother and baby often fall asleep. Usually the mother and father never forget this shared experience. It helps some parents to begin to attach to their real infant. We emphasize that this should be a private session. Keep in mind that many parents take days to fall in love with their infant and that this gradual process is entirely normal.

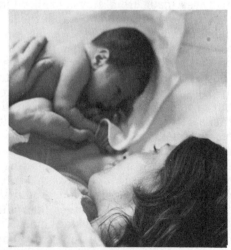

Figure 27–1. Mother receiving infant in the first minutes of life. (From Klaus, M. H., and Fanaroff, A. A.: Care of the High Risk Neonate, 2nd ed. Philadelphia, W. B. Saunders Co., 1979.)

Affectional bonds are further consolidated in the succeeding 4 to 5 days through continued close association of baby and mother, particularly when she cares for him. Close contact with her husband and other children is also obviously important.

7. If the baby must be moved to a hospital with an intensive care unit, we find it helpful to give the mother a chance to see and touch her infant, even if the baby has respiratory distress, is in an oxygen hood, and is being ventilated. The health care provider stops in the mother's room with the transport incubator and encourages her to touch her baby and look at him at close hand. A comment about the baby's strength and healthy features may be long remembered and appreciated. A picture of the infant given to the mother can help her remember her baby until she can see him again.

8. We encourage the father to follow the transport team to our hospital so he can see what is happening with his baby. He uses his own transportation so that he can stay in the premature unit for 3 to 4 hours. This extra time allows him to find out how the infant is being treated, to get to know the nurses and physicians in the unit, and to talk with them about what will happen to the baby in the succeeding days. We allow him to come into the nursery and explain in detail everything that is going on. We ask him to help act as a link between us and his family by carrying information back to his wife and request that he come to our unit before he visits his wife so that he can let her know how the baby is doing. We suggest that he take a Polaroid picture, even if the infant is on a respirator, so that he can show and describe to his wife in detail how the baby is being cared for. Mothers often tell us how valuable the picture is in keeping some contact with their infant, even while physically separated.

Parenting Considerations in High-Risk Postpartum Care

During the past several years, many changes have been made in the physical arrangements for mothers and obstetricians' approach to them. If the mother has not yet visited her baby we find it best to describe what the infant looks like and how the infant will appear to her physically. We do not talk about chances or survival rates or percentages but stress that most babies survive in spite of early and often worrisome problems. We do not emphasize problems that may occur in the future. We do try to anticipate common developments (e.g., the need for bilirubin reduction lights for jaundice in small premature infants). The following guidelines may be helpful.

1. A mother's room arrangements should be adjusted to her needs. Mothers are often best able to express themselves and work out their problems when they are alone, but some need companionship during this stressful period.

2. If at all possible, mother and infant should be kept near each other in the same hospital, ideally on the same floor.

3. It is useful to talk with the mother and father together whenever possible. When this is not possible, it is often wise to talk with one parent on the phone in the presence of the other. At least once a day we discuss with the parents how the child is doing; we talk with them at least twice a day if the child is critically ill. It is necessary to find out what the mother believes is going to happen or what she has read about the problem. We move at her pace during any discussion.

4. It is highly desirable for one professional (primary nurse or physician) to do most of the communicating with the family about the medical problem and the infant's progress. When more than one member of the hospital staff speaks with the parents, the parents often go on a stressful roller-coaster ride from optimism to pessimism as they receive varying information about the baby's problems and possible complications and interventions. Thus it is best for one individual to collect and synthesize the varied opinions of the members of the health care team and speak with one consistent voice.

5. The health care team should not relieve their own anxieties by adding their worries to those of the parents. If there is a possibility, for example, that the child has Turner's syndrome, it is not necessary to share this with the parents while the infant is still acutely ill with other problems and while affectional bonds are still weak. If the health care professionals are worried about a slightly high bilirubin level, it is not necessary to discuss kernicterus.

6. Before the mother comes to the neonatal unit, the nurse or physician should describe in detail what the baby and the equipment will look like. When she makes her first visit it is important to anticipate that she may become distressed when she looks at her infant. We always have a stool nearby so that she can sit down, and a nurse stays at her side during most of the visit, describing in detail the procedures being carried out such as the monitoring of respiration and heart rate.

7. The nurse should go into some detail in describing all the equipment surrounding the infant and should be nearby to answer questions and give support during the difficult period when the mother is first seeing her infant.

8. It is important to remember that feelings of love for the baby are often elicited through contact. Therefore, we turn off the lights and remove the eye patches from an infant under bilirubin lights so that the mother and infant can see each other.

9. In the past decade extended visiting for the mother of a normal full term infant from 1 to 7 P.M. when the mother is able to handle and completely care for her infant has been found to be a useful practice. This also pertains to the mother of a high-risk infant. In almost all intensive care units, visiting hours for parents and grandparents are unlimited. As soon as possible we describe to both the father and mother the value of touching the infant in helping them get to know him, reducing the number of apneic episodes (if this is a problem), increasing weight gain, and hastening the infant's discharge from the unit. This encourages them to visit the baby frequently for extended periods.

10. The nursery should keep a record of all phone calls and visits by parents. Our data reveal that when there are fewer than three phone calls or visits in a 2-week period, there is a high incidence of subsequent severe mothering disorders, such as failure-to-thrive, battering, or giving up the baby. This may vary with different units. Therefore, if the visiting pattern of the mother is less than that of most mothers, the mother is given extra help in adapting to the hospitalization. Unpublished information from an observational study at the University of Florida is consistent with other clinical observations and the child abuse studies of Margaret Lynch that suggest that prolonged antepartum hospitalization may interfere with the mother's bonding to her new baby. Some of these mothers have indicated a need to go home and be with their family and their other children. It is important to respect this need, which arises from a stressful separation and isolation. It is a reminder of the value of open visiting by the family during the mother's hospitalization. Keeping in mind the mother's emotional turmoil during this stressful period, and to provide follow-up care at the home when it might be necessary, health care professionals may find it helpful to encourage these mothers to visit and to go out of their way to call to keep them informed about the baby's progress.

11. To help the family during the infant's hospitalization, there must be a good working relationship among the health care professionals. Meetings with the nursery staff in the intensive care unit should be held every 2 weeks. This provides an opportunity for members of the team to express their concerns about a father's and mother's behavior and to work out a plan to assist them.

12. It may be possible to enhance normal attachment behavior in the mother several days or weeks following birth by permitting a special short nesting period of 3 or more days of close physical contact with privacy and virtual isolation during which the mother provides complete care for her small infant, with help and nursing support readily available nearby. If the safety and feasibility of early discharge of premature infants, as reported by Berg and others, are fully confirmed, we hypothesize that early discharge combined with a period of isolated physical contact with caretaking may help to normalize mothering behavior for infants discharged from intensive care nurseries.

13. Communicate with the mother about her condition and the baby's condition. This is important before, during, and after the birth. At times, this will be brief and incomplete, but communication is essential. For example, when there is evidence of fetal distress, the mother can be told, "We have evidence that your baby should be delivered quickly, so we are proceeding with this, and we will need your full cooperation." Or, when a baby shows stress or fails to breathe after birth, the parents can be told, "The baby has a problem. We will be working with the baby and will let you know more about this just as soon as we can."

Clinically, we have been impressed and

disturbed by the devastating and lasting untoward effects on the mothering capacity of women who have been frightened by the physician's pessimistic outlook about the chances of survival and normal development of an infant. For example, when a 3-lb premature baby is doing well but the mother is told that there is a reasonable chance that the baby may not survive, the mother will often show evidence of mourning (as if the baby were already dead) and reluctance to "become attached" to her baby. We have repeatedly observed that such mothers may refuse to visit or will show great hesitation about any physical contact.

When discussing such a situation with a physician who has spoken pessimistically with the mother, we have often been told that it is important to share all worries with a mother so that she will be prepared in case of a bad outcome. If there is a close and firm bond between the mother and infant (which occurs after an infant has been home for several months) there is no reason for the physician to withhold his concern. However, while the ties of affection are still forming, they can be easily retarded, altered, or permanently damaged. It is not easy to keep from sharing all the problems with a mother, but with the evidence available at present, it is our conviction that health care personnel should do their best to hold back. This does not mean that they should be untruthful, because parents will quickly sense their true feelings. They must base their statements on today's situation (infant mortality rates in low birth weight nurseries have decreased steadily year by year), not on yesterday's high mortality figures. Today many extremely immature babies live and are normal.

Caring for Parents of Infants with Congenital Malformations

PARENTAL REACTIONS AND ADAPTATIONS TO THE MALFORMED INFANT

The birth of an infant with a congenital malformation presents complex challenges to the health care providers who will care for the affected child and the family (Johns, 1971). Despite the relatively large number of infants with congenital anomalies, our understanding of how parents develop an attachment to a malformed child remains incomplete. Although previous investigators agree that the child's birth often precipitates major family stress, relatively few have described the process of family adaptation during the infant's first year of life (Hare et al., 1966; Johns, 1971; Roskies, 1972). Solnit and Stark's conceptualization of parental reactions emphasized that a significant aspect of adaptation is that parents must mourn the loss of the normal child they had expected, (Solnit and Stark, 1961). Other observers have noted pathologic aspects of family reactions, including the chronic sorrow that envelops the family of a defective child (Zuk, 1959; Olshansky, 1962). Less attention has been given to the more adaptive aspects of parental attachment to children with malformations.

Parental reactions to the birth of a child with a congenital malformation appear to follow a predictable course. For most parents, initial shock, disbelief, and a period of intense emotional upset (including sadness, anger, and anxiety) are followed by a period of gradual adaptation, which is marked by a lessening of intense anxiety and emotional reaction (Fig. 27–2). This adaptation is characterized by an increased satisfaction with and ability to care for the baby. These stages in parental reactions are similar to those reported in other crisis situations, such as those involving terminally ill children. The shock, disbelief, and denial reported by many parents seem to be an understandable attempt to escape the traumatic news of the baby's malformation, news so at variance with their expectations that it is impossible for it to register except gradually.

The intense emotional turmoil described by parents who have produced a child with a congenital malformation corresponds to a period of crisis (defined as "upset in a state of equilibrium caused by a hazardous event which creates a threat, a loss, or a challenge for the individual") (Bloom, 1963; Rappoport, 1965). A crisis consists of a period of impact, a rise in tension associated with stress, and finally a return to equilibrium. During such crisis periods, a person is, at least temporarily, unable to respond with his usual problem-solving activities. Roskies noted a similar "birth crisis" in her observations of mothers of children with birth defects caused by thalidomide (Roskies, 1972).

Solnit and Stark have likened the crisis of

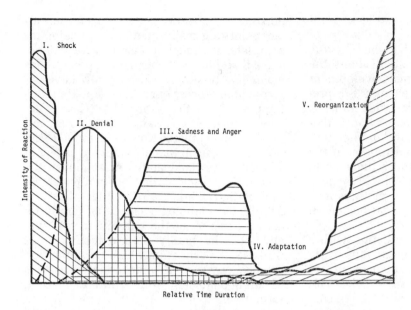

Figure 27–2. Hypothetical model of a normal sequence parental reactions to the birth of a malformed infant. (Adapted from Drotar, D., Baskiewicz, A., Irwin, N., Kennell, J., and Klaus, M.: Pediatrics 56:710–715, 1975. Copyright American Academy of Pediatrics 1975.)

the birth of a child with a malformation to the emotional crisis following the death of a child, in that the mother must mourn the loss of her expected normal infant (Solnit and Stark, 1961). In addition, she must become attached to her actual living, damaged child. However, the sequence of parental reactions to the birth of a baby with a malformation differs from that following the death of a child in another respect. Because of the complex issues raised by the continuation of the child's life and the demands of his physical care, the parents' sadness, which is initially important in their relationships with the child, diminishes in most instances once they take over the physical care. Parents reach a point at which they are able to adequately care for their child and effectively cope with disrupting feelings of sadness and anger.

The mother's initiation of the relationship with her child is a major step in reducing the anxiety and emotional upset associated with the trauma of the birth. As with normal children, the parents' caretaking experience with their infant seems to release positive feelings, which aid the mother-child relationship following the stresses associated with the news of the child's anomaly and, in many instances, the separation of mother and child in the hospital (Zuk, 1959). Lampe and coworkers noted significantly greater hospital visiting by the parents if an infant with an abnormality had been at home for a short while (Lampe et al., 1977).

PRACTICAL SUGGESTIONS FOR FACILITATING PARENTAL ATTACHMENTS TO THE MALFORMED INFANT

1. We have come to believe that, if medically feasible, it is far better to leave the infant with the mother for the first 2 to 3 days or discharge the baby home. If the child is rushed to the hospital where special surgery will eventually be done, the mother will not have enough opportunity to become attached to him. Even if immediate surgery is necessary, as in the case of bowel obstruction, it is best to bring the baby to the mother first, allow her to touch and handle him, and point out to her how normal he is in all other respects.

2. The parents' mental picture of the anomaly may often be far more alarming than the actual problem. Any delay in seeing the child greatly heightens their anxiety and causes their imaginations to run wild. Therefore we suggest that it is helpful to bring the baby to both parents when they are together as soon after delivery as possible.

3. We believe that parents should not be given tranquilizers, which tend to blunt their responses and slow their adaptation to the problem. However, a sedative at night is sometimes helpful.

4. Parents who are adapting reasonably well often ask many questions and indeed at times appear to be almost overinvolved in clinical care. We are pleased by this and are more concerned about the parents who ask

few questions, who appear stunned or over-whelmed by the problem, or who withdraw and visit infrequently. Parents who become involved in trying to find out what the best procedures are and who ask many questions about care are sometimes annoying but often make the best adaptation in the end.

5. Many anomalies are very frustrating to the physicians and nurses as well. There is a temptation for them to withdraw from the parents who ask many questions and then appear to forget and ask the same questions over and over.

6. We have found it best to move at the parents' pace. If we move too quickly, we run the risk of losing the parents along the way. It is beneficial to ask the parents how they view their infant.

7. Each parent may move through the sequence of shock, denial, anger, guilt, and adaptation at a different pace. If they are unable to talk with each other about the baby, their own relationship may be disrupted. Therefore, we use early crisis intervention and meet several times with the parents. During these discussions, we ask the mother how she is doing, how she feels her husband is doing, and how he feels about the infant. We then reverse the questions and ask the father how he is doing and how he thinks his wife is progressing. The hope is that they not only will think about their own reactions but will begin to consider each other's as well.

Summary of Care for Parents of Preterm, Sick, or Malformed Infants

1. When an infant weighs between 3 and 5 lb and appears to be doing well without grunting and retractions, we have found it useful and safe for the mother to have the baby placed in her bed for 20 to 30 minutes in the first hours of life with a heat panel above both of them. We do not recommend this unless the physician feels relaxed and sure about the infant's health.

2. When the long-term significance of early mother-infant contact is kept in mind, a modification of restrictions and territorial traditions can usually be arranged so that a mother and her infant can be kept near each other in the same hospital. It is helpful if the mother can have some private sessions with her infant in a separate room close to the unit.

3. Transporting the mother and baby together to the medical center that contains the intensive care nursery, either before or after delivery, is occurring more frequently now and should be encouraged for its immediate and long-term benefits.

4. The intensive care nursery should be open for parental visiting 24 hours a day and should have flexible rules about visits from others such as grandparents, supportive relatives, and, on certain occasions, siblings. Provided proper precautions are taken, infections will not be a problem.

5. A mother should be permitted to enter the premature nursery as soon as she is able to maneuver easily.

6. We also encourage grandparents, brothers, sisters, and other relatives to view the infant through the glass window of the nursery so that they will begin to feel attached to the infant.

7. If there is any chance that the infant will survive, we are optimistic in our talks with the parents from the beginning. There is no evidence that if a favorable prediction proves to be incorrect and the baby dies, the parents will be harmed by the early optimism. There is almost always time to prepare them before the baby actually dies. If the infant lives and the spokesperson for the health care team has been pessimistic, it is almost impossible for parents to become closely attached after they have figuratively dug a few shovelfuls of earth. We recognize that this recommendation is contrary to many old customs and places a heavy burden on the primary professional. It is our belief that if the infant does die, we must still work with the parents and help them with the mourning period.

8. Once the possibility that a baby has brain damage has been mentioned, the parents will not forget it. Therefore, unless we are 100 percent sure that the baby is damaged, we do not mention the possibility of any brain damage or retardation to the parents. On many occasions we have had neonates who have appeared to be brain damaged but who later were perfectly normal.

9. It is important to emphasize that if we have a clear objective finding, such as a cardiac abnormality or a specific congenital malformation, we see no reason to hide this

from the parents. We would never lie to a parent.

10. We should continue to study interventions such as rooming-in, nesting, and early discharge as well as transporting a healthy premature infant to be with his mother. It is necessary to try out these various interventions in different hospital settings and evaluate their ability to reduce the severe anxiety that many parents presently face during the prolonged hospitalization and the early days following discharge.

11. In all these interventions it is critical that nurses take mothers under their wings, especially supporting and encouraging them during these early days and weeks. The nurse's guidance in helping a mother with simple caretaking tasks can be extremely valuable in helping to overcome some of her anxiety. In this sense, the nurse assumes the role of the mother's own mother and contributes much more than merely teaching her basic caretaking techniques.

12. It is necessary to identify high-risk parents who are having special difficulties in adapting so that interventions can begin early. These parents often visit rarely and for short periods, appear frightened, and do not usually ask the medical staff questions about the infant's problems. Sometimes these mothers and fathers are hostile or irritable and show inappropriately low levels of anxiety.

13. As we develop a further understanding of the process by which normal mothers and infants interact with each other during the first months and the first year of life, it appears that recommendations for stimulation may be detrimental to normal development, at least at certain ages. Rather than suggesting stimulation, it may be important for a mother to naturally and unconsciously use imitation to learn about and find her own infant. The timing and appropriateness of this recommendation for different infants and mothers will require further study.

14. It has recently been reported that many infants weighing from 4 to 5 lb who were previously separated from their mothers immediately after birth and admitted to neonatal intensive care units can now be kept safely with their mothers on postpartum divisions. This requires special training for the nurses but proves to be popular with nurses and mothers (Whitby et al., 1982).

It is probable that in the future several of these interventions will be combined so that a mother may have early postdelivery contact with her premature infant if it is healthy, then have the baby stay with her on the postpartum division or, if smaller or sicker, brought to her bedside in the maternity unit from the NICU on several occasions early in the course of the infant's stay in the hospital and then before early discharge live in and nest with the mother for 3 or 4 days.

REFERENCES

Blau, A., Slaff, B., Easton, K., et al.: The psychogenic etiology of premature birth: a preliminary report. Psychosom. Med. 25:201, 1963.

Bloom, B.: Definitional concepts of the crisis concept. J. Consult. Psychol. 27:42, 1963.

Brown, G. W., and Harris, T.: Social Origins of Depression: A Study of Psychiatric Disorder in Women. New York, The Free Press, 1978.

Chappel, J.: Stresses Encountered by Hospitalized Antepartum Patients and Implications for the NICU Nurse. (Unpublished study report.) University of Florida, 1983.

Cohen, R.: Some maladaptive syndromes of pregnancy and the puerperium. Obstet. Gynecol. 27:562, 1966.

Hare, E., Lawrence, K., Paynes, H., et al.: Spina bifida cystica and family stress. Br. Med. J. 2:757, 1966.

Johns, N.: Family reactions to the birth of a child with a congenital abnormality. Med. J. Aust. 7:277, 1971.

Lampe, J., Trause, M., and Kennell, J.: Parental visiting of sick infants: the effects of living at home prior to hospitalization. Pediatrics 59:294, 1977.

Larson, C.: Efficacy of prenatal and postpartum home visits on child health and development. Pediatrics 66:191, 1980.

Merkatz, R.: Prolonged hospitalization of pregnant women: the effects on the family. Birth Family J. 5:204, 1978.

Moore, M. L.: Potential Alterations in Attachment: Maternal and/or Neonatal Illness. NAACOG Update Series. Princeton, NJ, Continuing Professional Education Center, Inc., 1983.

National Institutes of Health: Cesarean Childbirth Consensus Development Conference Summary, Bethesda, MD, 1980, Vol. 3, No. 6.

Olshansky, S.: Chronic sorrow: a response to having a mentally defective child. Soc. Case. 43:190, 1962.

Rappoport, L.: The state of crisis: Some theoretical considerations. In Parad, H. (ed.): Crisis Intervention. New York, Family Service Association, 1965.

Roskies, E.: Abnormality and Normality: The Mothering of Thalidomide Children. New York, Cornell University Press, 1972.

Solnit, A., and Stark, M.: Mourning and the birth of a defective child. Psychoanal. Study Child. 16:523, 1961.

Whitby, C., DeCates, C. R., and Roberton, N. R. C.: Infants weighing 1.8–2.5 kg: Should they be cared for in neonatal units or postnatal wards? Lancet 322, 1982.

Zuk, G.: Religious factor and the role of guilt in parental acceptance of the retarded child. Am. J. Ment. Defic. 64:145, 1959.

28

GRIEF COUNSELING

KENNETH R. KELLNER
MARIAN LAKE

The loss of a baby through stillbirth or neonatal death is a devastating experience for a woman. It precipitates intense emotional turmoil in the woman, her family and friends, and the medical professionals providing care during and after her pregnancy. If this emotional response is unrecognized and unattended, serious sequelae may develop.

The national perinatal death rate is 19.2 per 1000 live births (Vital Statistics, 1980). In most industrialized countries, the neonatal death rate equals the fetal death rate. Nurses, physicians, and other health care providers, although informed of the technologies to achieve fetal and neonatal survival, are often well-intentioned but ill-prepared to care for the woman and her family when perinatal death occurs.

Perinatal death causes a grief and mourning response as severe as, and perhaps even more disruptive than, that seen in families in whom adult members have died. Information presented here will allow readers to increase their awareness of the characteristics of normal grief and mourning, increase their appreciation of the significance and implications of the loss to the family, and assimilate methodologies designed to guide their care of the patient and her family.

Prenatal Maternal Attachment

It is often difficult for family members, friends, and medical professionals to understand the intensity of the woman's emotional response to the death of her fetus or newborn. It may be difficult to understand these emotions that seem to represent a deep, loving attachment to a baby that did not survive intrauterine life or never left the intensive care nursery. Unfortunately, the assumption may be made that since the baby was not, for example, full term or born alive or taken home and cared for by the mother, she has not been able to develop an attachment to the baby and therefore should be able to easily cope with the death, carry on with her life, and make a rapid, full recovery. In fact, an intense emotional attachment develops between the woman and her baby long before delivery and frequently long before conception.

The process involved in the development of the maternal-infant bond has been described in the work of Klaus and Kennell (1982). The attachment of mother to infant begins long before birth and physical care giving. As a young girl's socialization begins and she perceives a societal role as wife and mother, she may subconsciously begin the process of bonding to her baby through her fantasies of marriage, motherhood, and family, i.e., years before a pregnancy is actually conceived.

After conception, the bond between mother and fetus intensifies. Prior to the woman's detection of fetal movement, she may view the fetus as part of herself rather than as a separate individual. The perception of fetal movement allows and encourages her to identify the baby as an individual, now separate from her. Fantasizing about the baby's appearance and sex, the mother ascribes personality characteristics to the fetus, often giving the baby nicknames. The fetus now develops an individual identity. Long before delivery, the woman thinks about and plans for the baby's childhood, adolescence, and adult life. The death of a fetus or newborn cannot be viewed as the death of a baby whose identity and personality are unknown to the mother. It is the death of a perfect, idealized baby whose life has been long established for the woman and with whom she has developed an intense, loving relationship.

The existence of prenatal maternal attachment is further supported in the literature. The expression of grief after perinatal death may be viewed as evidence of that attachment (Kirkley-Best, 1981). The emotional expression of grief occurs irrespective of the woman's pleasure with being pregnant and the extent of parent-infant contact after delivery. In 1970, Kennell and colleagues, using "grief scores" to evaluate parental response to neonatal death, found that "clearly identifiable mourning" was present in each of the women interviewed, whether or not the pregnancy had been planned and whether or not the mother had touched the baby before or after death. Similar findings are reported in a study of 50 women experiencing neonatal death (Benfield et al., 1978). Both investigators found a grief response to be evident whether the baby was nonviable by weight or weighed over 4000 gm. Thus a woman, even one whose unplanned or unwanted pregnancy ends in the delivery of a nonviable fetus with whom she has had no physical contact, experiences a reaction demonstrating a preexisting emotional attachment to the baby.

The health professional must not assume that a woman will make a quick, full recovery from a perinatal death because she has had no opportunity to become attached to the baby. *Intense prenatal maternal attachment exists long before delivery* and is evident, irrespective of circumstances surrounding the pregnancy.

Grief and Mourning: Definitions

Information in the literature over the past few decades has increased our understanding of and sensitivity to the expression of grief following the loss of a loved one. Research concerning the survivor's grief after the death of an adult or child predominates. Although little attention has been directed to a systematic evaluation of the emotional

implications of a perinatal death, the available information clearly demonstrates that the family's response to this catastrophe parallels the descriptions of what families experience after the death of a child or adult. Experience with families after the delivery of a stillborn or the death of a neonate suggests to the authors that it may in fact be more disruptive.

Mourning is the process by which an individual reorganizes and adapts following the death of a loved one. The emotion that dominates this process is grief. Mourning is now recognized as a series of phases through which an individual passes after experiencing a loss (Lindemann, 1944; Bowlby, 1969; Parks, 1972). Although descriptions differ slightly, the process involves the following four phases:

1. Shock and disbelief
2. Yearning, searching, and anxiety
3. Disorganization, despair, and depression
4. Reorganization

The phase of *shock and disbelief* is characterized by a period of denial, usually short-lived. A sense of apathy, numbness, and unexpected calm typify this period. Concentration and the ability to make decisions are severely impaired. A typical response is to think a mistake has been made and that the loved one is still alive. The denial and inability to react are useful, self-protective defense mechanisms in that they allow the individual time to mobilize resources to cope with the shock. Patients relate that the emotions apparent in this phase are most intense during the first few weeks after the death. Denial that persists may constitute an abnormal response (Bowlby, 1961).

Yearning, searching, and anxiety make up the painful second phase of mourning. Preoccupied by thoughts and images of the deceased, the mourner cries, expresses anger and guilt, and often relates loneliness, sleeplessness, lack of strength and appetite, and a general loss in normal behavior patterns. This disruption in behavior results in confusion and anxiety. The grieving person is angry and needs to affix blame for the death. That blame may be directed at the survivor, the deceased, or, not uncommonly, health care professionals and those attempting to provide comfort. The intense emotional turmoil of this phase often prompts a feeling of profound personality changes and approaching insanity. The characteristics of this phase are most intense between the second week and fourth or fifth month after the death (Davidson, 1979).

Disorganization, despair, and depression predominate when the reality of the death becomes apparent and life is viewed without the relationship to the deceased. This phase, usually most intense 4 to 6 months after the death, may typically last several months. Previous meaningful aspects of life now carry little significance and activities are carried out only with effort. Work may be accomplished only by "going through the motions." Restlessness and aimless movements are common. Anorexia, insomnia, and malaise often prompt the mourner to make frequent calls to her physician seeking medical remedies.

Reorganization begins as time passes and preoccupation with the deceased wanes. The mourner is able to reenter activities of daily life without the oppressive feelings characteristic of the preceding three phases. Memory of the deceased is not gone; rather, it may be recalled but with feelings of sadness that do not disrupt daily functioning. Life is reorganized to allow the survivor to incorporate the severed relationship into her continuing life. The capacity to interact is no longer reduced. The emotional responses of each of the four phases are summarized in Table 28–1.

Health care providers coming in contact with grieving couples who have experienced a perinatal death must keep the following in mind:

1. *The process of mourning is both normal and painful.* The expression of grief is expected and the pain is inevitable.

2. *The process is not static.* Emotional responses typically intensify and wane over a period of 2 years with characteristics of each phase overlapping one another.

3. Although the process is presented in an orderly progression, *the individual's response may not be immutable.* The behavioral sequence may be described with the following progression: (a) anxiety, (b) anger, (c) pain, (d) despair, (e) hope. In reality, anger, for example, may precede anxiety, may not surface at all, or may persist through the whole process.

The length of time that passes before reorganization is reached varies. Full resolution may not be apparent for up to 2 years after the death. The duration of the response will be influenced by what has been described as "grief work," i.e., the ability to come to terms with the reality of the first three phases (Lindemann, 1944). To complete this difficult, often exhausting work, the bereaved must:

1. Accept the pain of the death,

2. Review their relationship with the deceased and emancipate themselves from it,

3. Readjust to their environment, and

4. Form new relationships.

Psychological sequelae of bereavement will be ameliorated by adequate grief work. Reorganization will be delayed if the process is impeded or in fact not encouraged.

Pathologic Grief Reactions

When the normal process of mourning and the expression of grief are blocked or suppressed, pathologic reactions can occur. In this instance, grief work is delayed, inhibited, or absent. The emotional expression of grief after perinatal death, vital to a healthy resolution, is often avoided by the woman and suppressed by those individuals with

Table 28–1. Characteristic Responses During the Phases of Mourning

Shock and Disbelief	Yearning, Searching, and Anxiety	Disorganization	Reorganization
Denial	Tears	Restlessness	Daily functioning not disrupted
Unexpected calm	Anger	Aimless movement	
Apathy	Guilt	Insomnia	Memories recalled with appropriate sadness
Numbness	Insomnia	Anorexia	
Impaired concentration	Anorexia	Malaise	
Impaired decision making	Need to affix blame	Life seems meaningless	Oppressive feelings have lifted
"There must be a mistake"	Confusion		Capacity to interact has returned
	Preoccupation with deceased		
	Loneliness		
	Disruption in normal patterns of behavior		

whom she comes into contact. Discussions of her pregnancy, her delivery, and the baby are avoided. Her need for support remains unmet. The silence and isolation she perceives may be interpreted as a lack of support, and attempts to review her relationship with the baby are thwarted. Often lacking any tangible evidence that the baby in fact ever existed, the woman's attempts to appreciate the reality of her baby's death are also blocked and she is placed at even further risk of developing a morbid grief response (Bowlby, 1961; Schoenberg, 1980).

Pathologic responses may be identified as either prolonged grief or absent, inhibited grief. Both have been described following perinatal death. Jensen and Zahourek (1972) found evidence of chronic depression, an aspect of prolonged grief, in six out of ten women 1 year after the death of a newborn. In a study of 56 women evaluated 1 to 2 years after a neonatal death, Cullberg (1971) found that 19 exhibited symptoms of a pathologic reaction. An additional study reports the incidence to be 26 percent of the population evaluated (Rowe et al., 1978).

Two groups of women seem to be at particular risk for an unsatisfactory outcome: women with pregnancies occurring within less than 6 months after a stillbirth, and women whose pregnancies involved a surviving twin. The British Stillbirth and Neonatal Death Association suggests that pregnancies occurring less than 6 months after a stillbirth can be associated with catastrophic grief reactions (Lockwood and Lewis, 1980). Additionally, in a group of nine women who either became pregnant within 5 months after a perinatal death or had a surviving twin, five developed morbid responses (Rowe et al., 1978). Although this study group is small, it is apparent that women in these circumstances need psychological follow-up.

As the phase of resolution is reached and the woman has incorporated the death of her baby as a part of her life, the symptoms of grief and mourning wane. This does not mean the baby's death will ever be perceived as fair or justifiable. Parents never "get over it" or forget the loss. It merely becomes less painful to remember. The dates of delivery, death, and/or funeral, in addition to certain holidays, are all anniversaries that may precipitate sadness and tears. This "shadow grief," as described by Peppers and Knapp (1980), may linger for a lifetime and does not constitute a morbid grief reaction. It is not a debilitating grief but rather represents the normal surfacing of memories and concomitant sadness.

Grief at the Event of Stillbirth

The concept of prenatal maternal attachment and a body of literature replete with anecdotal descriptions of parental responses allow us to appreciate the emotional impact of fetal and neonatal death (Kirkley-Best and Kellner, 1981). Health care providers caring for women experiencing stillbirth need to carefully consider several of this tragedy's special characteristics.

The sense of emptiness, typical of any mourning response, may be particularly acute in the case of fetal death in utero. The developing relationship between mother and fetus is abruptly terminated as evidenced by the fact that the growing, moving fetus is now quiet. In addition to losing a part of her body that had been relied on for recognition and gratification, the woman may experience profound disturbances in her body image. A sense of uncleanliness and loss of body integrity may predominate (Grubb, 1976; Kish, 1978).

Clearly, one of the most outstanding characteristics of the grief response at stillbirth is guilt. Both mother and father may experience it, but there is evidence to suggest that guilt is more intense and more prolonged in the woman (Helmrath and Steinitz, 1978). "What did I do that made my baby die?" and "What did I neglect to do?" are questions parents will repeatedly ask. A woman often spends extended periods of time reviewing the pregnancy to find where she was at fault. Often irrational or seemingly insignificant events are seen as the cause of death; for example, neglecting a prenatal vitamin, missing a prenatal visit, walking up a flight of stairs, contemplating an abortion early in the pregnancy. A father may assume guilt for leaving his partner home alone during the day, not insisting that she take her vitamins, or continuing sexual activities.

A woman's response to stillbirth has implications beyond her grief for the baby. A situation that has been described as a "double crisis" occurs (Quirk, 1979). The woman is confronted with not only the crisis of death but an implied inability to nurture and protect her baby. If the ability to complete a pregnancy and deliver a healthy infant is seen as proof of femininity and womanhood, the woman whose baby has been stillborn may grieve for lack of this proof. Pregnancy has been described as the fulfillment of a wish fantasy (Deutsch, 1944). If this wish is unfulfilled, intense feelings of anger, guilt, and depression can be expected.

Overcoming Obstacles to Parental Grief Work

Davidson (1977) studied 15 women and their families who had experienced a perinatal death. He identified three occasions when the mother seems most vulnerable to disorientation: (1) when she tries to confirm perceptually who died, (2) when she tries to get emotional support, and (3) when she compares her feelings with those of others. Although the work refers to mothers, fathers have similar problems. Each of these periods of vulnerability can be looked at as an obstacle to parental grief work. From this concept, methods to help families overcome each obstacle can be developed.

CONFIRMING PERCEPTUALLY WHO DIED

When an adult or older child dies, it is clear who that person was. There are memories, photographs, personal possessions, and mementos. Remembrances can be shared with relatives and friends. In contrast to this concrete, well-defined image of the person who has died, parents may be left with only vague feelings and images when perinatal death occurs. This is most pronounced with stillbirth, since the baby never existed as a separate, living human being outside its mother. Parents are left with hopes and dreams of the future that are unique to each individual and not easily shared. Mothers' memories of fetal movement and fathers' external perceptions of this may be the only physical contact with the baby. Parents who never see their dead baby and who are surrounded by silence from the medical staff know that something is missing but have difficulty conceptualizing what. Women who had stillbirths 20 or

30 years ago have asked, "How do I know my baby was dead? Maybe it was alive and they gave it to someone else." Such an occurrence has been reported in the lay press (LeBlanc, 1982). These women can be trapped in the phase of searching and yearning, never really believing their child is dead. Only when parents can believe and admit that the baby is dead can they progress to a satisfactory resolution of their grief.

These parents are also subject to disorientation because of the loss of control over their lives. All people need to feel that they have some control over their own destinies. When events occur over which we have no control, it can be very frightening. Since parents' plans and efforts are directed toward a healthy, normal baby, when this does not occur an overwhelming feeling of loss of control can take over that can make any further effort seem useless. To give back control, parents should be encouraged to make their own choices about the care of themselves and their baby. Letting parents make choices helps restore personal integrity (Lippman and Carlson, 1977) and removes responsibility from the staff who are usually anxious over their perceived responsibility for the tragedy.

Labor and delivery should be conducted as planned in order to help keep the parents oriented. There is no reason why the father cannot be present. Medical procedures such as episiotomy should be performed when indicated and not avoided "to spare the mother the discomfort." Above all, parents' individual wishes and desires must be respected. Davidson (1977) describes a woman with a previable baby who did not want to push at the end of her labor because she saw that as actively participating in the baby's death.

The simplest and probably most important way to help parents confirm who died is to let them *see the baby* (Lewis, 1971; Seitz and Warrick, 1974; Kowalski and Bowes, 1976; Davidson, 1977; Cohen et al., 1978; Kennell and Trause, 1978; O'Donohue, 1978; Bourne, 1979; Lewis, 1982). Davidson (1977) found no adverse reactions in mothers who had viewed their babies, and some seemed to adapt more easily to their loss. Cohen and coworkers (1978) found a higher percentage of nonviewers among mothers requiring psychiatric treatment than among those who resolved their grief satisfactorily. At the University of Florida, 91 percent of 164 parents chose to see their dead baby when offered the choice (Kellner et al., 1984). No correlation was found between the baby's appearance (maceration, malformation) and the desire to view the baby. This choice should be presented before delivery so that parents have time to decide. They should be told what the baby will look like. If they choose not to see the baby at delivery, it should be available at a later time. The normal, positive aspects of the baby's appearance should be pointed out, as this is what parents focus on and remember (Cohen et al., 1978; O'Donohue, 1978; Bourne, 1979). A majority of parents will also choose to *hold the baby* (Kellner et al., 1984), and they should be given time alone with it. They should be asked if there are other family or friends whom they would like to have view or hold the baby.

Naming the baby helps acknowledge the reality of the death and helps parents and others think and talk about the child. Parents are usually surprised when told that they can name a stillborn baby, and more than three fourths will do so when given the opportunity (Kellner et al., 1984).

Tangible evidence of the baby's existence is appreciated by parents. They may desire the baby's blanket, identification bracelet, or a lock of hair. A very simple memento is a set of the baby's *footprints* on the standard hospital form. In addition to confirming the actuality of the baby, the footprints reinforce the normality of the baby (normal feet and toes) and provide information about site, time, and staff involved, which can help the parents review events later.

Photographs are strongly desired by almost all families. These photographs should be good quality, as they are how parents will remember the child. Although instant photographs taken during labor and delivery may be adequate (Chez, 1982), photographs of the baby carefully wrapped in a blanket better facilitate acceptance (Kellner et al., 1981). Attempts should be made to avoid the harshness of typical pathology pictures and to photograph the baby in a manner that demonstrates compassionate care (Fig. 28–1). Davidson (1979) found that after being shown photographs of their babies, women who had not seen their babies previously stopped hearing phantom crying.

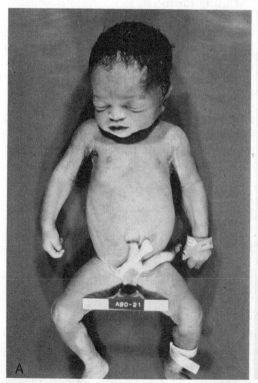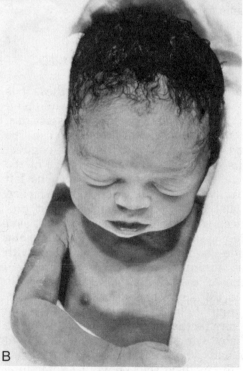

Figure 28–1. *A,* The harshness of the typical pathology photograph of a dead infant provides inadequate comfort to the family. *B,* When the baby is photographed in a manner that demonstrates compassionate care, acceptance is facilitated.

After delivery, patients should be given the choice of *where to recover*. Depending on the facilities, the value of being away from mothers and babies should be weighed against the expertise of the obstetric staff to handle the physical and emotional problems of the postpartum period. Lamb (1982) suggests using a color code on charts to signify mothers with sick or dead babies. She also presents a checklist form for the chart so that interventions and responses can be noted and not duplicated. Although there has been a traditional tendency to discharge these women as quickly as possible, many mothers, especially those with poor support systems at home, may benefit from longer contact with counseling personnel in the hospital.

Baptism may be requested (Kirkley-Best et al., 1982). This may be performed by the appropriate clergy either in the hospital or after discharge or by staff members familiar with the procedure. Religious practices vary (Hollingsworth and Pasnau, 1977) and should be considered when discussing choices.

An *autopsy* can help families in many ways. By providing a detailed description of the baby, it helps parents confirm that this was a real human being. Since almost all stillborns are completely normal, it can help restore feelings of value and self-esteem to the parents. An autopsy can also help answer the two questions that are central to the family's feelings: "Why did my baby die?" and "Will it happen again?" When a definite cause of death is found, parental guilt can be reduced and realistic recurrence risks given to relieve anxiety. Even when no cause of death is found, the normality of the child can be stressed and the low risk of recurrence reassuring. Such information can also be a comfort to the health care providers. A copy of the autopsy report should be given to the parents so that they can review it later when emotions have eased; it also serves as a sign that nothing is being held back or concealed. Several authors have reported that parents are interested in autopsy results and will return to get them (Cohen et al., 1978; Clyman et al., 1980; Kellner et al., 1984). The autopsy request, therefore, should be part of the care given the patient rather than an end in itself. Berger (1978) provides an excellent discussion of the value of the autopsy and how the request should be made. The request should come from the physician most involved with the patient's care, but he must be knowledgeable to answer the parents' questions about what will be done, when, where, and how much it will cost.

Information must also be available about options for disposition of the remains. An explanation of how the hospital will dispose of the body should be given if appropriate, since what happens to the body can be a source of long-lasting concern (Cohen et al., 1978). A *funeral* for a stillborn is perfectly appropriate, and the hospital should assist in facilitating this choice. A funeral can facilitate the grieving process in several ways. It formalizes the death as something real and important. It provides family and friends an opportunity to support the bereaved by sharing in this ritual. The grave provides a place the parents can visit to be with their baby and where sadness can be expressed. Even if cremation is chosen, a small service can be held. Parents remember the funeral as a positive experience and often see it as the time when the past was closed and they started looking toward the future.

Hospital staff often feel pressure to talk with parents about autopsy and disposition of remains in order to "get the paperwork over with." However, it must be appreciated by the staff, and it is helpful to acknowledge to the parents that they are being asked to make very difficult choices under circumstances where they would rather not be making any choices. There is rarely a circumstance in which parents cannot have several days to make these critical decisions about the care of their deceased baby.

Seeing, holding, and naming the baby; mementos; and the autopsy and funeral all help the parents confirm that this was indeed a baby, their baby who died, and serve as remembrances of the event. As Stack (1982) says, "The end point of the grieving process is not to help the person forget the lost loved one, but to remember without pain."

GETTING EMOTIONAL SUPPORT

Society, family, and friends often do not consider fetal loss to be a significant life event. Such solicitudes as "It's better the baby died before you got to know it," "You're young, you can have lots more babies,'' or ''You have other children at home so what's the big deal?'' are wrong and tend to isolate the bereaved from these often well-meaning people who do not understand what has happened.

Medicine has traditionally also shared this view and focused on the medical aspects of managing fetal death (ACOG, 1979). Health care providers are also hampered from giving support because the death raises their own anxieties. This will be discussed in greater detail later. Cullberg (1971) found that staff responded to the anxiety engendered by perinatal death by avoiding the situation, by projecting their feelings of anger and blame onto the parent, and by denial and ''magical repair.'' These strategies resulted in the staff's avoiding the family as much as possible or not being sensitive to their needs. Parents experiencing neonatal death report concern and many phone calls while the infant was ill, but once the baby died there was a ''conspiracy of silence'' around the parents as if they had never had a baby (Helmrath and Steinitz, 1978).

Families can be helped to overcome this obstacle by receiving support. First, health care providers must realistically evaluate their own anxieties and feelings so that they can help the family deal with theirs. Staff with special training or interest in this field can be very helpful. Second, professionals must *volunteer to help*. Families are quick to pick up both verbal and nonverbal cues that staff are uncomfortable and so tend to be silent and compliant to minimize distress. The staff interpret the parents' behavior as indicating that they do not want to talk, so they stay away, which completes the cycle of silence. Physicians and nurses must break the cycle by taking the initiative and going in to the patient's room. It is not necessary to spend a long time. Several 10- to 15-minute contacts during the day may be better than one long one, but this must be individualized. Shreiner and colleagues (1979) found that a simple, caring phone call to parents after the death of their newborn resulted in a decrease in the number and intensity of subsequent emotional problems.

The question that is always asked is ''What do I say?'' A simple statement that shows your feelings, acknowledges the reality of the event, and offers continuity of support is ideal, such as ''I'm sorry your baby died. Is there anything I can do for you?'' This also gives the parents permission to express

their feelings. Lippman and Carlson (1977) stress the concept of ''realistic support'' in this circumstance. This is a time when the staff person can purposely encourage the family to express themselves concerning the death and can listen patiently without having to ''do something.'' As they point out, this may be easier said than done for health care personnel accustomed to providing ''tangible'' care. However, the importance of listening as a therapeutic modality cannot be overemphasized. A mother of a stillborn said, ''I can understand why they avoided me, because they didn't know what to say . . . but sometimes you really don't have to say anything.''

It is also helpful to bring up certain topics that parents may be reticent to raise or have not anticipated because of the acute stress of the situation. Clyman and associates (1980) found that over half the mothers they interviewed had difficulty telling their other children of the death or in dealing with subsequent behavior problems such as nightmares. Discussions with siblings must be tailored to the children's age and previous experience and discussions about death. In general, though, it is recommended that parents explain that the child was in no way responsible for the death and that he is safe from a similar fate. This will be dealt with in more detail in a later section. Couples experiencing a first pregnancy are naturally concerned as to whether they will ever have a healthy baby. Although a definitive answer should not be given until all studies are complete, parents can usually be assured that stillbirth will not recur. Parents should also be warned that other people may not appreciate the magnitude of the tragedy that has occurred. Telling parents the type of things people may say and asking them to think about how they will respond is helpful preparation.

The mother may appreciate being able to discuss with a staff member how best to dispose of nursery items and baby clothes purchased before the loss of her child. It should be stressed, however, that the mother should handle this in a manner comfortable for her and not let others ''take care of things'' while she is in the hospital. As one mother said, ''Sometimes other people do your thinking for you and that's bad.'' There is no right or wrong. The mother may feel more comfortable having things put away before she gets home, doing it herself, or closing the nursery door and not going in for 6 months. It should be up to the parents alone.

It is beneficial to inquire, at a follow-up visit, about the couple's sexual relationship. This topic will rarely be raised by parents even when significant problems have developed as a result of the death. As with sexual problems under other circumstances, giving parents permission to talk about it may be beneficial in itself. Showing parents how this problem fits into their overall grieving reactions and explaining that this is an understandable and common problem is helpful.

Religion can be a very variable source of support (Kirkley-Best et al., 1982). Depending on ideology, parental participation, and formal support structures, religion may be a great comfort or a source of distress. Support should be given so parents can sort out their feelings and commitments.

In summary, parents have difficulty getting support because of a lack of understanding by society as well as health care professionals of their need for emotional support. The simplest way to help them overcome this obstacle is to volunteer our help and experience.

COMPARING THEIR FEELINGS WITH THOSE OF OTHERS

As has been stressed, parents will encounter many people who do not understand. These may be people whom the parents have formerly depended on for clues to appropriate behavior. In the case of perinatal death, the clues may be that parental mourning and feelings of grief are inappropriate and abnormal (Helmrath and Steinitz, 1978). The mother who tells her bereaved daughter to "eat to keep up her strength" and asks, "Why all the tears, it's been a month?" can cause very disorienting and uncomfortable feelings in the woman experiencing an acute and normal grief response. Likewise, the father who has just suffered the most devastating tragedy in his life and returns to work to find his friends silent and acting as if nothing has happened can become very confused (Davidson, 1977). He may react with anger and hostility, further alienating potential sources of support, or may convince himself that his feelings are abnormal and hold them within. The normal intense emotions of

grieving are difficult enough to bear without the added burden of feeling that those emotions are abnormal. "I feel like I'm going crazy" is a common complaint of the unprepared.

Problems also arise because of a lack of appreciation of the duration of mourning. Helmrath and Steinitz (1978) point out that the period of acute grief lasts 6 months to 1 year; Davidson (1979) feels that it takes a majority of adults 18 to 24 months to complete the mourning process. Although the overall intensity will gradually decrease and most couples may appear to be functioning normally in public at 6 months, it is common for mothers returning for gynecologic examinations a year or 2 later to cry when given permission to talk about the death. Unfortunately, this lengthy period can be a strain on family and friends who are not sharing these feelings and get "tired" of the sadness and mourning. This adds to the couple's alienation.

This obstacle can be overcome by discussions of what grieving will be like. *Education* should include not only the parents but also their family and friends whenever possible. Perinatal mortality counseling programs should have education as a major objective (Kellner et al., 1981).

It is tempting to describe normal grieving to couples so that it will not be perceived as abnormal and the distress intensified. However, such counseling may merely intellectualize the death and retard resolution. In addition, since each person will react according to his individual personality and emotional experiences, predictions of an individual's feelings and behaviors are highly inaccurate. One woman at the time of an early stillbirth was given a detailed list of the signs and symptoms of grieving and was disturbed later that she had not experienced all of them. One successful approach is to stress the individuality of responses to the death and introduce specific feelings with phrases such as "Some mothers have felt . . . ," "Some fathers have told us . . . ," "You may or may not feel that way. Whatever happens is right for you and O.K."

A discussion of "anniversaries," such as due date, confirmation of pregnancy, and the baby's death, as events that bring back painful memories can assuage the discomfort. It is like a deep wound, which, although healed, still hurts when traumatized.

Education and reassurance can do much

Table 28–2. Methods to Overcome the Obstacles to Normal Parental Grief

Confirming Perceptually Who Died	Getting Emotional Support	Comparing Feelings with Others'
See the baby	Volunteer time	Educate parents
Hold the baby	Volunteer topics	Educate family
Name the baby	Provide follow-up	Educate staff
Footprints		
Mementos		
Photographs		
Autopsy		
Funeral		

Data from Davidson, 1977.

to help parents understand and express their feelings. This can result in a healthier resolution of their grief. Obstacles to parental grief work and methods to help overcome these obstacles are summarized in Table 28–2.

Fathers

If the emotion at perinatal death is the "forgotten grief," then the father is certainly the "forgotten mourner." As one mother said, "After the baby died, all the cards and flowers were addressed to me." Several factors may conspire to make it even more difficult for the father to resolve his feelings in a healthy way than for the mother.

There can be no doubt that in almost all cases, prenatal maternal attachment to the baby is stronger than prenatal paternal attachment (Davidson, 1977). The physical intimacy shared by the woman and the baby developing within her can never be matched by the paternal experience. Peppers and Knapp (1980) have labeled this difference between the mother's and father's experience "incongruent bonding." Bugen (1977) proposed that the intensity and duration of a grieving response are directly proportional to the closeness of the relationship between the deceased and the bereaved. LaGrua (1979), studying families following perinatal death, found that grieving in this situation fits this model. It would, therefore, be expected that fathers, having a less intimate relationship with the fetus, would grieve less than mothers, and this seems to be the case (Helmrath and Steinitz, 1978; Benfield et al., 1978). Peppers and Knapp (1980) have called this "incongruent grieving."

Another important obstacle to paternal grief work is society's expectations that the man be strong and not show emotion. The father tries to give strength to his spouse and thereby denies his own feelings. While the mother is in the hospital and sheltered during the initial intense and overwhelming stages of grief, the father must go home and tell the children, tell the friends, arrange for the funeral, and interact with the hospital. The man is more likely to "purposely" not grieve, and when he does, he may be more upset by his emotions than the mother (Kennell et al., 1970). It is important to recognize, however, that the emotions of a father experiencing a stillbirth are also strong (Kotzwinkle, 1975).

The obstacles to paternal grief work not only increase the chances of a poor resolution of grief for the father but put his relationship with his wife at great risk. One third of the women studied by Cullberg (1971) reported marital difficulties. Feelings of anger and blame may be misdirected at a spouse, and the couple may be unable to accept each other as they did before. The "incongruent grieving" can easily lead to conflict as the husband quickly tires of his wife's intense emotions, whereas she accuses him of being unfeeling and not having loved the baby. This often affects their sexual relationship (Peppers and Knapp, 1980).

The solution is *support and education.* The father needs acknowledgement of his role in the pregnancy and his feelings about the death. He should be allowed to show his emotions, and other family members and friends should be encouraged to share the feelings with him and handle whatever personal affairs they can to lighten his burden. The husband and wife should be treated as a couple. The husband should be allowed to be with his wife as much as possible, and ideally they should be allowed to stay together continuously in the hospital. Communication between partners is the cornerstone of a satisfactory resolution of the crisis. The difference in grieving responses should be discussed and tolerance stressed. It can be very helpful to meet with the parents both together and separately to facilitate the expression of their feelings.

Siblings

In one perinatal mortality counseling program, almost half of the parents experiencing a perinatal death had living children (Kellner et al., 1981). These parents must face the problem of telling siblings about the death and appreciate help in doing so.

The age of the child is an important consideration. Grollman (1977) found that from ages 3 to 5, children deny that death is a regular or final process. From 5 to 9, they understand death to be final but do not recognize it as universal or something that will eventually happen to themselves. After age 9, the inevitability of death is acknowledged. This provides a general guideline to the type of information the child can process and may prepare parents for the child's responses. For example, young children, because they do not understand the finality of death, will repeatedly ask the parents where the baby is and when it is coming home. This can be very upsetting to the parents.

Difficulty also stems from the different feelings that parents and siblings have about the future child. Furman (1978) points out that whereas parents usually view the coming baby with anticipation as a happy addition to the family, a child may see it as a rival and feel jealousy and envy. It is easy to conceive of a child's having destructive fantasies about the baby. When the baby dies, the child may be faced with guilt over his wishes coming true coupled with his fear of what his parents may do if they find out. In addition, parents may interpret a child's short attention span as the child's lack of interest in the death and so not discuss it. Parents appreciate it when staff make them aware of these issues.

Parents may also wonder whether siblings should attend the funeral. Schowaiter (1980) feels the decision should be based on the child's level of development and the amount of environmental support available. Children less than 7 years old tend to be disruptive and should attend only if it is important to the parents. Those older than 7 should be allowed to be part of the decision after a discussion between the parents and child. If the child attends, the service should be conducted with his presence in mind; he should be allowed to leave at any time, and a specific person should be assigned to care for him (Schreiner et al., 1979).

The Next Pregnancy

Almost every woman asks, "When can I get pregnant again?" Becoming pregnant right away may seem to be a good strategy, but it is not.

Cain and Cain (1964), studying disturbed children of families who had experienced a previous child's death, found that one half of the physicians had suggested getting pregnant quickly as a means of forgetting the death or giving the mother something to do. Horowitz (1978) found that 38 of 40 mothers who had suffered a poor outcome in pregnancy either got pregnant again to replace the loss or purposely did not use contraception.

Unfortunately, *immediately replacing the dead child may have serious consequences.* Rowe and associates (1978) found that, in a sample of 26 mothers followed between 12 and 20 months after stillbirth, the only predictor of morbid grief reactions was the presence of a surviving twin or subsequent pregnancy within 5 months of the loss. Forrest and colleagues (1982) found that women who conceived within 6 months of their baby's death had a higher rate of detectable psychiatric disorders than those who conceived later. Jolly (1976) has likewise warned against replacing the dead infant with another child.

It must be remembered that the child who died was an ideal child. There was never a chance or the need to reconcile a real child with that image. In addition, the dead child represented hopes, dreams, plans, and perhaps an important part of his parents' identification and defense systems (Cain and Cain, 1964; Bourne, 1979). The "replacement child" must bear the burden of that image and those fantasies and a "lifelong sense of impossible destinies to fulfill."

Parents must have truly resolved their grief before they can successfully embark on having a new child who must be an individual in his own right (Klaus and Kennell, 1982). Parents must come to realize that yes, they can have another child, but no, they can never have the child that died. This should form the basis for counseling on this subject.

Physicians and Nurses

Health care personnel have feelings, too. The inability to appropriately recognize and deal with those feelings can interfere with the care of patients. A stillborn or neonatal death arouses strong emotions in physicians and nurses that may mirror those of the parents. The physician may have feelings of helplessness, defeat, guilt, resentment, and failure (Stack, 1982). Queenan (1978a) titled an editorial on fetal death, "The Ultimate Defeat."

Peppers and Knapp (1982) feel that because of their training, health care personnel and physicians in particular have difficulty dealing with death. "Death becomes something to work against, to avoid if possible, at any cost. It is not to be accepted; it is to be rejected. When death does occur it is considered the result of medical accident or technical error." Obstetricians and pediatricians dealing constantly with the beginning of life and so rarely with death may have particular problems accepting perinatal death. So too may nurses and social workers in areas where life begins.

Stillbirth arouses anxiety in the staff that, unless recognized, can be another contributing factor to parents not getting the support they need. Rowe and coworkers (1978) found that 60 percent of families were dissatisfied with the information they received or the way they received it and specifically with contacts with their physician. This is because of the way most physicians and nurses respond to anxiety (Cullberg, 1971; Stack, 1982). Reactions of health care personnel include avoidance of the situation, either by physical separation or dissociation, that is, separating one's feelings from the reality of the situation. They also project their personal feelings of guilt and anger onto the patient in the form of aggressive or accusing behavior and use denial to make believe nothing has happened by not showing the mother her dead baby and discharging her from the hospital early.

Just as these defenses may further isolate the parents and result in a cyclic degeneration of the relationship between them and the staff, the staff's recognition of their own feelings can be a positive factor in helping these families. As Queenan (1978b) says, "Never underestimate the help the obstetrician can offer bereaved parents." Peppers and Knapp (1980) offer practical advice for physicians in this difficult situation. When the time comes to talk with the family about what has happened or what will happen, it should be done in a quiet, private place. Appropriate family or friends may be present. It is helpful to plan ahead how the words will be spoken. It is best to keep the information simple and honest. Time should

be given for understanding and questions. It is important to note that parents may remember only some of what they are told but that they will remember forever. Physical contact, such as touching a hand or putting an arm around the father, can be very comforting. In one program, staff always sit down when in the room and remove their white coats (Kellner et al., 1981). Handing a box of tissues to the father gives him permission to express his emotions.

A plan for an ongoing relationship of contact and follow-up is needed. A phone call a week after the event (Schreiner et al., 1979) and an office visit for a discussion of autopsy reports should be the minimal contact. Contact with the family must be maintained until the parents feel it is no longer needed. Referral for professional counseling may be appropriate.

Physicians and nurses themselves also need support. They should share their feelings either in group discussion sessions (Scupholme, 1978) or individually with colleagues or professionals. It is a disservice to themselves and their patients for them to ignore their feelings.

Counseling and Support Programs

Just as the parents feel disoriented and overwhelmed after a perinatal death, so may individual physicians and nurses. The team approach can be very helpful in this situation. Several hospitals have developed formal programs, and these have been described in the literature (Lippman and Carlson, 1977; O'Donohue, 1978; Kennell and Trause, 1978; Davidson and Goldenberg, 1979; Kellner et al., 1981; Lake et al., 1983). 2901Formal support and counseling have been shown to shorten the duration of bereavement after perinatal death (Forrest et al., 1982).

A typical counseling team might be composed of an attending obstetrician, an obstetric resident on rotation, a pathologist, a nurse, and a social worker. It is believed that the interdisciplinary nature of this team is best suited to resolving the many problems these families have. Different family members often relate best to different team members, which facilitates the expression of feelings. In addition, the team allows a sharing of the emotional burden, which would be overwhelming for one person. Each member can not only give emotional support to other team members and hospital staff but also share his particular area of expertise. At the same time, each can pursue his own interests in this field, which include formal teaching of residents, students, nurses, and hospital staff.

Parents are seen at the time of diagnosis, at prenatal visits, at delivery, post partum in the hospital, at the postpartum visit, and at a final follow-up visit. This is the minimum contact, as additional telephone contacts are usually made. A data form is kept that serves two purposes: (1) noting of personal data so that at later interviews a personal relationship can be conveyed (Schreiner et al., 1979) and specific areas followed up, and (2) ensuring that interventions (such as giving footprints) are done and areas of counseling (such as what to tell siblings) are not unnecessarily repeated by different team members (Lamb, 1982).

These counseling programs were originally developed to aid families experiencing stillbirth, since these families did not fall into any already established program. However, proficiency in this field has grown, and they are now also providing aid to families with a congenital malformation diagnosed in utero and to pregnant patients with cancer who must make decisions about termination. Such teams now often function as a resource for hospital and community personnel faced with any poor outcome pregnancy.

The single most constant source of support for parents is another person who has been through the same experience. This is often a friend or relative who experienced a miscarriage or stillbirth many years ago, unbeknownst to the bereaved. Parents are amazed at the number of people who "come out of the closet" and share feelings that may have been suppressed for years. This can be very beneficial for both parents.

In an effort to capitalize on this source of support, several parent groups have been formed at local, national, and international levels. Peppers and Knapp (1980) provide an excellent discussion of the function and organization of these groups as well as addresses for additional information.

Conclusion

Perinatal death strikes the unprepared, the young, the inexperienced. It is, as Bourne (1979) says, "one of nature's obscenities."

How physicians and nurses deal with this situation can have lasting consequences for their patients and their families.

It is now clear that there is strong prenatal parental attachment to the baby. When that attachment is broken by perinatal death, intense grief is the appropriate, expected response. The resolution of this crisis is dependent on how health care providers respond to the grieving parents and family.

Learning what is helpful is only the first step. Professionals gladly share in their patients' joy when a healthy baby is born. They have an even stronger obligation to share in their patients' sorrow when the pregnancy ends in tragedy.

REFERENCES

ACOG: Diagnosis and management of missed abortion and antepartum fetal death. ACOG Tech. Bull., No. 55, November 1979.

Benfield, D. G., Leib, S. A., and Vollman, J. H.: Grief response of parents to neonatal death and parent participation in deciding care. Pediatrics 62:171, 1978.

Berger, L. R.: Requesting the autopsy: a pediatric perspective. Clin. Pediatr. 17:445, 1978.

Bourne, S.: Coping with perinatal death. Midwife Health Visit. Community Nurse 15:89, 1979.

Bowlby, J.: Processes of mourning. Int. J. Psychoanal. 42:317, 1961.

Bugen, L. A.: Human grief: a model for prediction and intervention. Am. J. Orthopsychiatry 47:196, 1977.

Cain, A. C., and Cain, B. S.: On replacing a child. J. Am. Acad. Child. Psychiatry 3:443, 1964.

Chez, R. A.: Symposium: Helping parents and doctors cope with perinatal death. Contemp. Ob/Gyn 20:98, 1982.

Clyman, R. I., Green, C., Rowe, J., et al.: Issues concerning parents after the death of their newborn. Crit. Care Med. 8:215, 1980.

Cohen, L., Zilkha, S., Middleton, J., et al.: Perinatal mortality: assisting in parental affirmation. Am. J. Orthopsychiatry 48:727, 1978.

Cullberg, J.: Mental reactions of women to perinatal death. In Psychosomatic Medicine in Obstetrics and Gynecology: Proceedings of Third International Congress, London, 1971. Basel, Karger, 1972, pp. 326–329.

Davidson, C. S., And Goldenberg, R. L.: Report on counseling elicited by symposiums on fetal death (equal time). Contemp. Ob/Gyn 13:13, 1979.

Davidson, G.: Death of the wished-for child: a case study. Death Educ. 1:265, 1977.

Davidson, G.: Understanding Death of the Wished-for Child. Springfield, IL, OGR Service Corporation, 1979.

Deutsch, H.: The Psychology of Women: A Psychoanalytic Interpretation; Vol. 2: Motherhood. New York, Grune & Stratton, 1944.

Forrest, G. C., Standish, E., and Baum, J. D.: Support after perinatal deaths: a study of support and counselling after perinatal bereavement. Br. Med. J. 285:1475, 1982.

Furman, E.: The death of a newborn: care of the parents. Birth Fam. J. 5:214, 1978.

Grollman, E. A.: Explaining death to children. J. School Health, June 1977, pp. 336–339.

Grubb, C. A.: Body image concerns of a multipara in the situation of intrauterine fetal death. Matern. Child Nurs. J. 5:93, 1976.

Helmrath, T. A., and Steinitz, E. M.: Death of an infant: parental grieving and the failure of social support. J. Fam. Pract. 6:785, 1978.

Hollingsworth, C. E., and Pasnau, R. O.: The Family in Mourning: A Guide for Health Professionals. New York, Grune & Stratton, 1977.

Horowitz, N. H.: Adolescent mourning reactions to infant and fetal loss. Soc. Casework, November 1978, pp. 551–559.

Jensen, J. S., and Zahourek, R.: Depression in mothers who have lost a newborn. Rocky Mountain Med. J., 71:61, 1972.

Jolly, H.: Family reactions to stillbirth. Proc. R. Soc. Med. 69:835, 1976.

Kellner, K. R., Kirkley-Best, E., Chesborough, S., et al.: Perinatal mortality counseling program for families who experience a stillbirth. Death Educ. 5:29, 1981.

Kellner, K. R., Donnelly, W. H., and Gould, S. D.: Parental behavior after perinatal death: lack of predictive variables. Obstet. Gynecol. 63:809, 1984.

Kennell, J. H., Sylter, H., and Klaus, M. H.: The mourning response of parents to the death of a newborn infant. N. Engl. J. Med. 283:344, 1970.

Kennell, J. H., and Trause, M. A.: Helping parents cope with perinatal death. Contemp. Ob/Gyn 12:53, 1978.

Kirkley-Best, E.: Grief in response to prenatal loss: an argument for the earliest maternal attachment. University of Florida (Gainesville), Doctoral Dissertation, 1981.

Kirkley-Best, E., and Kellner, K. R.: Grief at stillbirth: an annotated bibliography. Birth Fam. J. 8:91, 1981.

Kirkley-Best, E., and Kellner, K. R.: The forgotten grief: a review of the psychology of stillbirth. Am. J. Orthopsychiatry 52:420, 1982.

Kirkley-Best, E., Kellner, K. R., Gould, S., et al.: On stillbirth: an open letter to the clergy. J. Pastoral Care 36:17, 1982.

Kish, G.: Notes on C. Grubb's body image concerns of a multipara in the situation of intrauterine fetal death. Matern. Child Nurs. J. 7:111, 1978.

Klaus, M., and Kennell, J.: Parent-Infant Bonding, 2nd ed. St. Louis, C. V. Mosby Co., 1982.

Kotzwinkle, W.: Swimmer in the Secret Sea. New York, Avon Books, 1975.

Kowalski, K., and Bowes, W. A.: Parents' response to a stillborn baby. Contemp. Ob/Gyn 8:53, 1976.

LaGrua, P. M.: Grieving responses of parents to the death of their newborn infant. University of Florida (Gainesville), Master's Thesis, 1979.

Lake, M., Knuppel, R. A., Murphy, J., et al.: The role of a grief support team following stillbirth. Am. J. Obstet. Gynecol. 146:877, 1983.

Lamb, J. M.: In Chez, R.: Symposium: Helping parents and doctors cope with perinatal death. Contemp. Ob/Gyn 20:98, 1982.

LeBlanc, R. D.: My baby can't be dead. Readers Digest March 1982, pp. 73–77.

Lewis, E.: Reactions to stillbirth. In Psychosomatic Medicine in Obstetrics and Gynecology: Proceedings of Third International Congress, London, 1971. Basel, Karger, 1972, pp. 323–325.

Lewis, E.: Comments in Klaus, M. H., and Kennell, J. H.: Parent-Infant Bonding, 2nd ed. St. Louis, C. V. Mosby Co., 1982.

Lindemann, E.: Symptomatology and management of acute grief. Am. J. Psychiatr. 101:141, 1944.

Lippman, C., and Carlson, K.: In Hollingsworth, C. E., and Pasnau, R. O. (eds.): The Family in Mourning: A Guide for Health Professionals. New York, Grune & Stratton, 1977, pp. 17–28.

Lockwood, S., and Lewis, I. C.: Management of grieving after stillbirth. Med. J. Aust. 2:308, 1980.

O'Donohue, N.: Perinatal bereavement: the role of the health care professional. QRB, 4:30, 1978.

Parks, C. M.: Bereavement: Studies of Grief in Adult Life. New York, International University Press, 1972, pp. 13–26.

Peppers, L., and Knapp, R.: Motherhood and Mourning. New York, Praeger, 1980.

Queenan, J.: The ultimate defeat. (Letter from the Editor-in-Chief.) Contemp. Ob/Gyn 11:7, 1978a.

Queenan, J.: Never underestimate the help you can offer bereaved parents. (Letter from the Editor-in-Chief). Contemp. Ob/Gyn 12:9, 1978b.

Quirk, T. S.: Crisis theory, grief theory and related psychosocial factors: the framework for intervention. J. Nurse Midwife. 24:13, 1979.

Rowe, J., Clyman, R., Green, C., et al.: Follow-up of families who experience a perinatal death. Pediatrics 62:166, 1978.

Schoenberg, B. M. (ed.): Bereavement Counseling. Westport, CT, Greenwood Press, 1980, pp. 75–76.

Schowaiter, J.: Children and funerals. Pediatrics Rev. 1:337, 1980.

Schreiner, R. H., Gresham, E. L., and Green, M.: Physicians' responsibility to parents after death of an infant. Am. J. Dis. Child. 133:723, 1979.

Scupholme, A.: Who helps? Coping with the unexpected outcomes of pregnancy. JOGN Nurs. 7:36, 1978.

Seitz, P., and Warrick, L.: Perinatal death: the grieving mother. Am. J. Nurs. 74:2028, 1974.

Stack, J.: Reproductive casualties. Perinatal Press 6:29, 1982.

Vital Statistics of the United States 1978, Vol. II, Part A. DHHS Publ. No. (PHS) 83-1101. Washington, D.C., United States Public Health Service, U.S. Government Printing Office, 1982.

THE NATURE OF LAWSUITS RELATED TO OBSTETRIC CARE

STUART Z. GROSSMAN
J. B. SPENCE

In this chapter, we review those areas of obstetric care that engender the greatest number of medical negligence cases. From our collective experience of 40 years in dealing with medical-legal issues, we identify particular actions that physicians, nurses, and other hospital personnel can take to avoid serious legal consequences. Although some of these areas are controversial in regard to medical management, these recommendations are our opinions as to how the obstetric team can avoid lawsuits. It is not our intention to dictate management of the pregnant patient. The obstetric team should be aware of the constantly changing technology in the practice of obstetrics and should keep abreast of these changes as they reflect the national standards of patient care.

Why Obstetrics Has One of the Highest Malpractice Litigation Rates

The obstetric health care team practices in what is perhaps the most emotionally charged area of medicine. The arrival of the newborn is anticipated as a moment of joy rarely equalled in life. For most mothers, pregnancy is the first period of long-term contact with a physician. The close attention paid to her health and the well-documented physical and emotional changes undergone during pregnancy cause her to feel *deserving* of a healthy baby. The building anticipation includes only the expectation of a healthy baby.

The expectant father also has high hopes. He is relying on the medical profession to guide his wife through this period and feels at times awkward and helpless, yet proud and hopeful. The financial obligation that giving birth places on the father cannot be underestimated. In cases where the mother has been working prior to birth, an interruption in her career is often regarded as a personal sacrifice despite the fact that the child may have been very much wanted. Expectant parents are knowledgeable consumers, expecting that the fees charged them by all of the health care providers involved will have purchased appropriate care, often translated as a healthy baby.

Therefore, when a "bad baby" arrives and joy turns to despair, the much needed explanation as to "Why?" is often asked of a lawyer. The obstetric health care team is charged with the responsibility of practicing obstetrics within the accepted standard of care; their failure to do so will most assuredly result in litigation. In an attempt to define these areas of litigation (which is legalese for being sued for medical malpractice, often for millions of dollars), the health care team should pay particular attention to the following areas of practice.

WHY OBSTETRICIANS GET SUED

The Use of Oxytocin

The ground for litigation arising out of the use of oxytocin is usually divided into two categories: the injudicious use of the drug and the failure to appropriately monitor the patient during its administration.

Most of the cases involving the alleged negligent use of oxytocin occur when the obstetrician decides that oxytocin is needed to augment labor. However, arrest of labor is often an indication of a complication. All too commonly, this potent medication, joined with the forces of labor, causes some of the worst neonatal injuries seen.

Hopefully, a labor curve will be an indication to the obstetrician of his patient's condition and assist him in determining whether oxytocin should be used.

ADVICE TO THE PRACTITIONER
Every labor should be graphed using a Friedman labor curve or alternative graphing method so that the decision to use oxytocin can be shown to be a judicious one.

Once the decision to use oxytyocin is made, the obstetrician in attendance should be aware of the fact that oxytocin may cause hyperstimulation, which may in turn cause uteroplacental insufficiency. Knowledge of these effects, which can be adverse to the fetus, mandates that appropriate monitoring be ordered and done by the obstetrician. The American College of Obstetricians and Gynecologists (ACOG Bulletin No. 49, 1978) recommends that the physician be immediately available when oxytocin is used. This has been interpreted by some to mean in the hospital or at least within 10 minutes of the hopsital (Braun and Cefalo, 1983). Since it is well known that oxytocin can increase the duration, intensity, and frequency of uterine contractions and also elevate the baseline resting tone, internal electronic monitoring is mandated. External monitors, reliable only for measuring frequency and duration of contractions, are not deemed sufficient under these circumstances. Since oxytocin is used to augment a slow labor or to induce labor in high-risk patients, fetal heart rate changes can occur. Therefore, the internal fetal heart rate electrode should be used to most accurately observe the baseline, any decelerations, and any variability of the fetal heart rate. ACOG (Bulletin No. 44, 1977)

recognizes this, and it is therefore considered a national standard of care that internal monitoring be used when oxytocin is being administered.

ADVICE TO THE PRACTITIONER
Use of internal fetal monitoring during the administration of oxytocin is mandatory.

Difficult Vaginal Delivery

Three examples of difficult vaginal deliveries that spawn litigation are midforceps, breech, and multiple births. Years ago, high forceps deliveries were deleted from obstetric practice. Today, it has been shown that midforceps delivery can increase morbidity and mortality for the infant and cause trauma to the mother. In most cases where the infant cannot deliver spontaneously or by outlet (low) forceps, cesarean section is a safer alternative, especially for the infant.

ADVICE TO THE PRACTITIONER
(1) Beware of midforceps or difficult forceps deliveries. (2) After delivery, make a careful, complete record of what was done.

Some routine uses of cesarean section are being reevaluated. One such circumstance is some breech presentations. Breech deliveries present an increased risk of perinatal morbidity and mortality, even for skilled obstetricians. When cesarean section is used for premature breech deliveries, a low vertical uterine incision is most practical to ensure safe delivery of the after-coming head.

ADVICE TO THE PRACTITIONER
(1) Be sure of the presenting part prior to or in early labor. If there is a question, get an ultrasound or X-ray. (2) Avoid vaginal breech delivery. (3) Use a low vertical uterine incision in cesarean section of breech presentations in the premature.

With multiple births, most commonly twins, litigation concerning damage to the second baby is becoming increasingly common. Usually, the cause is either traumatic vaginal delivery or abruption of the placenta after delivery of the first infant.

ADVICE TO THE PRACTITIONER
Consider cesarean section when you are aware of multiple births. Recognize multiple births whenever possible, utilizing ultrasound in pregnancy either routinely or whenever clinical conditions suggest a multiple pregnancy.

Choice of Anesthesia

Traditionally, obstetricians took comfort in thinking that the choice of anesthesia and any untoward results would be the responsibility of the anesthesiologist. However, the lines of liability have merged, and an obstetrician can and will be held liable for the choice of anesthesia even though an anesthesiologist administers the drug and approves the decision. Specifically, general anesthesia has a significant risk for the pregnant patient, as the second leading cause of maternal death is aspiration during general anesthesia. This can occur even with a skilled anesthesiologist. If general anesthesia is used, intubation of the pregnant patient is mandatory.

ADVICE TO THE PRACTITIONER
(1) Know the propensities of anesthesia, and choose the safest method for cesarean delivery dictated by circumstances. (2) Avoid general anesthesia for vaginal deliveries.

Attendance

Due to the unpredictable events of birthing, physicians have been known to miss the labor and delivery of patients. Often, and unrealistically, a high level of responsibility is placed on the labor nurse to provide "coverage" for the absent obstetrician. If a disaster occurs, a lawsuit follows.

ADVICE TO THE PRACTITIONER
You have a legal duty to attend your patient. If attendance is impossible, coverage is mandatory. An organized group practice should be seriously considered to provide this coverage. It is best for an obstetrician to be present during labor.

Resuscitation

Every obstetrician has had the experience of delivering a child with an Apgar of 8 or higher who later turns blue somewhere between the delivery room and the nursery. Although most hospitals still do not have a pediatrician in attendance at the time of the delivery, the obstetrician should remain in attendance until the newborn is safely situated in the nursery or until a pediatrician is with the infant.

If a problem is noted before delivery it is a standard of care to request the presence of a pediatrician or resuscitation team at the delivery. Many salvageable newborns are further damaged by inappropriate resuscitation, especially (1) not using a DeLee suction when meconium is present as the fetal head delivers on the perineum (or through the uterine incision) before the chest is delivered; and (2) bagging the infant before suctioning has occurred.

ADVICE TO THE PRACTITIONER
(1) Stay with the newborn after birth. (2) If there are any indications that a medical complicaton will arise with this newborn prior to birth, make arrangements for a pediatrician to attend the delivery. (3) The baby is your patient also and must not be abandoned. Develop a good working relationship with the anesthesiologist or nurse anesthetist and establish a role for each of you when resuscitation is needed. (4) When meconium is present use DeLee suction with delivery of the head. (5) Always suction the infant before bagging is begun.

Prolonged Labor

The labor graph (discussed previously in conjunction with oxytocin) is a great source of information that will keep the obstetrician out of trouble. Since labor is a stress test for the baby, the internal monitor used in conjunction with the labor graph is an excellent way to follow the progress of the fetus and the mother.

ADVICE TO THE PRACTITIONER
Get in the habit of using a labor graph and become masterful at interpreting internal electronic fetal monitoring tracings. If your hospital has internal fetal monitoring available and you are not using it, you may encounter legal difficulties. The recognition and treatment of labor problems are important ways to prevent bad results.

Shoulder Dystocia

Cases of shoulder dystocia have emerged as a leading cause of malpractice suits. Obstetricians must avoid predisposing factors such as the injudicious use of oxytocin in patients with arrested labor due to cephalo-pelvic disproportion and difficult forceps deliveries. In addition, obstetricians should have a careful management plan, maneuver by maneuver, to avoid excessive downward traction on the fetal head, which can injure the brachial plexus. One often ignored maneuver that may result in successful delivery of the anterior shoulder is the knee-chest position (McRoberts maneuver) followed by manual suprapubic pressure. If this is also unsuccessful, the posterior arm should be delivered first.

The obstetrician should dictate a detailed summary of how he managed the problem, not just that there was "shoulder dystocia." This way, if his management was proper and the infant still sustained a brachial plexus injury, it can be defended better, as in some cases of severe shoulder dystocia these brachial plexus injuries cannot be avoided.

ADVICE TO THE PRACTITIONER
(1) Be mindful of predisposing factors; i.e., try not to use oxytocin in patients where an arrest in the active phase of labor may be due to cephalopelvic disproportion, and avoid difficult forceps deliveries. (2) Have a logical plan for management of shoulder dystocia and perform it systematically, keeping in mind the knee-chest positioning of the mother if needed. (3) Avoid excessive downward traction of the fetal head. (4) After the delivery, chart what you did in careful, well-organized detail.

Fetal Monitoring

The fetal monitor should be used to assess fetal status during labor. It can not only alert you to problems but can reassure you that the fetus is doing well. If an electronic monitor is not used, be certain that auscultation of the fetal heart rate is done properly every 15 to 30 minutes in the first stage of labor and more frequently in the second stage. Listening should take place through several contractions. Palpation of contractions through several contractions is also necessary to assess uterine activity properly.

ADVICE TO THE PRACTITIONER
(1) Auscultate appropriately when electronic monitoring is not used. (2) Use external monitoring when problems are not apparent, and do not rely on variability in this mode. (3) Use internal monitoring when any problems with the fetal heart rate or contractions are apparent. (4) Become masterful at interpretation of fetal heart rate tracings. (5) Continue fetal monitoring in the delivery room or operating room.

Charting

The patient's chart is a legal document. Just as important, the patient's chart documents the reasoning or rationale for the many obstetric decisions you make. During labor, the obstetrician must chart his own examinations and write progress notes. Likewise, nurses must chart their own observations and actions thoroughly. The patient's chart should be completed at the conclusion of each office visit and reviewed before it is sent to the hospital to be available in the labor and delivery suite prior to the patient's arrival.

ADVICE TO THE PRACTITIONER
The chart tells the whole story and will either back you up or sink you if your judgement and care are questioned. It must be understood by nurses who are going to assist you in the labor and delivery process. Never, under any circumstances, change your chart once it has come into issue in a legal forum. Even if there is a basis for making a change, you will look guilty.

Appropriate Prenatal Testing

The obstetrician should be aware of the increased use of amniocentesis and should recommend it to any appropriate obstetric candidate. Its use in screening chromosomal defects and other abnormalities should be available to all prospective parents regardless of their age if they elect additional screening.

In regard to the recognition of problems during pregnancy, patients must be observed carefully for any high-risk problems. If the mother becomes a high risk she should be seen more frequently, and appropriate tests, such as ultrasound and nonstress and contraction stress tests, should be performed.

ADVICE TO THE PRACTITIONER
Although some tests are routine, stay alert to the clinical signs that you are observing. Attempt to treat each patient individually by taking enough time to listen to her and follow up on her complaints, which are often subtle. Follow up complications appropriately.

Should This Procedure Be Done in the Hospital?

A recent trend in all medical fields is the increased use of the medical office for many medical procedures previously done in a hospital. Along with this "convenience" comes the concomitant responsibility to the patient should an untoward event occur. If a decision has been made not to perform a procedure in the hospital, be certain that your office is equipped with appropriate resuscitation facilities. Personnel must be educated for new procedures, such as the reading of a nonstress test or an ultrasound. Information regarding a contraction stress test or more sophisticated ultrasound could be missed owing to the level of the technician's education. The practitioner should be familiar with the limitations that a hospital has with respect to set-up time, operating room personnel, recovery room facilities, anesthesia service, ultrasound, and all other items that may be needed routinely as well as in an emergency.

ADVICE TO THE PRACTITIONER

You are responsible for knowing what is available in your medical community. Since you are responsible for ordering tests, be sure that you advise patients where these tests can be completed so that they can make arrangements in advance. Be conscious of the time it takes for your hospital to set up for emergency procedures, and always leave a margin of safety so that patients can receive the treatment they need at the hospital in a timely fashion. Finally, recognize the limitations of your office and your office staff in determining whether procedures should be performed there.

WHY OBSTETRIC NURSES GET SUED

The law no longer accepts the legal proposition that the nurse is a mere handmaiden, a mere servant of the physician. The nurse, unlike most physicians, is an employee of the hospital and is responsible to the hospital. The hospital assumes responsibility for the actions of the nurse. Thus, if a nurse is negligent, he or she can be sued independently and/or the hospital can be sued for the actions of its employee (vicarious liability).

Today the nurse is specialized and must attain the requisite level of knowledge and education for use in daily practice. With so many coexisting levels of nursing, from the technician to the clinical specialist, the level of practice can vary considerably. It should be clear that any patients at risk should be attended by a registered nurse. This is especially true in the labor and delivery areas. Today many hospitals provide exclusively RN coverage for their labor and delivery areas, since these have become intensive care areas where changes in even normal

patients can occur quickly and proper assessment is essential. Nevertheless, nurses who should be practicing appropriately in the following areas of knowledge and expertise are with relative frequency being sued for deficiencies.

Charting

If it is true that the chart is the documentation of antepartum progress, labor and delivery processes, and postpartum recovery, then it must follow that an incomplete chart is an indication of incomplete nursing care. With unfortunate frequency, charts left incomplete or blank in important areas provide an opportunity for the creation of a scenario that may not have occurred in the labor and delivery rooms. Items such as frequency of vital signs, labor progress, treatments and medications given, and notations of notifications to physicians are all important in terms of satisfying national standards and are uniformly demanded within individual institutions.

A nurse will not be faulted for caring for a patient and then completing the chart after the delivery has been accomplished or the complication resolved. Temporary nursing notes, which are later translated into a complete chart, should be kept.

ADVICE TO THE OBSTETRIC NURSE

Consider the chart the best evidence of what you did for the patient. Be sure your observations and actions are charted. If you did something for the patient and it is not charted, the assumption in court will probably be that it was not done.

Taking Vital Signs

The assumption that nurses are responsible for taking vital signs of patients and correlating these signs with the patient's underlying condition (or certainly reporting the vital signs to a physician if they are troubling) is a cornerstone of a nurse's duties to the patient and hence a cornerstone of that nurse's legal liability. The sources that a patient's attorney uses to determine whether the vital signs were taken with appropriate frequency are the hospital's, clinic's, and/or office's own regulations and national standards. Yet a surprising number of nurses remain unaware of these requirements concerning vital signs.

ADVICE TO THE OBSTETRIC NURSE

Be certain that you are aware of your own hospital's regulations and national standards concerning the taking (and charting) of vital signs. Do not be lulled into skipping the taking of vital signs because the patient "appears" to be okay.

Identification of High-Risk Patients

The identification of high-risk patients is often the responsibility of the nurse *because the high-risk status does not present itself until the patient has begun labor.* Frequently, the physician is not in attendance at that time and it may take him a while to arrive at the hospital. Unfortunately, sometimes patients become high risk with relatively subtle signs. This is, of course, another reason for diligence in monitoring both the mother and fetus. Knowledge of the predisposing factors and subtle signs of high risk and the appropriate treatment is a standard to which every nurse will be held responsible.

ADVICE TO THE OBSTETRIC NURSE

Know what constitutes a high-risk patient. If in doubt, ask a fellow nurse for assistance in making the diagnosis. Communicate this to the attending obstetrician as soon as possible and recommend that he come to the hospital or clinic/office if he is not there to see the patient. Chart your communication. Do not hesitate to ask the advice of another physician if the patient's own physician is unavailable. Finally, be sure that the person who attends a high-risk patient is a registered nurse and not an LPN.

Fetal Monitoring

The hospital purchases fetal monitoring equipment with the intention that it be used. Its very existence within the labor and delivery suite mandates that it be used properly. This, of course, means that electronic fetal monitoring tracings should be evaluated appropriately by the attending nurse and that this nurse should have the knowledge to undertake treatment when necessary. A nurse should feel free to call upon another nurse for consultation if there is any difficulty in interpreting the fetal tracing. Once any type of suspicious or ominous pattern is recognized, the attending obstetrician should be notified immediately and treatment instituted.

Unfortunately, not all physicians are experienced in electronic fetal monitoring, and some avoid the use of these monitors because of their lack of experience. Most hospitals have policies concerning when electronic fetal monitoring should be used, such as in conjunction with the use of oxytocin. However, it is imperative that the patient's well-being have the highest priority; therefore, the physician should be encouraged to allow the nurse to use the monitor. If the monitor is not used, specific procedures for auscultation should be used (see Fetal Monitoring section on page 578).

The fetal heart rate tracing is a permanent part of the patient's chart and should be treated as such. It should be retrievable.

The placement of the fetal heart rate electrode and intrauterine catheter by nurses is a subject of some dispute. Some institutions permit this and some do not. Certainly, this should only be attempted if the nurse has been educated and certified in its placement. In 1981 NAACOG recommendations stated that certified nurses could place the electrode but not the catheter (NAACOG, 1981). However, the 1986 NAACOG recommendations state that the qualified nurse can apply any of the fetal monitoring appliances (NAACOG, 1986). In 1981 the NAACOG standards stated that nurses could not rupture membranes, but this statement has been removed in the 1986 NAACOG standards. The nurse practice act for each state regulates this procedure, usually with broad statements that cover certified procedures. However, in Pennsylvania the nurse practice act disallows the placement of electrodes and catheters by nurses. In any event, if electronic fetal monitoring is mandatory, then the nurse must aggressively pursue the attending physician if he is responsible for attaching this electrode. It is suggested that the tracings be reviewed periodically by the nursing staff together with the physicians and that unique patterns be discussed freely and openly.

ADVICE TO THE OBSTETRIC NURSE

Labor nurses should be able to interpret fetal monitor tracings and treat fetal distress. Know how the fetal monitor functions and continuously update your knowledge and the knowledge of your colleagues by reviewing these tracings.

The Nurse as a Patient Advocate— Avoiding Fetal or Maternal Injury

This is currently the most sensitive area of litigation. The obstetrician used to be considered the "captain of the ship." It was his choice to attend or not attend the patient and his exclusive responsibility to make certain diagnoses. The ultimate responsibility for the pregnancy's outcome rested with the physician. This concept is now treated in the law like high forceps are treated in obstetrics: it is passé. Specialization among nurses is established and recognized (particularly in the fields of labor and delivery and newborn nursing), and the level of knowledge that the nurse is required to attain is significantly higher than in the past. Concomitant with this level of knowledge is the fact that the nurse is expected to communicate any untoward findings promptly so that fetal or maternal injury can be prevented. What does the nurse do when the obstetrician is not appropriately handling a situation or, perhaps, not even attending to a situation? There is always the chain of command. It should be the hospital's responsibility to provide a clear "chain of command" policy for nurses to follow when necessary. The hospital should encourage nurses to follow the policy without fear of penalty. If the nurse's assessments are inappropriate, then education should be undertaken.

In an emergency, however, the nurse may have to go to any source that is available to help the patient. You have a duty, as the patient's advocate, to be certain that the requisite standard of care is carried out.

ADVICE TO THE OBSTETRIC NURSE
Labor nurses should be assertive when they are in a situation in which fetal or maternal injury could occur. The chain of command should be used, but if it is not working in time to help the patient, then it should be abandoned and the patient's interests should receive top priority. The role of the nurse as a patient advocate is the modern trend in law; defense by the "captain of the ship" theory is outmoded.

Induction of Labor

National standards and hospital regulations often differ as to whether nurses can begin the induction of labor without the attending obstetrician. Indeed, questions concerning the management of the intravenous administration of oxytocin are also often left unresolved. Each nurse should be aware of the NAACOG standards and the regulations of the hospital where he or she works before attempting to induce labor and/or change the intravenous flow of oxytocin. Obviously, along with this, a complete

and thorough working knowledge of the propensities of oxytocin must be obtained, including the only appropriate route of administration, which is the intravenous route. (Please see previous discussion with respect to the use of electronic fetal monitoring in conjunction with oxytocin.)

ADVICE TO THE OBSTETRIC NURSE
Complete knowledge of the use of oxytocin involves not only the propensities of the drug but conjunctive use of monitoring and the treatment of oxytocin-induced complications. Chart the dose of oxytocin in mU/min, and know the appropriate dose and when to increase and stop it.

Resuscitation

Frequently babies are born in need of resuscitation; with even more frequency, pediatricians are not in attendance. This can often be avoided by notifying the pediatrician or resuscitation team when the first signs of fetal distress appear. Once they have been called, the nurse should be alert to their timely arrival. More than one notification may be necessary if delivery is about to occur and they have not arrived yet. The obstetrician is attending to the mother, and when the need for resuscitation arises it is the labor and delivery nurse who is left to carry out resuscitation if the pediatrician or resuscitation team has not arrived. Therefore, resuscitation should be learned and practiced with skill by each nurse who may be called upon to resuscitate an infant. Resuscitation mandates that an orderly procedure take place and that notes be kept on the chart. If a physician's assistance is required or is available, then an orderly system by which resuscitation will be carried out that crisply defines the role of each individual involved is necessary. Those not directly involved in resuscitation should assist by notifying a pediatrician and/or making whatever other arrangements are necessary.

ADVICE TO THE OBSTETRIC AND
NEWBORN NURSE
Learn how to resuscitate an infant and develop a system by which the resuscitation will be carried out in an orderly fashion, including the call for assistance and/or transfer of the infant when necessary.

Staffing

Hospital nurses and auxiliary staff are sometimes not optimal for the care of patients. This is particularly true in labor and delivery, where the number of patients can fluctuate greatly even within a 24-hour period. It is often difficult to pull nurses experienced in labor and delivery from another floor. Often the absence of a ward clerk or an aide can justify the placement of another nurse on the unit. "On call" staffing from within the department can be very helpful in solving this problem. One small hospital in Florida has its entire labor and delivery staff "on call." When labor patients come to the hospital, the nurse is called in and stays with the patient. Therefore, nurses are not in the hospital when there are no laboring patients.

ADVICE TO THE OBSTETRIC NURSE

Do not abandon your patients because of lack of staffing. Your help is better than no help. Document the lack of staffing to the hospital supervisor to avoid further problems.

Liability of Clinicians and Educators

Clinicians and nurse practitioners are expected to have more knowledge and experience than staff nurses, and their practice should reflect this advanced knowledge. Therefore, clinicians and nurse practitioners should take an active part in writing appropriate policies and procedures for the obstetric units to maintain optimal standard patient care. Educators should be active in preparing the staff for new policies and procedures as well as maintaining current policies and procedures. Obstetric educators should be responsible for the orientation of new employees. They should assess these new employees, who should not be allowed to practice independently until they are ready.

Nurse practitioners and clinicians also take on a more independent practice than a staff nurse. However, if there are any questions regarding patient care they must defer to the physicians. (However, educator and clinician/nurse practitioner litigation has rarely been seen.)

ADVICE TO EDUCATORS AND CLINICIANS/ NURSE PRACTITIONERS

Keep the staff well informed with educational programs. Provide current policies and procedures. Practice within the nurse's scope.

Conclusion

It is hoped that the foregoing discussion will be a practical tool for the health care provider to use in the obstetric setting. Our emphasis is the avoidance of malpractice and the desire to keep the reader from finding himself in the situation.

REFERENCES

ACOG: Intrapartum Fetal Monitoring. ACOG Technical Bulletin No. 44, January, 1977.

ACOG: Induction of Labor. ACOG Technical Bulletin No. 49, May, 1978.

ACOG/NAACOG: Electronic Fetal Monitoring. Joint statement by ACOG/NAACOG Task Force Committee, March, 1986.

Brann, A., Jr., and Cefalo, R. (eds.): Guidelines for Perinatal Care. Washington, D.C., AAP and ACOG, 1983.

Clark, D. M.: Oxytocin Guidelines (collective letters). International Correspondance Society of Obstetricians/Gynecologists, Vol. 24, No. 9, pp. 66–69, May, 1983.

Gilfix, M. G.: Electronic fetal monitoring: physician liability and informed consent. Vol. 10, No. 1 Spring 1984; Am. J. Law Med. 10:31, 1984.

Isil, O. A.: Legal Risks and Perinatal Health Care. NAACOG Update Series, Lesson 13, Vol. 1, 1984.

NAACOG: The Nurse's Role in Electronic Fetal Monitoring. NAACOG Technical Bulletin No. 7, July, 1980.

NAACOG: Obstetric, Gynecologic, and Neonatal Nursing Functions and Standards, 1981.

NAACOG: Obstetric, Gynecologic, and Neonatal Nursing Functions and Standards, 1986.

Parke, Davis & Co.: "Pitocin." Published by Parke, Davis & Co., a division of Warner-Lambert, Morris Plains, NJ, 1979.

Shane, J.: Medical-legal ramifications of difficult labor and delivery. Clin. Perinatol., 8:3, 1981.

Wiley, J.: The nurse's legal responsibility in obstetrical monitoring. JOGN Nurs., Vol. 5, No. 5. (Suppl.), Sept./Oct., 1976.

INDEX

Page numbers in *italics* indicate illustrations; those followed by t indicate tables.

Abdominal contractions, in second stage labor, 207
Abdominal diameter, fetal, *68*, 68–70, *71*
ABO incompatibility, 473
Abortion, spontaneous, and sexual intercourse, 194
  bleeding in, 419–423
  complete, 420, 420t
  etiology of, 419
  habitual, 422–423
  in idiopathic thrombocytopenic purpura, 451
  in multiple gestation, 347
  incomplete, 420–421, 420t
  inevitable, 420, 420t
  missed, 420t, 421–422
    ultrasound diagnosis of, 62–63, *63*
  previous, as risk factor, 15
  septic, 420t, 422
  signs and symptoms of, 420t
  threatened, 419–420, 420t
  therapeutic, saline, and disseminated intravascular coagulation, 448
Abruptio placentae, 18–19, 428–431, 436t-437t
  and disseminated intravascular coagulation, 447
  cesarean section in, 258
  in multiple gestation, 348
  in preeclampsia/eclampsia, 379
Absolute risk, of teratogenesis, 115
Acardia, 348
Acetaminophen, safety of, 121
Acetazolamide, in preeclampsia/eclampsia, 391t
Acetylsalicylic acid. See *Aspirin.*
Acid elution test, 472–473
Acid-base balance, fetal, assessment of, 249–251
  normal values for, 250, 250t
Acidosis, and fetal distress, 249–250
Acoustic impedance, 56
Acromial presentation, 215
Acute yellow atrophy, 170
Acyclovir, for genital herpes, 77
Adolescent pregnancy, diet in, 140

Adrenergic antagonists. See *Beta-adrenergic antagonists.*
Adrenergic receptors, 309–310
Adrenogenital syndromes, 543t
Age, gestational, determination of, 292–293, 325, 329–330
    prior to cesarean section, 260–293
    ultrasound, 67–70, 67t, *68*, *69*, *71*
  maternal, and chromosomal abnormalities, 524–525
    and congenital anomalies, 541, *542*
    and multiple gestation, *336*, 337
    and prolonged pregnancy, 329
    as risk factor, 14
  paternal, and chromosomal abnormalities, 524–525
Air insufflation, during cunnilingus, 196–197
Albumin, for neonatal resuscitation, 500t
  serum, reduction of, after jejunoileal bypass, 139
Albuterol, 310–313, 315t. See also *Beta-adrenergic antagonists.*
Alcohol, fetal effects of, 21, 308, 535–536
  for preterm labor, 308
  neonatal effects of, 513t
Aldomet, in preeclampsia/eclampsia, 386t
Alkaline phosphatase, normal changes in, 170
Alleles, 530
Alpha-fetoprotein determination, for prenatal neural tube defect diagnosis, 542–543
Alphaprodine, 280
  in labor, 232
Alternative insemination by donor, 548
Amenorrhea, in missed abortion, 421
Amino acids, in fetal aerobic metabolism, 125–126
Aminoaciduria, physiologic, 168
Aminoglycosides, safety of, 121
Aminophylline, safety of, 119
Amniocentesis, 496
  causing chorioamnionitis, 93
  for chorioamnionitis diagnosis, 94
  genetic, 541–543